Modern Drug Discovery and Development for the Treatment of Neurological Disorders

Modern Drug Discovery and Development for the Treatment of Neurological Disorders

Editor: Emmett Bentley

AMERICAN
MEDICAL PUBLISHERS
www.americanmedicalpublishers.com

AMERICAN
MEDICAL PUBLISHERS
www.americanmedicalpublishers.com

Cataloging-in-Publication Data

Modern drug discovery and development for the treatment of neurological disorders / edited by Emmett Bentley.
p. cm.
Includes bibliographical references and index.
ISBN 979-8-88740-274-1
1. Drugs--Design. 2. Drug development. 3. Nervous system--Diseases--Chemotherapy.
4. Nervous system--Diseases--Treatment. I. Bentley, Emmett.
RS420 .M63 2023
615.19--dc23

American Medical Publishers,
41 Flatbush Avenue,
1st Floor, New York,
NY 11217, USA

ISBN 979-8-88740-274-1 (Hardback)

Contents

Preface

Neurological disorders refer to the disorders that affect the nervous system, which includes spinal cord, brain, peripheral nerves, cranial nerves, autonomic nervous system, nerve roots, and neuromuscular junction. Alzheimer's disease, Parkinson's disease, epilepsy, depression, dementia, multiple sclerosis and brain tumors are some of the neurological disorders. These disorders occur due to electrical, structural and biochemical abnormalities occurring in the brain and spinal cord along with other nerves, which can result in a range of symptoms. The high biological and symptomatic heterogeneity of significant neurological disorders makes it a challenging task to develop efficient treatments that can manage all the symptoms. Majority of the drugs available currently are focused on reducing the symptoms, in place of amelioration of the cause that leads to the symptom. Thus, directing the focus on one major symptom that is well understood might result in a viable approach for the development and discovery of drugs for neurological disorders. This book contains some path-breaking studies in the discovery and development of drugs for treating neurological disorders. It will provide comprehensive knowledge to the readers.

This book is the end result of constructive efforts and intensive research done by experts in this field. The aim of this book is to enlighten the readers with recent information in this area of research. The information provided in this profound book would serve as a valuable reference to students and researchers in this field.

At the end, I would like to thank all the authors for devoting their precious time and providing their valuable contribution to this book. I would also like to express my gratitude to my fellow colleagues who encouraged me throughout the process.

Editor

1

Ginkgo biloba L. (Ginkgoaceae) Leaf Extract Medications from Different Providers Exhibit Differential Functional Effects on Mouse Frontal Cortex Neuronal Networks

*Benjamin M. Bader, Konstantin Jügelt, Luise Schultz and Olaf H.-U. Schroeder**

NeuroProof GmbH, Rostock, Germany

Correspondence:
Olaf H.-U. Schroeder
olaf.schroeder@neuroproof.com

Background: Details of the extraction and purification procedure can have a profound impact on the composition of plant-derived extracts, and thus on their efficacy and safety. So far, studies with head-to-head comparison of the pharmacology of *Ginkgo* extracts rendered by different procedures have been rare.

Objective: The objective of this study was to explore whether *Ginkgo biloba L. (Ginkgoaceae)* leaf extract medications of various sources protect against amyloid beta toxicity on primary mouse cortex neurons growing on microelectrode arrays, and whether the effects differ between different *Ginkgo* extracts.

Design: Our brain-on-chip platform integrates microelectrode array data recorded on neuronal tissue cultures from embryonic mouse cortex. Amyloid beta 42 (Aβ42) and various *Ginkgo* extract preparations were added to the networks *in vitro* before evaluation of electrophysiological parameters by multi-parametric analysis. A Multi-variate data analysis, called Effect Score, was designed to compare effects between different products.

Results: The results show that Ginkgo extracts protected against Aβ42-induced electrophysiological alterations. Different *Ginkgo* extracts exhibited different effects. Of note, the reference *Ginkgo biloba L. (Ginkgoaceae)* leaf medication Tebonin had the most pronounced rescuing effect.

Conclusion: Here, we show for the first time a side-by-side analysis of a large number of *Ginkgo* medications in a relevant *in vitro* system modeling early functional effects induced by amyloid beta peptides on neuronal transmission and connectivity. *Ginkgo biloba L. (Ginkgoaceae)* leaf extract from different manufactures exhibit differential functional effects in this neural network model. This in-depth analysis of functional phenotypes of neurons cultured on MEAs chips allows identifying optimal plant extract formulations protecting against toxin-induced functional effects *in vitro*.

Keywords: *Ginkgo biloba L. (Ginkgoaceae)*, microelectrode array, functional screening, Alzheimer's disease, *in vitro* model, amyloid beta 1-42

INTRODUCTION

Drugs and supplements containing various preparations from *Ginkgo biloba L. (Ginkgoaceae)* leaves are widely used in the elderly population (Gafner, 2018). There is a stunning number of various Ginkgo food supplements and medications, containing various leaf preparations or extracts. It is well established that it is not just the plant material that determines the nature, composition and effects of a plant extract, but that it is also highly dependent on the details of the extraction procedure (Itil et al., 1996). Considering the high popularity of Ginkgo extracts, it is an important question how different Ginkgo preparations compare to one another regarding their pharmacological properties. While for one specific extract, called EGb 761, the efficacy and safety for treatment of cognitive impairment, dementia, tinnitus, and vertigo has been demonstrated in multiple clinical studies (von Boetticher, 2011; Gauthier and Schlaefke, 2014; Basta, 2017), such scientific evidence is largely lacking for other Ginkgo products. Therefore, EGb 761 has often been considered the "gold standard" of Ginkgo extract, against which other Ginkgo preparations should be tested (Wohlmuth et al., 2014). EGb 761 decreases blood viscosity, thereby increasing microcirculation (Kellermann and Kloft, 2011); it affects neurotransmission (Yoshitake et al., 2010) and neuroplasticity (Tchantchou et al., 2007, 2009). It prevents oxidative stress (Brunetti et al., 2006; Mohamed and Abd El-Moneim, 2017) and most prominently it protects amyloid beta toxicity (Augustin et al., 2009; Shi et al., 2009, 2010; Tian et al., 2012, 2013; Liu et al., 2015, 2016; Zhang et al., 2015; Scheltens et al., 2016; Wan et al., 2016).

Protective effects against toxic amyloid protein species, especially the $Abeta_{1-42}$ form, are considered to suggest beneficial effects for Alzheimer's disease treatment (Selkoe and Hardy, 2016). Here, we have therefore chosen a cellular model for Amyloid beta toxicity to compare the neuroprotective potential of different Ginkgo preparations.

Functional *in vitro* analysis tools can bridge the gap between morphological and physiological *in vivo* readouts. The use of microelectrode arrays (MEAs) enables the recording of extracellular action potentials of a multitude of neurons cultured in a dish and thus elucidatation of the activity characteristics of neuronal networks. This technology has been used extensively for neurotoxicity studies (Gross et al., 1997; Gramowski et al., 2006b, 2011; Johnstone et al., 2010; Defranchi et al., 2011; Hogberg et al., 2011; Novellino et al., 2011; Frega et al., 2012; McConnell et al., 2012; Alloisio et al., 2015; Schultz et al., 2015) but also for functional phenotypic screening of pharmaceutical compounds to elucidate functional modes of action (Gramowski et al., 2004, 2006a; Johnstone et al., 2010; Parenti et al., 2013; Lantz et al., 2014; Hammer et al., 2015; Bader et al., 2017). Also, MEAs analyses have been used for testing food quality or for assessing functional effects of nutrients (Gramowski et al., 2006a; Nicolas et al., 2014; Allio et al., 2015). In the present study, we investigated the functional effects different commercial Ginkgo medications to rescue acute Aβ42-induced effects on primary cortical neuronal networks *in vitro*. To that end, we used neuronal cultures grown on microelectrode arrays. The compound's rescue effect on amyloid beta42 (Aβ42) pre-treated networks was investigated and the functional phenotypic effects assessed by multi-parametric analysis which finally were summarized into a single parameter, the effect score.

MATERIALS AND METHODS

Compounds

All test medications were purchased at local or internet-based pharmacies. Stock solutions were generated by grinding the tablets with pestel and mortar and dissolving tablet substance corresponding to 40 mg purified Ginkgo extract/ml in DMSO and diluted 1:2,000 to a final concentration of 20 μg /ml in the the cell culture medium. The stock solution for Tebonin was generated by using "Tebonin 120 mg bei Ohrgeräuschen," which contains EGb 761. EGb 761® is a dry extract from *G. biloba* leaves (35–67:1), extraction solvent: acetone 60% (w/w). The extract is adjusted to 22.0–27.0% ginkgo flavonoids calculated as ginkgo flavone glycosides and 5.0–7.0% terpene lactones consisting of 2.8–3.4% ginkgolides A, B, C, and 2.6–3.2% bilobalide, and contains $<$5 ppm ginkgolic acids. Amyloid beta peptides treated with Hexafluorisopropanol (HFIP) were purchased from r-peptide (A-1163-1).

Ethics

All neural tissue from animal were prepared according to the EU Directive 2010/63/EU on theprotection of animals used for scientific purposes (certification file number 7221.3 $\pm$ 2). In thisstudy no animal experiments were performed in accordance with the German Animal Protection §7/2 (Tierschutzgesetz). Time-pregnant animals were purchased and shipped by alicensed animal supplier Charles River, Germany. Animals were stored in a separate room for<24 h after arrival in their transport boxes including food and water equivalent. Animal storage is supervised by an animal welfare officer at NeuroProof GmbH, Germany. Short-term storage of animals in transport boxes is in agreement with Directive (EG) Nr. 1/2005 (Animal safety during transport). The mice were sacrificed by cervical dislocationaccording to the German Animal Protection Act §4.

Primary Cell Cultures

As previously published by our group (Gramowski et al., 2011; Gramowski-Voß et al., 2015; Bader et al., 2017) embryonic brain tissue was harvested from E15 NMRI mice (Charles River, Sulzfeld, Germany). Frontal cortex was dissociated enzymatically in DMEM10/10 (10% horse and 10% fetal calf serum) including papain and DNase I, cells were resuspended in DMEM10/10 containing 10 μg/ml laminin (Sigma) at a density of 7.5 $\times$ 10^6 cells/ml, and 150,000 cells were seeded onto each well of 48-well MEA neurochips (Axion Biosystems Inc., Atlanta, GA, USA). Each well contains an array of 16 embedded platinum electrodes resulting in a total of 768 channels. Prior to plating, MEAs were coated with freshly prepared 0.1% polyethyleneimine (PEI, Sigma, 181,978) dissolved in Borate buffer (Fisher Scientific, 28341). Cultures were kept at 37°C in a 10% CO_2 atmosphere. Half-medium changes were performed twice per week with DMEM containing 10% horse serum. The developing co-cultures were treated on day 5 *in vitro* with 5-fluoro-2′-deoxyuridine to prevent glial proliferation and overgrowth. After 4 weeks in culture, the activity pattern stabilizes and is composed of one coordinated main burst pattern with several coordinated sub-patterns (Gramowski et al., 2004, 2006b). In this study cultures between 28 and 30 div were used. Due to the serum used in the culture medium glia survival is supported in these cultures, and mainly because of proliferation of glia during the first 4 days after plating these neuron-glia co-cultures thus consist of approximately 20% neurons and 80% astrocytes including 1% microglia (Gramowski-Voß et al., 2015).

Multichannel Recordings

Multiwell MEA experiments were performed as described before (Gramowski-Voß et al., 2015). Briefly, recordings were executed with the Maestro recording system by Axion Biosystems Inc. (Atlanta, GA, USA) providing 1,200× amplification, sampling at 12.5 kHz, filtering, and spike detection, delivering whole channel neuronal spike data. Unit separation was performed using Spike Splitter (NeuroProof GmbH, Rostock, Germany) based on different waveform shapes yielding up to 2 units per electrode. For extracellular recordings, MEA cultures were maintained at 37°C and a pH of 7.4 through a continuous filtered and humidified airflow with 10% CO_2. Recordings were performed in DMEM with 10% horse serum.

Compound Treatment

After recording the native activity at 28 days *in vitro*, ultra pure recombinant amyloid beta peptides treated with Hexafluorisopropanol (HFIP) (rPeptide) were added at 100 nM and incubated for 4 h followed by addition of Ginkgo products corresponding to a final concentration of 20 μg purified extract/ml or 0.1% DMSO control which were incubated for 3 h (**Figure 1**). During the course of the experiment, extracts were prepared by a spearate person than conducting the experiments and data analysis. The test samples were numbered with consecutive numbers, and the experimenter was not aware which sample represented which number.

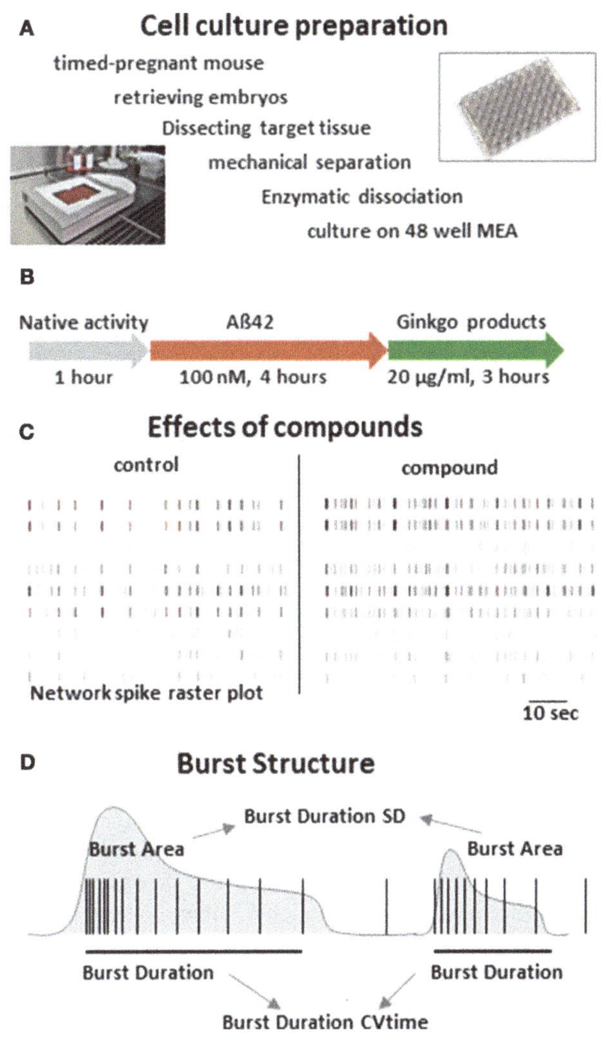

FIGURE 1 | Multi-parametric analysis of cortical neuron network activity. **(A)** Regime of culture preparation of primary mouse neurons. Smaller images: recording setup and 48 well MEA neurochip (Axion Biosystems). **(B)** Time scheme of recording and compound addition. **(C)** Spike raster plots of native cortical activity (control) and cortical activity after acute treatment an excitatory compound illustrating changes in activity patterns. **(D)** Scheme of two simplified bursts outlining some of the parameters extracted from the recordings in this study. SD = standard deviation. CVtime = coefficient of variation over time.

Data Analysis

A unit represents the activity originating from one recorded neuron. We analyzed the stable activity phase of the last 30 min. Action potentials (spikes) were recorded as spike trains, which are clustered in so-called bursts. Bursts were quantified via direct spike train analysis using the standard interspike interval (ISI) method in NPWaveX (NeuroProof GmbH). Bursts were defined by the following parameters: maximum ISI to start a burst: 40 ms, minimum ISI to end a burst: 200 ms, minimum interval between bursts: 100 ms, minimum duration of burst: 10 ms, and min number of spikes in a burst: 3. Data was normalized against the 4 h Aβ42 treatment phase. Integration of multi-parametric data in the Effect Score including selection of best describing parameters based on their Z'-factor was performed as described earlier (Kozak and Csucs, 2010; Kümmel et al., 2010). For demonstrating Aβ42 effects, data from 75 experiments were pooled in order to include the distribution of the Abeta effect sizes of the complete study into the calculation of the "Effect Score" which was built using 15 parameters with best Z'-factors. Blinded test groups were un-blinded after data analysis thereby reducing the bias.

Statistical Analysis

Time-response effects are shown as mean values ± SEM. Statistical analysis for single-parametric data: unpaired *t*-test with Bonferroni-Holm correction for time series: $p \leq 0.05$ are represented with $^*p \leq 0.01$ with ** and $p \leq 0.001$ with ***. For Effect Score measure ANOVA was used followed by Dunnett's test. Number of data points DMSO 5-18, Tebonin 7, Ginkgo-B 7, Ginkgo-C 7, Ginkgo-D 12, Ginkgo-E 8, Ginkgo-F 8.

RESULTS

Functional Acute Effects of Amyloid Beta 42 (Aβ42)

Aβ42 addition acutely affected the activity of frontal cortex neurons which is seen in multiple parameters. After 4 h of incubation with 100 nM synthethic HFIP-treated Aβ42, the overall spiking activity was slightly but statistically significantly reduced which was accompanied by reduction of "burstiness" indicated by the spike contrast (**Figure 2**). Aβ42 also affected the burst structure shown by reduced spike rate in burst (burst spike rate) and the maximal spike rate in bursts (burst spike max rate, **Figure 3**). The calculation of standard deviation (SD) and coefficient of variation over time (CVtime) of general activity or burst structure parameters reflect the regularity of periodic events, while increased values reflect increased variation and thus, lower regularity. Aβ42 increased burst structure variation (burst area SD, burst spike number CVtime, burst duration CVtime, **Figure 4**) indicating a subtle increase of irregularity of the normally regular cortex activity pattern. The neuronal phenotype affected by Aβ42 was used as the baseline to screen compound-induced effects.

Rescue of Aβ42 Effects by *Ginkgo biloba l. (Ginkgoaceae)* Exctract Tebonin

The reference compound Tebonin showed a rescue of Aβ42-mediated effects indicated by the return to activity levels of DMSO-treated networks within 3 h post-compound treatment. Noteworthy, some parameters showed a time-dependent increase of Aβ42 effects (e.g., burst duration CVtime). Tebonin stopped these effects after 3 h and reverted the activity values toward control condition. Some parameters (e.g., burst spike max rate) were instantly rescued within 1 h. All parameters had in common that Tebonin shifted the activity levels toward control condition, therefore, representing a rescue effect.

This feature of rescuing acute functional Aβ42 effects was also observed for other commercially available *Ginkgo biloba L. (Ginkgoaceae)* medications (ginkgo-B, -C, -D, -E, F) tested in this experimental regime. However, differences of rescue effects were observed: e.g., Ginkgo-C showed no rescue effects on spike rate (**Figure 2**); Ginkgo-D had no effects on burst spike max rate and smaller effects on burst duration, CVtime and burst spike number CVtime (**Figures 3**, **4**); Ginkgo-E had no effects on burst area SD (**Figure 4**).

This complex combination of different reactions complicates the comparison of rescue effects between the different compounds. Therefore, we used a linear combination of multiple parameters to enable ranking of rescue effects with one value.

Integration of Multi-Parametric Data and Ranking of Rescue Effects

To compare the rescue effects of acute functional Aβ42 effects between the test substances and positive control Tebonin, the 15 best-describing parameters from all 204 calculated were selected based on their Z'-factor using the method described earlier (Kozak and Csucs, 2010; Kümmel et al., 2010).

The result of this parameter integration of Aβ42 effects compared to DMSO control was termed the Effect Score. As described in the methods section, to calculate the Effect Score, values after 4 h Aβ42 treatment were set to 1, and the DMSO control was set to 0 (**Figure 5**). Using this calibration, the Effect Score was also calculated for 1, 2 and 3 h post-Aβ42 addition which showed a continuous increase from 1 to 3 h. The datasets of the Aβ42 + DMSO and Aβ42 + Ginkgo test compound combinations were then integrated using the Aβ42/DMSO calibration.

On the single parameter level, the Aβ42 + DMSO group showed an increase of Aβ42-specific parameters, indicating a time-dependent effect. In agreement, on the integrated parameter

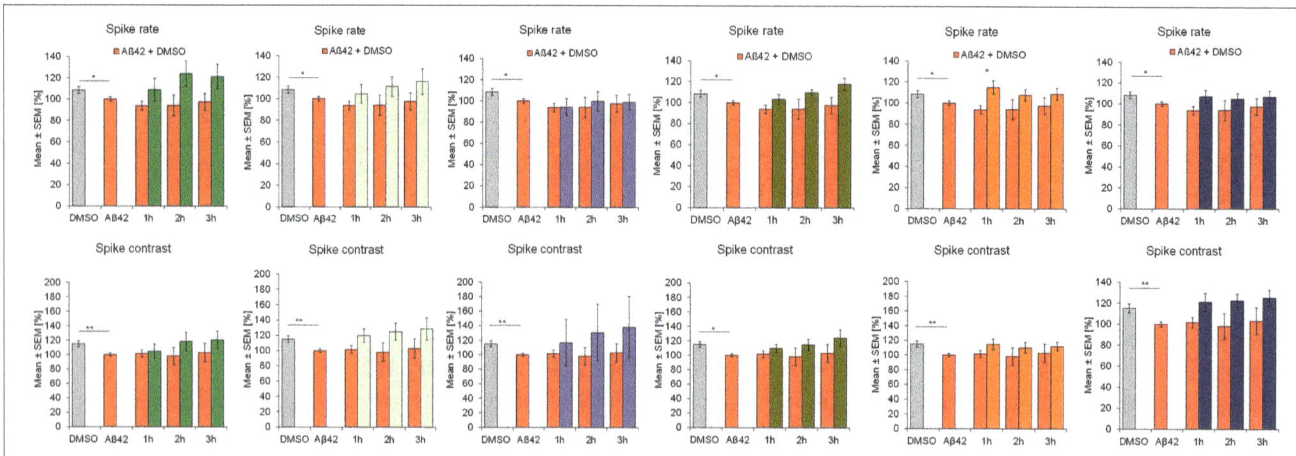

FIGURE 2 | Influence of 100 nM Aβ42 and combination of Aβ42 + 20 μg/ml Ginkgo medications solved in DMSO on **general activity** of cortex network activity *in vitro*. Acute addition of 100 nM Aβ42 induces measurable activity changes of spike rate and spike contrast (reflecting burstiness). Effects increases over time. DMSO control, Aβ42 + DMSO, Aβ42+Tebonin, Aβ42+Ginkgo B, Aβ42 + Ginkgo C, Aβ42 + Ginkgo D, Aβ42 + Ginkgo E, Aβ42 + Ginkgo F. Shown are mean values ± standard error, normalized to native activity. Student's *t*-test with Bonferroni-Holm correction with $^*p \leq 0.05$.

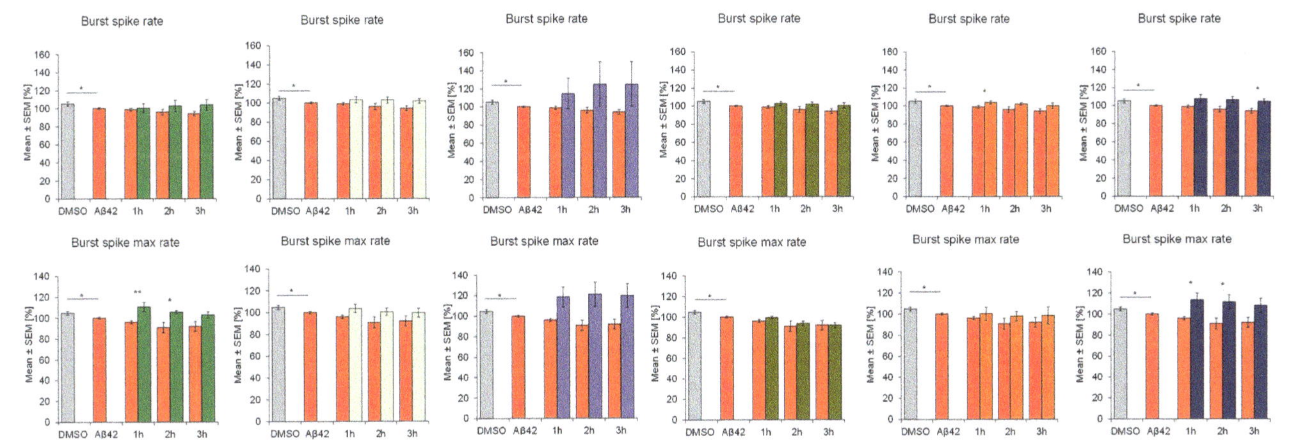

FIGURE 3 | Influence of 100 nM Aβ42 and combination of Aβ42 + 20 μg/ml Ginkgo medications on **burst structure** of cortex network activity *in vitro*. Acute addition of Aβ42 induces measurable activity changes of spike rate inburst and maximal spike rate in burst. DMSO control, Aβ42 + DMSO, Aβ42 + Tebonin, Aβ42 + Ginkgo B, Aβ42 + Ginkgo C, Aβ42 + Ginkgo D, Aβ42 + Ginkgo E, Aβ42 + Ginkgo F. Shown are mean values ± standard error, normalized to native activity. Student's *t*-test with Bonferroni-Holm correction with $^{*}p \leq 0.05$.

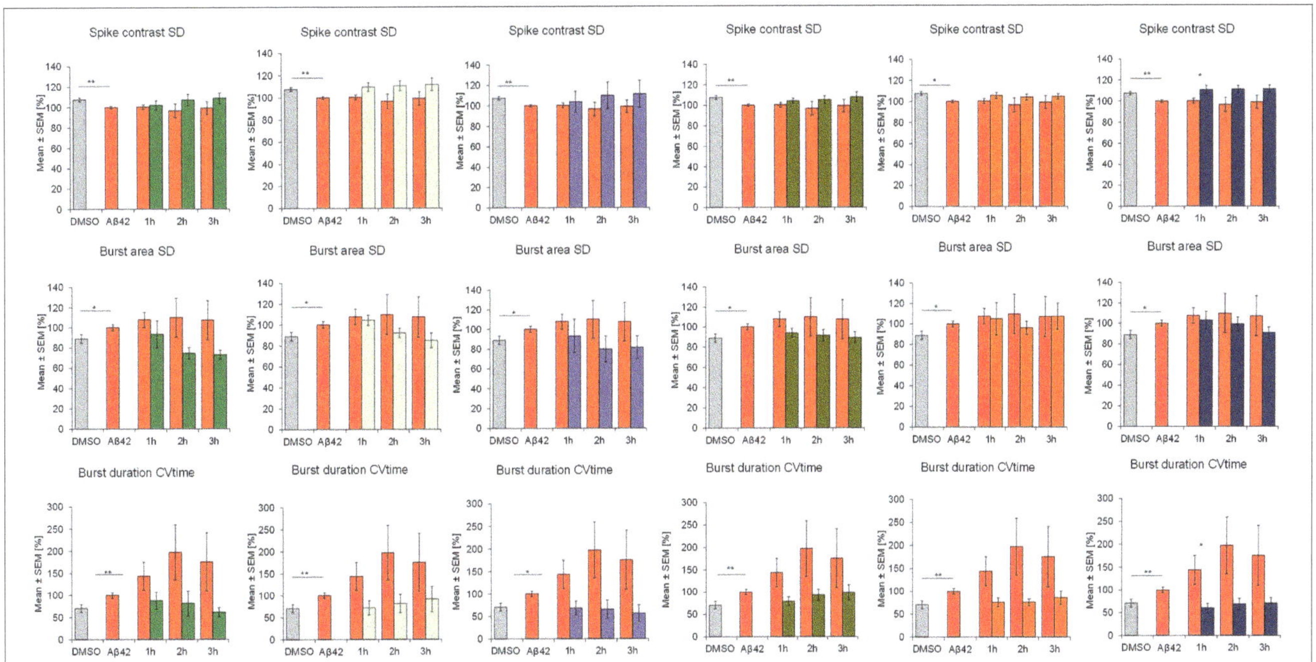

FIGURE 4 | Influence of 100 nM Aβ42 and combination of Aβ42 + 20 μg/ml Ginkgo medications on **regularity** of cortex network activity *in vitro*. Acute addition of Aβ42 induces measurable activity changes of spike contrast SD, burst area SD and burst duration CVtime reflecting the variation over time as an indicator for regularity. DMSO control, Aβ42 + DMSO, Aβ42 + Tebonin, Aβ42 + Ginkgo B, Aβ42 + Ginkgo C, Aβ42 + Ginkgo D, Aβ42 + Ginkgo E, Aβ42 + Ginkgo F. Shown are mean values ± standard error, normalized to native activity. Student's *t*-test with Bonferroni-Holm correction with $^{*}p \leq 0.05$.

levels the Effect Score also increased over time, but showed a more than 3.5-fold increase of the Effect Score within 3 h which is not as obvious when focusing on single parameters. The DMSO Effect Score maintained stable over time (**Figure 5**). Three hours after addition, Aβ42 showed the highest deviation from DMSO effects. This time point was therefore used to rank the test compounds for their rescue capacity. The rescue capacity is defined by the difference to DMSO which can be either below or above 0. Values below 0 represent compound effects which change parameter levels beyond DMSO levels. The effect score values of all tested compounds are listed in **Table 1**. Tebonin showed the strongest rescue directly followed by Ginkgo-B, which showed a negative Effect Score. Ginkgo-D showed a transient rescue at 1 h but lost the rescue efficacy thereafter, demonstrating the least rescuing effect at the 3 h time point.

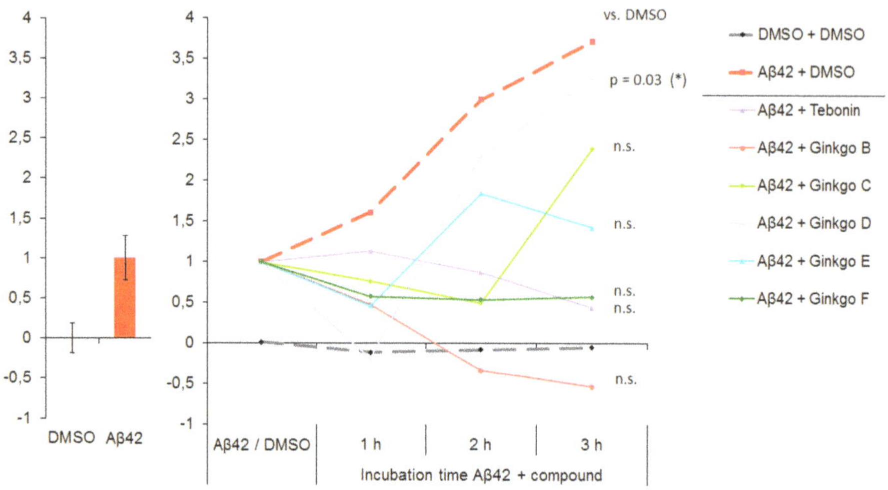

FIGURE 5 | Multi-parametric Aβ42 effects are integrated and presented as "NP Effect Score". **Left**: NP Effect Score for DMSO and Abeta normalized to "0" and "1", respectively. 15 best-describing parameters (partly including those showin in **Figure 2**) were integrated in the Effect Score. **Right**: NP Effect Score for all test compounds. Starting point is the intrinsic Aβ42 effect (set to 1). DMSO control is stable over time. The 3 h time point represents the time of highest resolution and thus the optimal time point for ranking compound efficacies to rescue Aβ42 effects toward DMSO control conditions. N-DMSO = 18, N-Aβ42 = 75. At 3 h time point: ANOVA with $p \leq 0.033$, Dunnett's test with $^*p \leq 0.05$.

TABLE 1 | Rescue efficacy of different Ginkgo medications.

	relative distance from DMSO control [%]	rank
Tebonin	12	1
Ginkgo B	14*	2
Ginkgo F	15	3
Ginkgo E	38	4
Ginkgo C	64	5
Ginkgo D	87	6

*The reference medication Tebonin showed with 12% the highest rescue indicated by relative disctance from DMSO [%]. * Ginkgo B showed a negative Effect Score value (compare **Figure 5**) highlighting the importance for using the distance from control as the most relevant rescue efficacy measure.*

DISCUSSION

Even when two extracts are derived from the same plant species, their composition, efficacy and tolerability can vary considerably. There is a large number of *Ginkgo* food supplements and medications on the market; their individual composition and effects are determined by the kind and quality of the plant material and, importantly, also by the extraction procedure (Itil et al., 1996). The most extensively examined extract, EGb 761, supports neurotransmission (Yoshitake et al., 2010) and neuroplasticity (Tchantchou et al., 2007, 2009) and protects against amyloid beta toxicity (Augustin et al., 2009; Shi et al., 2009; Tian et al., 2013; Liu et al., 2015; Scheltens et al., 2016; Wan et al., 2016) which includes prevention of oxidative stress (Brunetti et al., 2004, 2006; Mohamed and Abd El-Moneim, 2017) and is involved in improving neuro degeneration-induced downregulation of monoamine signaling (Chen et al., 2007; Ferrante et al., 2017). Protection against toxic amyloid protein species, especially the 1–42 forms, suggests potential beneficial effects for Alzheimer's disease (AD) treatment (Selkoe and Hardy, 2016). Therefore, a functional *in vitro* test system to analyze compound rescue efficacies against Aβ42-induced effects is valuable for evaluating treatments for AD. Functional electrophysiological readouts may be optimal for detecting early pathophysiological events which trigger cytotoxicity later on. Thus, a balance between detectable functional effects without pronounced cytotoxic influence is desirable. To establish AD-relevant *in vitro* models, primary neurons from adult diseased animals are the superior choice but difficult to culture for extended periods with goal to obtain a spontaneously active neuronal network. These neuronal networks can be formed using embryonic culture within days. Thus, brain slices and embryonic cultures are used for *in vitro* functional electrophysiological studies on the effects of Aβ which mostly are conducted using the patch clamp method (Lambert et al., 1998; Jhamandas et al., 2001; Gureviciene et al., 2003). However, *in vitro* microelectrode array (MEA) cell culture systems with primary embryonic rodent neuron cultures also provide a means to detect acute and chronic functional effects of Aβ42 peptides at sub-cytotoxic concentrations. Noteworthy, embryonic *in vitro* cultures mature over time and stabilize after 21 days *in vitro* (div) (Ito et al., 2013). We and others observed that bursting activity patterns of cortical neurons reach a plateau phase between 21 and 28 div and peak around 28 div (Chiappalone et al., 2006; Wagenaar et al., 2006). Therefore, we used 28 div cultures for this study. MEA experiments with 100 nM Aβ42–the concentration used in this study–showed specific effects including a reduction of general spiking activity, bursting strength and synaptic connectivity when applied to 28 div cortical neurons (Kirazov et al., 2008). This concentration was shown to be not accompanied by dramatic cytotoxic effects (Varghese et al., 2010). At concentrations above 5 μM, however, Aβ42 effects were shown to induce a more significant inhibition of network activity and connectivity which occurs within 4 h post-treatment and exhibits a time-dependent effect within 24 h (Kirazov et al., 2008; Charkhkar et al., 2015). These 5 μM tests were accompanied by significant cyto-toxic effects (Varghese et al., 2010; Charkhkar et al., 2015), which we wanted to avoid in the experiments described here. Therefore, we acutely treated mouse frontal cortex neurons with 100 nM human recombinant Aβ42 peptides and quantified the MEA readouts by multi-variate analyses. Several brain regions including hippocampus, hypothalamus and frontal cortex are affected in AD (Magalingam et al., 2018), thus, we selected frontal cortex cultures after 28 div for this study, also because in our hands cortical neurons showed a more assay-relevant reproducible phenotype compared to e.g., hippocampus (not shown). We show that 100 nM Aβ42-induced acute inhibitory effects increase in a time-dependent manner up to 7 h. We thereby extend previous reports (Varghese et al., 2010; Charkhkar et al., 2015) in a higher temporal resolution. Four h after Aβ42 was applied, different Ginkgo medications were added to investigate and compare their rescue efficacy. We show that the reference compound Tebonin reverted Aβ42-induced parameter changes toward control condition. Rescue was observed at different parameters within 3 h after Tebonin addition. The other tested Ginkgo products also showed rescue effects. Noteworthy, the parameter-specific rescue effects differed between the Ginkgo products, thereby complicating the comparison between the groups. For that reason we used a linear parameter combination (Kozak and Csucs, 2010; Kümmel et al., 2010) to integrate the Aβ42-affected parameters. This parameter, the Effect Score, allowed comparing the rescue effects between the *Ginkgo* products. One compound (i.e., Ginkgo-B) showed an Effect score below 0, suggesting an overshooting beyond the control profile. As the optimal Effect score is defined by DMSO control of 0, we defined the efficacy to rescue Aβ42-induced effects by the distance to the DMSO control functional profile which can be either below or above 0. In summary, the effect score values (**Table 1**) show that the reference medication Tebonin induced the strongest rescue with 12% distance to DMSO, directly followed by Ginkgo-B, which showed a negative Effect Score of −14% and Ginkgo-F with 15%. Ginkgo-C, -D and -E showed a lower rescue effects. The negative Effect Score value of Ginkgo B indicates that compounds can also affect the parametric shift beyond control levels and over compensate. The goal, however, was to find the Aβ42+compound mixture which resulted in a functional phenotype as similar to DMSO as possible which was the Aβ42+Tebonin combination.

Tebonin contains the Ginkgo extract EGb 761 was shown to be effective for treatment of cognitive impairment and dementia (von Boetticher, 2011; Gauthier and Schlaefke, 2014) and for affecting neurotransmission (Yoshitake et al., 2010) and neuroplasticity (Tchantchou et al., 2007, 2009). Here, for the first time, we systematically compare different commercially available Ginkgo products in one experimental *in vitro* approach and show that the different Ginkgo products with different extraction procedures (Itil et al., 1996) exhibit different functional effects.

AUTHOR CONTRIBUTIONS

BB and OS designed research; LS performed experiments, LS, BB, and KJ analyzed data; BB made the figures, BB wrote the paper.

REFERENCES

Allio, A., Calorio, C., Franchino, C., Gavello, D., Carbone, E., and Marcantoni, A. (2015). Bud extracts from Tilia tomentosa Moench inhibit hippocampal neuronal firing through GABAA and benzodiazepine receptors activation. *J. Ethnopharmacol.* 172, 288–296. doi: 10.1016/j.jep.2015.06.016

Alloisio, S., Nobile, M., and Novellino, A. (2015). Multiparametric characterisation of neuronal network activity for *in vitro* agrochemical neurotoxicity assessment. *Neurotoxicology* 48, 152–165. doi: 10.1016/j.neuro.2015.03.013

Augustin, S., Rimbach, G., Augustin, K., Schliebs, R., Wolffram, S., and Cermak, R. (2009). Effect of a short- and long-term treatment with *Ginkgo biloba* extract on amyloid precursor protein levels in a transgenic mouse model relevant to Alzheimer's disease. *Arch. Biochem. Biophys.* 481, 177–182. doi: 10.1016/j.abb.2008.10.032

Bader, B. M., Steder, A., Klein, A. B., Frølund, B., Schroeder, O. H. U., and Jensen, A. A. (2017). Functional characterization of GABAA receptor-mediated modulation of cortical neuron network activity in microelectrode array recordings. *PLoS ONE* 12:e0186147. doi: 10.1371/journal.pone.0186147

Basta, D. (2017). Schwindel im alter und vaskulär bedingter schwindel [presbyvertigo and vascular vertigo]., die medizinische *Welt* 68, 46–52.

Brunetti, L., Michelotto, B., Orlando, G., Recinella, L., Di Nisio, C., Ciabattoni, G., et al. (2004) Aging increases amyloid β-peptide-induced 8-iso-prostaglandin $F_{2\alpha}$ release from rat brain. *Neurobiol. Aging* 25, 125–129. doi: 10.1016/S0197-4580(03)00038-1

Brunetti, L., Orlando, G., Menghini, L., Ferrante, C., Chiavaroli, A., and Vacca, M. (2006). *Ginkgo biloba* leaf extract reverses amyloid beta-peptide-induced isoprostane production in rat brain *in vitro*. *Planta Med.* 72, 1296–1299. doi: 10.1055/s-2006-951688

Charkhkar, H., Meyyappan, S., Matveeva, E., Moll, J. R., McHail, D. G., Peixoto, N., et al. (2015). Amyloid beta modulation of neuronal network activity *In Vitro*. *Brain Res.* 1629, 1–9. doi: 10.1016/j.brainres.2015.09.036

Chen, L. W., Wang, Y. Q., Wei, L. C., Shi, M., and Chan, Y. S. (2007). Chinese herbs and herbal extracts for neuroprotection of dopaminergic neurons and potential therapeutic treatment of Parkinson's disease. *CNS Neurol. Disord. Drug Targets* 6, 273–281. doi: 10.2174/187152707781387288

Chiappalone, M., Bove, M., Vato, A., Tedesco, M., and Martinoia, S. (2006). Dissociated cortical networks show spontaneously correlated activity patterns during *in vitro* development. *Brain Res.* 1093, 41–53. doi: 10.1016/j.brainres.2006.03.049

Defranchi, E., Novellino, A., Whelan, M., Vogel, S., Ramirez, T., van Ravenzwaay, B., et al. (2011). Feasibility assessment of micro-electrode chip assay as a method of detecting neurotoxicity *in vitro*. *Front. Neuroeng.* 4:6. doi: 10.3389/fneng.2011.00006

Ferrante, C., Recinella, L., Locatelli, M., Guglielmi, P., Secci, D., Leporini, L., et al. (2017). Protective effects induced by microwave-assisted aqueous harpagophytum extract on rat cortex synaptosomes challenged with amyloid β-peptide. *Phytother Res.* 31, 1257–1264. doi: 10.1002/ptr.5850

Frega, M., Pasquale, V., Tedesco, M., Marcoli, M., Contestabile, A., Nanni, M., et al. (2012). Cortical cultures coupled to micro-electrode arrays: a novel approach to perform *in vitro* excitotoxicity testing. *Neurotoxicol. Teratol.* 34, 116–127. doi: 10.1016/j.ntt.2011.08.001

Gafner, S. (2018). "Adulteration of *Ginkgo biloba* leaf extract," in *BotanicalAdulterantsBulletin,* (American Botanical Council). Available

Online at: http://cms.herbalgram.org/BAP/pdf/BAP-BABs-Ginkgo-CC-V2b.pdf

Gauthier, S., and Schlaefke, S. (2014). Efficacy and tolerability of *Ginkgo biloba* extract EGb 761(R) in dementia: a systematic review and meta-analysis of randomized placebo-controlled trials. *Clin. Interv. Aging* 9, 2065–2077. doi: 10.2147/CIA.S72728

Gramowski, A., Jügelt, K., Stüwe, S., Schulze, R., McGregor, G. P., Wartenberg-Demand, A., et al. (2006a). Functional screening of traditional antidepressants with primary cortical neuronal networks grown on multielectrode neurochips. *Eur. J. Neurosci.* 24, 455–465. doi: 10.1111/j.1460-9568.2006.04892.x

Gramowski, A., Jügelt, K., Weiss, D. G., and Gross, G. W. (2004). Substance identification by quantitative characterization of oscillatory activity in murine spinal cord networks on microelectrode arrays. *Eur. J. Neurosci.* 19, 2815–1825. doi: 10.1111/j.0953-816X.2004.03373.x

Gramowski, A., Jügelt, K., Schroder, O. H., Weiss, D. G., and Mitzner, S. (2011). Acute functional neurotoxicity of lanthanum(III) in primary cortical networks. *Toxicol Sci.* 120, 173–183. doi: 10.1093/toxsci/kfq385

Gramowski, A., Stüwe, S., Jügelt, K., Schiffmann, D., Loock, J., Schröder, O., et al. (2006b). Detecting neurotoxicity through electrical activity changes of neuronal networks on multielectrode neurochips. *ALTEX* 23, 410–415. doi: 10.1289/ehp.0901661

Gramowski-Voß, A., Schwertle, H. J., Pielka, A. M., Schultz, L., Steder, A., Jugelt, K., et al. (2015). Enhancement of cortical network activity *in vitro* and promotion of gabaergic neurogenesis by stimulation with an electromagnetic field with a 150 mhz carrier wave pulsed with an alternating 10 and 16 hz modulation. *Front. Neurol.* 6:158. doi: 10.3389/fneur.2015.00158

Gross, G. W., Harsch, A., Rhoades, B. K., and Göpel, W. (1997). Odor, drug and toxin analysis with neuronal networks *in vitro*: extracellular array recording of network responses. *Biosens. Bioelectron.* 12, 373–393.

Gureviciene, I., Ikonen, S., Gurevicius, K., Sarkaki, A., van Groen, T., Pussinen, R., et al. (2003). Normal induction but accelerated decay of LTP in APP + PS1 transgenic mice. *Neurobiol. Dis.* 15, 188–195. doi: 10.1016/j.nbd.2003.11.011

Hammer, H., Bader, B. M., Ehnert, C., Bundgaard, C., Bunch, L., Hoestgaard-Jensen, K., et al. (2015). A multifaceted gabaa receptor modulator: functional properties and mechanism of action of the sedative-hypnotic and recreational drug methaqualone (quaalude). *Mol. Pharmacol.* 88, 401–420. doi: 10.1124/mol.115.099291

Hogberg, H. T., Sobanski, T., Novellino, A., Whelan, M., Weiss, D. G., and Bal-Price, A. K. (2011). Application of micro-electrode arrays (MEAs) as an emerging technology for developmental neurotoxicity: evaluation of domoic acid-induced effects in primary cultures of rat cortical neurons. *Neurotoxicology* 32, 158–168. doi: 10.1016/j.neuro.2010.10.007

Itil, T. M., Eralp, E., Tsambis, E., Itil, K. Z., and Stein, U. (1996). Central nervous system effects of ginkgo biloba, a plant extract. *Am. J. Ther.* 3, 63–73.

Ito, D., Komatsu, T., and Gohara, K. (2013). Measurement of saturation processes in glutamatergic and GABAergic synapse densities during long-term development of cultured rat cortical networks. *Brain Res.* 1534, 22–32. doi: 10.1016/j.brainres.2013.08.004

Jhamandas, J. H., Cho, C., Jassar, B., Harris, K., MacTavish, D., and Easaw, J. (2001). Cellular mechanisms for amyloid beta-protein activation of rat cholinergic basal forebrain neurons. *J. Neurophysiol.* 86, 1312–1320. doi: 10.1152/jn.2001.86.3.1312

Johnstone, A. F., Gross, G. W., Weiss, D. G., Schroeder, O. H., Gramowski, A., and Shafer, T. J. (2010). Microelectrode arrays: a physiologically based neurotoxicity testing platform for the 21st century. *Neurotoxicology* 31, 331–350. doi: 10.1016/j.neuro.2010.04.001

Kozak, K., and Csucs, G. (2010). Kernelized Z' factor in multiparametric screening technology. *RNA Biol.* 7, 615–620. doi: 10.4161/rna.7.5.13239

Kellermann, A. J., and Kloft, C. (2011). Is there a risk of bleeding associated with standardized *Ginkgo biloba* extract therapy? A systematic review and meta-analysis. *Pharmacotherapy* 31, 490–502. doi: 10.1592/phco.31.5.490.

Kirazov, E., Kirazov, L., Schroeder, O., Gramowski, A., Vssileva, E., Naydenov, C., et al. (2008). Amyloid beta peptides exhibit functional neurotoxicity to cortical network cultures. *Comptes Rendus de l'Acade'mie Bulgare des Sci.* 61, 905–910. Available Online at: http://www.proceedings.bas.bg/

Kümmel, A., Gubler, H., Gehin, P., Beibel, M., Gabriel, D., and Parker, C. N. (2010). Integration of multiple readouts into the z' factor for assay quality assessment. *J. Biomol. Screen* 15, 95–101. doi: 10.1177/1087057109351311

Lambert, M. P., Barlow, A. K., Chromy, B. A., Edwards, C., Freed, R., Liosatos, M., et al. (1998). Diffusible, nonfibrillar ligands derived from Abeta1-42 are potent central nervous system neurotoxins. *Proc. Natl. Acad. Sci. U.S.A.* 95, 6448–6453.

Lantz, S. R., Mack, C. M., Wallace, K., Key, E. F., Shafer, T. J., and Casida, J. E. (2014). Glufosinate binds N-methyl-D-aspartate receptors and increases neuronal network activity *in vitro*. *Neurotoxicology* 45, 38–47. doi: 10.1016/j.neuro.2014.09.003

Liu, L., Zhang, C., Kalionis, B., Wan, W., Murthi, P., Chen, C., et al. (2016). EGb761 protects against Abeta1-42 oligomer-induced cell damage via endoplasmic reticulum stress activation and Hsp70 protein expression increase in SH-SY5Y cells. *Exp Gerontol.* 75, 56–63. doi: 10.1016/j.exger.2016.01.003

Liu, X., Hao, W., Qin, Y., Decker, Y., Wang, X., Burkart, M., et al. (2015). Long-term treatment with *Ginkgo biloba* extract EGb 761 improves symptoms and pathology in a transgenic mouse model of Alzheimer's disease. *Brain Behav Immun.* 46, 121–131. doi: 10.1016/j.bbi.2015.01.011

Magalingam, K. B., Radhakrishnan, A., Ping, N. S., and Haleagrahara, N. (2018). Current concepts of neurodegenerative mechanisms in alzheimer's disease. *Biomed. Res. Int.* 2018:3740461. doi: 10.1155/2018/3740461

McConnell, E. R., McClain, M. A., Ross, J., Lefew, W. R., and Shafer, T. J. (2012). Evaluation of multi-well microelectrode arrays for neurotoxicity screening using a chemical training set. *Neurotoxicology* 33, 1048–1057. doi: 10.1016/j.neuro.2012.05.001

Mohamed, N. E., and Abd El-Moneim, A. E. (2017). *Ginkgo biloba* extract alleviates oxidative stress and some neurotransmitters changes induced by aluminum chloride in rats. *Nutrition* 35, 93–99. doi: 10.1016/j.nut.2016.10.012

Nicolas, J., Hendriksen, P. J., van Kleef, R. G., de Groot, A., Bovee, T. F., Rietjens, I. M., et al. (2014). Detection of marine neurotoxins in food safety testing using a multielectrode array. *Mol. Nutr. Food Res.* 58, 2369–2378. doi: 10.1002/mnfr.201400479

Novellino, A., Scelfo, B., Palosaari, T., Price, A., Sobanski, T., Shafer, T. J., et al. (2011). Development of micro-electrode array based tests for neurotoxicity: assessment of interlaboratory reproducibility with neuroactive chemicals. *Front. Neuroeng.* 4:4. doi: 10.3389/fneng.2011.00004

Parenti, C., Turnaturi, R., Aricò, G., Gramowski-Voss, A., Schroeder, O. H., Marrazzo, A., et al. (2013). The multitarget opioid ligand LP1's effects in persistent pain and in primary cell neuronal cultures. *Neuropharmacology* 71, 70–82. doi: 10.1016/j.neuropharm.2013.03.008

Scheltens, P., Blennow, K., Breteler, M. M., de Strooper, B., Frisoni, G. B., Salloway, S., et al. (2016). Alzheimer's disease. *Lancet.* 388, 505–517. doi: 10.1016/S0140-6736(15)01124-1

Schultz, L., Zurich, M. G., Culot, M., da Costa, A., Landry, C., Bellwon, P., et al. (2015). Evaluation of drug-induced neurotoxicity based on metabolomics, proteomics and electrical activity measurements in complementary CNS *in vitro* models. *Toxicol. In Vitro* 30(1 Pt A), 138–165. doi: 10.1016/j.tiv.2015.05.016.

Selkoe, D. J., and Hardy, J. (2016). The amyloid hypothesis of Alzheimer's disease at 25 years. *EMBO Mol. Med.* 8, 595–608. doi: 10.15252/emmm.201606210

Shi, C., Wu, F., and Xu, J. (2010). H_2O_2 and PAF mediate Abeta1-42-induced Ca^{2+} dyshomeostasis that is blocked by EGb761. *Neurochem Int.* 56, 893–905. doi: 10.1016/j.neuint.2010.03.016

Shi, C., Zhao, L., Zhu, B., Li, Q., Yew, D. T., Yao, Z., et al. (2009). Protective effects of *Ginkgo biloba* extract (EGb761) and its constituents quercetin and ginkgolide B against beta-amyloid peptide-induced toxicity in SH-SY5Y cells. *Chem Biol Interact.* 181, 115–123. doi: 10.1016/j.cbi.2009.05.010

Tchantchou, F., Lacor, P. N., Cao, Z., Lao, L., Hou, Y., Cui, C., et al. (2009). Stimulation of neurogenesis and synaptogenesis by bilobalide and quercetin via common final pathway in hippocampal neurons. *J. Alzheimers Dis.* 18, 787–798. doi: 10.3233/JAD-2009-1189

Tchantchou, F., Xu, Y., Wu, Y., Christen, Y., and Luo, Y. (2007). EGb 761 enhances adult hippocampal neurogenesis and phosphorylation of CREB in transgenic mouse model of Alzheimer's disease. *FASEB J.* 21, 2400–2408. doi: 10.1096/fj.06-7649com

Tian, X., Wang, J., Dai, J., Yang, L., Zhang, L., Shen, S., et al. (2012). Hyperbaric oxygen and *Ginkgo Biloba* extract inhibit Abeta25-35-induced toxicity and oxidative stress *in vivo*: a potential role in Alzheimer's disease. *Int. J. Neurosci.* 122, 563–569. doi: 10.3109/00207454.2012.690797

Tian, X., Zhang, L., Wang, J., Dai, J., Shen, S., Yang, L., et al. (2013). The protective effect of hyperbaric oxygen and *Ginkgo biloba* extract on Abeta25-35-induced oxidative stress and neuronal apoptosis in rats. *Behav Brain Res.* 242, 1–8. doi: 10.1016/j.bbr.2012.12.026

Varghese, K., Molnar, P., Das, M., Bhargava, N., Lambert, S., Kindy, M. S., et al. (2010). A new target for amyloid beta toxicity validated by standard and high-throughput electrophysiology. *PLoS ONE* 5:e8643. doi: 10.1371/journal.pone.0008643

von Boetticher, A. (2011). *Ginkgo biloba* extract in the treatment of tinnitus: a systematic review. *Neuropsychiatr. Dis. Treat.* 7, 441–447. doi: 10.2147/NDT.S22793

Wagenaar, D. A., Pine, J., and Potter, S. M. (2006). An extremely rich repertoire of bursting patterns during the development of cortical cultures. *BMC Neurosci.* 7:11. doi: 10.1186/1471-2202-7-11

Wan, W., Zhang, C., Danielsen, M., Li, Q., Chen, W., Chan, Y., et al. (2016). EGb761 improves cognitive function and regulates inflammatory responses in the APP/PS1 mouse. *Exp. Gerontol.* 81, 92–100. doi: 10.1016/j.exger.2016.05.007

Wohlmuth, H., Savage, K., Dowell, A., and Mouatt, P. (2014). Adulteration of *ginkgo biloba* products and a simple method to improve its detection. *Phytomedicine* 21, 912–918. doi: 10.1016/j.phymed.2014.01.010

Yoshitake, T., Yoshitake, S., and Kehr, J. (2010). The *ginkgo biloba* extract EGb 761(R) and its main constituent flavonoids and ginkgolides increase extracellular dopamine levels in the rat prefrontal cortex. *Br. J. Pharmacol.* 159, 659–668. doi: 10.1111/j.1476-5381.2009.00580.x

Zhang, L. D., Ma, L., Zhang, L., Dai, J. G., Chang, L. G., Huang, P. L., et al. (2015). Hyperbaric oxygen and *ginkgo biloba* extract ameliorate cognitive and memory impairment via nuclear factor kappa-b pathway in rat model of alzheimer's disease. *Chin. Med. J.* 128, 3088–3093. doi: 10.4103/0366-6999. 169105

2

Fatty Acids Rich Extract from *Clerodendrum volubile* Suppresses Cell Migration; Abates Oxidative Stress; and Regulates Cell Cycle Progression in Glioblastoma Multiforme (U87 MG) Cells

Ochuko L. Erukainure[1], Nadia Ashraf[2], Asma S. Naqvi[3], Moses Z. Zaruwa[4], Aliyu Muhammad[3,5], Adenike D. Odusote[6] and Gloria N. Elemo[1]*

[1] Nutrition and Toxicology Division, Federal Institute of Industrial Research Oshodi, Lagos, Nigeria, [2] Faculty of Pharmacy, Barrett Hodgson University, Karachi, Pakistan, [3] Dr. Panjwani Center for Molecular Medicine and Drug Research, International Center for Chemical and Biological Sciences, University of Karachi, Karachi, Pakistan, [4] Department of Biochemistry, Adamawa State University, Mubi, Nigeria, [5] Department of Biochemistry, Ahmadu Bello University, Zaria, Nigeria, [6] Analytical Division, Federal Institute of Industrial Research Oshodi, Lagos, Nigeria

***Correspondence:**
Ochuko L. Erukainure
loreks@yahoo.co.uk

Glioblastoma multiforme (GBM) is a malignant primary type of brain cancer with high proliferation and metastasis rates due to involvement of the microglial cell. It is resistant against available chemotherapy. Many strategic protocols have been developed but prognosis and patient life has not improved substantially. In this study, the anti-metastatic and antioxidant effect of fatty acids from *Clerodendrum volubile* leaves were investigated in U87-MG (Human Glioblastoma Multiforme) cell lines. The extracted fatty acids were incubated with U87-MG cells for 48 h. The anti-proliferative effect was determined by MTT assay, while apoptosis and cell cycle were analyzed with BD FACSCalibur. The transwell assay protocol was utilized in the analysis of cell migration and invasion. The treated cell lines were also assessed for reduced glutathione (GSH) level, catalase, superoxide dismutase (SOD) and lipid peroxidation. The fatty acid extract showed significant inhibitory activity on cell proliferation and cell cycle progression, mitigated oxidative stress, and suppressed migration and invasion in U-87 MG cell lines. These results give credence to the therapeutic potential of this plant against cancer, especially GBM.

Keywords: cancer, *Clerodendrum volubile*, oxidative stress, tumor migration, unsaturated fatty acids

INTRODUCTION

Glioblastoma multiforme (GBM) is a malignant primary brain tumor common amongst the young kids with range of age < 13 years, characterized by high rates of proliferation, metastasis, and resistance to chemotherapy protocols (Brada et al., 2001; Puli et al., 2006; Markiewicz-Żukowska et al., 2013). These therapeutic failures represent a great difficulty in its treatment and management, leading to short survival rate, and loss of patient's life quality (Puli et al., 2006). Its key epidemiologic risk includes age, sex, race, lifestyle behaviors, diet, and exposure to environmental factors including pollution from different sources (Efird, 2011).

Though epidemiology of glioblastoma has reported little or no occurrence in West Africa, changes in lifestyle particularly increased urbanization and adoption of western lifestyles and diet are however a major concern (Erukainure et al., 2016). An indigenous African diet often consists mainly of vegetable leaves, unrefined grains and spices, unlike the western counterpart consisting of sweetened desserts, saturated fats, and processed grains (Erukainure et al., 2016). Almost 30–40% of all cancers have been found to be preventive by healthy life style such as weight control, exercise, and physical activities (Potter and Potter, 1997; Jemal et al., 2011). Several studies have linked consumption of dietary fatty acids in diet with reduced brain cancer. Ketogenic diet characterized by high-saturated fats and low protein/carbohydrate, has proven to be effective during therapy and potent adjuvant management of malignancies in almost all types of cancers (Woolf and Scheck, 2015). Antal et al. (2014) reported increased sensitivity of glioblastoma cells to radiotherapy after treatment with arachidonic acid, docosahexaenoic acid, and γ-linolenic acid.

Clerodendrum volubile is among the common leafy vegetables in Southern part of Nigeria and it is well established for its medicinal use (Erukainure et al., 2010). It is indigenously known as *Obenetete* by the Itsekiris and Urhobos in the Delta of Niger. Commonly known as magic leaf, it is also used in the management and sometimes as adjunct for the treatment of diabetes mellitus, arthritis, rheumatism, ulcers, and many other diseases (Burkill, 1985). The phytochemicals of *C. volubile* and antioxidant activities have been reported (Adefegha and Oboh, 2010; Erukainure et al., 2011). Erukainure et al. (2014) isolated an iridoid glycoside from the leaves and reported its antioxidant activity in rats' brain and hepatic tissues. In our previous study, we extracted dietary fatty acids from the leaves and investigated its effect on breast cancer cells (Erukainure et al., 2016). The fatty acids arrested cell cycle progression and down-regulated matrix metalloproteinase-9 in the breast cancer cells (Erukainure et al., 2016). Furthermore, molecular studies are required to prove the proclaimed medicinal uses of the extract of *C. volubile* leaves.

This present study aims to report the anti-proliferative, anti-oxidative, and anti-migratory and/or anti-metastatic activity of the fatty acid rich extracts from leaves of *C. volubile* on U87-MG cancer cells.

MATERIALS AND METHODS

Plant Materials

Fresh *C. volubile* leaves, purchased from Ifon, Ondo State, Nigeria were identified and authenticated at the Department of Botany, University of Benin, Benin City, Nigeria (Voucher number: UBH_{C284}).

The leaves were dried under shed, blended, and stored in deoxygenated container for further analysis (chemical, biochemical, and biological activities).

Extraction of Fatty Acids

The blended leaves were subjected to methanol extraction, followed by fractionation with solvents of increasing polarity, as described by Erukainure et al. (2016).

The concentrated hexane fraction was subjected to methanolysis using the method described by Nickavar et al. (2003).

Cell Cultures and Treatments

U87-MG cells were procured from American Type Culture Collection (ATCC). On arrival the ATCC instructions were followed and cells were submitted to the Bio-Bank of PCMD; ICCBS, University of Karachi, Karachi, Pakistan.

These cells were cultured in DMEM medium, 10% (v/v) fetal Bovine Serum (Sigma), L-glutamine 1% (v/v), penicillin 100 U/mL and streptomycin 100 μg/mL.

These newly seeded cells were kept in humidified incubator with 5% CO_2.

Cellular Cytotoxicity Analysis Using MTT as a Dye

The anti-proliferative activity of the extracted fatty acids against U87-MG cancer cells was evaluated in a 96-well plate using standard MTT [3-(4,5-dimethylthiazole-2-yl)-2,5-diphenyltetrazolium bromide] colorimetric assay, as described by Mosmann (1983).

Cells (1×10^4 cells/mL) were seeded in 96-well plates.

After overnight incubation, the medium was replaced and 200 μL of fresh medium was added to each well, along with serial dilutions of the fatty acid extract (16, 32, 64, and 125 μg/mL, respectively).

Incubation at 48 h was done under same growth conditions, equal volume of the solution of dye MTT, 2 mg/mL, already prepared and preserved at −20°C was added to each well in triplicate manner.

After aspiration of nutrient media, 10% FBS and cell were then incubated for 4 h under same conditions as described for seeding the cells.

The nutrient media, 10% FBS 100 μL of DMSO were added to each well after aspiration of older media.

Absorbance was recorded at 570 nm wavelengths on a micro plate-reader (SoftMax PRO 4.3.1.LS, Molecular Devices, Sunnyvale, CA, United States).

The % inhibition was later calculated as follows:

$$\%\,\text{Inhibition} = 100 - \left(\frac{\text{Mean absorbance of sample}}{\text{Mean absorbance of control}}\right) \times 100 \quad (1)$$

Apoptotic Analysis by Propidium Iodide Flow Cytometry

Cells were seeded at 2×10^5/mL/well in 24-well plate.

These cells were then incubated (under same growth conditions as described above) at 37°C overnight.

These cells were incubated with the extracted fatty acids at 37°C under 5% CO_2 for 48 h. Cells treated with DMSO served as a negative control.

After incubations, cells were typsinized and centrifuged at 2500 rpm for 3–5 min. They were washed twice using phosphate buffer saline (PBS) before re-suspending in propidium iodide (PI) buffer.

One milliliter PI (0.5 mg/mL) was added for 1 min to the cells and their viability was analyzed with BD FACSCalibur.

Fluorescent Activated Cells' Cycle Analysis by Sorting (FACS)

U87-MG seeded in concentration of 1 million cells/mL/well using 6-well plate. The plate was incubated with the extracted fatty acid at 37°C for 48 h.

After incubation, the cells were then subjected to cell cycle analysis using flow cytometry on the BD Biosciences FACS machine, as described by Aliyu et al. (2013) and Erukainure et al. (2016).

The formula described by Pozarowski and Darzynkiewicz (2004) was used in calculating the duration of each phase.

Migration and Invasion Assay

This was carried out according to the method described by Yao et al. (2012) with slight modifications, as U87-MG is a sensitive cell line and requires gentle handling.

5×10^4 cells were seeded on top of the matrigel insert already prepared in top chamber with utmost care. Coating contained 150 μg matrigel on each membrane of top chamber.

The cells for both assays were trypsinized and resuspended in DMEM supplemented (700–900 μL) with 10% fetal bovine serum was gently pipetted down into the lower chambers. This was done in such a way that the surface of the media in lower chamber was just touching the lower side of the top matrigel-containing chamber.

The cells were incubated with the fatty acids extract of *C. volubile* in 120 μg/mL concentration at 37°C for 48 h for the migration and invasion assays, respectively. The cells at the top chambers were aspirated gently out.

Cells that adhered to the lower membrane of the inserts were fixed, and stained with solution of 20% methanol and 0.1% crystal violet.

They were subsequently counted and photographed with at 20–40× power-inverted microscope (Olympus Corp., Tokyo, Japan).

Determination of Oxidative Stress Parameters

For this analysis the U87-MG cells were specifically counted in concentration of 1 million cells/mL, and added to 24-well plate and were then treated with the fatty acid extract of *C. volubile* at a concentration of 120 μg/mL.

These cells were analyzed for total protein (Lowry et al., 1951), reduced glutathione (GSH) level (Ellman, 1959), catalase activity (Chance and Maehly, 1955), superoxide dismutase (SOD) (Kakkar et al., 1984) activity, and also malondialdehyde (MDA) level, (Chowdhury and Soulsby, 2002).

Inhibition of Chymotrypsin Activity

The α-chymotrypsin inhibitory activity of the extracted fatty acids was carried out as described by Cannell et al. (1988). Alpha-chymotrypsin (9 units/mL in 50 mM Tris-base buffer pH 7.6; Sigma Chemical Co., United States) was incubated with the fatty acid extract (2.5, 5.0, 10.0, and 20.0 μg/mL, respectively) for 20 min. A total of 100 pJ of substrate solution (*N*-Succinyl-phenylalanine-pnitroanilide, 1 mg/mL of 50 mM Tris-Base buffer pH 7.6) was added to start the enzyme reaction. The absorbance of released p-nitroaniline was read at 410 nm.

Statistics

To validate the significance of results, each experiment was repeated at least three times. Results were expressed as mean ± standard deviation (SD). One-way analysis of variance (ANOVA) was used in establishing statistical significance. While significant difference was established at $P < 0.05$ using LSD. Statistical analyses were carried out using SPSS for Windows, version 17.0 (SPSS Inc., Chicago, IL, United States).

RESULTS

A dose-dependent cytotoxic activity of the fatty acid extract was observed in U87-MG cell lines with an IC_{50} of ~120 μg/mL as shown in **Figure 1**, indicating a potent anti-proliferative effect.

Apoptosis analysis by PI flow cytometry (**Figure 2**) revealed high cell deaths as the concentration increased, which is an

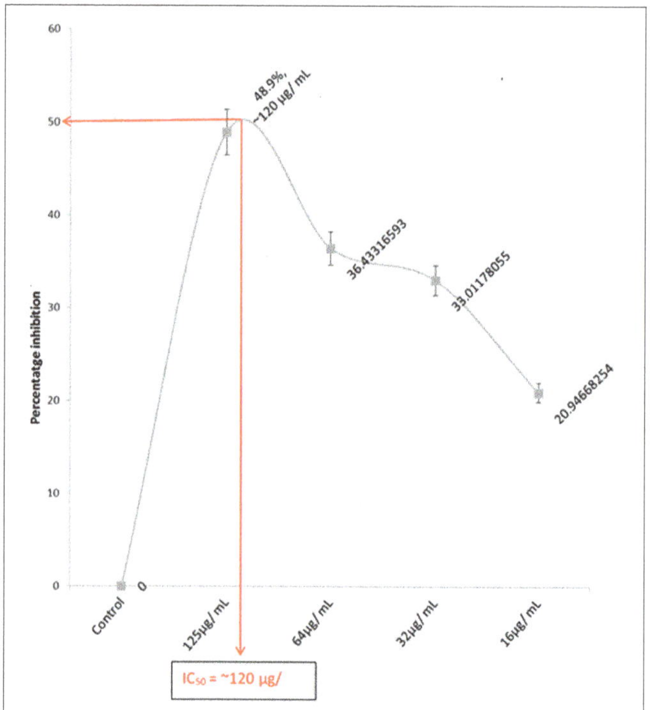

FIGURE 1 | IC_{50} of the anti-proliferation effect of extracted fatty acids on U87 MG cell lines. Values = mean ± SD; *n* = 3.

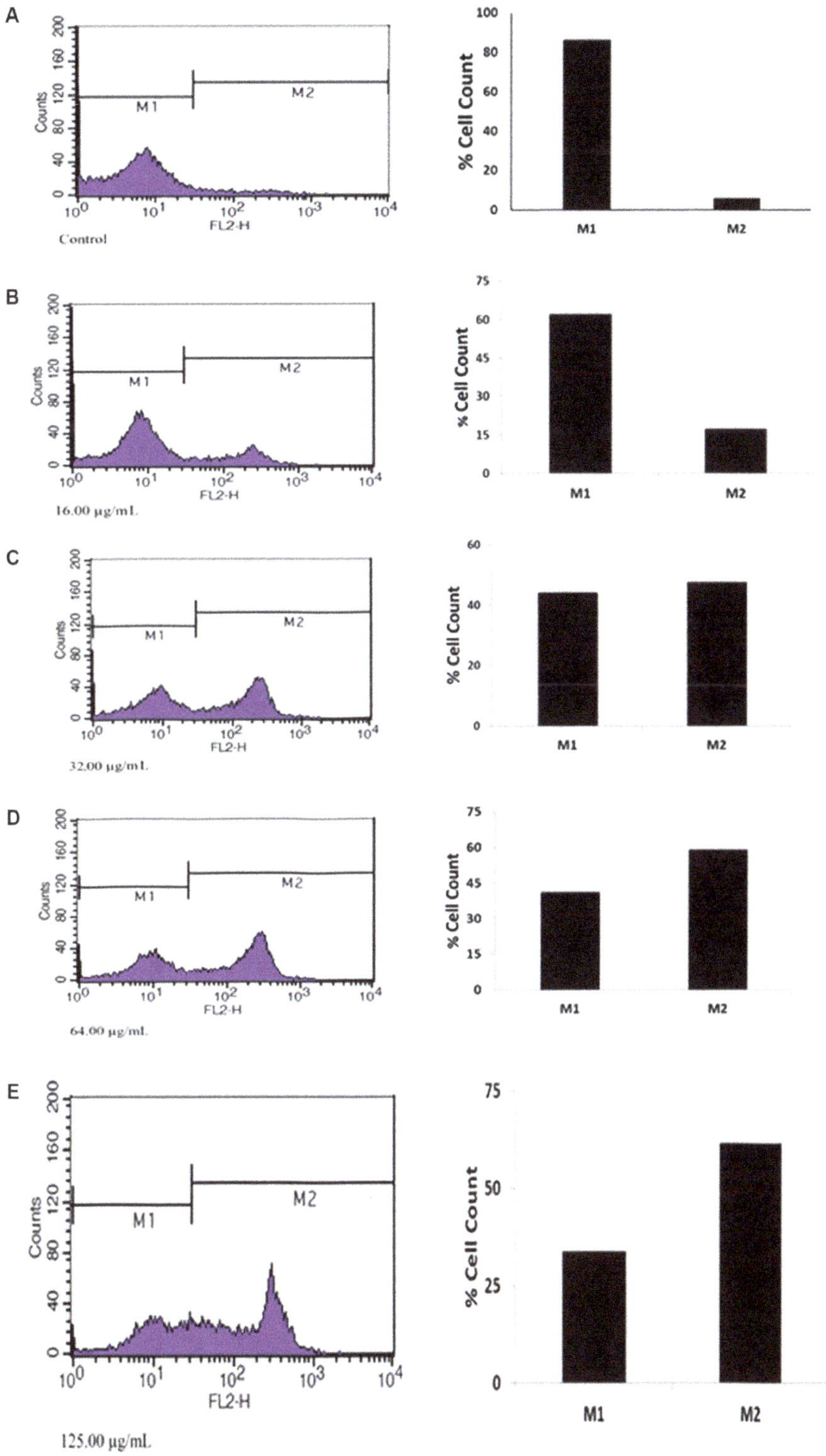

FIGURE 2 | Apoptotic effect of extracted fatty acids on U87 MG cell lines. **(A)** Contol; **(B)** 16.00 µg/mL; **(C)** 32.00 µg/mL; **(D)** 64.00 µg/mL; **(E)** 125.00 µg/mL.

indication of a dose-dependent anti-tumor activity of the fatty acid extract in U87-MG cancer cells.

The quantity of DNA in each cancer cell population in G0/G1 and G2/M phases were significantly depleted in the fatty acids treated cells, as depicted in **Figure 3**. This was also observed with the simultaneous arrest of S phase of the cell cycle.

Transwell migration analysis revealed the migration of the untreated cells in all six parts of the chamber of 24-well transwell

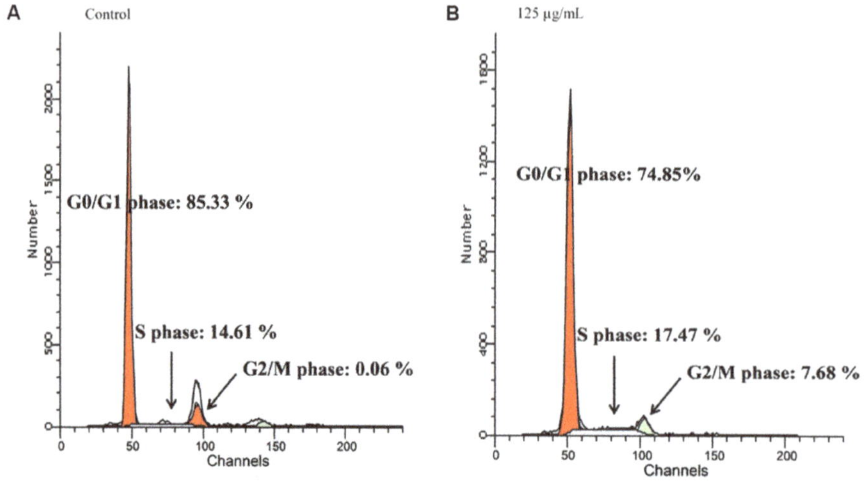

FIGURE 3 | Effect of extracted fatty acids on cell cycle phase distribution of U-87 MG cell lines. **(A)** Control; **(B)** 125 µg/mL.

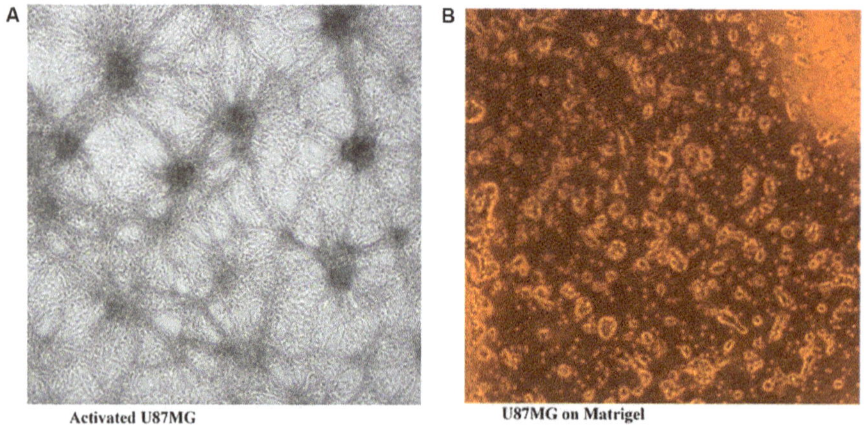

FIGURE 4 | U87MG cells seeded on Matrigel (20× [2 mm]). **(A)** activated U87MG; **(B)** U87MG.

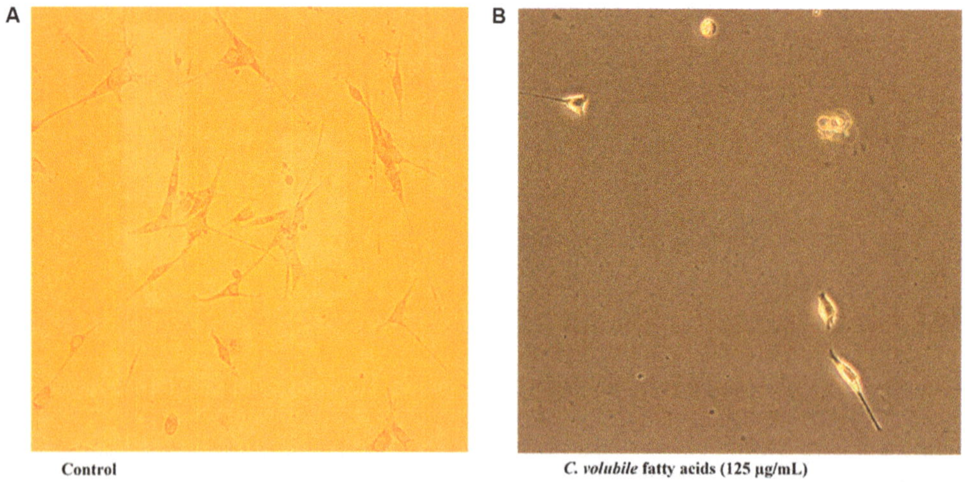

FIGURE 5 | Effect of *C. volubile* fatty acids on cell migration and invasion of U87-MG (Human Neuronal Glioblastoma) cell lines (20× [2 mm]). **(A)** Control; **(B)** Fatty acids.

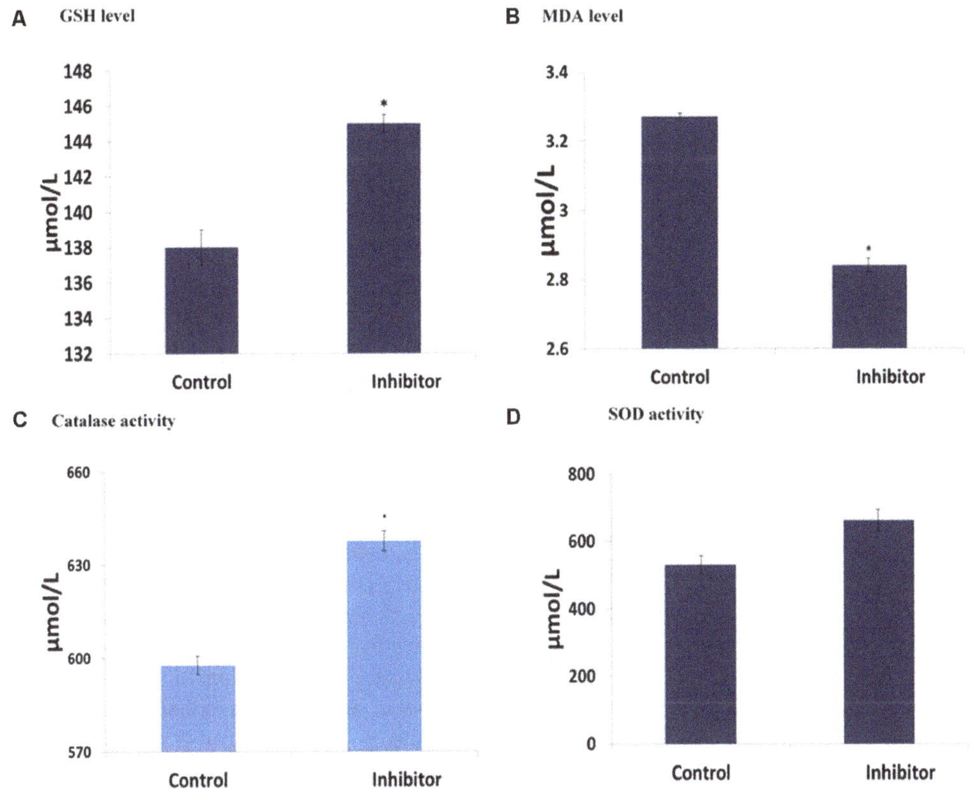

FIGURE 6 | Antioxidative activities of *C. volubile* fatty acids in U87-MG (Human Neuronal Glioblastoma) cell lines. Values = mean ± SD; $n = 3$. **(A)** GSH level; **(B)** MDA level; **(C)** Catalase activity; **(D)** SOD activity.

plate, as shown in **Figures 4, 5A**, indicating an occurrence of cell migration and/or invasion. However, the fatty acid treated cells showed little or no migration (**Figure 5B**), indicating a suppressive effect on cell migration and/or invasion.

Incubation of cells and fatty acid extract led to significant ($p < 0.05$) increase in GSH level with a concomitant decrease in MDA level, indicating an anti-oxidative activity as shown in **Figures 6A–D**. The significant ($p < 0.05$) increase as well as slight increase in catalase and SOD activities, respectively, further indicates the antioxidant potency of the fatty acids.

The fatty acids displayed a dose-dependent inhibitory effect on α-chymotrypsin activity and its kinetics as presented in **Figures 7A,B**.

DISCUSSION

Glioblastoma multiforme (GBM) has been recognized as a major brain tumor, and implicated in extensive invasion into neighboring brain tissue (Puli et al., 2006). This rapid invasion makes it difficult to treat especially while using surgical resection (Brada et al., 2001; Puli et al., 2006; Markiewicz-Żukowska et al., 2013). Hence, the need for an effective anti-proliferative agent that can suppress this invasion and/or migration with little or no side effects. In our previous study, we characterized the fatty acids extracted from *C. volubile* leaves using GC-MS to identify the fatty acid composition (Erukainure et al., 2016). Oleic acid was identified as the most abundant component, along with octadecanoic acid, n-hexadecanoic acid and 2-heptanone, 6-methyl in lesser quantities (Erukainure et al., 2016). In this present study, the suppressive effect of dietary fatty acids extracted from *C. volubile* was investigated on human glioblastoma multiforme cells with the aim of elucidating the possible molecular mechanism, along with its effect.

The cytotoxic effect of fatty acids on cancer cell lines has been reported in previous studies (Motaung et al., 1999). This corresponds with the observed cytotoxic effect of the extracted oil on U87-MG cells (**Figure 1**), thus indicating an anti-proliferative potential against GBM. This corresponds with our previous study of the anti-proliferative effect of *C. volubile* fatty against breast cancer, attributed to its high oleic acid concentration. The protective role of oleic acid against several cancers has been reported in previous epidemiological and animal studies (Carrillo et al., 2012). Thus, the observed anti-proliferative effect of the fatty acid extract, can be attributed to the high oleic acid content.

Novel natural therapies, targeted on induction of apoptosis in cancer cells, are gaining major interest. The role of apoptosis in cancer therapy is well emphasized in several studies. Most cancers manipulate and/or downregulates the antiapoptotic molecules, thereby evading this highly regulated program cell death (Koff

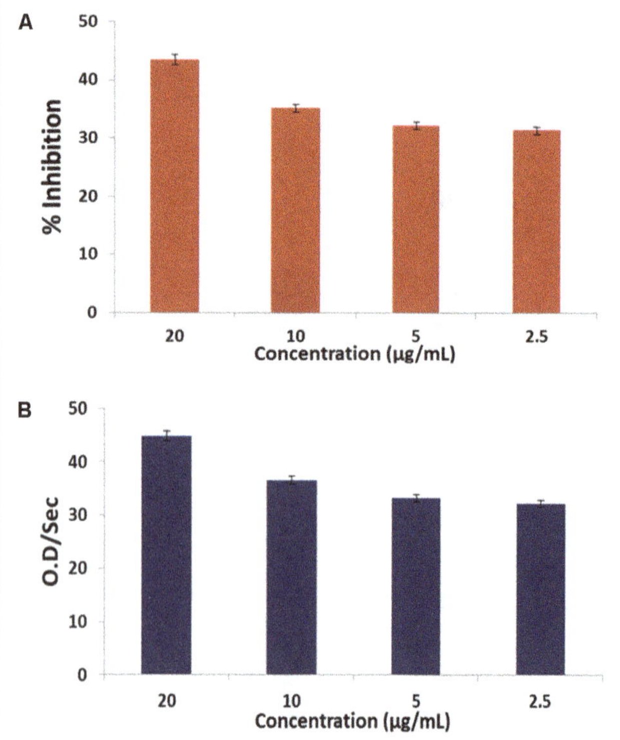

FIGURE 7 | (A) Inhibitory effect of *C. volubile* fatty acids on α-chymotrypsin activity; **(B)** Effect of *C. volubile* fatty acids on kinetics (V_{max}) of α-chymotrypsin. Values = mean ± SD; n = 3.

et al., 2015). The observed apoptotic activity of the fatty acid extract as evident by the increased cell death (**Figure 2**), further indicates the anticancer potency of the fatty acids. This can be attributed to the arrest of S phase with concomitant depopulation of the DNA contents/cell population in G0/G1 as well as G2/M phases of the cell cycle (**Figure 3**). Cell cycle arrest has been implicated in the induction of apoptosis (Aliyu et al., 2013). Fauser et al. (2013) reported the induction of cell cycle by fatty acids.

Cell migration and invasion have been associated with the pathophysiology of cancer and in fact a major characteristic of malignant tumors and one of the key causes of cancer death (Bozzuto et al., 2010). In this study, the observed anti-migration, and invasion activity of the fatty acid extract on U87-MG cancer cells indicates a suppressive effect (**Figure 5**). This can be associated with the ability of the fatty acid enriched extract to inhibit α-chymotrypsin *in vitro* (**Figure 7**). Alpha-chymotrypsin has been implicated in the activation of metalloproteinases, and degradation of the extracellular matrix (ECM proteins), thus plays a major role in tumor growth and metastasis (Novak and Trnka, 2005; Mu et al., 2012). ECM acts as a physical barrier to migrating cells and must be degraded before the metastasis can occur. The *in vitro* inhibition of α-chymotrypsin (**Figure 7**) by the fatty acids therefore indicates a protective potential against ECM degradation. It can thus be suggested that the anti-metastatic action of the fatty acid extract could be facilitated by lowering the ability of glioblastoma cells to degrade the extracellular matrix components, by inhibiting the activities of α-chymotrypsin.

The implication of oxidative stress in the etiology of cancer has been reported (Erukainure et al., 2016). Oxidative stress arises due to an imbalance in the production of free radicals and the cell's own antioxidant defenses (Erukainure et al., 2016). Often described as redox imbalance, it causes an impairment of normal cellular metabolism, which promotes malignancy, cancer initiation, and progression (Acharya et al., 2010). The observed reduced GSH level, SOD and catalase activities with concomitant increased MDA level in untreated U87-MG cells indicates an occurrence of oxidative stress (**Figures 6A–D**). Alteration of these enzymes has been reported in malignant cells and tumor tissues, thus suggesting an occurrence of redox imbalance in cancer cells (Barrera, 2012). The reversed levels and activities on following treatment with the fatty acids indicate an antioxidative potency against glioblastoma (**Figure 6**). Erukainure et al. (2016) reported a similar effect by same extract on MCF-7 cells, indicating the antioxidant protective effect of the leaf fatty acids against human invasive cancers. A remarkable association has been recognized between oxidative stress and increased uncontrollable drive of the G0/G1 and G2/M phases, leading to tumor metastasis and invasion (Pizarro et al., 2009; Chaudhary et al., 2013; Carrasco-Torres et al., 2017). This corresponds with the observed anti-oxidative activity, S phase arrest and concomitant depopulation of DNA contents/cell population in G0/G1 and G2/M phases of the cell cycle (**Figure 3**). This is also reflected by the decreased cell migration (**Figure 5**).

Fatty acids from *C. volubile* leaves could thus suppress tumor metastasis and/or invasion in human neuronal glioblastoma cells by the following mechanism: (1) attenuation of redox imbalance which inactivates the G0/G1 phase; (2) depopulation of DNA in the G0/G1 and G2/M phases with concurrent arrest of the S phase leading to inactivation of the cell cycle and apoptosis; and (3) Inhibition of α-chymotrypsin degradation of the extracellular matrix.

CONCLUSION

The results of the current study suggest a suppressive effect of the fatty acid extract of *C. volubile* leaves against tumor metastasis and/or invasion in human neuronal glioblastoma cells, thus demonstrating their preliminary therapeutic potential. This fatty acid rich extract may thus be proposed as dietary supplements for the treatment, and prevention of such ailments.

AUTHOR CONTRIBUTIONS

OE, NA, AN, AM, GE, and MZ: conceived and designed the project. OE, AN, and NA: performed the MTT, apoptosis, transwell migration, and cell cycle assays. OE and AM: performed the oxidative stress assay. OE, AM, AO, and MZ: performed the statistical analysis. All authors were involved in the interpretation of results. OE, AM, GE, and MZ wrote the manuscript. All authors revised the manuscript.

ACKNOWLEDGMENTS

We appreciate the consistent laboratory effort of Dr. Salman A. Khan from Molecular Oncology Laboratory, Dr. Panjwani Center for Molecular Medicine and Drug Research (PCMD), International Center for Chemical and Biological Sciences, University of Karachi, Karachi, Pakistan. OE acknowledges the World Academy of Sciences for the advancement of Science in Developing Countries (TWAS), Trieste, Italy, for ICCBS-TWAS Fellowship (2012) at the H.E.J. Research Institute of Chemistry, ICCBS, University of Karachi, Karachi, Pakistan.

REFERENCES

Acharya, A., Das, I., Chandhok, D., and Saha, T. (2010). Redox regulation in cancer: a double-edged sword with therapeutic potential. *Oxid. Med. Cell. Longev.* 3, 23–34. doi: 10.4161/oxim.3.1.10095

Adefegha, S., and Oboh, G. (2010). "Water Extractable Phytochemicals from some nigerian spices inhibit Fe2+-induced lipid peroxidation in Rat's brain – in vitro. *J. Food Process. Technol.* 2, 1–6.

Aliyu, M., Odunola, O. A., Farooq, A. D., Rasheed, H., Mesaik, A. M., Choudhary, M. I., et al. (2013). Molecular mechanism of antiproliferation potential of Acacia honey on NCI-H460 cell line. *Nutr. Cancer* 65, 296–304. doi: 10.1080/01635581.2013.756920

Antal, O., Hackler, L., Shen, J., Mán, I., Hideghéty, K., Kitajka, K., et al. (2014). Combination of unsaturated fatty acids and ionizing radiation on human glioma cells: cellular, biochemical and gene expression analysis. *Lipid. Health Dis.* 13, 142. doi: 10.1186/1476-511X-13-142

Barrera, G. (2012). Oxidative stress and lipid peroxidation products in cancer progression and therapy. *ISRN Oncol.* 2012:137289. doi: 10.5402/2012/137289

Bozzuto, G., Ruggieri, P., and Molinari, A. (2010). Molecular aspects of tumor cell migration and invasion. *Ann. Ist. Super. Sanita* 46, 66–80. doi: 10.1590/S0021-25712010000100009

Brada, M., Hoang-Xuan, K., Rampling, R., Dietrich, P., Dirix, L., Macdonald, D., et al. (2001). Multicenter phase II trial of temozolomide in patients with glioblastoma multiforme at first relapse. *Ann. Oncol.* 12, 259–266.

Burkill, H. M. (1985). *The Useful Plants of West Tropical Africa*, Edn 2, Vol. 1. Richmond, VA: Royal Botanic Gardens, Kew.

Cannell, R. J., Kellam, S. J., Owsianka, A. M., and Walker, J. M. (1988). Results of a large scale screen of microalgae for the production of protease inhibitors. *Planta Med.* 54, 10–14. doi: 10.1055/s-2006-962319

Carrasco-Torres, G., Baltiérrez-Hoyos, R., Andrade-Jorge, E., Villa-Treviño, S., Trujillo-Ferrara, J. G., and Vásquez-Garzón, V. R. (2017). Cytotoxicity, oxidative stress, cell cycle arrest, and mitochondrial apoptosis after combined treatment of hepatocarcinoma cells with maleic anhydride derivatives and quercetin. *Oxid. Med. Cell. Longev.* 2017:2734976. doi: 10.1155/2017/2734976

Carrillo, C., Cavia Camarero, M. D. M., and Alonso de la Torre, S. (2012). Antitumor effect of oleic acid; mechanisms of action. A review. *Nutr. Hosp.* 27, 1860–1865. doi: 10.3305/nh.2012.27.6.6010

Chance, B., and Maehly, A. (1955). Assay of catalases and peroxidases. *Method Enzymol.* 2, 764–775. doi: 10.1016/S0076-6879(55)02300-8

Chaudhary, P., Sharma, R., Sahu, M., Vishwanatha, J. K., Awasthi, S., and Awasthi, Y. C. (2013). 4-Hydroxynonenal induces G2/M phase cell cycle arrest by activation of the ataxia telangiectasia mutated and Rad3-related protein (ATR)/checkpoint kinase 1 (Chk1) signaling pathway. *J. Biol. Chem.* 288, 20532–20546. doi: 10.1074/jbc.M113.467662

Chowdhury, P., and Soulsby, M. (2002). Lipid peroxidation in rat brain is increased by simulated weightlessness and decreased by a soy-protein diet. *Annal. Clin. Lab. Sci.* 32, 188–192.

Efird, J. T. (2011). *Epidemiology of Glioma.* Rijeka: INTECH Open Access Publisher.

Ellman, G. L. (1959). Tissue sulfhydryl groups. *Arch. Biochem. Biophys.* 82, 70–77. doi: 10.1016/0003-9861(59)90090-6

Erukainure, L., Oke, O., Owolabi, F., and Adenekan, S. (2010). Antioxidant nutrient properties and antioxidant activities of obenetete (Clerodendrum volubile), a nonconventional leafy vegetable consumed in Nigeria. *Afric. J. Food Agric. Nutr. Dev.* 10, 4156–4167. doi: 10.4314/ajfand.v10i10.62893

Erukainure, O., Oke, O., Ajiboye, A., and Okafor, O. (2011). Nutritional qualities and phytochemical constituents of Clerodendrum volubile, a tropical non-conventional vegetable. *Int. Food Res. J.* 18, 1393–1399.

Erukainure, O. L., Ebuehi, O. A., Choudhary, I. M., Adhikari, A., Hafizur, R. M., Perveen, S., et al. (2014). Iridoid glycoside from the leaves of Clerodendrum volubile beauv. Shows potent antioxidant activity against oxidative stress in rat brain and hepatic tissues. *J. Diet. Suppl.* 11, 19–29. doi: 10.3109/19390211.2013.859213

Erukainure, O. L., Zaruwa, M. Z., Choudhary, M. I., Naqvi, S. A., Ashraf, N., Hafizur, R. M., et al. (2016). Dietary fatty acids from leaves of clerodendrum volubile induce cell cycle arrest, downregulate matrix metalloproteinase-9 expression, and modulate redox status in human breast cancer. *Nutr. Cancer* 68, 634–645. doi: 10.1080/01635581.2016.1156714

Fauser, J., Matthews, G., Cummins, A., and Howarth, G. (2013). Induction of apoptosis by the medium-chain length fatty acid lauric acid in colon cancer cells due to induction of oxidative stress. *Chemotherapy* 59, 214–224. doi: 10.1159/000356067

Jemal, A., Bray, F., Center, M. M., Ferlay, J., Ward, E., and Forman, D. (2011). Global cancer statistics. *CA Cancer J. Clin.* 61, 69–90. doi: 10.3322/caac.20107

Kakkar, P., Das, B., and Viswanathan, P. (1984). A modified spectrophotometric assay of superoxide dismutase. *Indian J. Biochem. Biophys.* 21, 130–132.

Koff, J. L., Ramachandiran, S., and Bernal-Mizrachi, L. (2015). A time to kill: targeting apoptosis in cancer. *Int. J. Mol. Sci.* 16, 2942–2955. doi: 10.3390/ijms16022942

Lowry, O. H., Rosebrough, N. J., Farr, A. L., and Randall, R. J. (1951). Protein measurement with the Folin phenol reagent. *J. Biol. Chem.* 193, 265–275.

Markiewicz-Żukowska, R., Borawska, M. H., Fiedorowicz, A., Naliwajko, S. K., Sawicka, D., and Car, H. (2013). Propolis changes the anticancer activity of temozolomide in U87MG human glioblastoma cell line. *BMC Complement. Altern. Med.* 13:50. doi: 10.1186/1472-6882-13-50

Mosmann, T. (1983). Rapid colorimetric assay for cellular growth and survival: application to proliferation and cytotoxicity assays. *J. Immun. Methods* 65, 55–63. doi: 10.1016/0022-1759(83)90303-4

Motaung, E., Prinsloo, S., Van Aswegen, C., Du Toit, P., Becker, P., and Du Plessis, D. (1999). Cytotoxicity of combined essential fatty acids on a human prostate cancer cell line. *Prostagl. Leukot. Essent. Fatty Acid* 61, 331–337. doi: 10.1054/plef.1999.0107

Mu, X.-M., Shi, W., Sun, L.-X., Li, H., Wang, Y.-R., Jiang, Z.-Z., et al. (2012). Pristimerin inhibits breast cancer cell migration by up-regulating regulator of G protein signaling 4 expression. *Asian Pac. J. Cancer Prev.* 13, 1097–1104. doi: 10.7314/APJCP.2012.13.4.1097

Nickavar, B., Mojab, F., Javidnia, K., and Amoli, M. A. R. (2003). Chemical composition of the fixed and volatile oils of *Nigella sativa* L. from Iran. *Z. Naturforsch. C* 58, 629–631. doi: 10.1515/znc-2003-9-1004

Novak, J. F., and Trnka, F. (2005). Proenzyme therapy of cancer. *Anticancer Res.* 25, 1157–1177.

Pizarro, J. G., Folch, J., Vazquez De la Torre, A., Verdaguer, E., Junyent, F., Jordán, J., et al. (2009). Oxidative stress-induced DNA damage and cell cycle regulation in B65 dopaminergic cell line. *Free Radic. Res.* 43, 985–994. doi: 10.1080/10715760903159188

Potter, J. D., and Potter, J. D. (1997). *Food, Nutrition and the Prevention of Cancer: A Global Perspective: Summary.* Washington, DC: American Institute of Cancer Research.

Pozarowski, P., and Darzynkiewicz, Z. (2004). Analysis of cell cycle by flow cytometry. *Methods Mol. Biol.* 281, 301–311. doi: 10.1385/1-59259-811-0:301

Puli, S., Lai, J. C., and Bhushan, A. (2006). Inhibition of matrix degrading enzymes and invasion in human glioblastoma (U87MG) cells by isoflavones. *J. Neuro Oncol.* 79, 135–142. doi: 10.1007/s11060-006-9126-0

Woolf, E. C., and Scheck, A. C. (2015). The ketogenic diet for the treatment of malignant glioma. *J. Lipid Res.* 56, 5–10. doi: 10.1194/jlr.R046797

Yao, J., Liang, L.-H., Zhang, Y., Ding, J., Tian, Q., Li, J.-J., et al. (2012). GNAI1 suppresses tumor cell migration and invasion and is post-transcriptionally regulated by mir-320a/c/d in hepatocellular carcinoma. *Cancer Biol. Med.* 9, 234–241. doi: 10.7497/j.issn.2095-3941.2012.04.003

3

In-Silico Characterization and *in-Vivo* Validation of Albiziasaponin-A, Iso-Orientin and Salvadorin Using a Rat Model of Alzheimer's Disease

Mahmood Rasool[1], Arif Malik[2], Sulayman Waquar[2], Qura Tul-Ain[2], Tassadaq H. Jafar[2], Rabia Rasool[2], Aasia Kalsoom[2], Muhammad A. Ghafoor[2], Sheikh A. Sehgal[3], Kalamegam Gauthaman[1], Muhammad I. Naseer[1], Mohammed H. Al-Qahtani[1] and Peter N. Pushparaj[1*]*

[1] *Center of Excellence in Genomic Medicine Research, Faculty of Applied Medical Sciences, King Abdulaziz University, Jeddah, Saudi Arabia,* [2] *Institute of Molecular Biology and Biotechnology, The University of Lahore, Lahore, Pakistan,* [3] *Institute of Zoology, Chinese Academy of Sciences, Beijing, China*

***Correspondence:**
Mahmood Rasool
mahmoodrasool@yahoo.com
Peter N. Pushparaj
peter.n.pushparaj@gmail.com

Alzheimer's disease (AD) is a neurodegenerative disorder characterized by dementia, excessive acetylcholinesterase (AChE) activity, formation of neurotoxic amyloid plaque, and tau protein aggregation. Based on literature survey, we have shortlisted three important target proteins (AChE, COX2, and MMP8) implicated in the pathogenesis of AD and 20 different phytocompounds for molecular docking experiments with these three target proteins. The 3D-structures of AChE, COX2, and MMP8 were predicted by homology modeling by MODELLER and the threading approach by using ITASSER. Structure evaluations were performed using ERRAT, Verify3D, and Rampage softwares. The results based on molecular docking studies confirmed that there were strong interactions of these phytocompounds with AChE, COX2, and MMP8. The top three compounds namely Albiziasaponin-A, Iso-Orientin, and Salvadorin showed least binding energy and highest binding affinity among all the scrutinized compounds. Post-docking analyses showed the following free energy change for Albiziasaponin-A, Salvadorin, and Iso-Orientin (−9.8 to −15.0 kcal/mol) as compared to FDA approved drugs (donepezil, galantamine, and rivastigmine) for AD (−6.6 to −8.2 Kcal/mol) and interact with similar amino acid residues (Pro-266, Asp-344, Trp-563, Pro-568, Tyr-103, Tyr-155, Trp-317, and Tyr-372) with the target proteins. Furthermore, we have investigated the antioxidant and anticholinesterase activity of these top three phytochemicals namely, Albiziasaponin-A, Iso-Orientin, and Salvadorin in colchicine induced rat model of AD. Sprague Dawley (SD) rat model of AD were developed using bilateral intracerebroventricular (ICV) injection of colchicine (15 μg/rat). After the induction of AD, the rats were subjected to treatment with phytochemicals individually or in combination for 3 weeks. The serum samples were further analyzed for biomarkers such as 8-hydroxydeoxyguanosine (8-OHdG), 4-hydroxynonenal (4-HNE), tumor necrosis factor-alpha (TNF-α), cyclooxygenase-2 (COX-2), matrix metalloproteinase-8 (MMP-8), isoprostanes-2 alpha (isoP-2α), and acetylcholine esterase (AChE) using conventional Enzyme Linked Immunosorbent

Assay (ELISA) method. Additionally, the status of lipid peroxidation was estimated calorimetrically by measuring thiobarbituric acid reactive substances (TBARS). Here, we observed a statistically significant reduction ($P < 0.05$) in the oxidative stress and inflammatory markers in the treatment groups receiving mono and combinational therapies using Albiziasaponin-A, Iso-Orientin, and Salvadorin as compared to colchicine alone group. Besides, the ADMET profiles of these phytocompounds were very promising and, hence, these potential neuroprotective agents may further be taken for preclinical studies either as mono or combinational therapy for AD.

Keywords: Alzheimer's disease, acetylcholinesterase (AChE), salvadorin, Albiziasaponin A, iso-orientin, *in silico* modeling, *in vivo* rat model, molecular docking

INTRODUCTION

Alzheimer's disease (AD) is a progressive and irreversible neurodegenerative disease characterized by dementia and afflicted individuals show a steady decline of memory and cognitive impairment (Zhang et al., 2011). The two pathogenic characteristics of AD are the neuritic plaques (NPs) of β-amyloid protein (Aβ) and insoluble twisted fibers called neurofibrillary tangles (NFTs) in the brain. These neurofibrillary tangles are the aggregates of "Tau" proteins involved in the stabilization of microtubules. Recognizable types of AD are often related with mutations in amyloid precursor proteins (APP) the presenilin-1 (PS1) or presenilin-2 (PS2). Sequential cleavage of APP by γ-secretases leads to the formation of amyloid beta (Aβ) protein, especially their longer isoforms ($A\beta_{40}$, $A\beta_{42}$) and especially $A\beta_{42}$ is more fibrillogenic and is associated with disease states (Yin et al., 2007). β-amyloid protein (Aβ) provokes synaptic disorganization, disturbs neural activity, and induces brain tissue damage. Accumulation and dispersal of Aβ in the brain is often associated with the clinical manifestation of AD (Muliyala and Varghese, 2010). The term AD was initially coined by Emil Kraepelin *in honor of Alois Alzheimer*, a German psychiatrist, who first identified this neurodegenerative disease in 1906 (Möller and Graeber, 1998). Presence of AD may be indicated by co-occurrences such as cognitive dysfunction, hallucinations, anxiety, depression, delusions, irritability, personality changes, sleep disturbance, agitation, restlessness, yelling, shredding paper, poor judgment and difficulty in learning and thoughts (Cummings et al., 1994). Aging Demographics and Memory Study (ADAMS) assessment indicates 16% of females and 11% of males aged 71 or more were suffering with AD (Plassman et al., 2007). The incidence of AD is projected to increase to 135 million by 2050 (He et al., 2016), and an estimate based on the United States 2010 census identified that out of about 5.3 million patients of AD of age group 65, amongst which 3.3 million are women and 2 million are men (Hebert et al., 2013).

AD is a multifactorial neurodegenerative disease due to the accumulation of Aβ plaques and NFTs in the brain. Various genes such as APP, BACE1, PS1/2, ApoE, NEP, IDE are found to be involved in the initiation and development of AD (Dong et al., 2012). Aging is one of the common causative factors for the development of AD. An array of factors are involved in the development and progression of AD like genetic mutation, polymorphism, irregular immune or inflammatory response, injury, oxidative stress, use of drugs, hormone replacement therapies, and also some environmental factors including education, low socio-economic status, nutrition and lack of social interactions (Small, 1998). Lethargy, violence and exertion may exist in these individuals (Förstl and Kurz, 1999). Cognitive dysfunction, diminished memory, difficulty in recognition, impaired speech and gait are predominant features in AD (Sperling et al., 2011). Molecular pathology of disease presents accumulation of amyloid plaques in different areas of brain. Various cutting edge laboratory techniques and tests are essential to understand the associated biological features. The structural and functional brain imaging approaches such as the use of computed tomography (CT), magnetic resonance imaging (MRI), positron emission tomography (PET), and single photon emission computed tomography (SPECT) enables the evaluation of brain activities in general and some also help in identification of pathological lacerations and abrasions in AD (Small, 2002).

Various factors contribute to the efficient treatment of AD and include both pharmacological and non-pharmacological therapies. Currently, there is no definitive therapy for AD. Acetylcholinesterase (AChE) inhibitors are the only licensed drug of various drugs used for the management and treatment of AD, and it helps to recover the symptoms of cognitive and neuropsychiatric impairments in AD. Some non-pharmacological therapies show positive response and attenuate the symptoms of disease (Grossberg et al., 2010). Non-pharmacologic treatments usually preserve and recover cognitive function. They help to maintain behavioral symptoms, personality changes, anxiety, depression, sleep disturbances (Grossberg et al., 2010). Bioactive and naturally occurring phytochemicals are reported to effectively reduce the risks of AD (Essa et al., 2012). Phytochemicals in general, are less toxic as compared to the synthetic drugs (Kim et al., 2014), have many beneficial effects including anti-oxidant activity (Kumar and Khanum, 2012) and therefore can be used for the treatment of AD (Venkatesan et al., 2015). There are some naturally occuring AChE/ butyrylcholinesterase (BChE) inhibitors as well-known as physostigmine and huperzine A

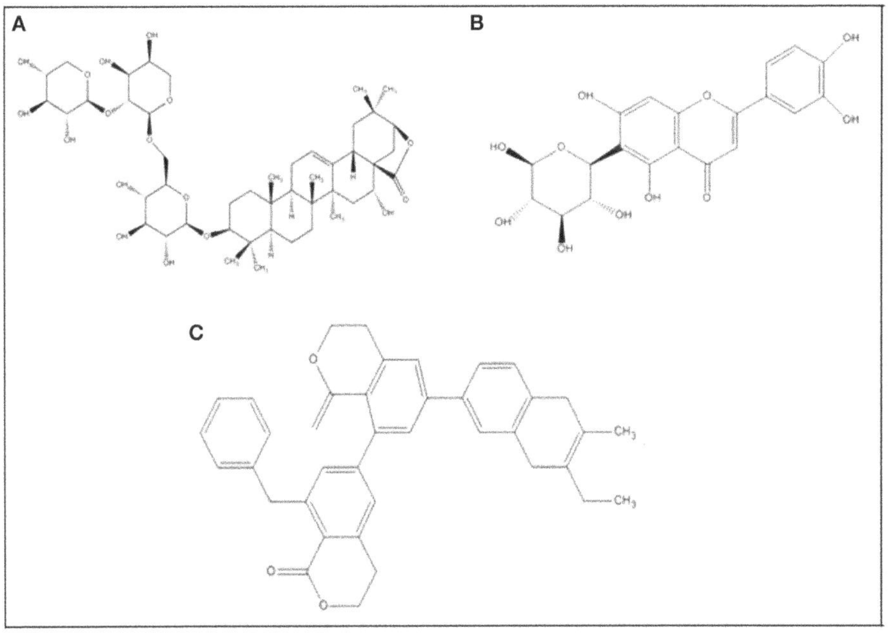

FIGURE 1 | 2D chemical structures of selected three top-ranked phytocompounds **(A)**, Albiziasaponin-A **(B)**, Iso-Orientin and **(C)**, Salavadorin.

TABLE 1 | Experimental design.

Groups (n=10)	Treatments	
	Cholchicine (15 μg, icv)	**Phytochemicals (100 mg/kg BW per oral)**
A	No (Sham Control)	Nil
B	Yes (Control)	Nil
C	Yes	Albiziasaponin-A
D	Yes	Iso-Orientin
E	Yes	Salvadorin
F	Yes	Albiziasaponin-A+Iso-Orientin
G	Yes	Albiziasaponin-A+Salvadorin
H	Yes	Iso-Orientin+Salvadorin
I	Yes	Albiziasaponin-A+Salvadorin+Iso-Orientin

from plant origin that show effective cognitive impairment (Essa et al., 2012).

MATERIALS AND METHODS

Drugs, Chemicals, Reagents and Assay Kits

The Salvadorin and Albiziasaponin A were prepared as described before and the isoorientin was purchased from Sigma (Yoshikawa et al., 2002; Mahmood et al., 2005). All other drugs, chemicals and reagents were purchased from Sigma Chemicals Co. (St. Louis Mo, USA).

In Silco Studies

The amino acid sequence of 3 target rat proteins (AChE 614 a.a.), COX2 (614 a.a), and MMP8 (158 a.a) were obtained from Uniprot database in FASTA format with their accession numbers (AChE (1Q83), COX2 (1PXX) respectively. All the proteins were subjected to PSI-BLAST (Altschul et al., 1990) against the Protein Data Bank (Sussman et al., 1998) to recognize the appropriate templates. MODELLER v9.18 (Fiser and Šali, 2003) was utilized to predict the 3D structures of proteins except of MMP8. Structures were further cross-validated with the help of ITASSER (Zhang, 2008). Three-dimensional (3D) structure of MMP8 was retrieved from RCSB (https://www.rcsb.org). Other validation tools used for the validation of protein structures include ERRAT (Colovos and Yeates, 1993), Verify3D (Eisenberg et al., 1997), and Rampage (Lovell et al., 2003). Obtained structures were then minimized using UCSF Chimera 1.112 (Meng et al., 2006) at 1000 steepest and 1000 conjugate gradient runs with Amber force field parameters.

After extensive survey of literature, 20 phytocompounds were selected from PubChem (Bolton et al., 2008) and were subjected to further structural optimization using ChemDraw Ultra. The energy-minimization, and geometry optimization of all compounds, was carried out by the help of UCSF Chimera v1.12 at 1,500 steepest and 1,500 conjugate gradient runs. The binding sites of all the target proteins were predicted using online tools like COACH (Yang et al., 2013), CASTP (Dundas et al., 2006), and 3D-ligand site (Wass et al., 2010). For comparison, three FDA approved drugs (Donepezil, Galantamine, and Rivastigmine) were administered to rats with AD. Two dimensional (2D) structures of these drugs were retrieved from PubChem (https://pubchem.ncbi.nlm.nih.gov/)

TABLE 2 | Response of albiziasaponin-a, salvadorin, iso-orientin in a rat model following colchicine (col) induced oxidative stress.

Groups	Mean ± SD (n = 10)							
	AChE µmol/min/mg Protein	4-HNE (ng/L)	8-OHdG (pg/ml)	TNF-α (ng/ml)	IsoP-2α (pg/ml)	MDA (nmol/ml)	COX-2 (ng/ml)	MMP-8 (ng/ml)
A	1.93 ± 0.03	1.29 ± 0.016	2.09 ± 0.16	18.29 ± 1.88	21.25 ± 2.19	0.99 ± 0.056	0.71 ± 0.012	33.25 ± 2.08
B	3.19 ± 0.95	18.26 ± 1.29	21.29 ± 3.29	92.26 ± 3.28	181.26 ± 5.26	8.28 ± 1.26	4.29 ± 1.07	115.26 ± 12.26
C	2.09 ± 0.62	12.29 ± 2.22	17.19 ± 2.28	45.29 ± 4.56	102.26 ± 7.28	4.29 ± 2.16	2.08 ± 0.99	65.26 ± 5.16
D	2.03 ± 0.19	16.19 ± 3.19	15.29 ± 3.29	56.23 ± 4.09	98.26 ± 6.25	5.99 ± 1.09	3.09 ± 0.19	71.26 ± 12.25
E	1.99 ± 0.23	13.29 ± 2.55	13.29 ± 2.18	32.26 ± 4.26	78.26 ± 7.26	6.66 ± 2.88	1.99 ± 0.166	52.26 ± 3.88
F	1.86 ± 0.13	10.26 ± 4.26	8.89 ± 1.28	35.26 ± 4.26	47.26 ± 5.26	4.19 ± 1.08	2.58 ± 0.19	46.26 ± 4.26
G	1.86 ± 0.11	12.26 ± 4.16	14.26 ± 3.29	27.19 ± 3.29	68.26 ± 4.44	3.29 ± 1.07	2.99 ± 0.198	51.26 ± 6.35
H	1.74 ± 0.18	9.28 ± 2.11	8.29 ± 3.26	28.26 ± 5.26	45.29 ± 4.23	4.19 ± 1.00	1.99 ± 0.165	50.26 ± 6.25
I	1.66 ± 0.32	2.16 ± 1.08	3.29 ± 1.99	15.26 ± 3.26	27.26 ± 4.277	1.09 ± 0.087	1.06 ± 0.047	40.22 ± 6.32
LSD (0.05)	0.34	3.02	6.29	10.26	8.16	2.09	1.25	7.16
p-VALUE	0.034	0.001	0.014	0.013	0.012	0.030	0.000	0.019

A-Control; B-Col alone; C-Col+Albiziasaponin-A; D-Col+Iso-Orientin; E-Col+Salvadorin; F-Col+Albiziasaponin-A+Iso-Orientin. G-Col+Albiziasaponin-A+Salvadorin; H-Col+Iso-Orientin+Salvadorin; I-Col+Albiziasaponin-A+Salvadorin+Iso-Orientin. Dose of Colchicine (Col) (15 µg Intracerebroventricular injection in each animal). Dose of Albiziasaponin-A, Salvadorin, Iso-Orientin (100 mg/kg BW per oral).

TABLE 3 | Pearson s' correlation coeeficients of different variables in rats under colchicine (col) stress receiving albiziasaponin-a, salvadorin, iso-orientin.

Variables	AchE	4-HNE	8-OHdG	TNF-α	IsoP-2α	MDA	COX-2	MMP-8
AchE	1.000	0.423	0.519	0.399	0.435	0.512*	0.423	0.823**
4-HNE		1.000	0.645*	0.715**	0.619**	0.774**	0.684**	0.659*
8-OhdG			1.000	0.648**	0.671**	0.719**	0.589*	0.726**
TNF-α				1.000	0.746*	0.659**	0.589**	0.865**
IsoP-2α					1.000	0.614**	0.741**	0.665
MDA						1.000	0.621*	0.596**
COX-2							1.000	0.619*
MMP-8								1.000

***Correlation is significant at the 0.01 level (two-tailed). *$p < 0.05$, **$p < 0.01$, ***$p < 0.001$.*

and were then configured by ChemDraw ultra (**Figure 1**). Finally, molecular docking studies were carried out by using Auto Dock Vina (Trott and Olson, 2010). The hydrogen polar atoms were added to all the selected receptor proteins. The total docking runs were sets to 100 for each docking experiment. The grid size was set at 126 × 126 × 126 Å in the x-, y-, and z-axis, respectively, with 0.575 Å grid spacing for all the selected 3 target proteins. The genetic algorithm implemented in Auto Dock Vina was utilized as the key search protocol, while other parameters were set to default values. Further it was visualized by UCSF Chimera v1.12 and ADMET properties of all compounds were calculated by admetSAR online tool (Cheng et al., 2012). The parameters of Lipinski RO5 were calculated by mCule server (Kiss et al., 2012).

In Vivo Animal Experiments

For the *In vivo* characterization of phytocompounds one hundred (n = 100) 6–8 weeks old male Sprague Dawley (SD) rats were categorized into ten different groups (n = 10) as A, B, C, D, E, F, G, H, I, and J. Ethical approval from the Institutional Review Board of the University of Lahore was obtained. All the animals were housed in the animal holding unit (AHU) and acclimatized for about 2 weeks under reversed light/dark (12 h each) cycle. Animals were fed on normal rat chow and had access to water *ad libitum.*

Development of Cochicine Induced AD Model

The SD rats were treated with intracerbroventricualr (icv) injection of cholchicine as described before (Kumar et al., 2009). Briefly, the rats were anasthetized with sodium pentobarbital 45 mg/kg body weight) and placed in stereotaxic apparatus. Through a midline sagittal incison the scalp was reflected and two drill holes made in the skull for placement of the injection canula in the lateral cerebral ventricle. The animals were given post-opeative antibiotic (gentamycin 5 mg/kg, intraperitoneally) to ward off sepsis. Rats were then administered cholchicine (15 µg dissolved in 5 µl of artificial cerebrospinal fluid) using Hamilton microsyringe. To facilitate drug diffusion, the canula was left in place for 2–3 min after the injection. The wound was then sealed with sterile wax and Neosporin powder sprayed externally as an additional antiseptic measure.

TABLE 4 | Binding affinities of all 20 phytocompounds and mCule properties.

Phytocompounds	Binding affinities (kcal/mol) against ache	Binding affinities (kcal/mol) against cox2	Binding affinities (kcal/mol) against MMP8	Mass	LOGP	HBA	HBD	PSA	RO5 Violations	Atoms	Rings
Salvadorin	−12.5	−12.1	−9.8	414.62	6.34	3.00	0	43.37	1	72.00	5
Albiziasaponin-A	−13.0	−15.0	−10.6	897.05	0.40	17	9	263.75	3	135	9
Epigallocatechin-3-gallate	−11.5	−10.6	−10.6	458.37	2.23	11	8	197.37	2	51	4
β-Sitosterol	−11.9	−8.7	−8.3	432.76	8.74	1	1	20.23	1	87	4
Iso-orientin	−12.5	−11.4	−10.0	434.34	−0.24	11	8	201.28	2	49	4
Melanoxetin	−9.9	−10.3	−7.9	302.23	1.98	7	5	131.36	0	32	3
Epicatechin	−9.2	−8.9	−7.8	290.26	1.54	6	5	110.38	0	35	3
Albigenin	−10.5	−9.8	−7.9	426.67	7.10	2	1	37.300	1	77	5
Lupeol	−9.6	−9.1	−7.3	426.71	8.02	1	1	20.23	1	81	5
Catechin	−10.0	−9.5	−8.5	290.26	1.54	6	5	110.38	0	35	3
Cabralealactone	−9.4	−10.1	−7.1	552.70	8.69	3.00	1.00	35.30	2.00	78.00	7.00
β-Amyrin	−8.9	−10.8	−7.5	426.71	8.16	1	1	20.23	1	81	5
Isovitexin	−9.9	−9.1	−9.3	132.37	0.09	10	7	181.05	1	51	4
Oleanolic acid	−9.4	−10.8	−8.2	456.69	7.23	3	2	57.53	1	81	5
Elliptone	−10.0	−9.1	−8.7	352.33	3.56	6	0	67.13	0	42	5
Genistein	−7.6	−9.4	−6.3	270.23	2.57	5	3	90.90	0	30	3
Kaempferol	−9.0	−8.1	−6.6	286.23	2.28	6	4	111.13	0	31	3
Solasodine	−8.1	−10.1	−7.1	429.68	5.57	3.00	1.00	32.70	1.00	78.00	6.00
Afzelechin	−7.1	−7.9	−7.5	274.26	1.84	5	4	90.15	0	34	3
Luteolin	−9.4	−10.3	−7.2	286.23	2.28	6	4	111.13	0	31	3

TABLE 5 | ADMET profile analyses of all 20 phytocompounds.

Phytocompounds	Bbb	Hia	CYP450 2C9 and 2D6 substrate	CYP450 2C9 and 2D6 inhibitor	CYP Inhibitory promiscuity (IP)	Ames toxicity	Carcinogens	Biodegradation	Acute oral toxicity	Aqueous solubility (LogS)	Rat acute toxicity (LD50, mol/kg)
Salvadorin	+	+	Non-substrate	Non-inhibitor	Low CYP IP	Non AMES toxic	Non-Carcinogens	Not readily biodegradable	III	−5.3955	2.0387
Albiziasaponin-A	+	+	Non-substrate	Non-inhibitor	Low CYP IP	Non AMES toxic	Non-Carcinogens	Not readily biodegradable	III	−4.2181	3.5521
Epigallocatechin-3-gallate	−	+	Non-substrate	Non-inhibitor	Low CYP IP	Non-AMES Toxic	Non-Carcinogens	Not readily biodegradable	IV	−3.3141	2.6643
β-Sitosterol	+	+	Non-substrate	Non-inhibitor	Low CYP IP	Non AMES toxic	Non-Carcinogens	Not readily biodegradable	I	−4.7027	2.6561
Iso-orientin	−	+	Non-substrate	Non-inhibitor	Low CYP IP	AMES Toxic	Non-Carcinogens	Not readily biodegradable	IV	−2.3978	2.3664
Melanoxetin	+	+	Non-substrate	Inhibitor for CYP450 2C9 and Non-inhibitor for CYP450 2D6	Low CYP IP	Non-AMES Toxic	Non-Carcinogens	Not readily biodegradable	II	−3.0804	3.1831
Epicatechin	−	+	Non-substrate	Non-inhibitor	Low CYP IP	Non-AMES Toxic	Non-Carcinogens	Not readily biodegradable	IV	−3.1015	1.8700
Albigenin	+	+	Non-substrate	Non-inhibitor	Low CYP IP	Non AMES toxic	Non-Carcinogens	Not readily biodegradable	III	−4.0877	2.0616
Lupeol	+	+	Non-substrate	Non-inhibitor	Low CYP IP	Non AMES toxic	Non-Carcinogens	Not readily biodegradable	III	−4.4139	3.3838
Catechin	−	+	Non-substrate	Non-inhibitor	Low CYP IP	Non-AMES Toxic	Non-Carcinogens	Not readily biodegradable	IV	−3.1015	1.8700
Cabralealactone	+	+	Non-substrate	Non-inhibitor	Low CYP IP	Non AMES toxic	Non-Carcinogens	Not readily biodegradable	III	−4.0522	2.4518
β-Amyrin	+	+	Non-substrate	Non-inhibitor	Low CYP IP	Non AMES toxic	Non-Carcinogens	Not readily biodegradable	III	−4.5209	2.0842
Isovitexin	−	+	Non-substrate	Non-inhibitor	Low CYP IP	AMES Toxic	Non-Carcinogens	Not readily biodegradable	IV	−2.3978	2.3664
Oleanolic acid	+	+	Non-substrate	Non-inhibitor	Low CYP IP	Non AMES toxic	Non-Carcinogens	Not readily biodegradable	III	−4.3883	2.3902
Elliptone	+	+	Non-substrate	Inhibitor	High CYP IP	Non AMES toxic	Non-Carcinogens	Not readily biodegradable	III	−3.2813	2.4560
Genistein	+	+	Non-substrate	Inhibitor for CYP450 2C9 and Non-inhibitor for CYP450 2D6	High CYP IP	Non AMES toxic	Non-Carcinogens	Not readily biodegradable	II	−3.0925	3.2988

(Continued)

TABLE 5 | Continued

Phytocompounds	Bbb	Hia	CYP450 2C9 and 2D6 substrate	CYP450 2C9 and 2D6 inhibitor	CYP Inhibitory promiscuity (IP)	Ames toxicity	Carcinogens	Biodegradation	Acute oral toxicity	Aqueous solubility (LogS)	Rat acute toxicity (LD50, mol/kg)
Kaempferol	+	+	Non-substrate	Inhibitor for CYP450 2C9 and Non-inhibitor for CYP450 2D6	High CYP IP	Non AMES toxic	Non-Carcinogens	Not readily biodegradable	II	−3.1423	3.0825
Solasodine	+	+	Non-substrate	Non-inhibitor	Low CYP IP	Non AMES toxic	Non-Carcinogens	Not readily biodegradable	III	−4.0047	1.9513
Afzelechin	+	+	Non-substrate	Non-inhibitor	Low CYP IP	Non AMES toxic	Non-Carcinogens	Not readily biodegradable	IV	−3.2332	2.0532
Luteolin	−	+	Non-substrate	Non-inhibitor	High CYP IP	Non AMES toxic	Non-Carcinogens	Not readily biodegradable	II	−2.9994	3.0200

Experimental Groups and Phytocompounds Treatment

The SD rats were randomly divided into 10 different groups (A, B, C, D, E, F, G, H, I, and J) (**Table 1**). The animals in Group A served as normal control and received no treatment with cholichicine. While the animals in Group B were injected with chochicine, but received no additional treatment and served as positive control. Group C to Group J were treated with the phytocompounds (Albiziasaponin-A, Iso-orientin and Salvadorian) which were selected earlier based on *in silico* screening studies (details provided in the next section). The phytocompounds were administered either individually or in combinations at a concentration of 100 mg/kg for each compound per orally for 3 weeks (see **Table 1** for details). Following the study period, all animals were sacrificed using inhalational overdose of carbon dioxide (CO_2). Blood samples were collected and allowed to clot for 60 min at room temperature. The blood samples were then centrifuged at 3,000 rpm for 10 min and the serum separated were stored as aliquots in −80°C until use in experiments.

Enzyme Linked Immunosorbent Assay (ELISA)

The serum samples from the control and treatment gorups were analyzed for the levels of 8-hydroxydeoxyguanosine (8-OHdG), 4-hydroxynonenal (4-HNE), tumor necrosis factor-alpha (TNF-α), cyclooxygenase-2 (COX-2), matrix metalloproteinase-8 (MMP-8), isoprostanes-2 alpha (isoP-2α) and acetylcholine esterase (AChE) using commercial ELISA kits according to the respective kit protocol following manufacturer's instructions.

Lipid Peroxidation Assay

The level of lipid peroxidation was estimated calorimetrically by measuring thiobarbituric acid reactive substances (TBARS) as described by Ohkawa et al. (1979). Briefly, to 0.2 ml of sample, 8.1% sodium dodecyl sulfate (0.2 ml), 20% acetic acid (1.5 ml) and 0.8% thiobarbituric acid (1.5 ml) were added. Following centrifugation (3,000 rpm for 10 min), the upper organic layer was aspirated, and the optical density (OD) was read at 532 nm using a spectrophotometer (Echelle, LTB Lasertechnik Berlin Gmbh). The levels of lipid peroxides were expressed as millimoles of TBARS/g.

STATISTICAL ANALYSES

The correlation analysis of the raw data for all the attributes was computed using COSTAT computer package (CoHort software, 2003, Monterey, California). The comparison of means was done by COSTAT computer package using Duncan's Multiple Range (DMR) test.

RESULTS

In Silico Characterization

After the *in-silco* analysis of all the proteins best suitable templates were selected on the basis of identity and query. After the generation of 3D structures of proteins overall identity and query coverage remained >65% in between selected templates and targets from end to end. The percentage was considered satisfactory for the prediction of 3D structure by homology modeling approach. The results were further cross-validated by other approaches using MODELLER V9.18 and ITASSER. Almost about 15 models for each protein were generated and evaluated showing favored, allowed and not-allowed regions. Furthermore, selected models were subjected for molecular docking. With the help of literature survey binding regions of proteins were identified and docked by current literature and various online tools. On basis of the score three best compounds were selected and were then compared with approved drugs for their efficacy.

One hundred runs (100) were done to generate docking complexes out of which top-ranked docked complex was selected for each protein based on the lowest binding affinity. It shows the overall binding energies of selected phytocompounds against AChE, COX2, and MMP8 remain (−6.3 to −15.0 Kcal/mol) as in **Table 1**. The lowest binding affinity of Albiziasaponin-A against targeted proteins was −13.0, −15.0, and −10.6 Kcal/mol respectively. While in the case of Iso-orientin and Salvadorin, the observed affinities were (−12.5, −11.4 and,−10.0 Kcal/mol) and (−12.5, −12.1, and −9.8 Kcal/mol) respectively. Moreover, these three phytocompounds have the lowest affinities to AChE similar to FDA approved drugs, Donepezil, Galantamine, and Rivastigmine, with binding affinities (−7.8, −8.2, and −6.6 Kcal/mol respectively) as shown in **Table 3**. All the selected compounds share common interactive residues as listed in **Table 4** (Tyr-103, Tyr-155, Trp-317, His-318, Leu320, Glu-323, Phe-328, and Tyr-372). The ADMET profiles (absorption, distribution, metabolism, excretion, and toxicity) also differed significantly as given in **Table 5**. The comparative molecular docking analyses of top 3 selected compounds and FDA approved drugs against AChE and the potential binding modes of these compounds with the interacting aminoacid residues at the atomic level with AChE were give in **Tables 6, 7** respectively. Besides, we have depicted the specific atoms of these three phytocompounds interacting with the aminoacid residues in the binding site of AChE in **Figure 5**.

IN VIVO STUDIES

The current study showed that use of phytocompounds individually or in combination have exerted significant improvements in biochemical parameters in the rat model of AD. Colchicine (Col) is responsible for the induction oxidative stress (**Table 2**) when compared to rats receiving colchicine presented the levels of AChE, 4-HNE, 8-OHdG, TNF-α, Iso-P2α, MDA, COX-2 and MMP-8 were significantly higher (3.19 ± 0.95 μmol/min/mg protein, 18.26 ± 1.29 ng/L, 21.29 ± 3.29 pg/ml, 92.26 ± 3.28 ng/ml, 181.26 ± 5.26 pg/ml, 8.28 ± 1.26 nmol/ml, 8.28 ± 1.26 nmol/ml, 4.29 ± 1.07 ng/ml, and 115.26 ± 12.26 ng/ml) as compared to the control group (1.93 ± 0.03 μmol/min/mg protein, 1.29 ± 0.016 ng/L, 2.09 ± 0.16 pg/ml, 18.29 ± 1.88 ng/ml, 21.25 ± 2.19 pg/ml, 0.99 ± 0.056 nmol/ml, 0.71 ± 0.01 ng/ml, and 33.25 ± 2.08 ng/ml). Furthermore, it shows that rats receiving Albiziasaponin-A, Iso-orientin and Salvadorian individually in Group C, D, and E reduced the levels of oxidative stress markers. Levels of 4-HNE and MDA were maximally reduced in the group C (receiving Albizasaponin-A) with (12.29 ± 2.22 ng/L) and (4.29 ± 2.16 nmol/ml) followed by group D and E (16.19 ± 3.19 ng/L, 5.99 ± 1.09 nmol/ml) and (13.29 ± 2.55 ng/L, 6.66 ± 2.88 nmol/ml) respectively. While levels of 8-OHdG, TNF-α and IsoP-2α were most improved in group E. Groups F, G and H were given different combinations of these phytocompounds. Results show a maximum synergism in the group H (group treated with combination of Iso-Orientin and Salvadorian, and results were significant as compared to all other groups (B, C, D, E, F, G). Finally in group I (treated with all three phytochemicals Albiziasaponin-A, Iso-orientin and Salvadorian) levels of different biochemical markers (4-HNE, 8-OHdG, TNF-α, IsoP-2α and MDA) were significantly reduced (2.16 ± 1.08 ng/L, 3.29 ± 1.99 pg/ml, 15.26 ± 3.26 ng/ml, 27.26 ± 4.277 pg/ml, and 1.09 ± 0.087 nmol/ml) as compared to group B (colchicine alone) and all the treatment groups C, D, E, F, G, and H. A significant positive correlation was observed among different variables, AChE vs. MMP-8 (r = 0.823**), TNF-α vs. MMP-8 (r = 0.865**), 8-OHdG vs. MDA (r = 0.719**), and 4-HNE vs. MDA (r = 0.774**) in rats experimentally induced with colchicine and administered with Albiziasaponin-A, Iso-Orientin and Salvadorin (**Table 3**).

DISCUSSION

The field of drug designing and development has progressed over last few years. It elucidates new and useful computational methods for the development of novel drugs (Kumar et al., 2011). In silico studies enabled the researchers to identify and develop less toxic herbal medicines as compared to that of conventional remedies (Taylor et al., 2001). The present study was designed to characterize the beneficial effects of different phytocompounds against AD using both *in silico* and *in vivo* strategies. Several phytocompounds with different active groups were screened and characterized using molecular docking studies. The top three phytocompounds, Albiziasaponin-A, Iso-Orientin, and Salvadorin, were selected for further validation in a rat model of AD based on least binding energy and highest binding affinity with target proteins, AChE, COX2, and MMP8, as compared to other phytocompounds. Moreover, Albiziasaponin-A, Iso-Orientin, and Salvadorin interact with the amino acid residues in the binding sites of AChE similar to the FDA approved drugs (donepezil, galantamine and rivastigmine) for AD treatment. Also, the cross validation of binding sites of the selected target proteins using literature mining precisely envisage the binding sites were similar to the binding pocket identified in our molecular docking analyses (Cheung et al., 2012, 2013; Caliandro et al., 2018). Besides, other phytocompunds, such as Epigallocatechin-3-Gallate (EGCG), and β-Sitosterol, strongly bind *in silico* with AChE, COX2, and MMP8. The EGCG has a very strong antioxidant activity, which is ascribed to the presence of B ring trihydroxy group and esterified gallate in C3 of the ring and it may cross the blood-brain barrier (BBB) in a time-dependent manner (Kim et al., 2014).

TABLE 6 | Comparative molecular docking analyses of top 3 selected compounds and FDA approved drugs against AChE.

TOP 3 selected phytocompounds from 20 phytocompounds and FDA approved drugs	BINDING affinities (kcal/mol) of top 3 selected phytocompounds and FDA approved drugs	INTERACTIVE residues in docked complexes of top 3 phytocompounds and FDA approved drugs
Albiziasaponin-A	−13.0 Kcal/mol	Asn-264, Pro-266, Thr-269, Ser-271, Arg-327, Thr-342, Asp-344, Trp-563, Asn-564, Pro-568, Leu-571
Iso-orientin	−12.5 Kcal/mol	**Tyr-103, Tyr-155, Trp-317, His-318, Leu320, Glu-323, Phe-328,** Tyr-368, Phe-369, **Tyr-372**
Salvadorin	−12.5 Kcal/mol	**Tyr-103, Tyr-155, Trp-317, His-318, Leu320, Glu-323, Phe-328, Tyr-372**
FDA APPROVED DRUGS		
Donepezil	−7.8 Kcal/mol	Pro-266, Asp-344, Gln-444, Pro-441, His-436, Trp-563, Pro-568
Galantamine	−8.2 Kcal/mol	Tyr-103, Tyr-155, Trp-317, Ser-324, Tyr-372
Rivastigmine	−6.6 Kcal/mol	Gly-45, Pro-83, Leu-209, Gln-212, Trp-213, Glu-216

TABLE 7 | The binding modes of these compounds with the interacting aminoacid residues at the atomic level with AChE.

Top 3 selected phytocompounds	Compounds interact with atoms of the active site residues of AChE
Albiziasaponin-	Asn-264: CA, CB, CG, OD1, HD21, ND2 Pro-266: 1C, CA, CG, N Thr-269: CA, CB, CG2, HG1, OG1 Ser-271: CA, CB, HG, OG Arg-327: CA, CB, CG, CZ, HE, HH11, HH12, H21, H22, NH1, NH2, NE Thr-342: CA, CB, HB, H1,H21, H22, H23, OG1, Asp-344: CA, CB, HB2, HB3, OD1, OD2 Trp-563: CA, CB, CD1, CD2, CE2, CE3, CH2, CG, CZ2, CZ3, HE1, NE1 Asn-564: CA, CB, CG, HB2, HB3, HD22, OD1, OE1, ND2 Pro-568: CB, CD, CG, HB2, HB3, HD2, HD3, HG2, HG3, N Leu-571: CA, CB, CG, CD1, CD2, HG, HB2, HB3, HD12, HD13, HD22, HD23
Iso-orientin	Tyr-103: CA, CB, CG, CD2, CE1, CE2, CZ, HH, OH Trp-317: CA, CB, CG, CD1, CD2, CE1, CE2, CE3, CH2, CZ2, CZ3, HB2, HB3, HD1, HE1, HE3, HH2, HZ2, HZ3 Tyr-155: CA, CB, CG, CD1, CD2, CE1, CE2, CZ, HH, OH His-318: CA, CB, CG, CD2, CE1, HB3, HE1, HE2, HD2, ND1, NE2 Leu320: CA, CB, CG, CD1, CD2, HG, HB2, HB3, HD11, HD12, HD13, HD21, HD22, HD23 Glu-323: CB, CG, CD, HB2, HB3, HG2, HG3, OE1, OE2 Phe-328: CA, CB, CG, CD1, CD2,CE1, CE2, CZ, HB2, HB3, HD1, HD2, HE1, HE2 Tyr-368: CA, CB, CG, CD1, CD2, CE1, CE2, CZ, HH, OH Phe-369: CB, CG, CA, CD1, CD2, CE1, CE2, CZ, HB2, HB3, HD1, HD2, HE1, HE2, Tyr-372: CB, CG, CD1, CD2, CE1, CE2, CZ, HB2, HB3, HD1, HD2, HE1, HE2, HH, OH
Salvadorin	Tyr-103: CA, CB, CG, CD1, CD2, CE1, CE2, CZ, HB2, HB3, HD1, HD2, HH, OH Tyr-155: CA, CB, CG, CD1, CD2, CE1, CE2, CZ, HH, OH Trp-317: CA, CB, CG, C, CD1, CD2, CE1, CE2, CE3, CH2, CZ2, CZ3, HB2, HB3, HD1, HE1, HE3, HH2, HZ2, HZ3, NE1 His-318: CA, CB, CG, CD2, CE1, HB2, HB3, HE1, HE2, HD2, ND1, NE2 Leu320: CA, CB, CG, CD1, CD2, HG, HB2, HB3, HD11, HD12, HD13, HD21, HD22, HD23 Glu-323: CA, CB, CG, CD, HB2, HB3, HG2, HG3, OE1, OE2 Phe-328: CA, CB, CG, CD1, CD2,CE1, CE2, CZ, HB2, HB3, HD1, HD2, HE1, HE2 Tyr-372: CA, CB, CG, CD1, CD2, CE1, CE2, CZ, HB2, HB3, HD1, HD2, HE1, HE2, HH, OH

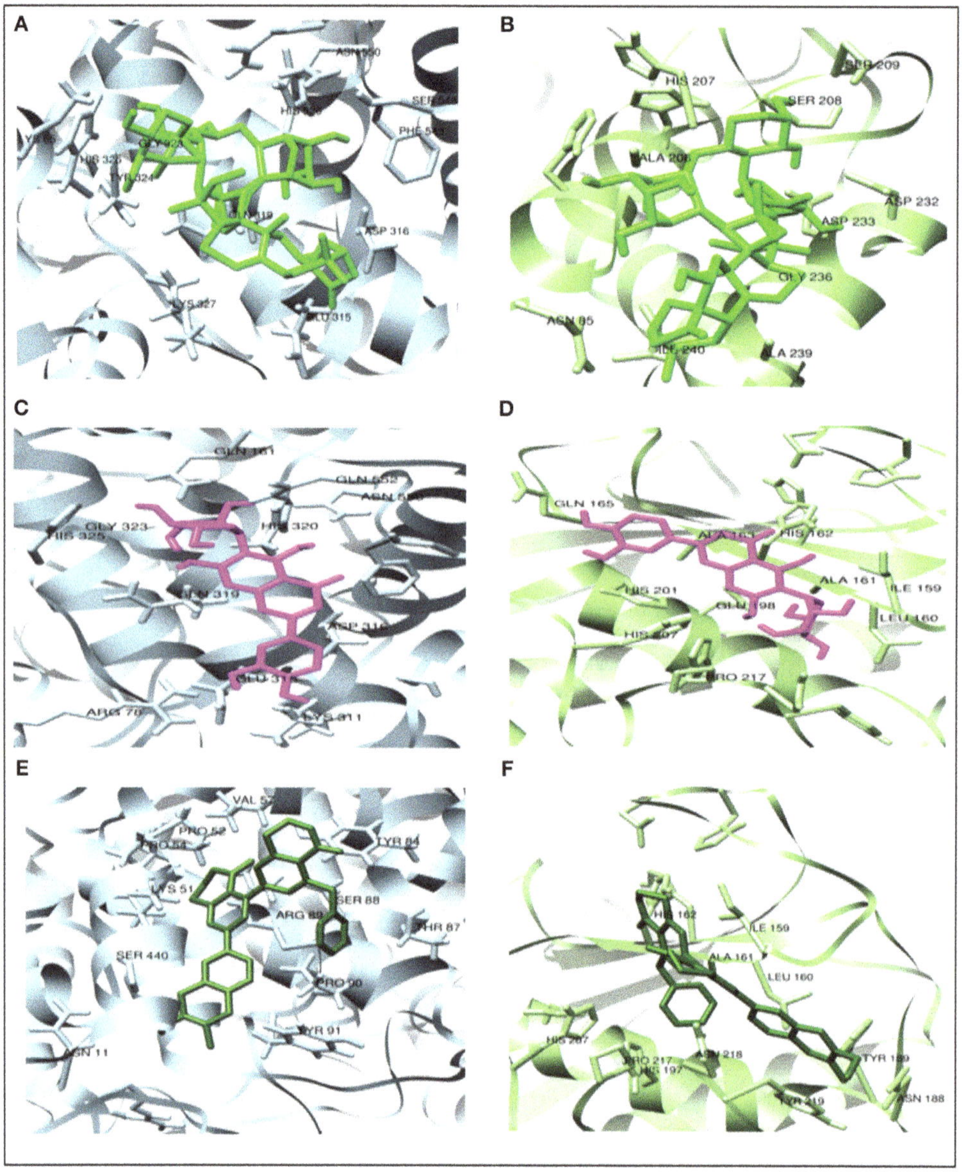

FIGURE 2 | The docked complexes of COX2 (light blue) and MMP2 (light green). Top-ranked 3 phytocompounds **(A,B)** Albiziasaponin-A (green), **(C,D)** Iso-orientin (magenta), and **(E,F)** Salvadorin (dark green).

The EGCG binds with proteins in the plasma membrane and modulates signal transduction pathways, expression of transcription factors, DNA methylation, mitochondrial function, and autophagy to cause its biological actions (Alam and Khan, 2014; Kim et al., 2014; Sehgal et al., 2016; Jamil et al., 2017; Yousuf et al., 2017). The signaling pathways regulated by EGCG include protein kinase C (PKC), NF-kB, and mitogen-activated protein kinase (MAPK) pathway (Kwon et al., 2012; Kim et al., 2014). The EGCG attenuates the activation of NF-kB, c-jun N-terminal kinase and MAPK p38 phosphorylation (Venkatesan et al., 2015). It was shown that the reduction in the release of nitric oxide (NO) by EGCG supresses the MAPK pathways in neuroblastoma cells leading to substantial decrease in both inflammation and oxidative stress levels (Kennedy et al., 2014).

Recent studies demonstrate the effects of phenolic compounds on APP in cell cultures through the inhibition of AChE and BChE to attenuate the formation of β amyloid plaques (Ahmad et al., 2017; Ayaz et al., 2017a,b). It was reported that β-sitosterol inhibits AChE activity both *in vivo* and *in vitro* (Ayaz et al., 2017a,b). It was further deduced that β-sitosterol can easily cross blood brain barrier and moves to the part of brain involved in cognition and inhibit the degradation of acetyl choline (Ach) mediated by AChE (Ayaz et al., 2017a,b). Hence, the inhibition of AChE and BChE may be considered as the primary reason for the degradation of

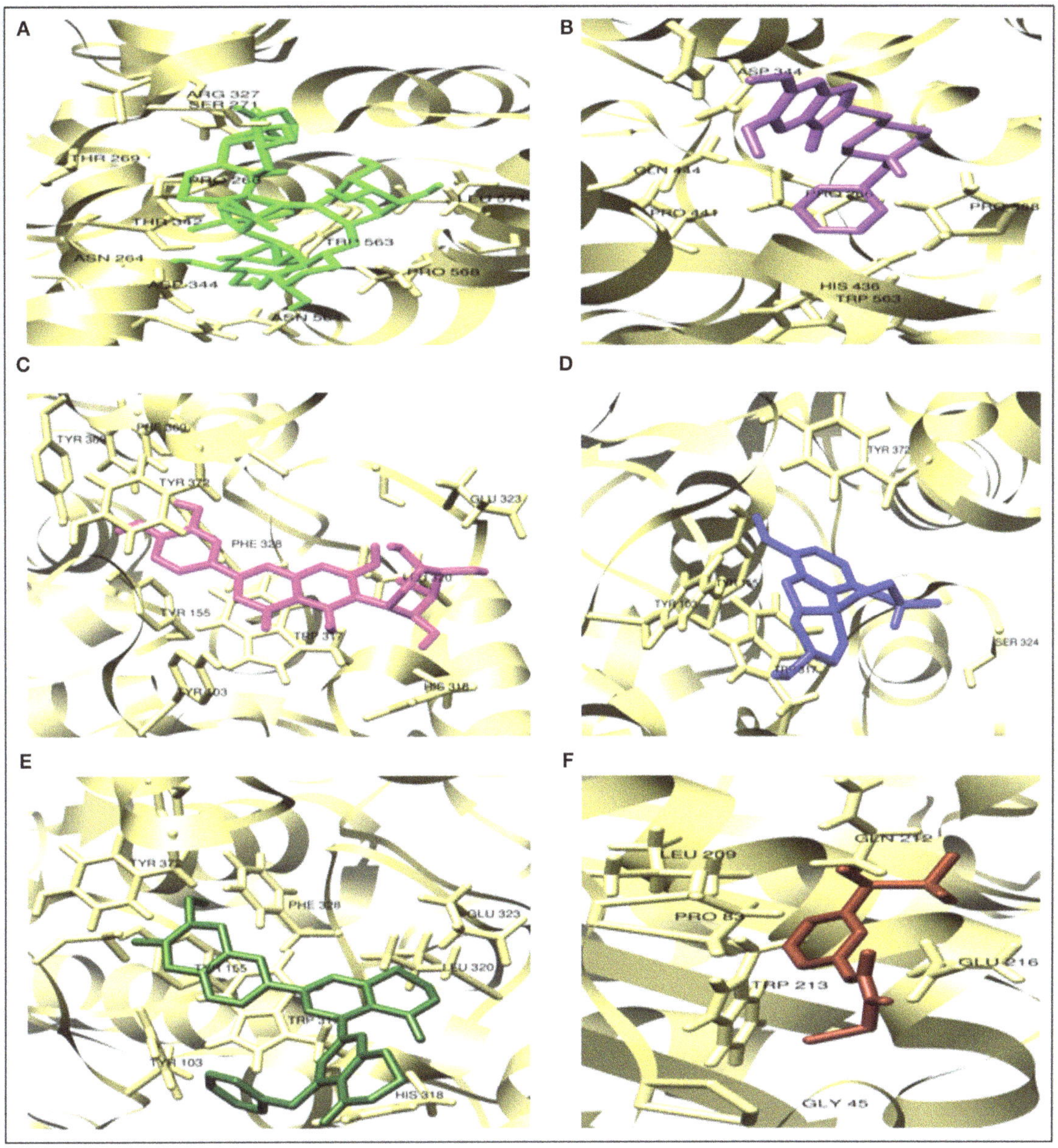

FIGURE 3 | The comparative docked complexes of AChE (khaki). Top-ranked 3 phytocompounds **(A)** Albiziasaponin-A (green), **(C)** Iso-orientin (magenta), **(E)** Salvadorin (dark green) and FDA approved drugs **(B)** donepezil (purple), **(D)** galantamine (blue) and **(F)** rivastigmine (dark red).

essential neurotransmitter (ACh) (Ali et al., 2017). Therefore, the development of drugs that inhibit AChE and BChE may serve as one of the most useful options to attenuate the progression of AD.

In the present study, Albiziasaponin-A, Iso-Orientin, and Salvadorin inhibit the activity of AChE in rats with experimentally induced AD. Furthermore, the inflammatory markers and oxidative stress levels were attenuated by these three compounds in the experimental rat model of AD. The serum levels of AChE, 4-HNE, 8-OHdG, TNF-α, Iso-P2α, MDA, COX-2, and MMP-8 were significantly reduced in the groups of rats treated with these compounds. Recent studies have further emphasized the importance of inhibiting the activity of AChE and BChE enzymes in AD patients (Ayaz et al., 2015, 2017a,b). After the screening of compounds by all possible dry and wet lab techniques it explains cognitive decline as necessary complication for the emergence of AD. It also tends to explain that increasing the cholinergic tone may help in reverting cognitive dysfunction either by the help of ACh precursors or by antagonizing nicotinic receptors as shown in **Figures 2–4**.

Here, we have further observed a strong and significant positive correlation among different variables, AChE vs. MMP-8 ($r = 0.823^{**}$), TNF-α vs. MMP-8 ($r = 0.865^{**}$), 8-OHdG vs.

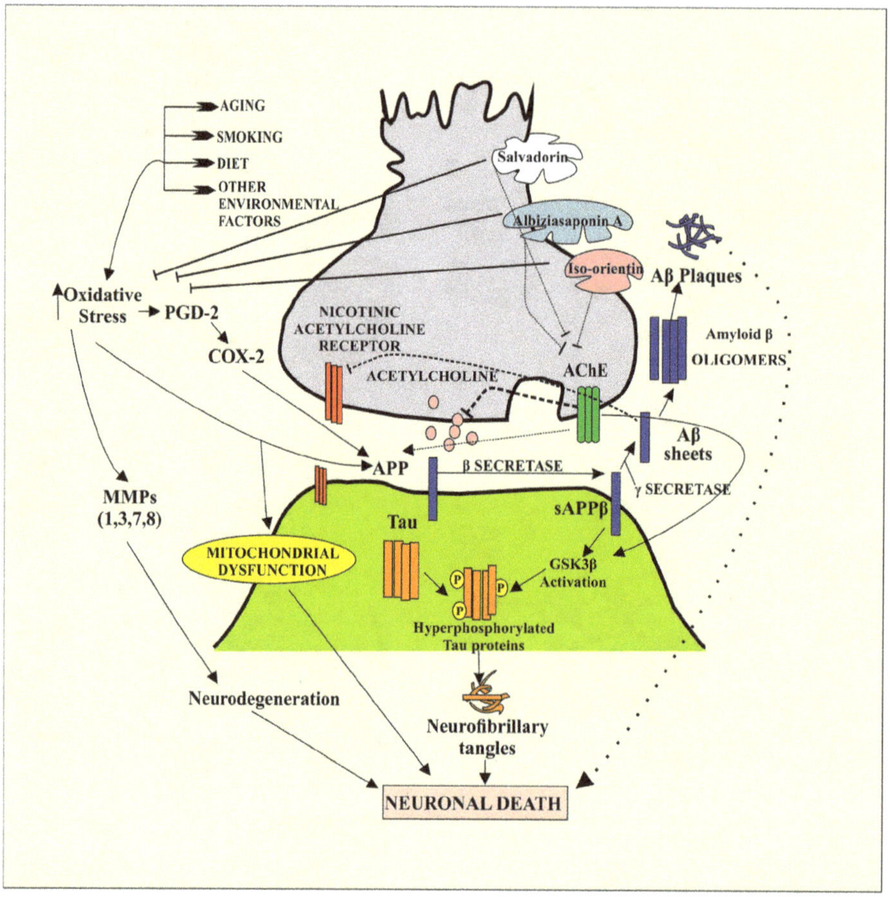

FIGURE 4 | The mechanism of Alzheimer's disease (AD). It shows the role of Acetylcholine Esterase (AchE) and oxidative stress in the neurodegeneration. Oxidative stress and AchE up-regulates the activity of Amyloid precursor proteins (APPs). Moreover, oxidative stress is involved in the activation of several MMPs and enzymes cyclooxygenase-2 (COX-2). MMPs are directly responsible for the degradation of extracellular membrane (ECM) that leads to neurodegeneration. Under the action of enzyme β-secretase APPs gets converted into serum APPβ that later with the action of γ-secretase is converted into amyloid-β sheets. These amyloid-β sheets ultimately form amyloid β plaques. Alzheimer disease is often characterized with the presence of amyloid β plaques, neurofibrillary tangles, and hyperphosphorylated tau proteins. Tau proteins are hyperphosphorylated under the action of GSK3β which is activated by the activity of sAPPβ. Cumulatively, all of the discussed factors are involved in the neurodegeneration, which leads to the Alzheimer disease. Most of the drugs used in the following case are AchE inhibitors. They halt the AchE so, there will be enough neurotransmission present for the proper neuronal functioning. Likewise, in the current study, salvadorin, albiziasaponin and iso-orientin, significantly blocked the activity of AchE to cause neuroprotection.

MDA ($r = 0.719^{**}$), and 4-HNE vs. MDA ($r = 0.774^{**}$) in rats experimentally induced with colchicine and administered with Albiziasaponin-A, Iso-Orientin and Salvadorin. Such correlations depict that if one of the variables is increased; it might cause the increase of other positively associated factors. As described, AChE is one of the primary enzymes responsible for the neurological dysfunctions therefore, depending upon the discussed correlations it may be stated as increased inflammatory status, oxidative stress, and DNA damage may potently increase the levels of AChEs. Albiziasaponin A, Iso-orientin, and Salvadorin have caused significant reduction in both inflammatory and oxidative levels by the upregulation of antioxidant enzymes and the inhibition of AChE. More notably, Iso-orientin is a polyphenolic compound contains ortho-dihydroxyl substituent over its aromatic ring (Brown et al., 1998). It works as an antioxidant by donating its hydrogen atom to free radicals present in the cells. The role of iso-orientin in the activation of several singling cascades such as PI3K, PKC, Nrf2 pathway, and MAPK is critical for its anti-oxidant properties. For example, PI3K activates the NQO1, which leads to the release of Nrf2 from Keapl through Nrf2-ARE cascade and subsequently increase the levels of antioxidant enzymes (Li et al., 2006) leading to neuroprotection. Such neuroprotective activities serve as an important treatment strategy for AD. Four out of five different therapies available for AD are primarily based on the inhibition of AChE. Activities of in rats experimentally induced with colchicine and administered with Albiziasaponin-A, Iso-Orientin and Salvadorin were also compared with the activity of FDA approved drugs such as donepezil, galantamine, and rivastigmine. Studies reported that galantamine binds to the nAChR that is a nicotinic receptor at the binding site, which is an additional

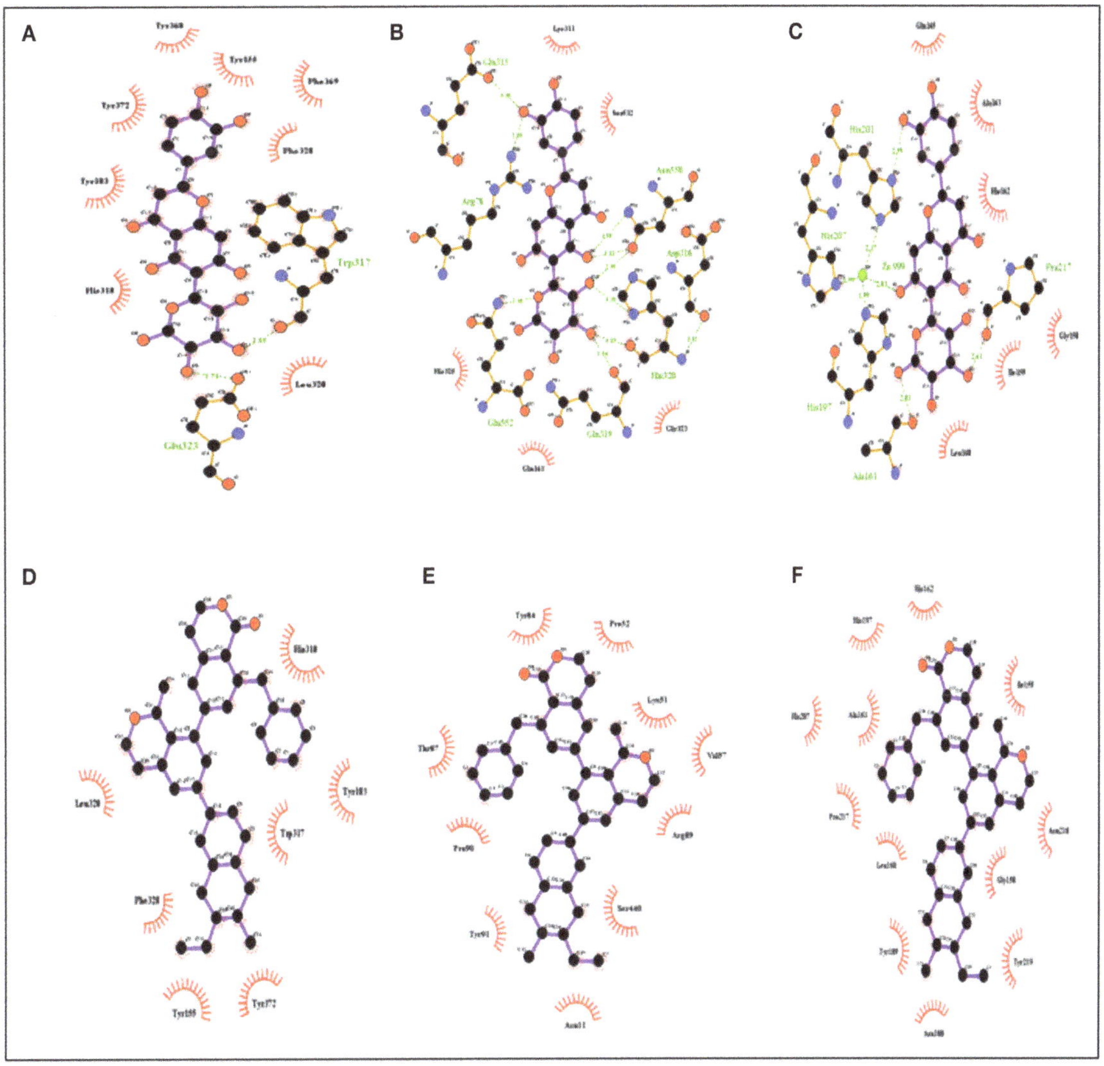

FIGURE 5 | Interactions of top ranked compounds against 3 targeted proteins **(A,B)** Albiziasaponin-A, **(C,D)** Iso-orientin, and **(E,F)** Salvadorin. Ligplot showed that Atoms of compounds and the interacting residues in the standard element colors respectively Iso-orientin and Salvadorin against AChE, Cox-2 and MMP8. The Ligplot did not show any Pi-Pi interactions of the selected compounds with the respective target proteins.

binding site of its natural agonist ACh. This binding causes the allosteric modulation of nicotinic receptor because of the co-binding of ACh and galantamine. An *in vivo* study demonstrated that donepezil, physostigmine, and tacrine also modulate the nicotinic ACh receptor allosterically. Hence, in the present study, the molecular docking and *in vivo* studies have uncovered the anti-AD properties of Albiziasaponin-A, Iso-Orientin and Salvadorin. These phytocompounds could be used to develop synthetic medicines such as rivastigmine (Howes and Houghton, 2012; Forbes-Hernandez et al., 2016) for the treatment of AD.

CONCLUSION

In the present study, both *in silico and in vivo* findings suggest potent neuroprotective roles of Albiziasaponin-A, Iso-orientin, and Salvadorin. The administration of these compounds in rats with experimentally induced AD result in the attenuation of AChE, oxidative stress, and inflammatory markers that play a significant role in the progression of AD. These results signify the potential of these phytocompounds as drugs against the progression of neurological disorders like AD. Further *in silico* and *in vivo* characterisation and validation of Albiziasaponin-A, Iso-orientin, and Salvadorin, against other important proteins implicated in the pathogenesis of AD may be essential to decipher novel mechanistic insights before taking these phytocompounds for preclinical studies.

AUTHOR CONTRIBUTIONS

AM, SW, QT-A, TJ, RR, AK, MG, SS, MR, and MN designed the

experiments. AM, SW, QT-A, TJ, RR, AK, MG, and SS conducted the experiments. MR, MN, PP, KG, and MA-Q analyzed the data. MR, MN, PP, AM, SW, QT-A, TJ, RR, AK, MG, SS, KG, and MA-Q wrote the paper. MR, MN, and PP proposed the research idea. All authors contributed to the editing of the paper and the scientific discussions.

ACKNOWLEDGMENTS

This work is funded by the National Plan for Science, Technology and Innovation (MAARIFAH)-King Abdulaziz City for Science and Technology-The Kingdom of Saudi Arabia-award number 12-BIO2267-03. The authors also acknowledge with thanks the Science and Technology Unit (STU), King Abdulaziz University for their excellent technical support.

REFERENCES

Ahmad, W., Ijaz, B., Shabbiri, K., Ahmed, F., and Rehman, S. (2017). Oxidative toxicity in diabetes and Alzheimer's disease: mechanisms behind ROS/RNS generation. *J. Biomed. Sci.* 24:76. doi: 10.1186/s12929-017-0379-z

Alam, S., and Khan, F. (2014). QSAR and docking studies on xanthone derivatives for anticancer activity targeting DNA topoisomerase IIα. *Drug Design Dev. Ther.* 8:183. doi: 10.2147/DDDT.S51577

Ali, M., Muhammad, S., Shah, M. R., Khan, A., Rashid, U., Farooq, U., et al. (2017). Neurologically potent molecules from *Crataegus oxyacantha*; isolation, anticholinesterase inhibition, and molecular docking. *Front. Pharmacol.* 8:327. doi: 10.3389/fphar.2017.00327

Altschul, S. F., Gish, W., Miller, W., Myers, E. W., and Lipman, D. J. (1990). Basic local alignment search tool. *J. Mol. Biol.* 215, 403–410. doi: 10.1016/S0022-2836(05)80360-2

Ayaz, M., Junaid, M., Ullah, F., Sadiq, A., Khan, M. A., Ahmad, W., et al. (2015). Comparative chemical profiling, cholinesterase inhibitions and anti-radicals properties of essential oils from *Polygonum hydropiper* L: a preliminary anti-Alzheimer's study. *Lipids Health Dis.* 14:141. doi: 10.1186/s12944-015-0145-8

Ayaz, M., Junaid, M., Ullah, F., Subhan, F., Sadiq, A., Ali, G., et al. (2017a). Anti-Alzheimer's Studies on β-Sitosterol Isolated from *Polygonum hydropiper* L. *Front. Pharmacol.* 8:697. doi: 10.3389/fphar.2017.00697

Ayaz, M., Sadiq, A., Junaid, M., Ullah, F., Subhan, F., and Ahmed, J. (2017b). Neuroprotective and anti-aging potentials of essential oils from aromatic and medicinal plants. *Front. Aging Neurosci.* 9:168. doi: 10.3389/fnagi.2017.00168

Bolton, E. E., Wang, Y., Thiessen, P. A., and Bryant, S. H. (2008). PubChem: integrated platform of small molecules and biological activities. *Annu. Rep. Comput. Chem.* 4, 217–241. doi: 10.1016/S1574-1400(08)00012-1

Brown, J. E., Khodr, H., Hider, R. C., and Rice-Evans, C. A. (1998). Structural dependence of flavonoid interactions with Cu2+ ions: implications for their antioxidant properties. *Biochem. J.* 330(Pt 3), 1173–1178.

Caliandro, R., Pesaresi, A., Cariati, L., Procopio, A., Oliverio, M., and Lamba, D. (2018). Kinetic and structural studies on the interactions of Torpedo californica acetylcholinesterase with two donepezil-like rigid analogues. *J. Enzyme Inhib. Med. Chem.* 33, 794–803. doi: 10.1080/14756366.2018.1458030

Cheng, F., Li, W., Zhou, Y., Shen, J., Wu, Z., Liu, G., et al. (2012). admetSAR: a comprehensive source and free tool for assessment of chemical ADMET properties. *J. Chem. Inf. Model.* 52, 3099–3105. doi: 10.1021/ci300367a

Cheung, J., Gary, E. N., Shiomi, K., and Rosenberry, T. L. (2013). Structures of human acetylcholinesterase bound to dihydrotanshinone I and territrem B show peripheral site flexibility. *ACS Med. Chem. Lett.* 4, 1091–1096. doi: 10.1021/ml400304w

Cheung, J., Rudolph, M. J., Burshteyn, F., Cassidy, M. S., Gary, E. N., Love, J., Height, J. J., et al. (2012). Structures of human acetylcholinesterase in complex with pharmacologically important ligands. *J. Med. Chem.* 55, 10282–10286. doi: 10.1021/jm300871x

Colovos, C., and Yeates, T. O. (1993). Verification of protein structures: patterns of nonbonded atomic interactions. *Protein Sci.* 2, 1511–1519. doi: 10.1002/pro.5560020916

Cummings, J. L., Mega, M., Gray, K., Rosenberg-Thompson, S., Carusi, D. A., and Gornbein, J. (1994). The Neuropsychiatric Inventory comprehensive assessment of psychopathology in dementia. *Neurology* 44, 2308–2308. doi: 10.1212/WNL.44.12.2308

Dong, S., Duan, Y., Hu, Y., and Zhao, Z. (2012). Advances in the pathogenesis of Alzheimer's disease: a re-evaluation of amyloid cascade hypothesis. *Transl. Neurodegener.* 1:18. doi: 10.1186/2047-9158-1-18

Dundas, J., Ouyang, Z., Tseng, J., Binkowski, A., Turpaz, Y., and Liang, J. (2006). CASTp: computed atlas of surface topography of proteins with structural and topographical mapping of functionally annotated residues. *Nucleic Acids Res.* 34(Suppl. 2), W116–W118. doi: 10.1093/nar/gkl282

Eisenberg, D., Lüthy, R., and Bowie, J. U. (1997). [20] Verify3D: assessment of protein models with three-dimensional profiles. *Meth. Enzymol.* 277, 396–404. doi: 10.1016/S0076-6879(97)77022-8

Essa, M. M., Vijayan, R. K., Castellano-Gonzalez, G., Memon, M. A., Braidy, N., and Guillemin, G. J. (2012). Neuroprotective effect of natural products against Alzheimer's disease. *Neurochem. Res.* 37, 1829–1842. doi: 10.1007/s11064-012-0865-3

Fiser, A., and Šali, A. (2003). Modeller: generation and refinement of homology-based protein structure models. *Methods Enzymol.* 374, 461–491. doi: 10.1016/S0076-6879(03)74020-8

Forbes-Hernandez, T. Y., Gasparrini, M., Afrin, S., Bompadre, S., Mezzetti, B., Quiles, J. L., et al. (2016). The healthy effects of strawberry polyphenols: which strategy behind antioxidant capacity? *Crit. Rev. Food Sci. Nutr.* 56, S46–S59. doi: 10.1080/10408398.2015.1051919

Förstl, H., and Kurz, A. (1999). Clinical features of Alzheimer's disease. *Eur. Arch. Psychiatry Clin. Neurosci.* 249, 288–290.

Grossberg, G. T., Christensen, D. D., Griffith, P. A., Kerwin, D. R., Hunt, G., and Hall, E. J. (2010). The art of sharing the diagnosis and management of Alzheimer's disease with patients and caregivers: recommendations of an expert consensus panel. *Prim. Care Compan. J. Clin. Psychiatry* 12:09cs00833. doi: 10.4088/PCC.09cs00833oli

He, W., Goodkind, D., and Kowal, P. (2016). *US Census Bureau, International Population Reports*. P95/16-1, An Aging World: 2015.

Hebert, L. E., Weuve, J., Scherr, P. A., and Evans, D. A. (2013). Alzheimer disease in the United States (2010–2050) estimated using the 2010 census. *Neurology* 80, 1778–1783. doi: 10.1212/WNL.0b013e31828726f5

Howes, R. M. J., and Houghton, P. J. (2012). Ethnobotanical treatment strategies against Alzheimer's disease. *Curr. Alzheimer Res.* 9, 67–85. doi: 10.2174/156720512799015046

Jamil, F., Ali, A., and Sehgal, S. A. (2017). Comparative modeling, molecular docking, and revealing of potential binding pockets of RASSF2; a candidate cancer gene. *Interdiscip. Sci. Comput. Life Sci.* 9, 214–223. doi: 10.1007/s12539-016-0145-z

Kennedy, K., Tucci, M. A., and Benghuzzi, H. A. (2014). Comparison of potential preventive therapeutic agents green tea, thymoquinone, and dilinoleoylphosphatidylcholine on human neuroblastoma cells. *Biomed. Sci. Instrum.* 50, 132–139.

Kim, M. H., Kim, S. H., and Yang, W. M. (2014). Mechanisms of action of phytochemicals from medicinal herbs in the treatment of Alzheimer's disease. *Planta Med.* 80, 1249–1258. doi: 10.1055/s-0034-1383038

Kiss, R., Sandor, M., and Szalai, F. A. (2012). Mcule.com: a public web service for drug discovery. *J. Chem. Inform.* 4:P17. doi: 10.1186/1758-2946-4-S1-P17

Kumar, A., Dogra, S., and Prakash, A. (2009). Neuroprotective effect of Cantella Asiatica against intrecerebroventricular colchicine-induced cognitive impairment and oxidative stress. *Int. J. Alzheimers Dis.* 2009:972178. doi: 10.4061/2009/972178

Kumar, G. P., and Khanum, F. (2012). Neuroprotective potential of phytochemicals. *Pharmacogn. Rev.* 6:81. doi: 10.4103/0973-7847.99898

Kumar, P., Pillay, V., Choonara, Y. E., Modi, G., Naidoo, D., and Du'Toit, L. C. (2011). In silico theoretical molecular modeling for Alzheimer's disease: the nicotine-curcumin paradigm in neuroprotection and neurotherapy. *Int. J. Mol. Sci.* 12, 694–724. doi: 10.3390/ijms12010694

Kwon, O. W., Moon, E., Chari, M. A., Kim, T. W., Kim, A. J., Lee, P., et al. (2012). A substituted 3, 4-dihydropyrimidinone derivative (compound D22) prevents inflammation mediated neurotoxicity; role in microglial activation in BV-2 cells. *Bioorg. Med. Chem. Lett.* 22, 5199–5203. doi: 10.1016/j.bmcl.2012.06.082

Li, W., Yu, S. W., and Kong, A. N. T. (2006). Nrf2 possesses a redox-sensitive nuclear exporting signal in the Neh5 transactivation domain. *J. Biol. Chem.* 281, 27251–27263. doi: 10.1074/jbc.M602746200

Lovell, S. C., Davis, I. W., Arendall, W. B., de'Bakker, P. I., Word, J. M., Prisant, M. G., et al. (2003). Structure validation by Cα geometry: φ, ψ and Cβ deviation. *Proteins Struct. Funct. Bioinformatics* 50, 437–450. doi: 10.1002/prot.10286

Mahmood, T., Ahmed, E., and Malik, A. (2005). Structure determination of salvadorin, a novel dimeric dihydroisocoumarin from Salvadora oleoides, by NMR spectroscopy. *Magn. Reson. Chem.* 43, 670–672. doi: 10.1002/mrc.1607

Meng, E. C., Pettersen, E. F., Couch, G. S., Huang, C. C., and Ferrin, T. E. (2006). Tools for integrated sequence-structure analysis with UCSF Chimera. *BMC Bioinformatics* 7:339. doi: 10.1186/1471-2105-7-339

Möller, H. J., and Graeber, M. B. (1998). The case described by Alois Alzheimer in 1911 Historical and conceptual perspectives based on the clinical record and neurohistological sections. *Eur. Arch. Psychiatry Clin. Neurosci.* 248, 111–122.

Muliyala, K. P., and Varghese, M. (2010). The complex relationship between depression and dementia. *Ann. Indian Acad. Neurol.* 13(Suppl. 2), S69–S73. doi: 10.4103/0972-2327.74248

Ohkawa, H., Ohishi, N., and Yagi, K. (1979). Assay for lipid peroxides in animal tissues by thiobarbituric acid reaction. *Anal. Biochem.* 95, 351–358.

Plassman, B. L., Langa, K. M., Fisher, G. G., Heeringa, S. G., Weir, D. R., Ofstedal, M. B., et al. (2007). Prevalence of dementia in the United States: the aging, demographics, and memory study. *Neuroepidemiology* 29, 125–132. doi: 10.1159/000109998

Sehgal, S. A., Mannan, S., and Ali, S. (2016). Pharmacoinformatic and molecular docking studies reveal potential novel antidepressants against neurodegenerative disorders by targeting HSPB8. *Drug Des. Dev. Ther.* 10, 1605–1618. doi: 10.2147/DDDT.S101929

Small, G. W. (1998). The pathogenesis of Alzheimer's disease. *J. Clin. Psychiatry* 59, 7–14.

Small, G. W. (2002). "Structural and functional brain imaging of alzheimer disease," *Neuropsychopharmacology: The Fifth Generation of Progress*, eds K. L. Davis, D. Charney, J. T. Coyle, and C. Nemeroff (Philadelphia, PA: American College of Neuropsychopharmacology), 2080.

Sperling, R. A., Aisen, P. S., Beckett, L. A., Bennett, D. A., Craft, S., Fagan, A. M., et al. (2011). Toward defining the preclinical stages of Alzheimer's disease: recommendations from the National Institute on Aging-Alzheimer's Association workgroups on diagnostic guidelines for Alzheimer's disease. *Alzheimer's Dement.* 7, 280–292. doi: 10.1016/j.jalz.2011.03.003

Sussman, J. L., Lin, D., Jiang, J., Manning, N. O., Prilusky, J., Ritter, O., et al. (1998). Protein Data Bank (PDB): database of three-dimensional structural information of biological macromolecules. *Acta Crystallogr. Sec. D Biol. Crystallogr.* 54, 1078–1084. doi: 10.1107/S0907444998009378

Taylor, J. L. S., Rabe, T., McGaw, L. J., Jäger, A. K., and Van Staden, J. (2001). Towards the scientific validation of traditional medicinal plants. *Plant Growth Regul.* 34, 23–37. doi: 10.1023/A:1013310809275

Trott, O., and Olson, A. J. (2010). AutoDock Vina: improving the speed and accuracy of docking with a new scoring function, efficient optimization and multithreading. *J. Comput. Chem.* 31, 455–461. doi: 10.1002/jcc.21334

Venkatesan, R., Ji, E., and Kim, S. Y. (2015). Phytochemicals that regulate neurodegenerative disease by targeting neurotrophins: a comprehensive review. *BioMed. Res. Int.* 2015:814068. doi: 10.1155/2015/814068

Wass, M. N., Kelley, L. A., and Sternberg, M. J. (2010). 3DLigandSite: predicting ligand-binding sites using similar structures. *Nucleic Acids Res.* 38(suppl. 2), W469–W473. doi: 10.1093/nar/gkq406

Yang, J., Roy, A., and Zhang, Y. (2013). Protein–ligand binding site recognition using complementary binding-specific substructure comparison and sequence profile alignment. *Bioinformatics* 29, 2588–2595. doi: 10.1093/bioinformatics/btt447

Yin, Y. I., Bassit, B., Zhu, L., Yang, X., Wang, C., and Li, Y. M. (2007). {gamma}-secretase substrate concentration modulates the Aβ42/Aβ40 Ratio: implications for alzheimer disease. *J. Biol. Chem.* 282, 23639–23644. doi: 10.1074/jbc.M704601200

Yoshikawa, M., Morikawa, T., Nakano, K., Pongpiriyadacha, Y., Murakami, T., and Matsuda, H. (2002). Characterization of new sweet triterpene saponins from *Albizia myriophylla. J Nat Prod.* 65, 1638–1642. doi: 10.1021/np020220l

Yousuf, Z., Iman, K., Iftikhar, N., and Mirza, M. U. (2017). Structure-based virtual screening and molecular docking for the identification of potential multi-targeted inhibitors against breast cancer. *Breast Cancer Targets Ther.* 9, 447–459. doi: 10.2147/BCTT.S132074

Zhang, Y. (2008). I-TASSER server for protein 3D structure prediction. *BMC Bioinformatics* 9:40. doi: 10.1186/1471-2105-9-40

Zhang, Y. W., Thompson, R., Zhang, H., and Xu, H. (2011). APP processing in Alzheimer's disease. *Mol. Brain* 4:3. doi: 10.1186/1756-6606-4-3

4

Rhodiola rosea L. Improves Learning and Memory Function: Preclinical Evidence and Possible Mechanisms

Gou-ping Ma[1], Qun Zheng[2], Meng-bei Xu[2], Xiao-li Zhou[2], Lin Lu[3], Zuo-xiao Li[4]* and Guo-Qing Zheng[2]**

[1] Tongde Hospital of Zhejiang province, Hangzhou, China, [2] Department of Neurology, The Second Affiliated Hospital and Yuying Children's Hospital of Wenzhou Medical University, Wenzhou, China, [3] School of Chinese Medicine, Hong Kong Baptist University, Hong Kong, China, [4] Department of Neurology, Affiliated Hospital of Southwest Medical University, Luzhou, China

***Correspondence:**
Lin Lu
lulinlc@126.com
Zuo-xiao Li
lzx3235@sina.com
Guo-Qing Zheng
gq_zheng@sohu.com

Rhodiola rosea L. (*R. rosea* L.) is widely used to stimulate the nervous system, extenuate anxiety, enhance work performance, relieve fatigue, and prevent high altitude sickness. Previous studies reported that *R. rosea* L. improves learning and memory function in animal models. Here, we conducted a systematic review and meta-analysis for preclinical studies to assess the current evidence for *R. rosea* L. effect on learning and memory function. Ultimately, 36 studies involving 836 animals were identified by searching 6 databases from inception to May 2018. The primary outcome measures included the escape latency in Morris water maze (MWM) test on behalf of learning ability, the frequency and the length of time spent on the target quadrant in MWM test representing memory function, and the number of errors in step down test, dark avoidance test and Y maze test on behalf of memory function. The secondary outcome measures were mechanisms of *R. rosea* L. for learning and/or memory function. Compared with control, the pooled results of 28 studies showed significant effects of *R. rosea* L. for reducing the escape latency ($P < 0.05$); 23 studies for increasing the frequency and the length of time spent on the target quadrant ($P < 0.05$); and 6 studies for decreasing the number of errors ($P < 0.01$). The possible mechanisms of *R. rosea* L. are largely through antioxidant, cholinergic regulation, anti-apoptosis activities, anti-inflammatory, improving coronary blood flow, and cerebral metabolism. In conclusion, the findings suggested that *R. rosea* L. can improve learning and memory function.

Keywords: *Rhodiola rosea L.*, salidroside, learning and memory, cognition, preclinical evidence, possible mechanisms

INTRODUCTION

Lasting changes in behavior resulting from prior experience can be characterized as the result of learning, memory, and retrieval processes (Thompson, 1986). However, memory is vulnerable across the adult lifespan. A decrease in learning and memory functions is the most common complaint in normal aging process. In a large number of organic diseases, in which there is a physical change in the structure of an organ or part, such as amnesia, Alzheimer's disease (AD) and vascular dementia, the most prominent sign is memory impairment (Thompson, 1986). Currently, there is no valid treatment for cognition impairment in western medicine, although many potential agents exist through novel mechanisms (Parihar and Hemnani, 2004). Cholinesterase inhibitors

(ChEIs) and N-methyl-D-aspartate (NMDA) receptor antagonists are first-line pharmacotherapy for mild-to-moderate AD in clinical, with high non-response rate 50–75% (Johnson et al., 2004). Thus, it is urgent to seek new strategies to improve function of memory and cognition.

Rhodiola rosea L. (*R. rosea* L.), also known as Rhodiola, Roseroot, Arctic Root, and Golden Root, belongs to the plant family of Crassulaceae, subfamily of sedoideae and genus Rhodiola (Farhath et al., 2005). *R. rosea* L. and its ingredients replenish qi (vital energy), activate blood circulation, unblock blood vessels, enhance mental function, and smooth asthmatic conditions in traditional Chinese medicine (TCM) (Pharmacopoeia Committee of the People's Republic of China Ministry of health, 2005). Salidroside, p-tryosol, rosavin, pyridrde, rhodiosin, and rhodionin are the most unique active ingredients in the Rhodiola species, but vary in the amounts (Zhang et al., 2006). Of the Rhodiola species, *R. rosea* L. has been extensively studied on its phytochemical and toxicological properties (Kurkin and Zapesochnaya, 1985). Modern pharmacological studies indicate that its extracts can increase neurotransmitter level, central nervous system activity, and cardiovascular function. Current studies reported that *R. rosea* L. ingestion can improve cognitive function (Spasov et al., 2000), reduce mental fatigue (Shevtsov et al., 2003), promote free radical mitigation, and exists anti-oxidative (Zhang et al., 2007) and neuroprotective effect (Yu et al., 2008), increase endurance performance (De Bock et al., 2004), and treat symptoms of asthenia subsequent to intense physical and psychological stress (Lazarova et al., 1986). However, the current evidence of *R. rosea* L. for learning and memory function still lack systematic analysis. Thus, we conduct a preclinical systematic review of Rhodiola on learning and memory function to clarify its effectiveness and potential mechanisms on animal models.

METHODS

Preferred Reporting Items for Systematic Review and Meta-Analyses (PRISMA) statement (Stewart et al., 2015) and the Guidelines for reporting systematic reviews and meta-analyses of animal studies (Sena et al., 2014) were abided.

Database And Literature Search Strategy

Six databases of PubMed, EMBASE, Web of Science, Chinese National Knowledge Infrastructure (CNKI), Wanfangdatabase and VIP information database were electronically searched from the inception up to May 2018. Studies reporting the use of *R. rosea* L. and/or its bioactive ingredients for learning and memory function in animals were identified. Our literature search strategy was as following: 1. Rhodiola (s); 2. *Rhodiola rosea* (s); 3. Roseroot (s); 4. rhodioloside; 5. salidroside; 6. OR/1-5; 7. Memory; 8. Learning; 9. Cognitive function; 10. 6 AND (7 OR 8 OR 9); 11. Animals NOT humans; 12. 10 AND 11.

Study Selection

Two investigators independently screened the titles and/or abstracts based on the search strategy. Of the search results, we assessed the full-text articles for eligibility. Any uncertainty eligibility was resolved by discussion. Studies were eligible for our systematic review if they met: (1) Animal models were established for learning and memory injury; (2) Analyzed interventions were received *R. rosea* L. and/or its bioactive ingredients as monotherapy at any dose. Comparator interventions were isosteric non-functional liquid (normal saline) or no treatment; (3) the primary measured outcomes were indexes of learning and/or memory function tests, including Morris water maze (MWM), Y maze, step down test, dark avoidance test, active avoidance reaction and one step through test. The secondary outcome measures were mechanisms of *R. rosea* L. for learning and/or memory function. Pre-specified exclusion criteria were as follows: *R. rosea* L. was treated in conjunction with other compounds or *R. rosea* L.-based prescriptions, or without predetermined outcome index, or without *in vivo* model, or without control group, or duplicate publications. In the case of multiple publications from one study, we choose the articles with the largest sample or the earliest publication.

Data Extraction

The following details were extracted from each included study: (1) the first author's name, publication year; (2) individual data for each study, including animal species, number, sex, and weight; (3) type of animal model and anesthetic used in the model; (4) intervention characteristics, including timing for initial treatment, dosage and method of treatment, duration of treatment, and comparable treatment of control group;(5) main outcome measures on behavior tests and its corresponding *p*-value. For each comparison, we extracted data of mean value and standard deviation from each treatment and control group of every study. If the data for meta-analysis were missing or only expressed graphically, we tried to contact authors for further information or calculated by ourselves if available. Otherwise we only performed qualitative analysis. The data of highest dose was selected when the treatment group included various doses of the target drug. The result of the peak time point was included when the data were expressed at different times.

Quality Assessment

Two authors independently assessed the methodological quality of the included articles according to the Collaborative Approach to Meta-Analysis and Review of Animal Data from Experimental Studies (CAMARADES) 10-item checklist (Sena et al., 2007): (1) peer-reviewed publication; (2) statements of temperature control; (3) randomization to treatment or control group; (4) blinded induction of model; (5) blinded assessment of outcome; (6) use of anesthetic without significant intrinsic neuroprotective activity; (7) appropriate animal model; (8) sample size calculation; (9) compliance with animal welfare regulations; and (10) declaration of potential conflict of interests. Each study was given an aggregate quality score based on one-point awarding for each item. Discrepancies were resolved by discussion or consultation with corresponding author.

Statistical Analysis

Meta-analyses and sub-analyses were performed using RevMan 5.3 software. Outcome measures were all considered as continuous data and given an estimate of the combined overall effect sizes utilizing standard mean difference (SMD) with the random effects model. SMD with its 95% confidence interval (CI) was used to assess the strength of efficacy of *R. rosea* L. and/or its bioactive ingredients for learning and memory function. Publication bias was assessed with a funnel plot. To clarify the impact of factors potentially modifying the outcome measures, we also conducted sensitivity analyses and subgroup analyses according to the following variables: animal species, anesthetic used, type of animal model and the treatment time. The I^2 statistic was used for assessment of heterogeneity among individual studies. Probability value $P < 0.05$ was considered significant.

RESULTS

Study Inclusion

We identified 760 potentially relevant articles from the six databases. After removal of duplicates and irrelevant articles, 150 records remained. After going through the titles and abstracts, 55 were excluded because they were case reports, clinical trials or review articles. By reading the remaining full-text articles, 59 articles were excluded if: (1) not predetermined outcome index; (2) not published in peer-review journals; (3) compared with other medicine; (4) no *in vivo* model; (5) no control group; (6) conjunction with other compounds or *R. rosea* L.-based prescriptions. Finally, 36 eligible studies (You et al., 2000; Jiang et al., 2001; Liu et al., 2003, 2017a,b; Xie, 2003; Wu et al., 2004; Deng, 2006; Shi et al., 2006; Chen, 2008; Wang et al., 2008, 2012, 2013; Cao, 2009; Ji et al., 2009; Liu, 2009; Qu et al., 2009; Zou et al., 2009; Mao et al., 2010; Zhao et al., 2010; Yang et al., 2011a,b, 2017; Sun et al., 2012; Zhang S. et al., 2012; Zhang X.X. et al., 2012; Qi et al., 2013; Zhang et al., 2013; Barhwal et al., 2015; Yan et al., 2015; Vasileva et al., 2016; Ge et al., 2017; Guo et al., 2017; Wei, 2017; Xiong and Gao, 2017; Yang, 2017) involving 836 animals were identified (**Figure 1**).

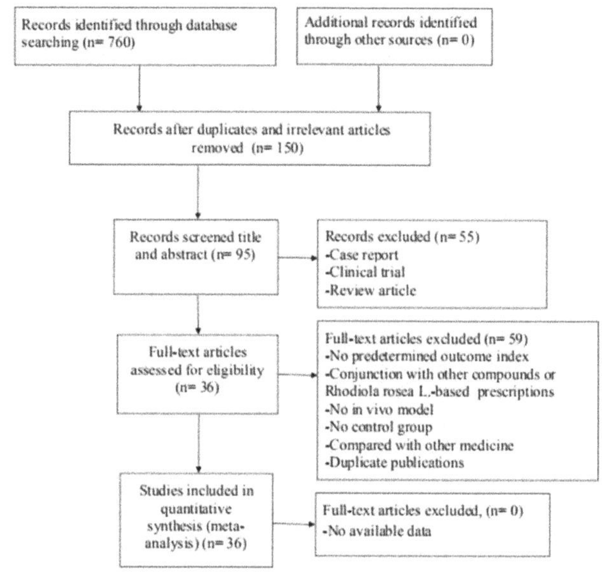

FIGURE 1 | Summary of the process for identifying candidate studies.

Characteristics of Included Studies

The basic characteristics of the included studies are summarized in **Table 1**. Thirty-six studies included were published between 2000 and 2017 and described comparisons based on three main outcome measures of learning and memory function. For animal species, 27 studies used rats including Sprague-Dawley (SD) rats (Wang et al., 2008; Cao, 2009; Ji et al., 2009; Liu, 2009; Qu et al., 2009; Zou et al., 2009; Yang et al., 2011a,b, 2017; Zhang X.X. et al., 2012; Qi et al., 2013; Zhang et al., 2013; Barhwal et al., 2015; Yan et al., 2015; Liu et al., 2017a,b; Wei, 2017) and Wistar rats (Jiang et al., 2001; Xie, 2003; Chen, 2008; Zhao et al., 2010; Sun et al., 2012; Wang et al., 2012; Vasileva et al., 2016; Ge et al., 2017; Xiong and Gao, 2017; Yang, 2017) as animal models. Eight studies used mice including C57BL/6J (Mao et al., 2010), ICR (Deng, 2006; Zhang X.X. et al., 2012), BALB/C (Liu et al., 2003), Kunming mice (You et al., 2000; Wu et al., 2004; Wang et al., 2013; Ge et al., 2017). The remaining 1 study used mice without mentioning its species (Shi et al., 2006). Seventeen studies (You et al., 2000; Jiang et al., 2001; Liu et al., 2003, 2017a; Xie, 2003; Wu et al., 2004; Deng, 2006; Shi et al., 2006; Wang et al., 2008; Cao, 2009; Ji et al., 2009; Qu et al., 2009; Mao et al., 2010; Sun et al., 2012; Zhang X.X. et al., 2012; Zhang et al., 2013; Yang et al., 2017) induced cognitive impairment by Alzheimer's disease (AD) model, 8 studies (Chen, 2008; Liu, 2009; Zou et al., 2009; Zhang X.X. et al., 2012; Wang et al., 2013; Yan et al., 2015; Liu et al., 2017b; Xiong and Gao, 2017) by vascular dementia (VD) model, 5 studies (Yang et al., 2011b; Qi et al., 2013; Barhwal et al., 2015; Ge et al., 2017; Guo et al., 2017) by hypobaric hypoxia model, 2 studies (Wang et al., 2012; Zhang X.X. et al., 2012) by sleep deprivation model, 2 studies (Zhao et al., 2010; Yang, 2017) by diabetes mellitus (DM) model, 1 study by status epileptics (SE) model (Yang et al., 2011b), 1 study (Wei, 2017) by posttraumatic stress disorder, and the remaining 1 study (Vasileva et al., 2016) by using scopolamine. For anesthesia chosen in experiments, 6 studies (Cao, 2009; Liu, 2009; Zou et al., 2009; Wang et al., 2013; Liu et al., 2017b; Xiong and Gao, 2017) used chloral hydrate, 8 studies (Xie, 2003; Chen, 2008; Qu et al., 2009; Zhang X.X. et al., 2012; Zhang et al., 2013; Wei, 2017; Yang, 2017; Yang et al., 2017) used pentobarbital sodium, 1 study (Yan et al., 2015) used isoflurane,1 study (Wang et al., 2012) used ethyl ether, 3 studies (Liu et al., 2003; Deng, 2006; Zhao et al., 2010) needn't use it because of only neurobehavioral tests being conducted in rats/mice, and the remaining 17 studies did not report it. Thirty-four studies were conducted in China, 1 study (Vasileva et al., 2016) in Bulgaria, and the remaining one (Barhwal et al., 2015) in India. For outcome measures, 28 studies of comparisons reported learning data as escape latency in MWM (Jiang et al., 2001; Liu et al., 2003, 2017a,b; Wu et al., 2004; Deng, 2006; Shi et al., 2006; Chen, 2008; Wang et al., 2008, 2012; Cao, 2009; Ji et al., 2009; Liu, 2009; Qu et al., 2009; Zou et al., 2009; Zhao et al., 2010; Yang et al., 2011a,b, 2017; Sun et al., 2012; Zhang et al., 2013; Barhwal et al., 2015; Yan et al., 2015; Ge et al., 2017; Guo et al., 2017; Wei, 2017; Xiong and Gao, 2017; Yang, 2017), 23 studies

TABLE 1 | Characteristics of included 36 studies.

Study	Species (Sex, n = trial/control group)	Weight	Modeling approach	Anesthetic	Intervention: Trial group	Intervention: Control group	Outcome measure	Intergroup Differences
1. You et al., 2000	Kunming mice (male,10/10)	25 ± 2 g	Cognitive impairment induced by i.p. SCOP (1 mg/kg); by i.g. 30% ethanol (0.1 ml/10 g); by s.i. sodium nitrite (120 mg/kg)	NR	*R. rosea* L., i.g. 200 mg/kg/day for 30 days before the model	Normal saline	1. Error latency in SDT 2. Error latency in DAT	1. $P < 0.01$ 2. $P < 0.01$
2. Jiang et al., 2001	Wistar rats (male, 8/8)	445.35 ± 625.73 g	Cognitive Impairment induced by i.p SCOP (2 mg/kg)	NR	*R. rosea* L., i.m. 15 mg/kg/day for 4 weeks before the model	Normal saline	1. Escape latency in MWM 2. The number of errors in SDT 3. Ach, ChAT 4. LPO, SOD	1. $P < 0.05$ 2. $P < 0.05$ 3. $P < 0.05$ 4. $P < 0.05$
3. Liu et al., 2003	BALB/c mice (male, 10/10)	20–25 g	Cognitive impairment induced by i.p SCOP;	No need	Rhodiola henryi Extract, i.g. 0.1, 0.3, 0.5 g/kg/day for 30 days before the model	Distilled water	1. Escape latency in MWM 2. The number of errors in DAT	1. $P < 0.05$ 2. $P < 0.01$
	BALB/c mice (male, 10/10)	20–25 g	Pre-treatment with normal mice	No need	Rhodiola henryi Extract, i.g. 0.1, 0.3, 0.5 g/kg/day for 30 days	Distilled water	1. Escape latency in MWM 2. The number of errors in DAT 3. The number of errors in SDT	1. $P < 0.05$ 2. $P > 0.05$ 3. $P > 0.05$
4. Xie, 2003	Wistar rats (male, 10/10)	131.7 ± 12.2 g	AD model induced by bilateral hippocampal injection Aβ_{1-40} and i.p. D-gal	2.5% pentobarbital sodium (40 nmg/kg)	*R. rosea* L., i.p. 15 mg/kg/day for 4 weeks accompanying the model	Normal saline	1. Reaction time in Y maze 2. Escape latency in one step through test 3. AchE	1. $P < 0.05$ 2. $P < 0.05$ 3. $P < 0.01$
5. Wu et al., 2004	Kunming mice (male and female, 12/12)	18–20 g	Cognitive impairment induced by i.p SCOP (2 mg/kg)	NR	R. rosea L. extract, i.g. 1.27, 3.81, 11.41 g/kg/day for 2 weeks before the model	CMC-Na	1. Escape latency in MWM 2. AchE	1. $P < 0.05$ 2. $P < 0.01$
6. Shi et al., 2006	mice (male, 10/10)	NR	Cognitive impairment induced by i.p SCOP (5 mg/kg)	NR	R. rosea L. extract, i.g. 3.81 g/kg/day for 3 weeks before the model	CMC-Na	1. Escape latency in MWM 2. AchE 3. SOD, MDA, MAO	1. $P < 0.01$ 2. $P < 0.01$ 3. $P < 0.01$
7. Deng, 2006	ICR mice (male and female, 27/28)	20 ± 2 g	Cognitive impairment induced by i.p SCOP (2 mg/kg)	No need	*R. rosea* L., i.g. 0.1, 0.6 g/kg/day for 15 days before the model	Distilled water	1. Escape latency in MWM 2. The number of errors in SDT	1. $P < 0.01$ 2. $P < 0.01$
8. Chen, 2008	Wistar rats (male, 8/8)	250 g	Bilateral permanent occlusion of the common carotid arteries	0.4% pentobarbital sodium (1 ml/100 g)	*R. rosea* L., i.g. 5 g/kg/day for 28 days after the model	Distilled water	1. Escape latency in MWM 2. The number of target platform crossings 3. Time spent in target quadrant 4. SOD, MDA 5. AchE 6. Neuronal apoptosis	1. $P < 0.05$ 2. $P < 0.05$ 3. $P < 0.05$ 4. $P < 0.05$ 5. $P < 0.05$ 6. $P < 0.05$

(Continued)

TABLE 1 | Continued

Study	Species (Sex, *n* = trial/control group)	Weight	Modeling approach	Anesthetic	Intervention: Trial group	Intervention: Control group	Outcome measure	Intergroup Differences
9. Wang et al., 2008	SD rats (male, 12/11)	250–300 g	AD model induced by D-gal +$AlCl_3$+SCOP	NR	*R. rosea* L., i.g. 5 g/kg/day for 4 weeks after the model	Normal saline	1. Escape latency in MWM 2. The number of target platform crossings 3. Time spent in target quadrant 4. CAT, GSH-Px	1. $P < 0.05$ 2. $P < 0.05$ 3. $P < 0.05$ 4. $P < 0.05$
10. Cao, 2009	SD rats (male, 12/12)	250 ± 20 g	AD model induced by D-gal +$AlCl_3$ +SCOP	10% chloral hydrate (3.5 ml/kg)	*R. rosea* L., i.g. 5 g/kg/day for 28 days after the model	Normal saline	1. Escape latency in MWM 2. The number of target platform crossings 3. Time spent in target quadrant 4. AchE 5. NOS 6. Bax, Bcl-2	1. $P < 0.01$ 2. $P < 0.01$ 3. $P < 0.01$ 4. $P < 0.01$ 5. $P < 0.01$ 6. $P < 0.01$
11. Ji et al., 2009	SD rats (male,12/11)	250–300 g	AD model induced by D-gal +$AlCl_3$ +SCOP	NR	*R. rosea* L., i.g. 10 g/kg/day for 4 weeks after the model	Distilled water	1. Escape latency in MWM 2. The number of target platform crossings 3. Time spent in target quadrant	1. $P < 0.05$ 2. $P < 0.05$ 3. $P < 0.05$
12. Liu, 2009	SD rats (male, 11/11)	240–300 g	Cerebralhypoperfusion by MCAO for 3 h	4% chloral hydrate (1 ml/100 g)	R. rosea L.,i.p. 12 mg/day for 10 days before the model	Normal saline	1. Escape latency in MWM 2. Time spent in target quadrant 3. Ach	1. $P > 0.05$ 2. $P > 0.05$ 3. $P < 0.01$
13. Qu et al., 2009	SD rats (male, 12/12)	240–260 g	AD model induced by bilateral ICV with STZ (1.5 mg/kg)	1% pentobarbital sodium (40 mg/kg)	R. rosea L. crenulate extracts, i.g. 1.5, 3.0, 6.0 mg/kg, twice a day for 21 days before the model	CMC-Na	1. Escape latency in MWM 2. Time spent in target quadrant 3. GSH, GR, MDA 4. ATP, COX 5. Neuronal apoptosis 6. Caspase-3, NeuN	1. $P < 0.05$ 2. $P < 0.05$ 3. $P < 0.05$ 4. $P < 0.05$ 5. $P < 0.05$ 6. $P < 0.05$
14. Zou et al., 2009	SD rats (male, 15/15)	300 ± 20 g	VD model induced by bilateral CCAO for 10 min	10% chloral hydrate (400 mg/kg)	R. rosea L., i.p. 12 mg/kg/day for 7 days before surgery	Normal saline	1. Escape latency in MWM 2. Time spent in target quadrant 3. SOD, MDA 4. TNF-α	1. $P < 0.05$ 2. $P < 0.05$ 3. $P < 0.05$ 4. $P < 0.05$
15. Mao et al., 2010	C57BL/6J mice (female, 10/10)	5-month-old mice	Aging model induced by s.i. D-gal (50 mg/kg)	NR	*R. rosea* L., i.g. 1 g /kg/day for 8 weeks accompanying the model	PBS	1. The number of errors in SDT 2. GFAP, NT-3 3. Splenic T Lymphocyte 4. Proliferation and IL-2 Activity	1. $P > 0.05$ 2. $P < 0.01$ 3. $P < 0.01$

(Continued)

TABLE 1 | Continued

Study	Species (Sex, *n* = trial/control group)	Weight	Modeling approach	Anesthetic	Intervention: Trial group	Intervention: Control group	Outcome measure	Intergroup Differences
16. Zhao et al., 2010	Wistar rats (male, 10/10)	200–250 g	DM model induced by i.p. STZ	No need	R. rosea L., i.g., 50 mg/kg for 12 weeks after the model	Normal saline	1. Escape latency in MWM 2. The number of target platform crossings 3. Time spent in target quadrant	1. $P < 0.01$ 2. $P > 0.05$ 3. $P < 0.05$
17. Yang et al., 2011b	SD rats (male, 8/8)	190–250 g	Status epilepticus model induced by i.p. lithium chloride + pilocarpine	NR	*R. rosea* L., i.p. 1 g/kg/day for 7 days (1 day before the model)	Normal saline	1. Escape latency in MWM 2. Time spent in target quadrant 3. SOD, MDA, GSH,GSH-Px	1. $P < 0.05$ 2. $P < 0.05$ 3. $P < 0.05$
18. Yang et al., 2011a	SD rats (male, 10/10	180–220 g	Hypobaric hypoxia	NR	*R. rosea* L., i.p. 1 g/kg/day for 34 days accompanying the model	Normal saline	1. Escape latency in MWM 2. Time spent in target quadrant 3. SOD, MDA, GSH, GSH-Px	1. $P < 0.05$ 2. $P < 0.05$ 3. $P < 0.05$
19. Sun et al., 2012	Wistar rats (male, 9/8)	350 ± 20 g	AD model induced by D-gal+$AlCl_3$+SCOP	NR	*R. rosea* L., i.g. 5 g/kg/day for 4 weeks after the model	Distilled water	1. Escape latency in MWM 2. The number of target platform crossings 3. Time spent in target quadrant	1. $P < 0.05$ 2. $P < 0.05$ 3. $P < 0.05$
20. Wang et al., 2012	Wistar rats (male, 5/5)	190–230 g	Sleep deprivation induced by MMPM	Ethyl ether	*R. rosea* L., i.g. 180 mg/kg/day until sacrifice (10 days before the model)	Normal saline	1. Reaction time in Y maze	2. $P < 0.05$
21. Zhang S. et al., 2012	ICR mice (male and female, 10/10)	21.4 ± 2 g	Cognitive impairment induced by i.p. SCOP (1 mg/kg); by i.g. 40% ethanol (0.2 ml)	NR	*R. rosea* L. compound i.g. 1.2 g/kg/day for 28 days before the model	Normal saline	1. Time spent in target quadrant of MWM 2. SOD, NO	1. $P < 0.05$ 2. $P < 0.05$
22. Zhang X.X. et al., 2012	SD rats (male, 6/6)	240–270 g	Sleep deprivation induced by MMPM	0.4% pentobarbital sodium (40 mg/kg)	*R. rosea* L., i.p. 10 ml/kg/day for 3 days before the model	Normal saline	1. Reaction time in Y maze 2. The number of errors 3. SOD, MDA 4. Neuronal apoptosis 5. AchE	1. $P < 0.05$ 2. $P < 0.05$ 3. $P < 0.05$ 4. $P < 0.05$ 5. $P < 0.05$
23. Zhang et al., 2013	SD rats (male, 8/8)	300 ± 15 g	AD model induced by bilateral hippocampal injection A β_{1-40} with 10 ug	1% pentobarbital sodium (40 mg/kg)	*R. rosea* L., i.p. 25, 50, 75 mg/kg/day for 21 days after the model	Normal saline	1. Escape latency in MWM 2. The number of target platform crossings 3. Time spent in target quadrant 4. SOD, MDA, GSH-Px 5. Ach, AchE 6. NADH/NADPH 7. nuclear factor κB	1. $P < 0.01$ 2. $P < 0.01$ 3. $P < 0.01$ 4. $P < 0.01$ 5. $P < 0.01$ 6. $P < 0.01$ 7. $P < 0.01$

(Continued)

TABLE 1 | Continued

Study	Species (Sex, *n* = trial/control group)	Weight	Modeling approach	Anesthetic	Intervention		Outcome measure	Intergroup Differences
					Trial group	Control group		
24. Qi et al., 2013	SD rats (male, 10/10)	180–200 g	Hypobaric hypoxia	NR	*R. rosea* L., i.g. 1 g/100 g, twice a day for 2 weeks before the model	Normal saline	1. AAR retention 2. Neuronal apoptosis	1. $P < 0.05$ 2. $P < 0.05$
25. Wang et al., 2013	Kunming mice (male and female, 10/10)	18–22 g	VD model by bilateral CCAO for 20 min*2	4%chloralhydrate (400 mg/kg)	*R. rosea* L., i.g. 60 mg/kg/day for 25 days after the model	Distilled water	1. Escape latency in MWM 2. The number of errors in SDT 3. NOS, NO	1. $P < 0.01$ 2. $P < 0.01$ 3. $P < 0.01$
26. Yan et al., 2015	SD rats (male, 12/12)	240 ± 20 g	VD model by bilateral permanent CCAO	isoflurane	*R. rosea* L., i.p. 20 mg/kg/day for 35 days (1 day before the model)	Normal saline	1. Escape latency in MWM 2. Time spent in target quadrant 3. Caspase-3 4. Bax/Bcl-2	1. $P < 0.05$ 2. $P < 0.05$ 3. $P < 0.05$ 4. $P < 0.05$
27. Barhwal et al., 2015	SD rats (male, 12/12)	220 ± 10 g	Hypobaric hypoxia	NR	*R. rosea* L., i.g. 25 mg/kg/day for 22 days (8 days before the model)	Normal saline	1. Escape latency in MWM 2. The number of target platform crossings 3. Time spent in target quadrant 4. NADH/NADPH	1. $P < 0.01$ 2. $P < 0.01$ 3. $P < 0.01$ 4. $P < 0.01$
28. Vasileva et al., 2016	Wistar rats (male, 10/10)	160–200 g	Scopolamine-impaired memory model	No need	*R. rosea* L., i.g., 50, 100 mg/kg for 12 days after the model	Normal saline	1. Escape times in AAR 2. Number of intertrial crossings in AAT	1. $P > 0.05$ 2. $P > 0.05$
29. Ge et al., 2017	Wistar rats (male, 9/9)	NR	Hypobaric hypoxia	No need	*R. rosea* L., i.g., 40 mg/kg for 28 days after the model	Normal saline	1. Escape latency in MWM 2. The number of target platform crossings	1. $P < 0.05$ 2. $P < 0.05$
30. Liu et al., 2017a	SD rats (male, 10/10)	260 ± 20 g	AD model induced by i.h. NaN_3	NR	*R. rosea* L., i.g., 15 mg/kg for 28 days after the model	Normal saline	1. Escape latency in MWM 2. Time spent in target quadrant 3. AKT, GSK-3β 4. (p-AKT, p-GSK-3β) 5. Bax, Bcl-2	1. $P < 0.05$ 2. $P < 0.05$ 3. $P < 0.05$ 4. $P < 0.05$
31. Liu et al., 2017b	SD rats (male, 10/10)	260 ± 20 g	VD model induced by CCAO	10% chloral hydrate	*R. rosea* L., i.g., 15 mg/kg for 28 days after the model	Normal saline	1. Escape latency in MWM 2. Time spent in target quadrant 3. SOD, MDA 4. p38 5. Caspase-3	1. $P < 0.05$ 2. $P < 0.05$ 3. $P < 0.05$ 4. $P < 0.05$ 5. $P < 0.05$

(Continued)

TABLE 1 | Continued

Study	Species (Sex, *n* = trial/control group)	Weight	Modeling approach	Anesthetic	Intervention: Trial group	Intervention: Control group	Outcome measure	Intergroup Differences
32. Wei, 2017	SD rats (male, 10/10)	230 ± 25 g	PTSD model induced by single prolonged stress	1% pentobarbital sodium	*R. rosea* L., i.g., 25, 50, 75 mg/kg for 14 days after the model	Normal saline	1. Escape latency in MWM 2. The number of target platform crossings 3. Neuronal apoptosis 4. SOD, MDA 5. Bax, Bcl-2, Synapsin I, p-CREB	1. $P < 0.01$ 2. $P < 0.05$ 3. $P < 0.05$ 4. $P < 0.05$ 5. $P < 0.05$
33. Yang et al., 2017	SD rats (male, 16/16)	250 ± 24 g	AD model induced by bilateral hippocampal injection $A\beta_{1-40}$	1% pentobarbital sodium (40 mg/kg i.p.)	*R. rosea* L., i.g., 25, 50, 100 mg/kg for 21 days after the model	Normal saline	1. Escape latency in MWM 2. The number of target platform crossings 3. Aβ 4. p75NTR, p-JNK	1. $P < 0.01$ 2. $P < 0.01$ 3. $P < 0.01$ 4. $P < 0.01$
34. Guo et al., 2017	Kunming mice (male/female, 30/30)	21.4 ± 2.2 g	Hypobaric hypoxia	No need	*R. rosea* L., i.g., 200 mg/kg for 56 days after the model	Normal saline	1. Escape latency in MWM 2. Time spent in target quadrant 3. Bax, Bcl-2	1. $P < 0.05$ 2. $P < 0.05$ 3. $P < 0.05$
35. Yang, 2017	Wistar rats (male, 10/10)	200–250 g	DM model induced by i.p. STZ	1% pentobarbital sodium	*R. rosea* L., i.g., 50 mg/kg for 84 days after the model	Normal saline	1. Escape latency in MWM 2. The number of target platform crossings 3. SOD, MDA	1. $P < 0.05$ 2. $P < 0.05$ 3. $P < 0.05$
36. Xiong and Gao, 2017	Wistar rats (male,15/15)	257 ± 29 g	VD model induced by CCAO	10% chloral hydrate	*R. rosea* L., i.g., 10 mg/kg for 28 days after the model	Normal saline	1. Escape latency in MWM 2. The number of target platform crossings 3. Time spent in target quadrant 4. SOD, MDA, MAO 5. COX-2, NF- κB	1. $P < 0.05$ 2. $P < 0.05$ 3. $P > 0.05$ 4. $P < 0.05$ 5. $P < 0.05$

AAR, active avoidance reaction; Ach, acetylcholine; AchE, Acetyl cholinesterase;AD, Alzheimer's disease; AlCl3, aluminum trichloride; CCAO, common carotid artery occlusion; ChAT, acetylcholine transferase; CMC-Na, sodium carboxymethylcellulose; DAT, dark avoidance test; D-gal, D-galactose; DM:Diabetes mellitus; ICV, intracerebroventricular injection; i.g., intra-gastrical injection; i.m.:intramuscular injection; i.p., intra-peritoneal injection; i.h., hypodermic injection; LPO, lipid peroxide; MWM, Morris water maze; MCAO, middle cerebral artery occlusion; MDA, Malondialdehyde; MMPM, modified multiple platform method; NR, not report; SCOP:scopolamine; MCAO:middle cerebral artery occlusion; PBS, phosphate buffer saline; PTSD, posttraumatic stress disorder; SDT, step down test; s.i., subcutaneous injection; STZ, streptozotocin; SOD, superoxide dismute; VD, vascular dementia.

of comparisons presented the frequency and/or the length of time spent on the target quadrant in MWM as the indicator of memory ability (Chen, 2008; Wang et al., 2008; Cao, 2009; Ji et al., 2009; Liu, 2009; Qu et al., 2009; Zou et al., 2009; Zhao et al., 2010; Yang et al., 2011a,b, 2017; Sun et al., 2012; Zhang S. et al., 2012; Zhang et al., 2013; Barhwal et al., 2015; Yan et al., 2015; Ge et al., 2017; Guo et al., 2017; Liu et al., 2017a,b; Wei, 2017; Xiong and Gao, 2017; Yang, 2017), and 7 studies (Jiang et al., 2001; Liu et al., 2003; Deng, 2006; Liu, 2009; Zhang X.X. et al., 2012; Wang et al., 2013; Vasileva et al., 2016) of comparisons reported memory outcome measure by the number of errors in step down test, dark avoidance test, the active avoidance test and/or Y maze. Additionally, 3 studies (Wu et al., 2004; Wang et al., 2012; Zhang X.X. et al., 2012) report the reaction time in Y maze. Glutathione (GSH) was reported in 5 studies (Wang et al., 2008; Qu et al., 2009; Yang et al., 2011a,b; Zhang et al., 2013); NADH/NADPH in 2 studies (Zhang et al., 2013; Barhwal et al., 2015); superoxide dismutase (SOD) and/or malondialdehyde (MDA) in 14 studies (Jiang et al., 2001; Shi et al., 2006; Chen, 2008; Qu et al., 2009; Zou et al., 2009; Yang et al., 2011a,b; Zhang S. et al., 2012; Zhang X.X. et al., 2012; Zhang et al., 2013; Liu et al., 2017b; Wei, 2017; Xiong and Gao, 2017; Yang, 2017); NO and/or NOS in 3 studies (Deng, 2006; Chen, 2008; Wang et al., 2013); acetylcholine (Ach) and/oracetylcholinesterase (AchE) in 7 studies (Jiang et al., 2001; Xie, 2003; Wu et al., 2004; Shi et al., 2006; Chen, 2008; Cao, 2009; Zhang et al., 2013); caspase-3 in 3 studies (Qu et al., 2009; Yan et al., 2015; Liu et al., 2017b); tumor necrosis factor-α(TNF-α) in 1 study (Zou et al., 2009); nuclear factor κB (NF-κB) in 1 study (Zhang et al., 2013); Bcl-2 and/or Bax protein in the hippocampus in 5 studies (Cao, 2009; Yan et al., 2015; Guo et al., 2017; Liu et al., 2017a; Wei, 2017).

Study Quality

The score of study quality checklist items ranged from 1/10 to 6/10 in **Table 2**. Of which, 1 study (Vasileva et al., 2016) obtained 6 points, 10 studies obtained 5 points (Chen, 2008; Zou et al., 2009; Wang et al., 2012, 2013; Zhang X.X. et al., 2012; Zhang et al., 2013; Barhwal et al., 2015; Yan et al., 2015; Xiong and Gao, 2017; Yang et al., 2017), 9 studies (Liu et al., 2003, 2017b; Deng, 2006; Cao, 2009; Liu, 2009; Qu et al., 2009; Mao et al., 2010; Zhao et al., 2010; Guo et al., 2017) obtained 4 points, 8 studies (Jiang et al., 2001; Xie, 2003; Wu et al., 2004; Ji et al., 2009; Ge et al., 2017; Liu et al., 2017a; Wei, 2017; Yang, 2017) obtained 3 points, 7 studies (Shi et al., 2006; Wang et al., 2008; Yang et al., 2011a,b; Sun et al., 2012; Zhang S. et al., 2012; Qi et al., 2013) obtained 2 points, and the remaining one (You et al., 2000) obtained 1 point. Seven studies (Xie, 2003; Deng, 2006; Chen, 2008; Cao, 2009; Liu, 2009; Qu et al., 2009; Wei, 2017) are master's or doctoral thesis, and remaining studies were published in peer-reviewed journals or databases. Twenty-one studies (Liu et al., 2003, 2017a,b; Xie, 2003; Deng, 2006; Chen, 2008; Cao, 2009; Ji et al., 2009; Liu, 2009; Qu et al., 2009; Zou et al., 2009; Wang et al., 2012, 2013; Zhang X.X. et al., 2012; Zhang et al., 2013; Barhwal et al., 2015; Yan et al., 2015; Vasileva et al., 2016; Wei, 2017; Xiong and Gao, 2017; Yang et al., 2017) described control of the room temperature. Except six studies (You et al., 2000; Yan et al., 2015; Liu et al., 2017a,b; Xiong and Gao, 2017; Yang, 2017), the remaining studies declared that they had random allocation to treatment and control groups. Twenty-one studies (Liu et al., 2003, 2017b; Xie, 2003; Deng, 2006; Chen, 2008; Cao, 2009; Liu, 2009; Qu et al., 2009; Zou et al., 2009; Zhao et al., 2010; Wang et al., 2012, 2013; Zhang X.X. et al., 2012; Zhang et al., 2013; Yan et al., 2015; Vasileva et al., 2016; Guo et al., 2017; Wei, 2017; Xiong and Gao, 2017; Yang, 2017; Yang et al., 2017) used anesthetic without significant intrinsic vascular protection activity. Animal model with aged rats/ mice was used in 2 studies (Jiang et al., 2001; Mao et al., 2010), with DM rats in 2 studies (Zhao et al., 2010; Yang, 2017). Thirteen studies (Wu et al., 2004; Chen, 2008; Zou et al., 2009; Mao et al., 2010; Wang et al., 2012, 2013; Zhang X.X. et al., 2012; Zhang et al., 2013; Barhwal et al., 2015; Yan et al., 2015; Vasileva et al., 2016; Xiong and Gao, 2017; Yang et al., 2017) mentioned compliance with animal welfare regulations. Thirteen studies (Deng, 2006; Chen, 2008; Cao, 2009; Liu, 2009; Qu et al., 2009; Barhwal et al., 2015; Yan et al., 2015; Vasileva et al., 2016; Ge et al., 2017; Guo et al., 2017; Liu et al., 2017a,b; Xiong and Gao, 2017) contained statements on potential conflict of interests. There was neither study reporting that if the model establishment and outcome assessment were conducted in double-blind trial or not, nor calculating sample size in the animal experiment.

Effectiveness

Twenty-eight studies reported the escape latency in MWM as the outcome measure of learning ability included in the analysis. We pooled the whole data to process and found a significant difference in favor of *R. rosea* L. treatment compared with control groups ($P < 0.00001$; SMD $= -1.83$, 95% CI $[-2.03, -1.64]$; Heterogeneity: $\chi^2 = 174.39$, df $= 28$ ($P < 0.00001$); $I^2 = 84\%$, **Figure 2**). Twenty-three studies reported the frequency and/or the length of time spent on the target quadrant as the indicator of memory ability. The pooled result showed that *R. rosea* L. significantly increased the frequency and the length of time spent on the target quadrant in MWM ($P < 0.00001$; SMD $= 1.79$, 95% CI $[1.60, 1.98]$; Heterogeneity: $\chi^2 = 131.87$, df $= 32$ ($P < 0.00001$); $I^2 = 76\%$, **Figure 3**). Seven studies reported memory outcome measure by the number of errors in step down test, dark avoidance test, the active avoidance test and Y maze. The pooled data showed that *R. rosea* L. resulted in a significant depression on the number of errors when comparing to that in control groups ($P < 0.00001$; SMD $= -1.04$, 95% CI $[-1.35, -0.72]$; Heterogeneity: $\chi^2 = 6.93$, df $= 8$ ($P = 0.54$); $I^2 = 0\%$, **Figure 4**).

Mechanisms of *Rhodiola rosea* for Learning and Memory Function

Compared with controls, meta-analysis of 5 studies (Wang et al., 2008; Qu et al., 2009; Yang et al., 2011a,b; Zhang et al., 2013) showed that *R. rosea* L. significantly increased the level of GSH ($n = 50$, SMD 1.67, 95% CI [1.20 to 2.14], $P < 0.00001$; heterogeneity: $\chi^2 = 2.09$, df $= 4$ ($P = 0.72$); $I^2 = 0\%$), (**Figure 5**); 2 studies (Zhang et al., 2013; Barhwal et al., 2015) for increasing the level of NADH and/or NADPH, ($P < 0.05$); meta-analysis of 12 studies (Shi et al., 2006; Chen, 2008; Zou et al., 2009; Yang et al., 2011a,b; Zhang S. et al., 2012; Zhang X.X. et al., 2012; Zhang et al., 2013; Liu et al., 2017b; Wei, 2017; Xiong and Gao, 2017; Yang, 2017) for increasing SOD level ($n = 115$, SMD 2.12,

TABLE 2 | Risk of bias of the included studies.

Study	A	B	C	D	E	F	G	H	I	J	Total
1. You et al., 2000	√										1
2. Jiang et al., 2001	√		√				√				3
3. Liu et al., 2003	√	√	√			√					4
4. Xie, 2003		√	√			√					3
5. Wu et al., 2004	√		√						√		3
6. Shi et al., 2006	√		√								2
7. Deng, 2006		√	√			√				√	4
8. Chen, 2008		√	√			√			√	√	5
9. Wang et al., 2008	√		√								2
10. Cao, 2009		√	√			√				√	4
11. Ji et al., 2009	√	√	√								3
12. Liu, 2009		√	√			√				√	4
13. Qu et al., 2009		√	√			√				√	4
14. Zou et al., 2009	√	√	√			√			√		5
15. Mao et al., 2010	√		√				√		√		4
16. Zhao et al., 2010	√		√			√	√				4
17. Yang et al., 2011b	√		√								2
18. Yang et al., 2011a	√		√								2
19. Sun et al., 2012	√		√								2
20. Wang et al., 2012	√	√	√			√			√		5
21. Zhang S. et al., 2012	√		√								2
22. Zhang X.X. et al., 2012	√	√	√			√			√		5
23. Zhang et al., 2013	√	√	√			√			√		5
24. Qi et al., 2013	√		√								2
25. Wang et al., 2013	√	√	√			√			√		5
26. Yan et al., 2015	√	√				√			√	√	5
27. Barhwal et al., 2015	√	√	√						√	√	5
28. Vasileva et al., 2016	√	√	√			√			√	√	6
29. Ge et al., 2017	√		√							√	3
30. Liu et al., 2017a	√	√								√	3
31. Liu et al., 2017b	√	√				√				√	4
32. Wei, 2017		√	√			√					3
33. Yang et al., 2017	√	√	√			√			√		5
34. Guo et al., 2017	√		√			√				√	4
35. Yang, 2017	√					√	√				3
36. Xiong and Gao, 2017	√	√				√			√	√	5

Studies fulfilling the criteria of: A, peer reviewed publication; B, control of temperature; C, random allocation to treatment or control; D, blinded induction of model; E, blinded assessment of outcome; F, use of anesthetic without significant intrinsic neuroprotective activity; G, animal model (aged, diabetic, or hypertensive); H, sample size calculation; I, compliance with animal welfare regulations; J, statement of potential conflict of interests.

95% CI [1.77 to 2.47], P < 0.00001; heterogeneity: $\chi^2 = 22.11$, df= 11 ($P = 0.02$); $I^2 = 50\%$), (**Figure 6**); meta-analysis of 12 studies (Shi et al., 2006; Chen, 2008; Qu et al., 2009; Zou et al., 2009; Yang et al., 2011a,b; Zhang X.X. et al., 2012; Zhang et al., 2013; Liu et al., 2017b; Wei, 2017; Xiong and Gao, 2017; Yang, 2017) for reducing MDA level ($n = 117$, SMD−1.89, 95% CI [−2.22 to −1.56], $P < 0.00001$; heterogeneity: $\chi^2 = 18.08$, df= 11 ($P = 0.08$); $I^2 = 39\%$), (**Figure 7**); 3 studies (Deng, 2006; Chen, 2008; Wang et al., 2013) for enhancing the expression of NO and/or NOS ($P < 0.05$); meta-analysis of 2 studies (Jiang et al., 2001; Zhang et al., 2013) increasing the activity of Ach ($n = 13$, SMD 1.22, 95% CI [0.34 to 2.10], $P < 0.00001$; heterogeneity: $\chi^2 = 0.6$, df = 1 ($P = 0.44$); $I^2 = 0\%$), (**Figure 8A**); meta-analysis of 5 studies (Wu et al., 2004; Shi et al., 2006; Chen, 2008; Cao, 2009; Zhang et al., 2013) down-regulating the activity of AchE ($n = 46$, SMD −1.61, 95% CI [−2.11 to −1.12], P < 0.00001; heterogeneity: $\chi^2 = 6.86$, df = 4 ($P = 0.14$); $I^2 = 42\%$), (**Figure 8B**); 3 studies (Chen, 2008; Qu et al., 2009; Qi et al., 2013) for reducing the amount of calcium in nerve cells, ($P < 0.05$); meta-analysis of 3 studies (Qu et al., 2009; Yan et al., 2015; Liu et al., 2017b) for down-regulating the expression of caspase-3 ($n = 23$, SMD −3.57, 95% CI [−4.62 to −2.52], $P <$ 0.00001; heterogeneity: $\chi^2 = 3.59$, df = 2 ($P = 0.17$); $I^2 = 44\%$), (**Figure 9**); 5 studies (Cao, 2009; Yan et al., 2015; Guo

Study or Subgroup	Experimental Mean	Experimental SD	Experimental Total	Control Mean	Control SD	Control Total	Weight	Std. Mean Difference IV, Fixed, 95% CI
Barhwal 2015	7.901	0.956	12	17.342	1.435	12	0.6%	-7.48 [-9.92, -5.03]
Cao 2009	12.69	1.85	12	29.54	3.36	12	1.0%	-6.00 [-8.02, -3.98]
Chen 2008	9.827	5.34	8	25.09	4.47	8	1.7%	-2.93 [-4.46, -1.40]
Deng 2006	31.4	32.6	26	78.5	72.9	28	12.5%	-0.81 [-1.37, -0.25]
Ge 2017	32.31	0.47	3	52.98	4.21	3	0.1%	-5.52 [-11.09, 0.05]
Guo 2017	36.35	12.53	30	45.72	16.02	30	14.4%	-0.64 [-1.16, -0.12]
Ji 2009	12.69	11.85	12	36.54	8.36	12	3.5%	-2.25 [-3.31, -1.19]
Jiang 2001	19.255	5.149	8	25.875	4.794	8	3.2%	-1.26 [-2.36, -0.16]
Liu 2017	52.12	7.03	10	76.34	5.98	10	1.7%	-3.55 [-5.06, -2.04]
Liu 2003	48.1	39.5	10	92.1	37	10	4.3%	-1.10 [-2.06, -0.15]
Liu 2003A	53.8	36.7	10	99.3	36.4	10	4.1%	-1.19 [-2.16, -0.22]
Liu 2009	34.75	19.27	4	37.69	12.95	4	2.0%	-0.16 [-1.55, 1.23]
Liu 2017A	46.34	8.82	10	68.55	8.69	10	2.6%	-2.43 [-3.64, -1.22]
Qu 2009	10.45	2.08	8	39.91	4.82	8	0.4%	-7.50 [-10.65, -4.35]
Shi 2006	107.2	22.966	10	226.1	28.815	10	1.3%	-4.37 [-6.12, -2.62]
Sun 2012	12.66	1.85	9	27.42	3.7	8	0.9%	-4.89 [-6.99, -2.79]
Wang 2008	12.69	11.85	12	36.54	8.36	11	3.3%	-2.22 [-3.30, -1.14]
Wang 2013	77.9	12.6	10	109.6	16.7	10	3.1%	-2.05 [-3.18, -0.92]
Wei 2017	7.44	1.22	10	28.83	8.15	10	1.7%	-3.52 [-5.01, -2.02]
Wu 2004	66.4	32.4	12	100.55	32.98	12	5.3%	-1.01 [-1.87, -0.15]
Xiong 2017	28.5	6.9	15	37.8	8.2	15	6.3%	-1.19 [-1.98, -0.41]
Yan 2015	17.641	6.691	12	41.808	5.758	12	2.0%	-3.74 [-5.14, -2.33]
Yang 2011	18.462	7.215	8	42.605	5.483	8	1.3%	-3.56 [-5.29, -1.84]
Yang 2011A	25.538	5.037	10	42.156	5.551	10	2.1%	-3.00 [-4.36, -1.64]
Yang 2017	15.73	3.82	16	48.81	7.38	16	1.5%	-5.49 [-7.08, -3.89]
Yang 2017A	19.43	2.77	10	28.32	4.04	1028	9.8%	-2.20 [-2.83, -1.57]
Zhang 2013	21.1	4.1	8	29.1	6.2	8	3.0%	-1.44 [-2.57, -0.30]
Zhao 2010	19.45	1.75	10	27.18	6.11	10	3.6%	-1.65 [-2.69, -0.60]
Zou 2009	8	3	15	23	5	15	2.7%	-3.54 [-4.74, -2.34]
Total (95% CI)			**330**			**1348**	**100.0%**	**-1.83 [-2.03, -1.64]**

Heterogeneity: Chi² = 174.39, df = 28 (P < 0.00001); I² = 84%
Test for overall effect: Z = 18.22 (P < 0.00001)

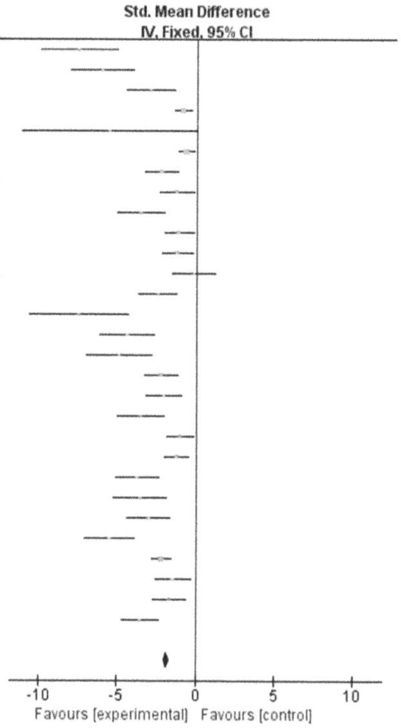

FIGURE 2 | The forest plot: effects of *Rhodiola rosea* L. for decreasing the escape latency in MWM compared with control group.

et al., 2017; Liu et al., 2017a; Wei, 2017) for increasing the expression of Bcl-2 and reducing the expression of Bax protein in the hippocampus,($P < 0.05$); 1 study (Zou et al., 2009) for inhibiting the expression of TNF-α; 1 study (Zhang et al., 2013) for inhibiting the expression of nuclear factor κB (NF-κB).

Subgroup Analysis and Sensitivity Analysis

To explore potential confounding factors which affected the outcome measures, we stratified analysis of the escape latency based on variables including animal species, animal model, the duration of treatment, and the quality of study. In the subgroup analysis of these factors, the effect size of rat species was larger than mice (SMD $= -2.09$ vs. SMD $= -1.08$, **Figure 10A**). Animal model showed great discrepancy in the overall effect of outcome measure, which the model of hypobaric hypoxia with scale of 16.4% weight accounted for smaller effect size than any other model (SMD $= -1.18$ vs. SMD $_{\text{pooled}} = -1.96$, **Figure 10B**). The longer period of *R. rosea* L. treatment also showed greater effect size than the shorter treatment with 2 weeks or less (SMD $= -1.92$ vs. SMD $= -1.83$, **Figure 10C**). Notably, the lower quality studies did not exhibit larger effect size than the higher ones (SMD $= -1.65$ vs. SMD $= -2.55$, **Figure 10D**).

Sensitivity analyses showed that the results did not substantially alter after removing any one trial. However, when we only include studies using mice as animal models, meta-analysis of 5 studies (Liu et al., 2003; Wu et al., 2004; Deng, 2006; Wang et al., 2013; Ge et al., 2017) showed a small difference in favor of *R. rosea* L. treatment compared with control groups with lower heterogeneity ($n = 61$, SMD $= -1.08$, 95%CI $[-1.47, -0.68]$, $P < 0.00001$; Heterogeneity: $\chi^2 = 6.22$, df $= 4$ ($P < 0.00001$); $I^2 = 36\%$).

DISCUSSION

Summary of Evidence

In this meta-analysis, we assessed *R. rosea* L. treatment on learning and memory function based on 36 eligible studies. The results revealed that *R. rosea* L. could evidently reduce the escape latency, improve the frequency and the length of time spent in MWM and decrease the number of errors in step down test, dark avoidance test, and Y maze when comparing with control groups in animal models.

Limitations

Some limitations should be considered while interpreting this study. First, the methodological quality of the included studies was considerably variable and inferior. Nearly all of the included studies had an overall assessment as "high risk of bias," so we could not exclude that our results may be biased. Second, calculation of sample size and blindness of model establishment and outcome measurement are pivotal in quality control of research, yet no studies provided these critical information in this systematic review. Third, it's not worthy that almost all the included studies declared random allocation to treatment and control groups, while the detailed procedure was not supported at all. Additionally, gender

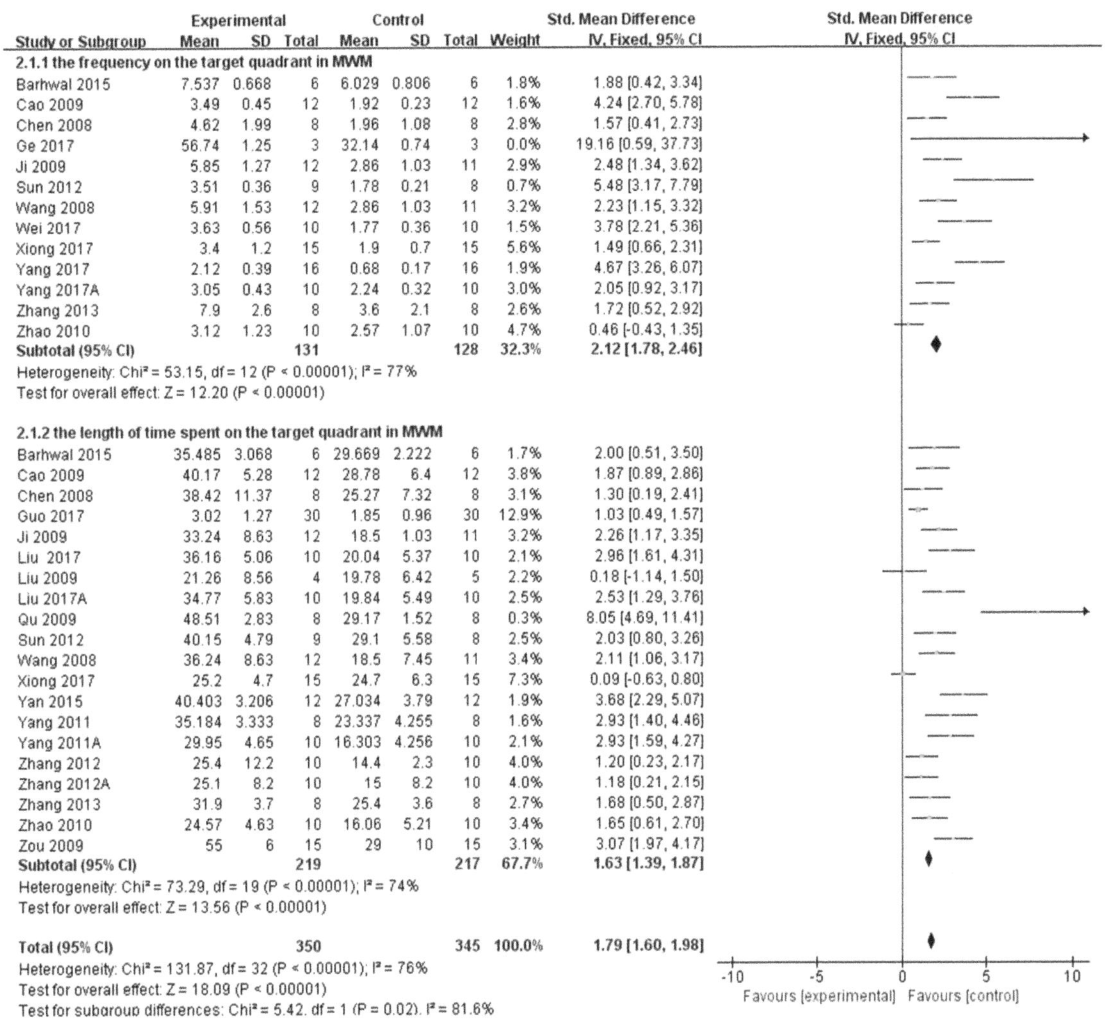

FIGURE 3 | The forest plot: effects of *Rhodiola rosea* L. for decreasing the frequency and the length of time spent on the target quadrant in MWM compared with control group.

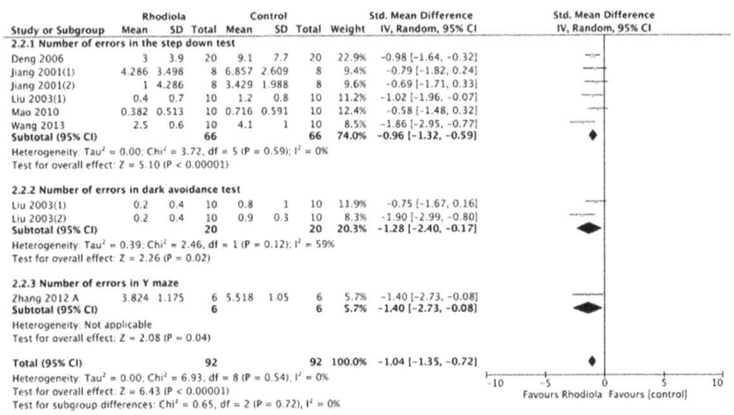

FIGURE 4 | The forest plot: effects of *Rhodiola rosea* L. For decreasing the number of errors compared with control group.

Study or Subgroup	Experimental Mean	Experimental SD	Experimental Total	Control Mean	Control SD	Control Total	Weight	Std. Mean Difference IV, Fixed, 95% CI
Qu 2009	11.86	1.34	12	8.18	1.79	12	19.9%	2.25 [1.19, 3.31]
Wang 2008	141.46	13.1	12	124.24	13.05	12	28.1%	1.27 [0.38, 2.16]
Yang 2011	25.45	5.42	8	16.63	4.83	8	16.2%	1.62 [0.45, 2.80]
Yang 2011A	28.57	7.88	10	15.98	7.76	10	21.2%	1.54 [0.52, 2.57]
Zhang 2013	26.5	4.2	8	18.6	3.7	8	14.6%	1.89 [0.65, 3.12]
Total (95% CI)			**50**			**50**	**100.0%**	**1.67 [1.20, 2.14]**

Heterogeneity: Chi² = 2.09, df = 4 (P = 0.72); I² = 0%
Test for overall effect: Z = 6.93 (P < 0.00001)

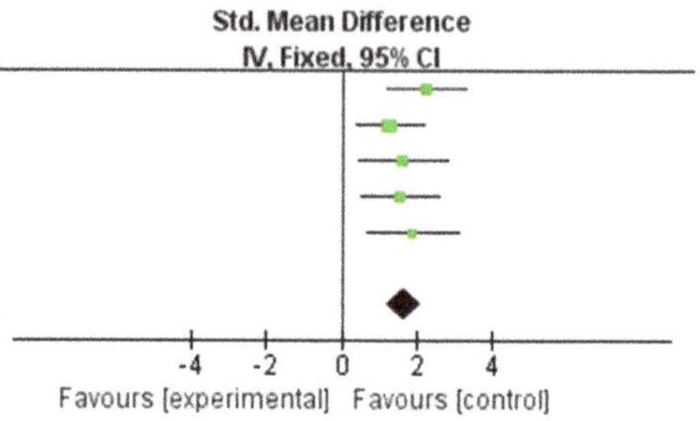

FIGURE 5 | The forest plot: effects of *Rhodiola rosea* L. for increasing glutathione compared with control group.

Study or Subgroup	Experimental Mean	Experimental SD	Experimental Total	Control Mean	Control SD	Control Total	Weight	Std. Mean Difference IV, Fixed, 95% CI
Chen 2008	118.86	9.556	8	91.42	13.702	8	7.1%	2.20 [0.88, 3.51]
Liu 2017A	7.13	0.91	5	3.95	0.64	5	2.1%	3.65 [1.25, 6.05]
Shi 2006	154.27	5.84	10	146	8.8	10	13.5%	1.06 [0.11, 2.01]
Wei 2017	82	20	10	30	10	10	6.3%	3.15 [1.75, 4.55]
Xiong 2017	45	4.23	15	35	4.37	15	13.7%	2.26 [1.32, 3.21]
Yang 2011	62.72	7.36	8	34.78	4.87	8	3.2%	4.23 [2.28, 6.19]
Yang 2011A	62.33	8.47	10	38.66	4.77	10	5.9%	3.30 [1.86, 4.74]
Yang 2017A	132.45	18.92	10	103.65	14.78	10	11.3%	1.62 [0.58, 2.67]
Zhang 2012	197.9	16.8	10	150.3	17.7	10	7.6%	2.64 [1.38, 3.91]
Zhang 2012A	157	29	6	118	22	6	7.0%	1.40 [0.08, 2.72]
Zhang 2013	112	12	8	68	13	8	4.5%	3.33 [1.68, 4.98]
Zou 2009	74.38	20.43	15	45.24	15.83	15	17.7%	1.55 [0.72, 2.38]
Total (95% CI)			**115**			**115**	**100.0%**	**2.12 [1.77, 2.47]**

Heterogeneity: Chi² = 22.11, df = 11 (P = 0.02); I² = 50%
Test for overall effect: Z = 11.90 (P < 0.00001)

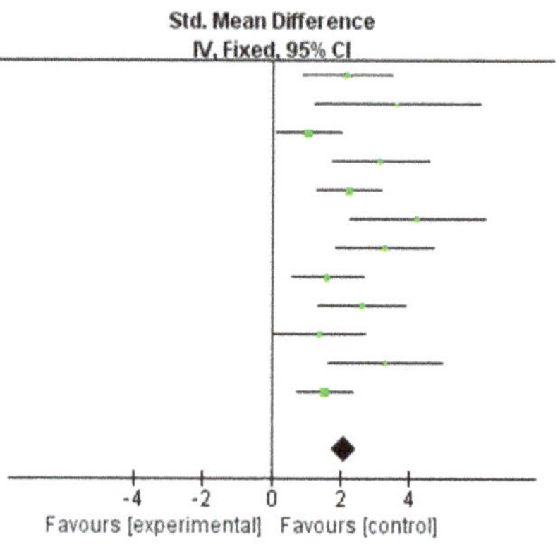

FIGURE 6 | The forest plot: effects of *Rhodiola rosea* L. for increasing superoxide dismutase compared with control group.

Study or Subgroup	Experimental Mean	Experimental SD	Experimental Total	Control Mean	Control SD	Control Total	Weight	Std. Mean Difference IV, Fixed, 95% CI
Chen 2008	0.884	0.184	8	1.21	0.274	8	8.7%	-1.32 [-2.43, -0.21]
Liu 2017A	1.06	0.19	5	1.53	0.24	5	3.9%	-1.96 [-3.62, -0.30]
Qu 2009	0.68	0.1	12	0.86	0.14	12	12.9%	-1.43 [-2.34, -0.51]
Shi 2006	7.646	0.923	10	8.611	0.716	10	11.7%	-1.12 [-2.08, -0.16]
Wei 2017	13.2	4.2	10	23.9	1.2	10	5.2%	-3.32 [-4.76, -1.87]
Xiong 2017	3.47	1.13	15	7.51	2.11	15	11.8%	-2.32 [-3.28, -1.37]
Yang 2011	2.97	0.2	8	4.99	0.83	8	4.2%	-3.16 [-4.76, -1.57]
Yang 2011A	3.57	0.46	10	5.87	1.23	10	7.5%	-2.37 [-3.57, -1.17]
Yang 2017A	6.43	0.91	10	7.64	1.09	10	11.6%	-1.15 [-2.12, -0.19]
Zhang 2012A	1.71	0.33	6	3	0.59	6	3.9%	-2.49 [-4.15, -0.83]
Zhang 2013	6.9	0.7	8	8.1	0.9	8	8.4%	-1.41 [-2.54, -0.28]
Zou 2009	3.92	0.17	15	4.8	0.41	15	10.2%	-2.73 [-3.76, -1.70]
Total (95% CI)			**117**			**117**	**100.0%**	**-1.89 [-2.22, -1.56]**

Heterogeneity: Chi² = 18.08, df = 11 (P = 0.08); I² = 39%
Test for overall effect: Z = 11.29 (P < 0.00001)

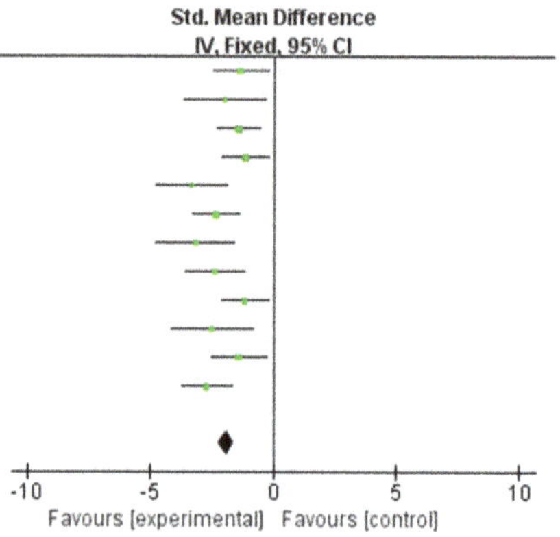

FIGURE 7 | The forest plot: effects of *Rhodiola rosea* L. for decreasing malondialdehyde compared with control group.

difference was overlooked in the included study. Male/female mice models were used in the two studies (Wu et al., 2004; Wang et al., 2013) for cognitive experiments. Although the mechanism is unclear, a male advantage for working memory and a female advantage for visual memory and social cognition in rodent models were highlighted (Leger and Neill, 2016). Moreover, funnel plots (**Figure 11**) showed potential publication bias existed in this research field, suggesting studies with null effect are missing. Studies achieved statistically significant outcomes have been shown to be three times more likely to be published than that with null outcomes (Dickersin et al., 1987). Publication bias is due to multiple factor such as researchers and journal editors prefer positive results rather than negative or inconclusive results (Wolfgang, 2007). Thus, the effect of *R. rosea* L. on learning and memory function cannot be excluded from overall over estimation of effect sizes and efficacy, which may weaken the validity of conclusions.

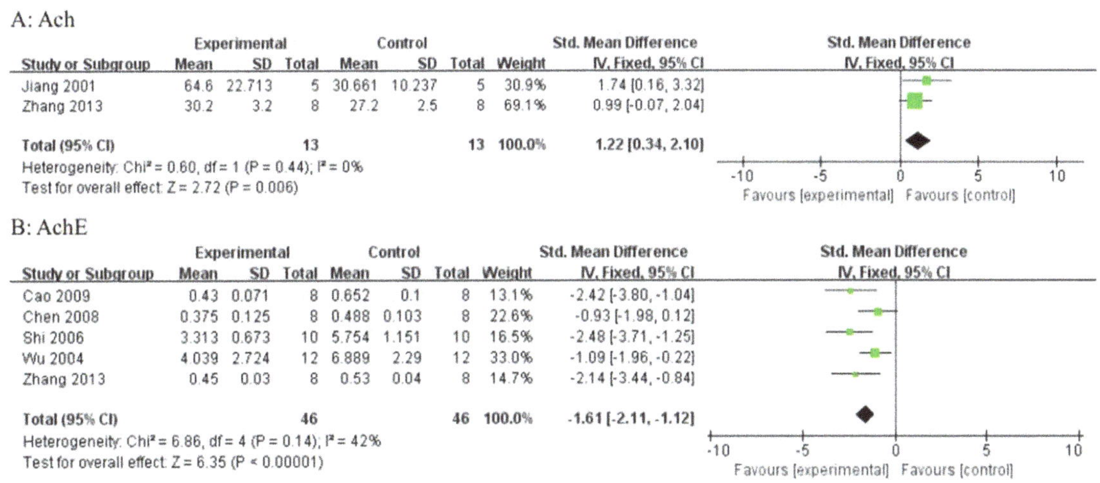

FIGURE 8 | (A) The forest plot: effects of textitRhodiola rosea L. for increasing acetylcholine; **(B)** The forest plot:effects of *Rhodiola rosea* L. for decreasing acetylcholinesterase compared with control group.

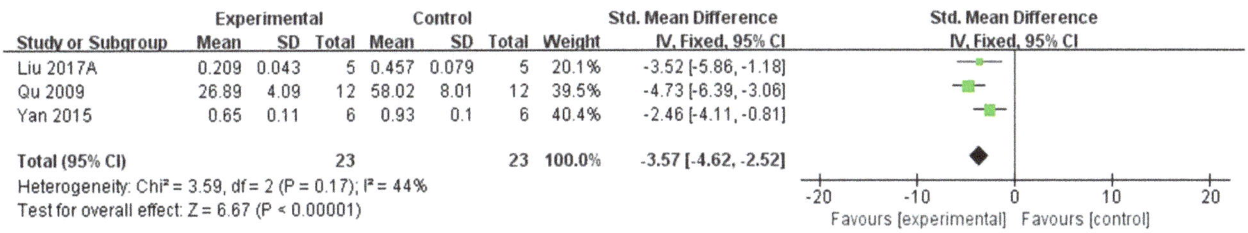

FIGURE 9 | The forest plot: effects of *Rhodiola rosea* L. for decreasing caspase-3 compared with control group.

Interpretation of the Results

Considerably high heterogeneity was present in this meta-analysis, the summary positive results should be interpreted with caution. Given that there are many potential sources of heterogeneity in the outcome, several means are taken into consideration for the finding of the causes. Firstly, random-effects models are used in our study. Heterogeneity is a key condition for the execution of meta-regression, but it can also cause confusion if confounding factors are not well-balanced. As small number of studies were included in this meta-analysis, we made the meta-regression with reservations and did subgroup analysis based on four potential confounding factors including animal species, animal model, the duration of treatment, and the quality of study. The results of subgroup analyses suggested that the first three factors were very likely to be the sources of heterogeneity in this research, while the poor quality of methodology still could not be exempted from the excuses for high heterogeneity. Sensitivity analyses have also been adopted to detect the effects of studies identified as being aberrant result, or being highly influential in the analysis (Haidich, 2010). While no studies identified as being aberrant result or being highly influential in the analysis from the results of sensitivity analyses in this review.

Implication for Further Studies

While mice models are increasing used for cognitive experiments involving learning and memory process that were originally designed for rat species, the stability of spatial cognitive representation in rats changes more slightly over time than in mice (Hok et al., 2016). In the subgroup analyses, rat species also showed greater effect size in depression of escape latency than that of mice. Thus, rat species were considered as suitable cognitive experiments involving learning and memory process. In addition, the impact of gender on cognitive function deserves attention. In the present study, male rats models and male/female mice models were used in the included studies of our review for working memory process, while no significant difference existed in the pooled result of meta-analysis in escape latency of MWM test after discarding two studies with male/female mice (Wu et al., 2004; Wang et al., 2013). However, a male advantage for working memory and a female advantage for visual memory and social cognition in rodent models were highlighted in recent systematic review (Leger and Neill, 2016). Thus, using a single sex animal model is considered more reasonable for study learning and memory function in future experiments.

Two dementia models of AD and vascular dementia (VaD) are most commonly approached for learning and memory

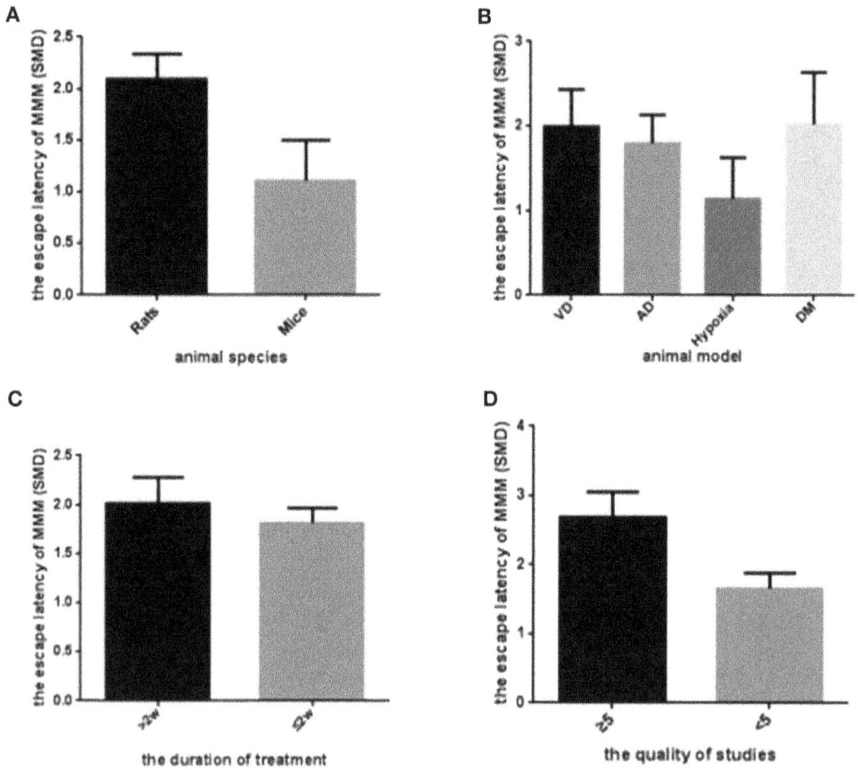

FIGURE 10 | Subgroup analyses of the escape latency. **(A)** The animal species on the effect size of the outcome measure; **(B)** the animal model on the effect size of the outcome measure; **(C)** the duration of the treatment on the effect size of the outcome measure; **(D)** the quality of studies on the effect size of the outcome measure. The magnitude of absolute value SMD reflected the effect size.

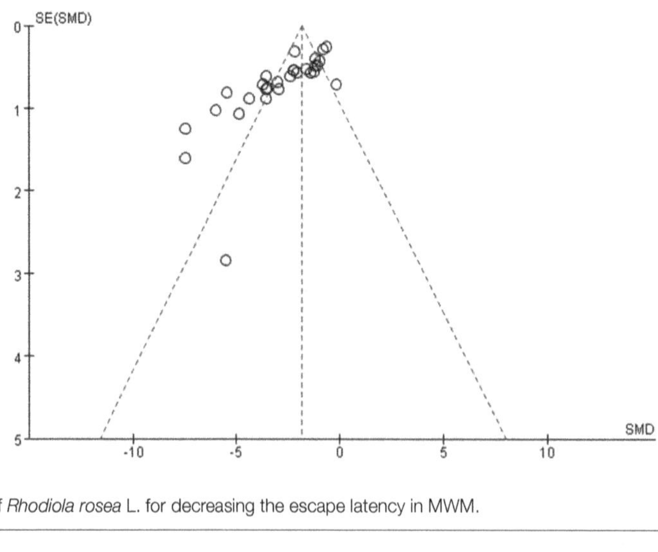

FIGURE 11 | The funnel plot: effects of *Rhodiola rosea* L. for decreasing the escape latency in MWM.

research (Kalaria et al., 2008). However, there are several model methods for inducing these two dementia types and their differences of effectiveness and robustness are not investigated. For this systematic review, intra-peritoneal injection with scopolamine, combination with aluminum trichloride, D-galactose and scopolamine, intracerebroventricular injection with streptozotocin, and hippocampal injection with $A\beta_{1-40}$ were the most approaches for AD models in the included studies. Different time scales of artery occlusion and different arteries selected for blood blocking were adopted for VaD models. In the subgroup analyses, six animal models including AD, VaD, hypoxia, sleep deprivation, epilepsy, and diabetes mellitus models

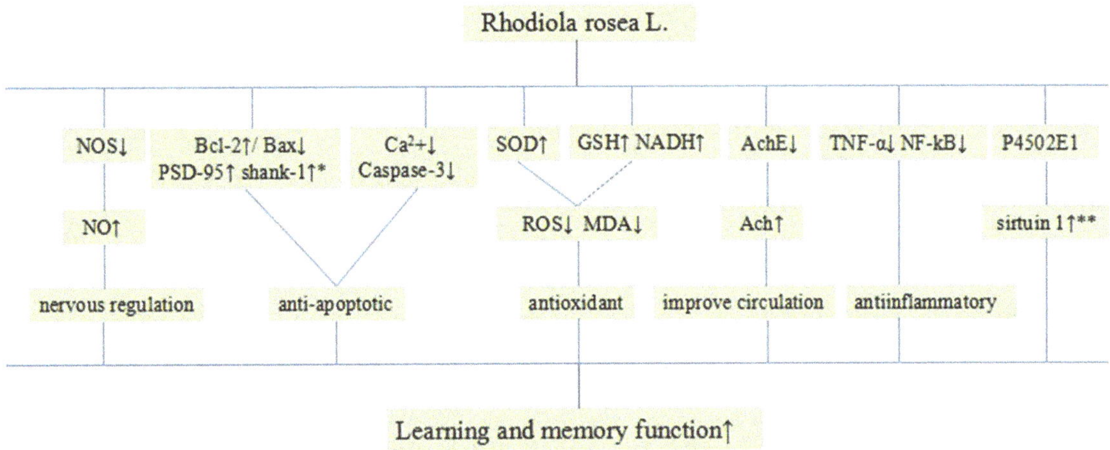

FIGURE 12 | A schematic representation of possible mechanisms of *Rhodiola rosea* L. for improving learning and memory function. Solid lines indicate established effects, whereas dashed lines represent putative mechanisms. *The expression of Bcl-2, Bax protein, PSD-95 and shank-1 protein in the hippocampus; **The activity of sirtuin 1.

were conducted for cognitive impairment, of which AD models accounted for 38.7% weight and VaD models accounted for 17.7% weight. These two most weight of models showed no significant difference in effect size on escape latency of MWM test, which can indirectly reflect the effectiveness and robustness of the two dementia models for cognitive impairment.

A lower-quality study trends toward better outcomes, leading to the global estimated effect overstated (García-Bonilla et al., 2012). In the present study, many domains had flaws in aspects of randomization, allocation concealment, and blinding and sample size calculation, which are the core standards of study design (Moher et al., 2015). Thus, we recommended that the experimental research of *R. rosea* L. for learning and memory function need be promoted by means of incorporating the ARRIVE guidelines (Kilkenny et al., 2012).

Long-term treatment for dementia progression with Gingko biloba showed great effect on prevention of cognitive decline (Dodge et al., 2008). In parallel, treatment with *R. rosea* L. more than 2 weeks showed greater effect size in the escape latency of MWM test than that of <2 weeks' treatment in the subgroup analyses, suggesting that long-term treatment with *R. rosea* L. has a greater benefit for cognitive function. In view of the number of studies in subgroup analyses was relatively small and may lack of statistical power to detect smaller effect sizes. Therefore, we recommend that future studies involving this problem are conducted strictly complying with standards of research methodology and report their adequate information clearly.

Systemic review of animal studies plays a critical role in drug development and the clarification of physiological and pathological mechanisms of clinical research. In this systematic review, some included studies speculated on how *R. rosea* L. enhanced learning and memory function and the possible mechanisms are summarized as follows: (1) antioxidant through increasing the level of GSH (Wang et al., 2008; Qu et al., 2009; Yang et al., 2011a,b; Zhang et al., 2013), NADH/NADPH (Zhang et al., 2013; Barhwal et al., 2015), and enhancing SOD-induced antioxidant via attenuating chondriokinesis to reduce the release of MDA (Jiang et al., 2001; Shi et al., 2006; Chen, 2008; Qu et al., 2009; Zou et al., 2009; Yang et al., 2011a,b; Zhang S. et al., 2012; Zhang X.X. et al., 2012; Zhang et al., 2013; Liu et al., 2017b; Wei, 2017; Xiong and Gao, 2017; Yang, 2017); (2) improvement of the circulation by enhancing the expression of NO via up-regulating the expression of NOS (Deng, 2006; Chen, 2008; Wang et al., 2013); (3) cholinergic regulation through increasing the activity of Ach via down-regulating the activity of AchE (Jiang et al., 2001; Xie, 2003; Wu et al., 2004; Shi et al., 2006; Chen, 2008; Cao, 2009; Zhang et al., 2013); (4) inhibition of apoptosis through reducing the amount of calcium in nerve cells (Chen, 2008; Qu et al., 2009; Qi et al., 2013) and down-regulating the expression of caspase-3 (Qu et al., 2009; Yan et al., 2015; Liu et al., 2017b); (5) anti-inflammatory through inhibiting the expression of TNF-α (Zou et al., 2009) and NF-κB (Zhang et al., 2013); (6) increasing sirtuin 1 (SIRT1) activity through a cytochrome P4502E1 (CYP2E1)-regulated mechanism (Cao, 2009); (7) increasing the expression of Bcl-2 and reducing the expression of Bax protein in the hippocampus (Cao, 2009; Yan et al., 2015; Guo et al., 2017; Liu et al., 2017a; Wei, 2017) and improving the expression of PSD-95 and shank-1 protein in the hippocampus (Wang et al., 2008), alleviating apoptosis in the hippocampal CA1 area. The possible mechanisms of *R. rosea* L. for learning and/or memory function are through antioxidant, cholinergic regulation, anti-apoptosis activities, anti-inflammatory, improving coronary blood flow, and cerebral metabolism (**Figure 12**).

CONCLUSION

We have provided a first-ever comprehensive preclinical systematic review of *R. rosea* L. for cognitive behavior in animal studies and our findings indicate that *R. rosea* L. improves learning and memory function in experimental models.

AUTHOR CONTRIBUTIONS

GM, QZ, MX, XZ, ZL, LL, and GZ designed the study. GM and QZ collected the data. GM and MX performed all analyses. GM, QZ, ZL, LL, and GZ wrote the manuscript. All authors contributed to writing of this manuscript.

ACKNOWLEDGMENTS

This project was supported by the grant of National Natural Science Foundation of China (81573750/81473491/81173395/H2902).

REFERENCES

Barhwal, K., Das, S. K., Kumar, A., Hota, S. K., and Srivastava, R. B. (2015). Insulin receptor A and Sirtuin 1 synergistically improve learning and spatial memory following chronic salidroside treatment during hypoxia. *J. Neurochem.* . 135, 332–346. doi: 10.1111/jnc.13225

Cao, J. (2009). *The Experimental Study of the Effect of Rhodiola Herb Against Activity of AchE, NOS and the Expression Bcl-2, Bax Proteinin the Hippocampus Tissue of Alzheimer's Disease in Rats.* , MDthesis. Available online at: http://kns.cnki.net/KCMS/detail/detail.aspx?dbcode=CMFD&dbname=CMFD2009&filename=2009123437.nh&uid (Accessed March 5, 2016)

Chen, Y. Q. (2008). *The Experimental Study of the Effete of Rhodiola Against Vaseular Dementia Rats on Activity of SOD, Content of MDA, Activity of AchE and Apoptosis of Neurons in Hippocampus Tissue.* , MDthesis. Available online at: http://kns.cnki.net/KCMS/detail/detail.aspx?dbcode=CMFD&dbname=CMFD2009&filename=2008138185.nh&uid (Accessed July 5, 2016)

De Bock, K., Eijnde, B. O., Ramaekers, M., and Hespel, P. (2004). Acute *Rhodiola rosea* intake can improve endurance exercise performance. *Int. J. Sport Nutr. Exerc. Metab.* 14, 298–307. doi: 10.1123/ijsnem.14.3.298

Deng, S. M. (2006). *Study on the Quality Standard and Pharmacological Activity Process, Extraction of Total Tannins Inrhodiola.* Ph.D. thesis. Available online at: http://kns.cnki.net/KCMS/detail/detail.aspx?dbcode=CDFD&dbname=CDFD9908&filename=2006194899.nh&uid (Accessed July 5, 2016).

Dickersin, K., Chan, S., and Chalmers, T. C. ,(1987). Publication bias and clinical trials. *Control. Clin. Trials.* 8, 343–353. doi: 10.1016/0197-2456(87)90155-3

Dodge, H. H., Zitzelberger, T., Oken, B. S., Howieson, D., and Kaye, J. (2008). A randomized placebo-controlled trial of Ginkgo biloba for the prevention of cognitive decline. *Neurology.* 70, 1809–1817. doi: 10.1212/01.wnl.0000303814.13509.db

Farhath, K., Amarinder, S. B., and Brahm, S. (2005). *Rhodiola rosea*: a versatile adaptogen. *Compr. Rev. Food Sci. F.* 4, 55–62. doi: 10.1111/j.1541-4337.2005.tb00073.x

García-Bonilla, L., Campos, M., Giralt, D., Salat, D., Chacón, P., Hernández-Guillamon, M., et al. (2012). Evidence for the efficacy of statins inanimal stroke models: a meta-analysis. *J. Neurochem.* 122, 233–243.doi: 10.1111/j.1471-4159.2012.07773.x

Ge, Y. L., Li, L. Q., Wang, H. Y., Zhang, J. B., Zhang, P. P., and Zhuang, Y. J. (2017). Effect of Herba Rhodiolae on learning and memory abilities and morphology of hippocampus in rats with intermittent hypoxia. *Chinese J. Gerontol.* 37, 4978–4979 doi: 10.3969/j.issn.1005-9202.2017.20.010

Guo, T. X., Liu, S., Zhang, L., Liu, D. X., Yang, Z. L., and Liu, S. Y. (2017). Effects of salidroside on learning and memory dysfunction in chronic hypoxic mice. *Chin. J. Gerontol.* 37, 6029–6031. doi: 10.3969/j.issn.1005-9202.2017.24.011

Haidich, A. B. (2010). *Meta-Analysis in Medical Research.* Hippokratia.14, 29-–37. Available online at: http://xueshu.baidu.com/s?wd$=$paperuri%3A%2812aad278fcfead385616bbb203ebe932%29&filte, (Accessed March 5, 2016)

Hok, V., Poucet, B., Duvelle, É., Save, É., and Sargolini, F. (2016). Spatial cognition in mice and rats: similarities and differences in brain and behavior. *Wiley Interdiscip. Rev. Cogn. Sci.* 7, 406–421. doi: 10.1002/wcs.1411

Ji, J. H., Dong, L. L., Cao, J., Yang, F. M., and Wang, J. (2009). Effects of Integripetal Rhodiola Herb on Ethology and Anti-OxydatiOn Potential of Brain Tissue of Alzheimer's Disease model Rats. *Chin. J. Inf. Tradit. Chin. Med.* 2, 38–40. doi: 10.3969/j.issn.1005-5304.2018.02.014

Jiang, W. H., Meng, X. T., Hao, L. M., Cui, L., Dong, Z. Y., and Wang, S. L. (2001). Study of anti-aging and anti-dementia effects of Rhodosin on aging rats and experimental dementia rats. *J. N. Bethune Univ. Med. Sci.* 2, 127–129. doi: 10.13481/j.1671-587x.2001.02.010

Johnson, C. N., Roland, A., and Upton, N. (2004). New symptomatic strategies in Alzheimer's disease. *Drug Discovery Discov. Today Therapeutic Ther. Strategies..* 1, 13–19. doi: 10.1016/j.ddstr.2004.08.003

Kalaria, R. N., Maestre, G. E., Arizaga, R., Friedland, R. P., Galasko, D., and Hall, K. (2008). Alzheimer's disease and vascular dementia in developing countries: prevalence, management, and risk factors. *Lancet Neurol.* 7, 812–826. doi: 10.1016/S1474-4422(08)70169-8

Kilkenny, C., Browne, W. J., Cuthill, I. C., Emerson, M., and Altman, D. G. (2012).Improving bioscience research reporting: the ARRIVE guidelines for reportinganimal research. *Osteoarth. Cartil.* 20, 256–260. doi: 10.1016/j.joca.2012.02.010

Kurkin, V. A., and Zapesochnaya, G. G. (1985). Chemical composition and pharmacological characteristics of *Rhodiola rosea*. *J. Med. Plants* 10, 1231–1245.

Lazarova, M. B., Petkov, V. D., and Markovska, V. L. (1986). Effects of meclofenoxate and Extr. Rhodiolae roseae L. on electroconvulsive shock-impaired learning and memory in rats. *Methods Find. Exp. Clin. Pharmacol.* 8, 547–552.

Leger, M., and Neill, J. C. (2016). A systematic review comparing sex differences in cognitive function in schizophrenia and in rodent models for schizophrenia, implications for improved therapeutic strategies. *Neurosci. Biobehav.* 68, 979–1000. doi: 10.1016/j.neubiorev.2016.06.029

Liu, B. B. (2009). *Effects of RSGS on Learning/Memory and the BLOOD Ach Content in Vascular Dementia Rats.* MD thesis. Available online at: http://kns.cnki.net/KCMS/detail/detail.aspx?dbcode=CMFD&dbname=CMFD2010&filename=2009206173.nh&uid (Accessed March 5, 2016)

Liu, N., Xu, M., Wang, H. L., Wang, W. T., Wang, Y. Y., and Wang, M.W. (2017b). The effects of Rhodosin on cognition in rats with vascular demetia. *J. Hebei Med. Univ.* 38, 621–624. doi: 10.3969/j.Issn.1007-3205.2017.06.001

Liu, N.,Wang, J. H., Wang, H. L., Qiu, H. Q., Wang, Y. Y., and Wang, M. W. (2017a). The therapeutic effects of Rhodosin on cognition in AD rats. *J. Hebei Med. Univ.* 38, 133–137. doi: 10.3969/j.Issn.1007-3205.2017.02.003

Liu, Z. W., Wu, M. C., and Chen, P. (2003). Effects of *Rhodiola henryi* extract on learning memory and antihypoxia in mice. *Acta Nutrimenta Sinica.* 01, 101–104. doi: 10.13325/j.cnki.acta.nutr.sin

Mao, G. X., Deng, H. B., Yuan, L. G., Li, D. D., Li, Y. Y., and Wang, Z. (2010). Protective role of salidroside against aging in a mouse model induced by D-galactose. *Biomed. Environ. Sci.* 23, 161–166. doi: 10.1016/s0895-3988(10)60047-5

Moher, D., Avey, M., Antes, G., and Altman, D. G. (2015). Erratum: the nationalinstitutes of health and guidance for reporting preclinical research. *BMC Med.* .13, 1741-7015. doi: 10.1186/s12916-015-0321-8

Parihar, M. S., and Hemnani, T. (2004). Alzheimer's disease pathogenesis and therapeutic interventions. *J. Clin. Neurosci.* 11, 456–467. doi: 10.1016/j.jocn.2003.12.007

Pharmacopoeia Committee of the People's Republic of China Ministry of health (2005). *Pharmacopoeia of People's Republic of China Part I.* Beijing: Chemical Industry Press.

Qi, C. F., Dong, M. Y., Li, C. X., Zhang, J. F., Zhang, J. S., Li, F. X., et al. (2013). The mechanisms and effects of rhodiola on expression of parvalbumin in rat brains after hypobaric hypoxia injury. *J. Qinghai Med. Coll.* 3, 167–172. doi: 10.13452/j.cnki.jqmc.2013.03.001

Qu, Z. Q., Zhou, Y., Zeng, Y. S., Li, Y., and Chung, P. (2009). Pretreatment with *Rhodiola rosea* extract reduces cognitive impairment induced by intracerebroventricular streptozotocin in rats: implication of anti-oxidative and neuroprotective effects. *Biomed. Environ. Sci.* 22, 318–326. doi: 10.1016/S0895-3988(09)60062-3

Sena, E., van der Worp, H. B., Howells, D., and Macleod, M. (2007). How can we improve the pre-clinical development of drugs for stroke? *Trends Neurosci.* 30, 433–439. doi: 10.1016/j.tins.2007.06.009

Sena, E. S., Currie, G. L., McCann, S. K., Macleod, M. R., and Howells, D. W. (2014). Systematic reviews and meta-analysis of preclinical studies: why perform them and how to appraise them critically. *J. Cereb Blood Flow Metab.* 34:737-–742. doi: 10.1038/jcbfm.2014.28

Shevtsov, V. A., Zholus, B. I., and Shervarly, V. I. (2003). A randomized trial of two different doses of a SHR-5 Rhodiola rosea extract versus placebo and control of capacity for mental work. *Phytomedicine* 10, 95–105. doi: 10.1006/phrs.1998.0410

Shi,. J., Li, X. X., Yao, W. B.,Wang, H., Guo, H., and Gao, X. D. (2006). Study on the synergistic effects of the extract of Rhodiola rosea L. and CoQ10 on improving the ability of learning and memory in mice. *Chin. J. Bio. Pharm.* 1, 15-–18. doi: 10.3969/j.issn.1005-1678.2006.01.005

Spasov, A. A., Wikman, G. K., Mandrikov, V. B., Mironova, I. A., and Neumoin, V. V. (2000). A double-blind, placebo-controlled pilot study of the stimulating and adaptogenic effect of Rhodiola rosea SHR-5 extract on the fatigue of students caused by stress during an examination period with a repeated low-dose regimen. *Phytomedicine*. 7, 85–89. doi: 10.1016/S0944-7113(00)80078-1

Stewart, L. A., Clarke, M., Rovers, M., Riley, R. D., Simmonds, M., Stewart, G., et al. (2015). Preferred reporting items for systematic review and meta-analyses of individual participant data: the PRISMA-IPD Statement. *JAMA* 313, 1657–1665. doi: 10.1001/jama.2015.3656

Sun, H. Y., Dong, L. L., Cui, H. Y., and Cao, J. (2012). The Influence of Integripetal R hod iola Herb on Behavior and the Expression of Synapse—associated Protein in H ippocam pus of M od el Rats with Alzheimer's Disease. *Chin. J. Integra. Med. Cardio-/Cerebrovasc Dis.* 4, 455–456. doi: 10.3969/j.issn.1672-1349.2012.04.039

Thompson, R. F. (1986). The neurobiology of learning and memory. *Science* 233, 941–947. doi: 10.1016/0010-0277(89)90010-3

Vasileva, L. V., Getova, D. P., Doncheva, N. D., Marchev, A. S., and Georgiev, M. I. (2016). Beneficial effect of commercial Rhodiola extract in rats with scopolamine-induced memory impairment on active avoidance. *J. Ethnopharmacol.* 193, 586–591. doi: 10.1016/j.jep.2016.10.011

Wang, J., Li, L., Cao, J., Ji, J. H., and Yang, F. M. (2008). Effects of integripetal rhodiola herb on spatial learning and memory abilities of AD-like rats as well as protein expression of CAT and GSH-Px in hippocamps of AD-like rats. *J. Emerg. Tradit. Chin. Med.* 12, 1725–1749. doi: 10.3969/j.issn.1004-745X.2008.12.040

Wang, J. T., Zhou, H. R., Wu, D. M., Xu, H., Wang, B. X., Qiu, H. B., et al. (2012). Effect of riodiola extra on learning and memory and ultramicrostructure of cells in sleep deprivation rats. *Progr. Anat. Sci.* 4, 337–340. doi: 10.1016/B978-0-08-034186-6.50031-1

Wang, Y., Liu, Y. G., and Chen, Z. F. (2013). Effects of salidroside on learning and memory ability of vascular dementia in mice. *Hebei. Med. J.* 16, 2416–2418. doi: 10.3969/j.issn.1002-7386.2013.16.005

Wei, J. X. (2017). *Effects of Salidroside on Behavior and its Underlying Mechanisms in PTSD Rats.* MD thesis. Available online at: http://kns.cnki.net/KCMS/detail/detail.aspx?dbcode=CMFDanddbname=CMFD201801andfilename=1017237742.nhanduid (Accessed May 10, 2018)

Wolfgang, V. (2007). Publication bias in meta-analysis: prevention, assessment and adjustments. *Psychometrika* 72, 269–271. doi: 10.1007/s11336-006-1450-y

Wu, Y. Q., Yao, W. B., Gao, X. D., and Wang, H. (2004). Effects of the extracts of *Rhodiola rosea* L. on improving the ability of learning an memory in mice. *J. Chin. Pharm. Univ.* 1, 71–74. doi: 10.3321/j.issn:1000-5048.2004.01.018

Xie, G. Q. (2003). *Experimental Study on Rhodiosin and Melatonin for Senile Dementia Senile Dementia in Rats and its Possible Mechanism.* MD thesis. Available online at: http://kns.cnki.net/KCMS/detail/detail.aspx?dbcode=CMFDanddbname=CMFD9904andfilename=2003091197.nhanduid (Accessed March 5, 2016).

Xiong, Y., and Gao, L. L. (2017). Salidroside affects spatial memory,NF-κB and COX-2 expressions in vascular dementia rats. *Chin. Arch. Tradi. Chin. Med.* 35, 402–404. doi: 10.13193/j.issn.1673-7717.2017.02.040

Yan, Z. Q., Chen, J., Xing, G. X., Huang, J. G., Hou, X. H., and Zhang, Y. (2015). Salidroside prevents cognitive impairment induced by chronic cerebral hypoperfusion in rats. *J. Int. Med. Res.* 43, 402–411. doi: 10.1177/0300060514566648

Yang, D. S., Gan, G. P., Le, H. H., Ji, G. J., Chen, S. L., and Hou, S. (2017). Effect of Salidroside on Learning and Memory Abilities and Expression of p75NTR Signal Transducers and Aβ in Hippocampus of AD Rat. *Her. Med.* 36, 141–144. doi: doi: 10.3837/j.Issn.1004-0781.2017.02.006

Yang, J., H., Wei, M., Zhang, R., Li, H., Yan, Z. Q., and Liu, S.M. (2011b). Salidroside for epilepticus-induced cognitive deficits in rats and its possible m echanism. *Progr. Modern Biomed.* 15, 2868–2871. doi: 10.13241/j.cnki.pmb.2011.15.014

Yang, J. H., Li, H., Xiu, B. H., Yan, Z. Q., and Liu, S. M. (2011a). Salidroside for Hypobaric Hypoxia—induced cognitive deficits in rats and its possible mechanism. *Progr. Modern Biomed.* 11, 2026–2029. doi: 10.13241/j.cnki.pmb.2011.11.013

Yang, N. (2017). Effect of the learning and memory ability and oxidative stress by rhodioside in diabetic model rats. *ACTA Chin. Med.* 32, 1426–1429. doi: 10.16368/j.issn.1674-8999.2017.08.376

You, D. Q., Zou, R. F., Cheng, Q., and Cheng, K. M. (2000). Studies on the Effects of Rhodiola crenulata Compound on the Grade of Learning and Memory and Antihypoxia in Mice. *Lishizhen Med. Mater. Med. Res.* 5, 392–393. doi: 10.3969/j.issn.1008-0805.2000.05.007

Yu, S., Liu, M., Gu, X., and Ding, F. (2008). Neuroprotective effects of salidroside in the PC12 cell model exposed to hypoglycemia and serum limitation. *Cell. Mol. Neurobiol.* 28, 1067–1078. doi: 10.1007/s10571-008-9284-z

Zhang, J., Zhen, Y. F., Ren, P. C. B., Song, L. G., Kong, W. N., and Shao, T. M., et al. (2013). Salidroside attenuates beta amyloid-induced cognitive deficits via modulating oxidative stress and inflammatory mediators in rat hippocampus. *Behav. Brain Res.* 1, 70–81. doi: 10.1016/j.bbr.2013.01.037

Zhang, L., Yu, H., Sun, Y., Lin, X., Chen, B., and Tan, C., et al. (2007). Protective effects of salidroside on hydrogen peroxide-induced apoptosis in SH-SY5Y human neuroblastoma cells. *Eur. J. Pharmacol.* 564, 18–25. doi: 10.1016/j.ejphar.2007.01.089

Zhang, S., Zeng, Z. F., Chu, Z. Y., and Wang, J. C. (2012). The improving effect and mechanisms of Rhodiola compound on memory-damaged mice. *Chin. J. Behav. Brain Sci.* 9, 797–799. doi: 10.3760/cma.j.issn.1674-6554.2012.09.010

Zhang, X. D., Yu, Z. Y., and Zhang, R. (2006). Progress in the chemical composition of Rhodiola. *Aerosp. Med.* 17, 61–63. doi: 10.3969/j.issn.2095-1434.2006.01.060

Zhang, X. X., Zheng, H., Ma, Z. S., Shi, L. X., and Zeng, S. L. (2012). Effects of *Rhodiola rosea* on learning and memory in rats after sleep deprivation and the dissection of its mechanism. *Chin. J. Clin. Pharm. Ther.* 6, 634–639. Available online at: http://www.wanfangdata.com.cn/details/detail.do?_type=perio&id=zglcylxyzlx201206006

Zhao, L. Y., Cheng, Y. J., and Zhang, Y. (2010). Cognitive function Effect of Salidroside on Diabetic Encephalopathy Rats. *Chin. J. Labora Diag.* 11, 1722–1724. doi: 10.3969/j.issn.1007-4287.2010.11.012

Zou, Y. Q., Cai, Z. Y., Mao, Y. F., Li, J. B., and Deng, X. M., et al. (2009). Effects of salidroside-pretreatment on neuroethology of rats after global cerebral ischemia-reperfusion. *J. Chin. Integr. Med.* 2, 130–134. doi: 10.3736/jcim20090207

5

Da-Bu-Yin-Wan Improves the Ameliorative Effect of DJ-1 on Mitochondrial Dysfunction Through Augmenting the Akt Phosphorylation in a Cellular Model of Parkinson's Disease

Yi Zhang[1†], Xiao-Gang Gong[1,2†], Hong-Mei Sun[1*], Zhen-Yu Guo[1], Jing-Hong Hu[3], Yuan-Yuan Wang[1], Wan-Di Feng[1], Lin Li[4], Ping Li[5], Zhen-Zhen Wang[6] and Nai-Hong Chen[6,7]*

[1] Department of Anatomy, School of Traditional Chinese Medicine, Beijing University of Chinese Medicine, Beijing, China, [2] College of Special Education, Beijing Union University, Beijing, China, [3] Center for Scientific Research, School of Traditional Chinese Medicine, Beijing University of Chinese Medicine, Beijing, China, [4] Key Laboratory for Neurodegenerative Diseases of Ministry of Education, Capital Medical University, Beijing, China, [5] Beijing Key Lab for Immune-Mediated Inflammatory Diseases, Institute of Clinical Medical Science, China-Japan Friendship Hospital, Beijing, China, [6] State Key Laboratory of Bioactive Substances and Functions of Natural Medicines, Neuroscience Center, Institute of Materia Medica, Chinese Academy of Medical Sciences, Peking Union Medical College, Beijing, China, [7] College of Pharmacy, Hunan University of Chinese Medicine, Changsha, China

***Correspondence:**
Yi Zhang
zy_dalian@yahoo.com;
yzhang@bucm.edu.cn
Hong-Mei Sun
hm.sun@yahoo.com

[†] These authors have contributed equally to this work

Da-Bu-Yin-Wan (DBYW) is recorded originally in China over six centuries ago, and it is used to treat Parkinson's disease (PD) clinically in recent decades. DJ-1 is a homodimeric protein linked to early-onset PD, and found in the mitochondria. In addition, DJ-1 could protect the cells by regulating gene transcription and modulating the Akt signal pathways. Therefore, in this research, we aimed to investigate the ameliorative effect of DBYW on mitochondria in the view of the DJ-1 and Akt signaling. Rat adrenal pheochromocytoma cell line PC-12 was transfected with the plasmid pcDNA3-Flag-DJ-1 (pDJ-1). Subsequently, PC-12 cells were exposed to the PD-related mitochondrial toxin (1-methyl-4-phenylpyridinium) without/with the DBYW. After transfected with the plasmid pDJ-1, the 1-methyl-4-phenylpyridinium-induced toxicity was decreased, and the DJ-1 expression in protein level was increased. DJ-1 overexpression not only increased the mitochondrial mass, but also improved the total ATP content. Moreover, Akt phosphorylation was augmented by DJ-1 overexpression. Additionally, DBYW enhanced the above effects. Conclusively, these findings indicate that DBYW promotes the ameliorative effects of DJ-1 on mitochondrial dysfunction at least through augmenting the Akt phosphorylation in 1-methyl-4-phenylpyridinium-treated PC-12 cells.

Keywords: Da-Bu-Yin-Wan, Parkinson's disease, DJ-1, Akt, mitochondrial function

INTRODUCTION

Parkinson's disease (PD) is a highly debilitating neurodegenerative disorder that induces body rigidity, tremor, bradykinesia, and postural instability (Kalia and Lang, 2015). The PD pathology is characterized by gradual loss of dopaminergic neurons in the substantia nigra (Pagonabarraga et al., 2015), the underlying mechanisms still need to be clarified even though the disease was first described 200 years ago (Przedborski, 2017). Compelling evidence from molecular studies and experimental animal models has demonstrated that mitochondrial dysfunction was associated with the pathogenesis of PD (Mattson et al., 2008). Given the critical role of mitochondria in cellular function, it is convincing that mitochondrial dysfunction has appeared as an important mechanism at the coincidence of genetic, environmental and neurotoxin threatens to PD (Dagda et al., 2009).

DJ-1, namely PARK7 (Parkinson protein 7), is a homodimeric protein highly conserved in divergent organisms and linked to early-onset PD (Bonifati et al., 2003). DJ-1 is detected in both the nucleus and cytoplasm, and found in the mitochondria (Zhang et al., 2005; Junn et al., 2009). DJ-1 could prevent the fragmentation of mitochondria (Blackinton et al., 2009), while DJ-1 mutations damage mitochondrial dynamics and lead to mitochondrial dysfunction (Wang et al., 2012). In addition, DJ-1 could protect the cells by regulating gene transcription and modulating cell signal pathways, e.g., Akt signaling (Wilson, 2011). Akt, a downstream protein of phosphoinositide 3-kinase (PI3K), is the essential mediator of neuron survival (Dudek et al., 1997). Akt exerts its neuroprotective effect on neuronal cells by phosphorylation (Franke et al., 2003), whereas Akt signaling defection has partly linked to the pathological process of PD (Burke, 2007; Levy et al., 2009). In addition, DJ-1 is important for Akt phosphorylation enhancement on oxidative stress in the models of PD (Aleyasin et al., 2010).

Da-Bu-Yin-Wan (DBYW) was originally interpreted in a traditional Chinese medicine (TCM) monograph *Dan Xi Xin Fa* authored by Dan-Xi Zhu, an outstanding TCM professionalist and physician during China Yuan Dynasty. DBYW is also recorded in the updated edition of *Pharmacopeia of People's Republic of China* issued in the year of 2015 (Chinese Pharmacopoeia Commission, 2015). In China Ming Dynasty, Yi-Kui Sun (A.D. 1522–1619) firstly defined the disease dominated by body tremor as "Tremor Disease" in his literature *Chi Shui Xuan Zhu*. He considered by TCM theory that the tremor syndrome in the aged people resulted from multiple deficiencies in the human body, e.g., low Yin essence (Zhang et al., 2006). Accordingly, DBYW was employed as a TCM intervention to treat PD clinically in recent decades (Jia et al., 2010). Our previous studies demonstrate that DBYW increases the expression of tyrosine hydroxylase (TH) in SN, induces the ultrastructure change, and raises the level of monoamine neurotransmitters in the mice model of PD (He et al., 2010; Zhang et al., 2013). In addition, DBYW lessens the DNA damage of mitochondria, and increases the mitochondrial subunit NADH dehydrogenase 1 expression (Zhang et al., 2013). Moreover, DBYW up-regulates cellular adenosine 5′-triphosphate (ATP) content in the midbrain, and decreases the expression of ATP-sensitive potassium channel subunit (Gong et al., 2014). Additionally, DBYW could reduce the mitochondrial fragmentation induced by the PD-related mitochondrial toxin (1-methyl-4-phenylpyridinium) in human derived neuroblastoma cell line (Ma et al., 2015). However, the cellular mechanisms by which DBYW exerts its protective effect on mitochondria are not totally interpreted. Therefore, in this research, we examined the possible link between DBYW and mitochondria from DJ-1 and Akt signaling in the cellular model of PD.

MATERIALS AND METHODS

Chemical Reagents and Antibodies

All reference standard chemicals were obtained from National Institutes for Food and Drug Control, China[1], including berberine hydrochloride ($C_{20}H_{18}ClNO_4$, PubChem CID: 12456, Lot No.: 111895–201504), mangiferin ($C_{19}H_{18}O_{11}$, PubChem CID: 5281647, Lot No.: 111607–201503), and phellodendrine chloride ($C_{20}H_{24}ClNO_4$, PubChem CID: 59818, Lot No.: 110713–201212). Lipofectamine 2000 and MitoTracker Green (MTG) were purchased from Invitrogen (Grand Island, NY, United States). 1-methyl-4-phenylpyridinium (MPP^+) were obtained from Sigma-Aldrich (St. Louis, MO, United States). The bicinchoninic acid kit, protease and phosphatase inhibitors, and enhanced chemiluminescence kit were bought from Applygen (Beijing, China). The used antibodies as the following: rabbit anti-DJ-1, rabbit anti-PI3K, rabbit anti-Akt, rabbit anti-Akt phosphorylation^{Thr308}, rabbit anti-Akt phosphorylation^{Ser473} were obtained from Cell Signaling (Beverly, MA, United States). Mouse anti-beta-action primary antibody and all secondary antibodies were obtained from Zhong-Shan (Beijing, China).

Preparation and Analysis for the Decoction

All components of DBYW were listed as the following (with Pharmacopoeia and local names) and described previously (Zhang et al., 2013, 2016a): Amur corktree bark (*Phellodendron chinense Cortex*; Huang-Bai) 12 g, Common anemarrhena rhizome (*Anemarrhenae Rhizoma*; Zhi-Mu) 12 g, Prepared rehmannia root (*Radix Rehmanniae Praeparata*; Shu-Di-Huang) 18 g, and Tortoise shell (*Carapax et Plastrum Testudinis*; Gui-Jia) 18 g. All components were obtained from Beijing Tong-Ren-Tang Nature Pharmacy (Beijing, China) and authenticated by the pharmacognosy professionals in the pharmacy. Briefly, the preparation method for the decoction was described previously (Chan et al., 2012). After treatment, final dose of the decoction extract was condensed to 1 g/ml (equivalent to dry weight of the component raw materials) by water bath. The extract was passed through a 0.22 μm filter (Millipore, Billerica, MA, United States), then divided and stored as the stock solution at −70°C.

Identification and quantification of the marker compounds in DBYW decoction were performed according to the method

[1] http://www.nifdc.org.cn

described in the updated *Pharmacopeia of People's Republic of China* (Chinese Pharmacopoeia Commission, 2015), with minor modifications relating to the instrument and chromatographic conditions. Briefly, the marker compounds were analyzed using high performance liquid chromatography (Agilent 1100) with the diode-array detection (HPLC-DAD, Agilent, Santa Clara, CA, United States), respectively. Chromatographic separations were carried out using a Diamonsil C18 column (250 mm × 4.6 mm, 5-μm particle size, Dikma, Beijing, China), and appropriate mixture of acetonitrile/phosphoric acid /HPLC-grade water as the mobile phase. The mobile phase was filtered through a membrane (0.45-μm pore size) and degassed by ultrasonication before use. All measurements were made at a flow-rate of 1 mL/min, and detector was set for various compounds at different wavelength according to the China Pharmacopeia, respectively. The injection volume was 1 μL with analyte concentrations of 10–100 μg/mL, respectively. Analyte concentrations were adjusted to avoid overload of the columns. The integration of the chromatograms was performed with the Clarity software (Version 2.6.3, DataApex, Prague, Czechia). Peak areas in the chromatograms of DBYW were quantitated by external standard technique using solutions of the relative reference standards as described previously (Zhang et al., 2013).

Cell Line and Culture Conditions

Rat PC-12 cells (adrenal gland, pheochromocytoma) were obtained from Institute of Materia Medica, Chinese Academy of Medical Sciences and Peking Union Medical College. PC-12 cells were grown in a culture mixture of Dulbecco's modified Eagle's medium (HyClone, Logan, UT, United States) containing 6% horse serum (Invitrogen, Grand Island, NY, United States) and 6% fetal bovine serum (Sijiqing, Hangzhou, China), supplemented with 1% streptomycin/penicillin (Gibco, Grand Island, NY, United States), in 5% CO_2 humidified chamber at 37°C. The culture procedures were in strict compliance with proper cell density for all the following experiments.

Transient Transfection and Treatments

The simplified structure of plasmid for expression of DJ-1 as described previously (Zhang et al., 2016b), pcDNA3-Flag-DJ-1 (pDJ-1), is displayed in **Figure 1**. The plasmid was validated by DNA sequencing and purified by the GoldHi plasmid kit (CoWin, Beijing, China) to remove endotoxin contamination. Cells were seeded at a density of 8 × 10^4/well 24 h prior to transfection. For each well in 6-well plate, cells were transfected with pDJ-1 by the polycationic liposome-mediated transfection method, using the optimum amount of Lipofectamine 2000. Twenty-four hours post transfection, cells were exposed to the medium containing MPP^+ (1 mM) with/without different doses of DBYW for 48 h, respectively. Experimental treatments are shown in **Table 1**.

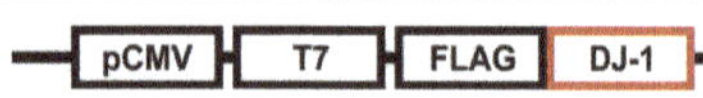

FIGURE 1 | The plasmid pcDNA3-Flag-DJ-1 simplified structure.

TABLE 1 | Experimental groups and treatments.

Groups	pDJ-1 transfection	MPP^+ (1 mM)	DBYW (μg/ml)
Control	–	–	–
Model	–	+	–
Overexpression of DJ-1	+	+	–
DBYW at low concentration	+	+	20
DBYW at medium concentration	+	+	100
DBYW at high concentration	+	+	500

DBYW, Da-Bu-Yin-Wan; MPP^+, 1-methyl-4-phenylpyridinium.

Cell Viability Determination

Cell viability was assessed by using the Cell Counting Kit-8 (CCK-8) colorimetric assay (Dojindo, Kumamoto, Japan) (Ishiyama et al., 1997). Briefly, 24 h after previous cell transfection, PC-12 cells were seeded at a density of 8 × 10^4 cells/mL in a 96-well plate and incubated for 24 h. Then various concentrations of DBYW were added with or without MPP^+ (final concentrations mentioned in **Table 1**), respectively. Cells were incubated for a further 24 h, 10 μl of CCK-8 reagent was added to each well in a 96-well plate. After 1.5 h of incubation at 37°C, the absorbance was measured at a wavelength of 450 nm using the Safire2 microplate reader (Tecan, Männedorf, Switzerland). All results were expressed as compared to the control, which was defined as the baseline (100%).

Western Blot Analysis

Cells were washed with phosphate-buffered saline solution, followed by lysis with radioimmunoprecipitation assay buffer containing protease and phosphatase inhibitors. The extract of total protein was run and separate on sodium dodecyl sulfate polyacrylamide gel electrophoresis, then transferred onto polyvinylidene difluoride membrane (Millipore, Billerica, MA, United States). Different blots were incubated overnight with primary antibodies against DJ-1 (1:1000 dilution), PI3K (1:1000), Akt (1:1000), β-action (1:2000), Phospho-Akt (Thr308) (1:500), Phospho-Akt (Ser473) (1:500), respectively; followed by horseradish peroxidase-conjugated secondary antibodies (1:2000) for 1 h. Then complexes were visualized with enhanced chemiluminescence kit. Signals on the Flims were quantified by densitometry performed with the Bio-Rad Quantity One software, Version 4.62 (Hercules, CA, United States). Beta-actin served as an internal control for DJ-1, PI3K, and Akt, respectively; whereas the total Akt as loading control for the Akt phosphorylation.

Confocal Fluorescence Microscopy

To assess the mitochondrial mass, mitochondrial labeling was carried out using a cell-permeable fluorescent dye (MTG) based on the activity of mitochondria and involves minimal manipulation (Pendergrass et al., 2004). For visualization of mitochondria, cells were primarily treated with MTG (100 nM) for 15 min. Fluorescence was detected (490 nm/516 nm) by the confocal microscope FV1000 with the software Olympus FluoView Viewer, Version 3.1.2 (Olympus, Tokyo, Japan). Digital

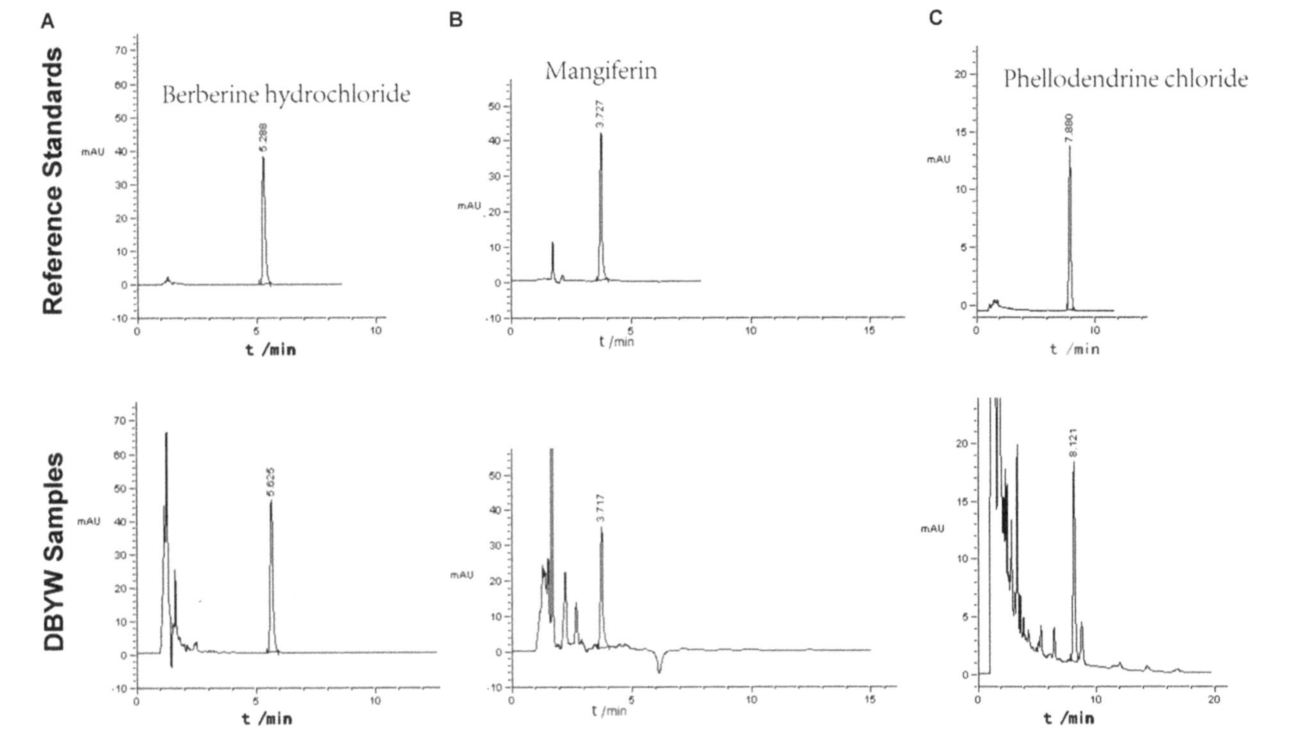

FIGURE 2 | HPLC-DAD analysis of the DBYW decoction. Three reference standards were used for identifying and quantifying the marker compounds for DBYW. Panel **(A)** for berberine hydrochloride, panel **(B)** for mangiferin, and panel **(C)** for phellodendrine chloride.

pictures were processed with the Image-Pro Plus software, Version 6.0 (Media Cybernetics, Bethesda, MD, United States).

Total ATP Content Detection

Total ATP content was detected by the Stay Brite ATP bioluminescence assay kit (BioVision, Milpitas, CA, United States) according to the manufacturer's protocol, based on the measurement for the firefly luciferase bioluminescence (Crouch et al., 1993). Briefly, PC-12 cells were subcultured in 96-well plates at a density of 8×10^4 cells/ml. Twenty-four hours after various concentrations of DBYW treatment with or without MPP^+ (1 mM), respectively. Then, 100 μl of ATP detection working solution was added to each well and incubated for 1 h at room temperature after lysed from the cells in the lysate buffer. The mixtures were centrifuged at 12,000 *g* for 30 s. The luminescence in the supernatant was recorded according to ATP-dependent luciferase activity, using the microplate reader Safire2 (Tecan, Männedorf, Switzerland). The bioluminescence value was normalized by the protein concentration that measured using bicinchoninic acid kit (Gong et al., 2014).

Statistical Analysis

All result data are expressed as the mean ± standard deviation. Statistically significant differences among means were determined by one-way analysis of variance followed by Newman–Keuls' *post hoc* tests, using the GraphPad Prism software, Version 6.02 (GraphPad, San Diego, CA, United States). A typical level at which the threshold of *P*-value is taken at 0.05.

RESULTS

Analysis of Marker Compounds of DBYW

The marker compounds in DBYW were analyzed with HPLC-DAD. By referring to reference standard chemicals, HPLC-DAD analysis indicated that the decoction contained the following marker compounds ($n = 3$): berberine hydrochloride (1.760 ± 0.033 mg/mL), mangiferin (0.501 ± 0.009 mg/mL), and phellodendrine chloride (0.476 ± 0.011 mg/mL). Chromatograms of the DBYW analyzed with relative reference standards are shown in **Figure 2**.

DBYW Affects the Cell Viability

The cells were exposed to MPP^+ (1 mM) with/without different doses of DBYW, respectively. As illustrated in **Figures 3A,B**, MPP^+ significantly inhibited the cell viability ($P < 0.05$). However, cytotoxic effect of MPP^+ was ameliorated in PC-12 cells transfected with pDJ-1. Moreover, this effect was promoted by DBYW dose-dependently ($P < 0.05$; **Figures 3A,B**).

DBYW Affects the DJ-1 Expression

To examine the effect of DBYW on the DJ-1 expression, western blot was performed. The results displayed that MPP^+ (1 mM) treatment decreased the DJ-1 expression (**Figure 4**).

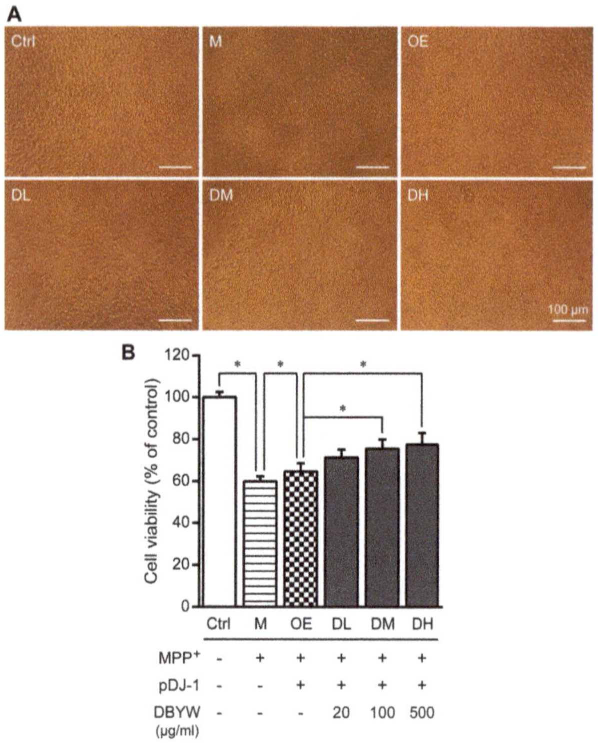

FIGURE 3 | Cell viability detection. **(A)** Representative images showed treatment with MPP^+ (1 mM) with/without DBYW in the PC-12 cells transfected with pDJ-1. **(B)** Cell viability was detected by CCK-8 assay. Ctrl, the control group; M, the MPP^+-treated group; OE, the DJ-1 overexpression group; DL/DM/DH, DBYW low/medium/high dose groups; pDJ-1, the plasmid pDJ-1 transfection group. Analysis of variance, $P < 0.05$, *post hoc* *$P < 0.05$ versus compared group.

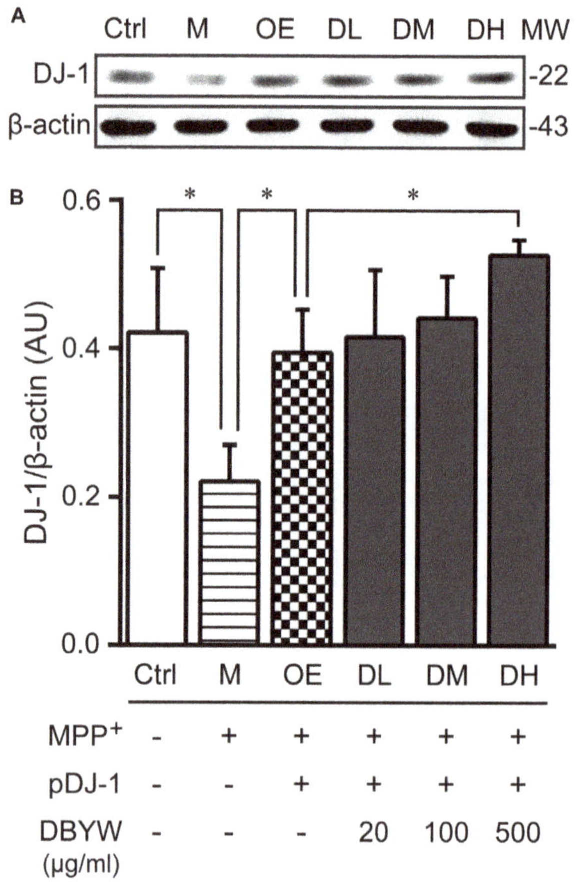

FIGURE 4 | DJ-1 expression detection. **(A)** Representative expressions for DJ-1/internal control are demonstrated. **(B)** The graph displays the analysis from three independent bolts for the expression ratio of DJ-1/beta-actin. AU, arbitrary unit; Ctrl, the control group; M, the MPP^+-treated group; MW, molecular weight (kDa); OE, the DJ-1 overexpression group; DL/DM/DH, DBYW low/medium/high dose groups; pDJ-1, the plasmid pDJ-1 transfection group. Analysis of variance, $P < 0.05$, *post hoc* *$P < 0.05$ versus compared group.

The plasmid pDJ-1 transfection inhibited the MPP^+-induced DJ-1 decreased expression in PC-12 cells. Similarly, DBYW at various concentrations attenuated the MPP^+-induced decrease of DJ-1 in PC-12 cells with pDJ-1 transfected, in comparison with only pDJ-1 transfection ($P < 0.05$; **Figure 4**). The combined results demonstrated that pDJ-1 could overexpress the protein of DJ-1, and DBYW could promote the DJ-1 expression.

DBYW Ameliorated the Mitochondrial Dysfunction

Confocal fluorescence images evidenced that treatment with MPP^+ (1 mM) has decreased mitochondrial mass significantly, while pDJ-1 transfection prevented the loss of mitochondrial mass ($P < 0.05$; **Figure 5**). Moreover, different doses of DBYW promoted the mitochondrial mass dose-dependently in the PC-12 cells transfected with pDJ-1, compared to the cells only transfected with pDJ-1 ($P < 0.05$; **Figure 5**).

Subsequently, we measured changes in the total ATP content. The data displayed that MPP^+ (1 mM) treatment significantly reduced the level of total ATP. Similarly, pDJ-1 transfection reversed the reduction in MPP^+-treated PC-12 cells. Additionally, DBYW at different doses considerably increased total ATP content in a dose-dependent manner in the PC-12 cells transfected with pDJ-1, compared to the cells only transfected with pDJ-1 ($P < 0.05$; **Figure 6**).

Effect of DBYW on the PI3K/Akt Signaling

Western blot results showed that expressions of PI3K or Akt were not affected by MPP^+ treatment or transfection with pDJ-1. Additionally, DBYW at different doses (20, 100, and 500 μg/ml) could not statistically change the expressions of PI3K or total Akt in the transfected PC-12 cells ($P > 0.05$; **Figure 7**), suggesting that DJ-1 or DBYW could not affect the PI3K and total Akt expressions in MPP^+-treated PC-12 cells.

Subsequently, threonine 308 (Thr308) and serine 473 (Ser473), two residues of Akt phosphorylation (Sarbassov et al., 2005), were investigated by western blot. MPP^+ (1 mM) treatment significantly decreased the expression of Akt

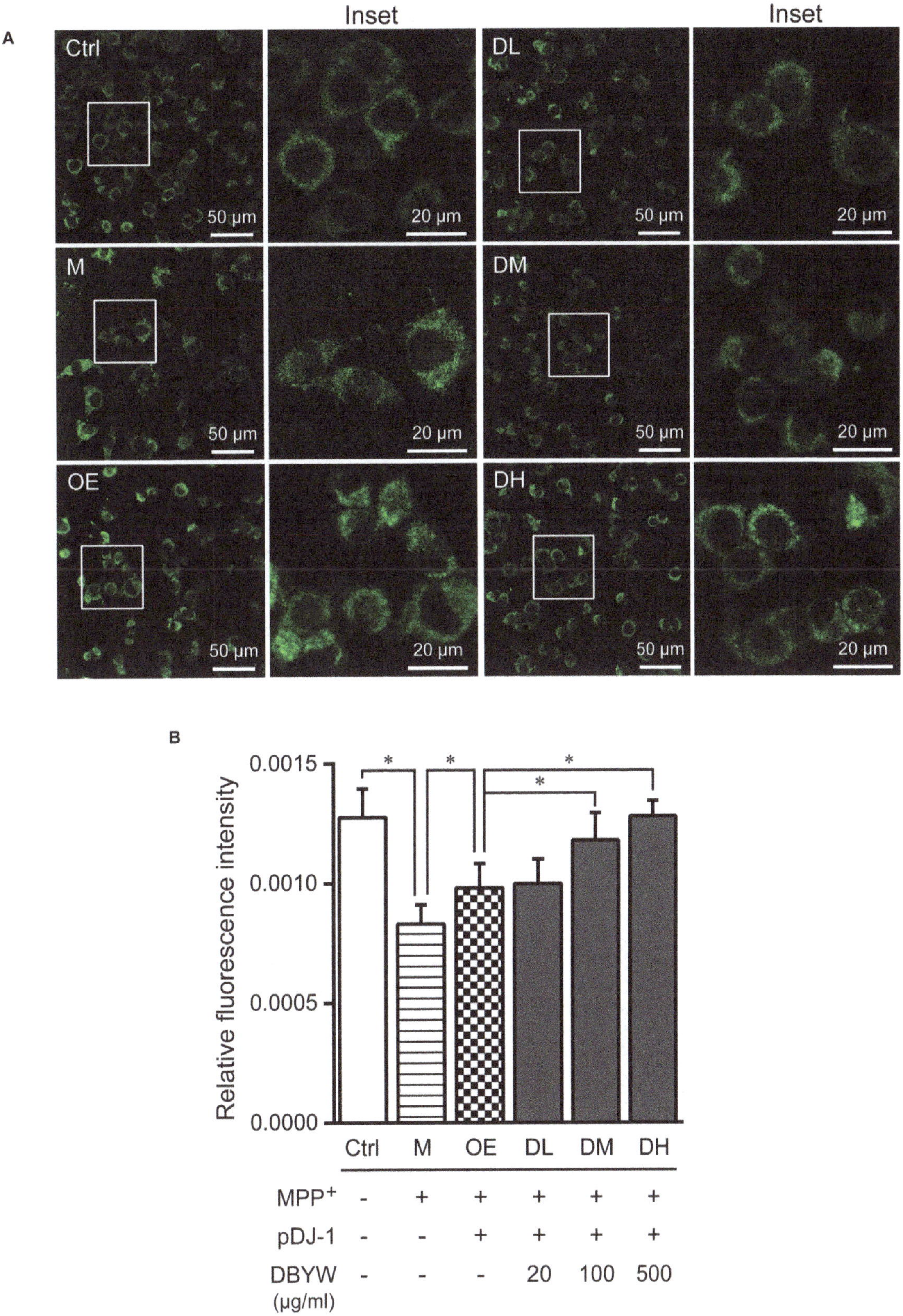

FIGURE 5 | Mitochondrial mass assessment. **(A)** Representative images taken by the confocal microscopy in the different groups. **(B)** Results are the mean ± standard deviation of ten replicates. Ctrl, the control group; M, the MPP^+-treated group; OE, the DJ-1 overexpression group; DL/DM/DH, DBYW low/medium/high dose groups; pDJ-1, the plasmid pDJ-1 transfection group. Analysis of variance, $P < 0.05$, *post hoc* $^*P < 0.05$ versus compared group.

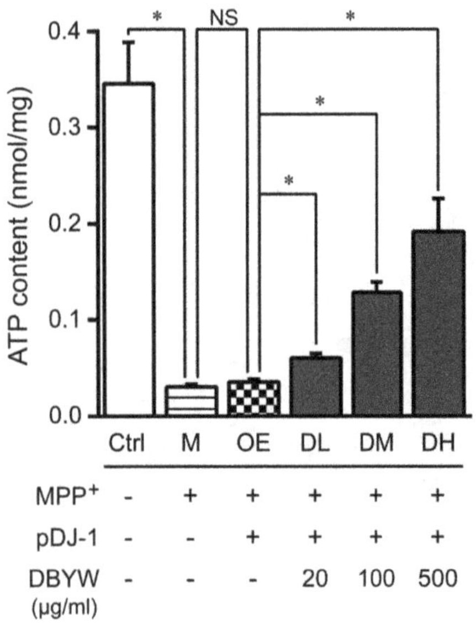

FIGURE 6 | Total ATP content detection. Ctrl, the control group; M, the MPP$^+$-treated group; OE, the DJ-1 overexpression group; DL/DM/DH, DBYW low/medium/high dose groups; pDJ-1, the plasmid pDJ-1 transfection group. Analysis of variance, P < 0.05, *post hoc* *P < 0.05 versus compared group.

phosphorylation on these two residuses, while pDJ-1 transfection reversed the decrease. Furthermore, different doses of DBYW enhanced the Akt phosphorylation on these two residues dose-dependently, respectively, in the PC-12 cells transfected with pDJ-1 (P < 0.05; **Figure 8**), compared to the cells only transfected with pDJ-1. The results displayed that DJ-1 could augment the Akt phosphorylation; and the treatment with DBYW enhanced the effects.

DISCUSSION

In our previous research, we exposed PC-12 cells to various doses of MPP$^+$ for different time periods, respectively. We found a significant loss of PC-12 cells treated with 1 mM MPP$^+$ for 48 h. Therefore, we used this condition for PC-12 cells in present research. Additionally, PC-12 cells have been widely served as a cellular model system for investigating PD (Hatanaka, 1981; Westerink and Ewing, 2008), because they have the enzymes for dopamine synthesis, metabolism and transportation (Hatanaka, 1981; Tuler et al., 1989). Our recent research demonstrated that DJ-1 could protect the mitochondria through enhancing the phosphorylation of Akt in MPP$^+$-untreated PC-12 cells (Zhang et al., 2016b).

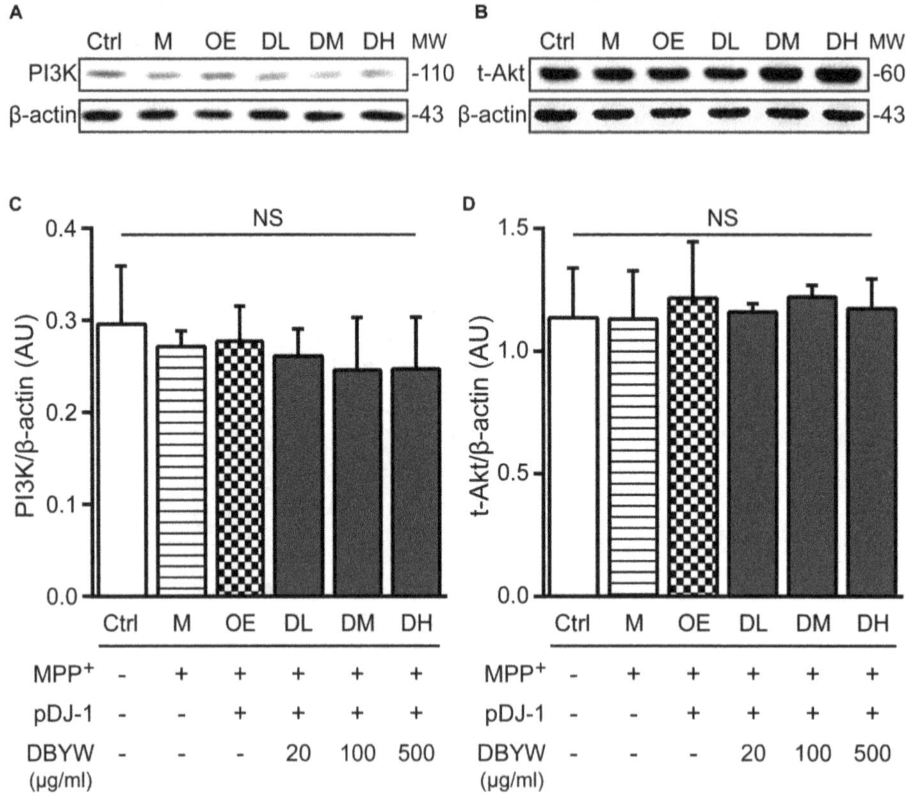

FIGURE 7 | PI3K and total Akt expressions detection. **(A,B)** Representative expressions for PI3K, total Akt, and beta-actin are demonstrated. **(C,D)** The graph shows the analysis in from three independent blots for the expression ratios of PI3K or total Akt, normalized to beta-actin. AU, arbitrary unit; Ctrl, the control group; M, the MPP$^+$-treated group; MW, molecular weight (kDa); OE, the DJ-1 overexpression group; DL/DM/DH, DBYW low/medium/high dose groups; pDJ-1, the plasmid pDJ-1 transfection group; NS, not significant statistically.

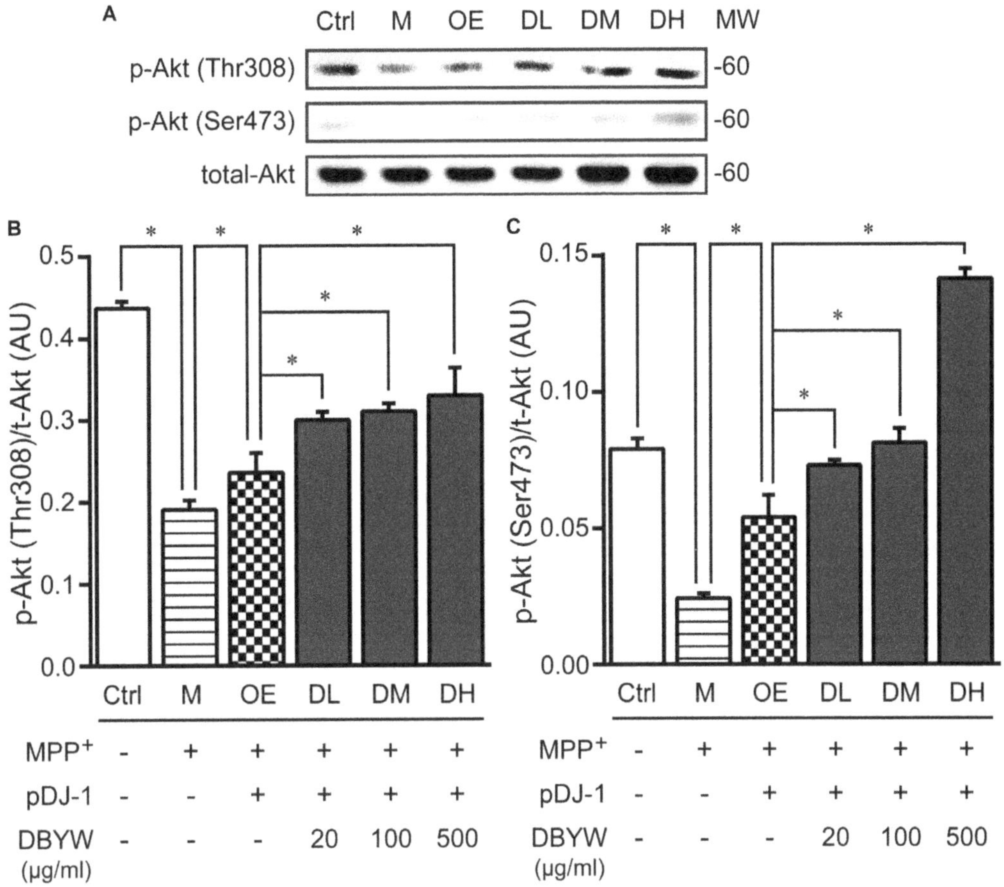

FIGURE 8 | Akt phosphorylation detection. (A) Representative expressions for p-Akt^{Thr308}, p-Akt^{Ser473}, and total Akt are demonstrated. **(B,C)** The graph demonstrates the analysis from three independent blots for the expression ratios of p-Akt^{Thr308} or p-Akt^{Ser473}, normalized to total Akt. AU, arbitrary unit; Ctrl, the control group; M, the MPP$^+$-treated group; MW, molecular weight (kDa); OE, the DJ-1 overexpression group; DL/DM/DH, DBYW low/medium/high dose groups; pDJ-1, the plasmid pDJ-1 transfection group. Analysis of variance, $P < 0.05$, *post hoc* $^*P < 0.05$ versus compared group.

Traditional Chinese medicine formulas or other natural medicines are complex mixtures of many chemical compounds that have diverse pharmacological properties (Zhang Y. et al., 2014). *Anemarrhena asphodeloides* Bge., native to China, Korea, and Mongolia (Wang et al., 2014), is one component of DBYW. Mangiferin is a natural C-glucoside xanthone commonly encountered in *Anemarrhena asphodeloides* Bge. (Vyas et al., 2012). Mangiferin also increases the superoxide dismutase activity and glutathione levels, and prevents depletion of dopamine and its metabolites (3-methoxy-4-hydroxyphenylacetic acid and homovanillic acid) in the striatum of MPTP-induced mice (Kavitha et al., 2013; Feng et al., 2014). Catalpol, an ingredient abundant in the *Radix Rehmanniae* Praeparata, exerts protective effects on PC-12 cells injured by L-glutamate and Aβ_{25-35} (Wang et al., 2008). In addition, catalpol reverses intracellular calcium level, mitochondrial membrane potential, and reactive oxygen species (ROS) accumulation in MPTP-treated mesencephalic neuron-astrocyte cultures and inhibits the activity of monoamine oxidase B in MPP$^+$-treated astrocytes (Bi et al., 2008). The antioxidant α-tocopherol (vitamin E) also significantly increases the synthesis rate and the levels of monoaminergic neurotransmitters in the hippocampus and striatum, brain regions involved in memory processing and motor coordination (Ramis et al., 2016). Additionally, the aqueous extract of *Harpagophytum procumbens* could reduce amyloid β-peptide stimulation of malondialdehyde and 3-hydroxykynurenine and blunt the decrease of dopamine, norepinephrine, and serotonin, in the cortex (Ferrante et al., 2017). Catalpol protects dopaminergic neurons against lipopolysaccharide-induced neurotoxicity dose-dependently, through reducing the release of ROS, nitric oxide, and tumor necrosis factor-α, and attenuating the expression of inducible nitric-oxide synthase in mesencephalic neuron-glia cultures (Tian et al., 2006). Moreover, catalpol could protect mitochondrial function through inhibiting ROS production and nitric oxide synthase activity, increasing activities of mitochondrial complexes and level of mitochondrial membrane potential in the cortex and hippocampus mitochondria of D-galactose injected mouse (Zhang et al., 2010). Furthermore, catalpol improves the locomotor ability dose-dependently and raises the TH neuron number in SN, the density of striatal dopamine transporter, and the protein level of striatal glial cell derived neurotrophic factor in MPTP-treated mice (Xu et al., 2010). Catalpol also attenuates chronic cerebral hypoperfusion-induced white matter lesions by promoting oligodendrocyte survival and oligodendrocyte progenitor differentiation through the Akt signaling in Wistar rats (Cai et al., 2014). Additionally, tetrahydroberberine, an alkaloid isolated from *Phellodendron chinense* Schneid., protects neurons against degeneration through blocking neuronal ATP-sensitive potassium channels in SN of rat (Wu et al., 2010). The extracted decoction of Plastrum Testudinis (Tortoise shell), another component of DBYW, could substantially reduce the rotational behavior (Li et al., 2004; Deng et al., 2008) and increase the TH-positive neurons in the compact zone of substantia nigra (Deng et al., 2008), and also increase the levels of dopamine, 3,4-dihydroxyphenylacetic acid (DOPAC), and homovanillic acid (HVA) in the striatum of the PD model rats (Li et al., 2004). In addition, treatment with the combination of Plastrum Testudinis and β-asarone could improve the behavior of PD rats and increased TH-positive neurons, while decrease α-synuclein level in the corpus striatum (Zhang S. et al., 2014). Additionally, Plastrum Testudinis is one of the main components of Gui-Ling-Pa-An Capsule (GLPAC), a TCM formula that is used in the treatment for PD clinically. A multicenter, randomized, double-blind, controlled clinical trial has demonstrated that GLPAC shows obvious effects in improving the motor syndrome and quality of life of PD patients, and also reduces the required dosage of levodopa (Zhao et al., 2009).

Akt signaling defection has partly involved in the neurodegenerative progression of Alzheimer's and Huntington's diseases (Colin et al., 2005; Griffin et al., 2005). In addition, Akt signaling has a crucial role in mediating the dopaminergic receptor (Beaulieu et al., 2007) and redistributing the dopaminergic transporters (Garcia, 2005). Moreover, some PD treatment drugs (e.g., bromocriptine and ropinirole) that targeting the dopaminergic system had demonstrated the neuroprotective effects via Akt signaling (Lim et al., 2008; Nair and Olanow, 2008). Akt activation could induce various biological responses, such as insulin metabolic function, oncogenic signal transduction, higher brain function linked to cognition (Franke, 2008). Phosphorylation is a crucial modulatory mechanism that occurs both in prokaryotic and eukaryotic organisms (Barford et al., 1998), and the significant post-translational determinant of Akt activity (Sarbassov et al., 2005). Rasagiline, a selective monoamine oxidase B inhibitor, could up-regulate the Akt phosphorylation on Ser473 in midbrain dopamine neurons in MPTP-induced mice (Sagi et al., 2007). Furthermore, both gain-of-function and loss-of-function experiments have demonstrated that DJ-1 promotes cell survival *via* Akt phosphorylation on Ser473 in *Drosophila* (Kim et al., 2005). Additionally, using the DJ-1 null mouse model of PD, reduced Akt phosphorylation on Ser473 is associated with gradual loss of neurons in SN (Aleyasin et al., 2010). Further studies *in vivo* should be performed to better understand these *in vitro* findings.

In summary, these results demonstrate that DJ-1 could ameliorate the mitochondrial dysfunction at least through medicating the Akt phosphorylation in the rat adrenal pheochromocytoma PC-12 cells treated with MPP^+. Additionally, our findings also suggest that DBYW promotes the ameliorative effect of DJ-1 in the MPP^+-treated PC-12 cells.

AUTHOR CONTRIBUTIONS

YZ and HMS conceptualized the study. YZ, XGG, ZZW, and HMS analyzed the data. YZ, XGG, ZYG, JHH, YYW, and WDF performed the experiments. YZ drafted and finalized the paper. ZZW, HMS, LL, PL, and NHC were the contributors in writing and revising the manuscript.

FUNDING

This study was supported by grants from the National Natural Science Foundation of China (Nos. 81473376, 81573773, and 81774110), Follow-Up Research Project of Beijing University of Chinese Medicine (No. 81202939), and Open Program of Key Laboratory of Neurodegenerative Diseases of Ministry of Education (Capital Medical University) (No. 2016SJBX03).

ACKNOWLEDGMENTS

We thank everyone who contributed to this manuscript.

REFERENCES

Aleyasin, H., Rousseaux, M. W., Marcogliese, P. C., Hewitt, S. J., Irrcher, I., Joselin, A. P., et al. (2010). DJ-1 protects the nigrostriatal axis from the neurotoxin MPTP by modulation of the AKT pathway. *Proc. Natl. Acad. Sci. U.S.A.* 107, 3186–3191. doi: 10.1073/pnas.0914876107

Barford, D., Das, A. K., and Egloff, M. (1998). The structure and mechanism of protein phosphatases: insights into catalysis and regulation. *Annu. Rev. Biophys. Biomol.* 27, 133–164. doi: 10.1146/annurev.biophys.27.1.133

Beaulieu, J., Gainetdinov, R. R., and Caron, M. G. (2007). The Akt-GSK-3 signaling cascade in the actions of dopamine. *Trends Pharmacol. Sci.* 28, 166–172. doi: 10.1016/j.tips.2007.02.006

Bi, J., Wang, X., Chen, L., Hao, S., An, L., Jiang, B., et al. (2008). Catalpol protects mesencephalic neurons against MPTP induced neurotoxicity via attenuation of mitochondrial dysfunction and MAO-B activity. *Toxicol. Vitro* 22, 1883–1889. doi: 10.1016/j.tiv.2008.09.007

Blackinton, J., Lakshminarasimhan, M., Thomas, K. J., Ahmad, R., Greggio, E., Raza, A. S., et al. (2009). Formation of a stabilized cysteine sulfinic acid is critical for the mitochondrial function of the Parkinsonism protein DJ-1. *J. Biol. Chem.* 284, 6476–6485. doi: 10.1074/jbc.M806599200

Bonifati, V., Rizzu, P., van Baren, M. J., Schaap, O., Breedveld, G. J., Krieger, E., et al. (2003). Mutations in the DJ-1 gene associated with autosomal recessive early-onset parkinsonism. *Science* 299, 256–259. doi: 10.1126/science.1077209

Burke, R. (2007). Inhibition of mitogen-activated protein kinase and stimulation of Akt kinase signaling pathways: two approaches with therapeutic potential in the treatment of neurodegenerative disease. *Pharmacol. Ther.* 114, 261–277. doi: 10.1016/j.pharmthera.2007.02.002

Cai, Q., Yao, Z., and Li, H. (2014). Catalpol promotes oligodendrocyte survival and oligodendrocyte progenitor differentiation via the Akt signaling pathway in rats with chronic cerebral hypoperfusion. *Brain Res.* 1560, 27–35. doi: 10.1016/j.brainres.2014.03.001

Chan, K., Shaw, D., Simmonds, M. S., Leon, C. J., Xu, Q., Lu, A., et al. (2012). Good practice in reviewing and publishing studies on herbal medicine, with special emphasis on traditional Chinese medicine and Chinese materia medica. *J. Ethnopharmacol.* 140, 469–475. doi: 10.1016/j.jep.2012.01.038

Chinese Pharmacopoeia Commission (2015). *"Da-Bu-Yin-Wan," in Pharmacopoeia of the People's Republic of China (Part 1).* Beijing: Chinese Medical Science Press, 498.

Colin, E., Régulier, E., Perrin, V., Dürr, A., Brice, A., Aebischer, P., et al. (2005). Akt is altered in an animal model of Huntington's disease and in patients. *Eur. J. Neurosci.* 21, 1478–1488. doi: 10.1111/j.1460-9568.2005.03985.x

Crouch, S. P., Kozlowski, R., Slater, K. J., and Fletcher, J. (1993). The use of ATP bioluminescence as a measure of cell proliferation and cytotoxicity. *J. Immunol. Methods* 160, 81–88. doi: 10.1016/0022-1759(93)90011-U

Dagda, R. K., Zhu, J., and Chu, C. T. (2009). Mitochondrial kinases in Parkinson's disease: converging insights from neurotoxin and genetic models. *Mitochondrion* 9, 289–298. doi: 10.1016/j.mito.2009.06.001

Deng, R. D., Li, Y. W., Chen, D. F., Li, H., Zhang, S. X., Zhao, D., et al. (2008). Protective effect of *Plastrum testudinis* on the apoptosis of dopamine neurons of rats with Parkinson's disease. *Chin. J. Neuroanat.* 3, 301–306.

Dudek, H., Datta, S. R., Franke, T. F., Birnbaum, M. J., Yao, R., Cooper, G. M., et al. (1997). Regulation of neuronal survival by the serine-threonine protein kinase Akt. *Science* 275, 661–665. doi: 10.1126/science.275.5300.661

Feng, G., Zhang, Z., Bao, Q., Zhang, Z., Zhou, L., Jiang, J., et al. (2014). Protective effect of chinonin in MPTP-induced C57BL/6 mouse model of Parkinson's disease. *Biol. Pharm. Bull.* 37, 1301–1307. doi: 10.1248/bpb.b14-00128

Ferrante, C., Recinella, L., Locatelli, M., Guglielmi, P., Secci, D., Leporini, L., et al. (2017). Protective effects induced by microwave-assisted aqueous harpagophytum extract on rat cortex synaptosomes challenged with amyloid beta-peptide. *Phytother. Res.* 31, 1257–1264. doi: 10.1002/ptr.5850

Franke, T. F. (2008). PI3K/Akt: getting it right matters. *Oncogene* 27, 6473–6488. doi: 10.1038/onc.2008.313

Franke, T. F., Hornik, C. P., Segev, L., Shostak, G. A., and Sugimoto, C. (2003). PI3K/Akt and apoptosis: size matters. *Oncogene* 22, 8983–8998. doi: 10.1038/sj.onc.1207115

Garcia, B. (2005). Akt is essential for insulin modulation of amphetamine-induced human dopamine transporter cell-surface redistribution. *Mol. Pharmacol.* 68, 102–109. doi: 10.1124/mol.104.009092

Gong, X. G., Sun, H. M., Zhang, Y., Zhang, S. J., Gao, Y. S., Feng, J., et al. (2014). Da-Bu-Yin-Wan and Qian-Zheng-San to neuroprotect the mouse model of Parkinson's disease. *Evid. Based Complement. Alternat. Med.* 2014:729195. doi: 10.1155/2014/729195

Griffin, R. J., Moloney, A., Kelliher, M., Johnston, J. A., Ravid, R., Dockery, P., et al. (2005). Activation of Akt/PKB, increased phosphorylation of Akt substrates and loss and altered distribution of Akt and PTEN are features of Alzheimer's disease pathology. *J. Neurochem.* 93, 105–117. doi: 10.1111/j.1471-4159.2004.02949.x

Hatanaka, H. (1981). Nerve growth factor-mediated stimulation of tyrosine hydroxylase activity in a clonal rat pheochromocytoma cell line. *Brain Res.* 222, 225–233. doi: 10.1016/0006-8993(81)91029-5

He, X., Sun, H. M., Wu, H. X., Xu, H., Wang, Y. Y., Gao, Y. S., et al. (2010). Neuroprotective effect of Dabuyin Pill, Qianzheng powder and combined formula on Parkinson's disease mice brain. *Liaoning J. Tradit. Chin. Med.* 37, 2098–2101.

Ishiyama, M., Miyazono, Y., Sasamoto, K., Ohkura, Y., and Ueno, K. (1997). A highly water-soluble disulfonated tetrazolium salt as a chromogenic indicator for NADH as well as cell viability. *Talanta* 44, 1299–1305. doi: 10.1016/S0039-9140(97)00017-9

Jia, Y. Q., Zhang, L. Z., Feng, L. Y., and Zhen, W. L. (2010). Overview of Chinese medicine treatment for Parkinson's disease. *Chin. J. Tradit. Med. Sci. Technol.* 17, 183–184.

Junn, E., Jang, W. H., Zhao, X., Jeong, B. S., and Mouradian, M. M. (2009). Mitochondrial localization of DJ-1 leads to enhanced neuroprotection. *J. Neurosci. Res.* 87, 123–129. doi: 10.1002/jnr.21831

Kalia, L. V., and Lang, A. E. (2015). Parkinson's disease. *Lancet* 386, 896–912. doi: 10.1016/S0140-6736(14)61393-3

Kavitha, M., Nataraj, J., Essa, M. M., Memon, M. A., and Manivasagam, T. (2013). Mangiferin attenuates MPTP induced dopaminergic neurodegeneration and improves motor impairment, redox balance and Bcl-2/Bax expression in experimental Parkinson's disease mice. *Chem. Biol. Interact.* 206, 239–247. doi: 10.1016/j.cbi.2013.09.016

Kim, R. H., Peters, M., Jang, Y., Shi, W., Pintilie, M., Fletcher, G. C., et al. (2005). DJ-1, a novel regulator of the tumor suppressor PTEN. *Cancer Cell* 7, 263–273. doi: 10.1016/j.ccr.2005.02.010

Levy, O. A., Malagelada, C., and Greene, L. A. (2009). Cell death pathways in Parkinson's disease: proximal triggers, distal effectors, and final steps. *Apoptosis* 14, 478–500. doi: 10.1007/s10495-008-0309-3

Li, Y. W., Zhou, J. H., Chen, D. F., Li, H., and Du, S. H. (2004). Effect of tortoises shell on behavior and striatum levels of dopamine in rat model of Parkinson's disease. *Anat. Res.* 26, 17–21.

Lim, J. H., Kim, K., Kim, S. W., Hwang, O., and Choi, H. J. (2008). Bromocriptine activates NQO1 via Nrf2-PI3K/Akt signaling: novel cytoprotective mechanism against oxidative damage. *Pharmacol. Res.* 57, 325–331. doi: 10.1016/j.phrs.2008.03.004

Ma, L., Sun, H. M., Gong, X. G., He, X., Gao, Y. S., Zhang, Y., et al. (2015). Protective effect of Qianzheng san plus dabuyin wan on mitochondria in SH-SY5Y cells in Parkinson's disease model induced by MPP +. *World J. Integr. Tradit. West. Med.* 10, 487–492.

Mattson, M. P., Gleichmann, M., and Cheng, A. (2008). Mitochondria in neuroplasticity and neurological disorders. *Neuron* 60, 748–766. doi: 10.1016/j.neuron.2008.10.010

Nair, V. D., and Olanow, C. W. (2008). Differential modulation of Akt/glycogen synthase kinase-3 pathway regulates apoptotic and cytoprotective signaling responses. *J. Biol. Chem.* 283, 15469–15478. doi: 10.1074/jbc.M707238200

Pagonabarraga, J., Kulisevsky, J., Strafella, A. P., and Krack, P. (2015). Apathy in Parkinson's disease: clinical features, neural substrates, diagnosis, and treatment. *Lancet Neurol.* 14, 518–531. doi: 10.1016/S1474-4422(15)00019-8

Pendergrass, W., Wolf, N., and Poot, M. (2004). Efficacy of mitotracker green and CMXrosamine to measure changes in mitochondrial membrane potentials in living cells and tissues. *Cytometry A* 61, 162–169. doi: 10.1002/cyto.a.20033

Przedborski, S. (2017). The two-century journey of Parkinson disease research. *Nat. Rev. Neurosci.* 18, 251–259. doi: 10.1038/nrn.2017.25

Ramis, M. R., Sarubbo, F., Terrasa, J. L., Moranta, D., Aparicio, S., Miralles, A., et al. (2016). Chronic alpha-tocopherol increases central monoamines synthesis and improves cognitive and motor abilities in old rats. *Rejuvenation Res.* 19, 159–171. doi: 10.1089/rej.2015.1685

Sagi, Y., Mandel, S., Amit, T., and Youdim, M. B. H. (2007). Activation of tyrosine kinase receptor signaling pathway by rasagiline facilitates neurorescue and restoration of nigrostriatal dopamine neurons in post-MPTP-induced parkinsonism. *Neurobiol. Dis.* 25, 35–44. doi: 10.1016/j.nbd.2006.07.020

Sarbassov, D. D., Guertin, D. A., Ali, S. M., and Sabatini, D. M. (2005). Phosphorylation and regulation of Akt/PKB by the rictor-mTOR complex. *Science* 307, 1098–1101. doi: 10.1126/science.1106148

Tian, Y., An, L., Jiang, L., Duan, Y., Chen, J., and Jiang, B. (2006). Catalpol protects dopaminergic neurons from LPS-induced neurotoxicity in mesencephalic neuron-glia cultures. *Life Sci.* 80, 193–199. doi: 10.1016/j.lfs.2006.09.010

Tuler, S. M., Hazen, A. A., and Bowen, J. M. (1989). Release and metabolism of dopamine in a clonal line of pheochromocytoma (PC12) cells exposed to fenthion. *Fundam. Appl. Toxicol.* 13, 484–492. doi: 10.1016/0272-0590(89)90284-4

Vyas, A., Syeda, K., Ahmad, A., Padhye, S., and Sarkar, F. H. (2012). Perspectives on medicinal properties of mangiferin. *Mini Rev. Med. Chem.* 12, 412–425. doi: 10.2174/138955712800493870

Wang, J. H., Zhu, S. H., Sun, S. M., Zhong, Y. M., and Qu, H. M. (2008). Compare of the protective effect of catalpol on PC12 cells injury induced by L-glutamate and Aβ25-35. *Chin. Prac. Med.* 3, 25–26.

Wang, X., Petrie, T. G., Liu, Y., Liu, J., Fujioka, H., and Zhu, X. (2012). Parkinson's disease-associated DJ-1 mutations impair mitochondrial dynamics and cause mitochondrial dysfunction. *J. Neurochem.* 121, 830–839. doi: 10.1111/j.1471-4159.2012.07734.x

Wang, Y., Dan, Y., Yang, D., Hu, Y., Zhang, L., Zhang, C., et al. (2014). The genus *Anemarrhena* Bunge: a review on ethnopharmacology, phytochemistry and pharmacology. *J. Ethnopharmacol.* 153, 42–60. doi: 10.1016/j.jep.2014.02.013

Westerink, R. H. S., and Ewing, A. G. (2008). The PC12 cell as model for neurosecretion. *Acta Physiol.* 192, 273–285. doi: 10.1111/j.1748-1716.2007.01805.x

Wilson, M. A. (2011). The role of cysteine oxidation in DJ-1 function and dysfunction. *Antioxid. Redox Signal.* 15, 111–122. doi: 10.1089/ars.2010.3481

Wu, C., Yang, K., Liu, Q., Wakui, M., Jin, G. Z., Zhen, X., et al. (2010). Tetrahydroberberine blocks ATP-sensitive potassium channels in dopamine neurons acutely-dissociated from rat substantia nigra pars compacta. *Neuropharmacology* 59, 567–572. doi: 10.1016/j.neuropharm.2010.08.018

Xu, G., Xiong, Z., Yong, Y., Wang, Z., Ke, Z., Xia, Z., et al. (2010). Catalpol attenuates MPTP induced neuronal degeneration of nigral-striatal dopaminergic pathway in mice through elevating glial cell derived neurotrophic factor in striatum. *Neuroscience* 167, 174–184. doi: 10.1016/j.neuroscience.2010.01.048

Zhang, L., Shimoji, M., Thomas, B., Moore, D. J., Yu, S. W., Marupudi, N. I., et al. (2005). Mitochondrial localization of the Parkinson's disease related protein DJ-1: implications for pathogenesis. *Hum. Mol. Genet.* 14, 2063–2073. doi: 10.1093/hmg/ddi211

Zhang, S., Gui, X. H., Huang, L. P., Deng, M. Z., Li, L., and Fang, Y. Q. (2014). Neuroprotective effect and mechanism of Carapax et *Plastrum testudinis* combined with β-asarone against rat model of Parkinson's disease. *Tradit. Chin. Drug Res. Clin. Pharmacol.* 25, 264–268.

Zhang, X., Liu, W., Niu, X., and An, L. (2010). Systemic administration of catalpol prevents D-galactose induced mitochondrial dysfunction in mice. *Neurosci. Lett.* 473, 224–228. doi: 10.1016/j.neulet.2010.02.054

Zhang, Y., Gong, X. G., Wang, Z. Z., Sun, H. M., Guo, Z. Y., Gai, C., et al. (2016a). Protective effects of DJ-1 medicated Akt phosphorylation on mitochondrial function are promoted by Da-Bu-Yin-Wan in 1-methyl-4-phenylpyridinium-treated human neuroblastoma SH-SY5Y cells. *J. Ethnopharmacol.* 187, 83–93. doi: 10.1016/j.jep.2016.04.029

Zhang, Y., Gong, X. G., Wang, Z. Z., Sun, H. M., Guo, Z. Y., Hu, J. H., et al. (2016b). Overexpression of DJ-1/PARK7, the Parkinson's disease-related protein, improves mitochondrial function via Akt phosphorylation on threonine 308 in dopaminergic neuron-like cells. *Eur. J. Neurosci.* 43, 1379–1388. doi: 10.1111/ejn.13216

Zhang, Y., Sun, H. M., He, X., Wang, Y. Y., Gao, Y. S., Wu, H. X., et al. (2013). Da-Bu-Yin-Wan and Qian-Zheng-San, two traditional Chinese herbal formulas, up-regulate the expression of mitochondrial subunit NADH dehydrogenase 1 synergistically in the mice model of Parkinson's disease. *J. Ethnopharmacol.* 146, 363–371. doi: 10.1016/j.jep.2013.01.005

Zhang, Y., Wang, Z. Z., Sun, H. M., Li, P., Li, Y. F., and Chen, N. H. (2014). Systematic review of traditional Chinese medicine for depression in Parkinson's disease. *Am. J. Chin. Med.* 42, 1035–1051. doi: 10.1142/S0192415X14500657

Zhang, Z. X., Dong, Z. H., and Roman, G. C. (2006). Early descriptions of Parkinson disease in ancient China. *Arch. Neurol.* 63, 782–784. doi: 10.1001/archneur.63.5.782

Zhao, G. H., Meng, Q. G., Yu, X. D., Bai, J. Y., Luo, X. D., Yuan, C. X., et al. (2009). Gui-Ling-Pa-An Capsule in the treatment of Parkinson's disease: a multicenter double-blind randomized controlled trial. *Chin. J. Integr. Tradit. West. Med.* 29, 590–594.

6

Anti-Parkinson Potential of Silymarin: Mechanistic Insight and Therapeutic Standing

Hammad Ullah[†] and Haroon Khan[*†]

Department of Pharmacy, Abdul Wali Khan University Mardan, Mardan, Pakistan

***Correspondence:**
Haroon Khan
hkdr2006@gmail.com
[†] These authors have contributed equally to this work.

Parkinson's disease (PD) involves aggregation of α-synuclein and progressive loss of dopaminergic neurons. Pathogenesis of PD may also be related to one's genetic background. PD is most common among geriatric population and approximately 1–2% of population suffers over age 65 years. Currently no successful therapies are in practice for the management of PD and available therapies tend to decrease the symptoms of PD only. Furthermore, these are associated with diverse range of adverse effects profile. The neuroprotective effects of polyphenols are widely studied and documented. Among phytochemicals, silymarin is one of the most widely used flavonoids because of its extensive therapeutic properties and has been indicated in pathological conditions of prostate, CNS, lungs, skin, liver, and pancreas. Silymarin is a mixture of flavonolignans (silybin, isosilybin, and silychristin), small amount of flavonoids (taxifolin), fatty acids, and other polyphenolic compounds extracted from the dried fruit of *Silybum marianum* and is clinically used for hepatoprotective effects since ancient times. Neuroprotective effects of silymarin have been studied in various models of neurological disorders such as Alzheimer's disease, PD, and cerebral ischemia. The aim of the present study is to provide a comprehensive review of the recent literature exploring the effects of silymarin administration on the progression of PD. Reducing oxidative stress, inflammatory cytokines, altering cellular apoptosis machinery, and estrogen receptor machinery are mechanisms that are responsible for neuroprotection by silymarin, as discussed in this review. Additionally, because of poor aqueous solubility, the bioavailability of silymarin is low and only 23–47% of silymarin reaches systemic circulation after oral administration. Our primary focus is on the chemical basis of the pharmacology of silymarin in the treatment of PD and its mechanisms and possible therapeutic/clinical status while addressing the bioavailability limitation.

Keywords: silymarin, neuroprotective effects, anti-Parkinson's activity, mechanistic insights, drug of future

INTRODUCTION

Parkinson's disease is the most common neurodegenerative movement disorder characterized by progressive loss of dopaminergic neurons in substantia nigra pars compacta (SNpc) along with widespread intracellular aggregates of the protein α-synuclein (Thome et al., 2016; Pinto et al., 2018). Twenty genetic variants have been identified by human genetic studies, which are linked to PD pathogenesis (Pan et al., 2017). Currently monogenetic PD accounts for 3–5% of total cases of PD (Ben-David and Tu, 2015). PARK genes are most commonly linked to pathogenesis of PD and the inheritance patterns may be autosomal dominant such as in case of PARK 1, 3, 5, and 8 or autosomal recessive as in case of PARK 2, 6, and 7 (Hamza et al., 2010). The basic features of PD include tremors at rest, rigidity, bradykinesia, gait, and balance dysfunction (Patel et al., 2014). It has been observed that PD is found in all ethnic groups but geographical differences exist is prevalence of disease. Approximately 1–2% of the population suffers from PD over the age of 65 years and this figure increases to 3–5% in people of 85 years and older (De Lau and Breteler, 2006; Alves et al., 2008). The incidence rate of PD is 8–18 per 100,000 person-years. The rate of incidence is lower in Asian countries than in western countries (Tan, 2013; Lee and Gilbert, 2016). It is also documented that prevalence of PD will be almost double by 2030 and the burden of disease will also shift from developed western countries to developing eastern nations (Dorsey et al., 2007).

Although no successful therapies are currently available that can modify the disease. However, dopaminergic medications are the mainstay of treatment for symptomatic relief of motor symptoms (AlDakheel et al., 2014; Rizek et al., 2016). The available medications that are currently in practice for management of PD include levodopa, dopamine agonists (ropinirole, bromocriptine, cabergoline), MAOIs (selegiline), amantadine, anticholinergics (trihexyphenidyl), carbidopa, and entacapone (Nakaoka et al., 2014; Pagano et al., 2015). Levodopa is the most efficacious to control motor symptoms of the disease and is drug of choice to initiate first in course of treatment (Connolly and Lang, 2014). Other medications indicated for control of non-motor symptoms are clozapine and quetiapine for psychotic symptoms, SSRIs, TCAs, and SNRIs for depression, rivastigmine for dementia, BZs and non-BZ hypnotics for insomnia, and fiber-rich diet for constipation (Todorova et al., 2014). There are certain limitations to the use of anti-Parkinson's medications especially to efficacious classes of drugs. Dopaminergic medications including levodopa are most commonly associated with psychosis, motor complications, and impulsive compulsive disorder (Rascol et al., 2003; Weiss and Marsh, 2012). Most of the patients with PD develop motor complications and dyskinesia within 5–10 years of levodopa treatment (Băjenaru et al., 2016).

Polyphenols are most abundant antioxidant phytochemicals present in human diet. They are secondary metabolites present in foods and beverages of plant origin including fruits, vegetables, cereals, herbs, spices, legumes, nuts, olives, chocolate, tea, coffee, and red wine (Fantini et al., 2015). Polyphenols possess antimicrobial, anti-inflammatory, antiviral, anticancer, and immunomodulatory activities (Marzocchella et al., 2011; Benvenuto et al., 2013). Polyphenols could be divided in different classes depending on chemical skeleton of compound including phenolic acids, flavonoids, stilbenes, and lignans (Li et al., 2014; Kim et al., 2016). Polyphenols are capable of crossing blood–brain barrier and control neuronal disease pathogenesis at molecular and symptomatic level (Bhullar and Rupasinghe, 2013). The neuroprotective effects of polyphenols/natural compounds have been documented in various neurological disorders (Ayaz et al., 2015, 2017a,b; Ahmad et al., 2016; Patel et al., 2017; Rauf et al., 2017a,b; Farooq et al., 2018; Khan et al., 2018) including cerebral ischemia, brain edema, PD, amyotrophic lateral sclerosis, brain tumors, and cognitive impairments (Jagla and Pechanova, 2015). Their neuroprotective activities are attributed to their antioxidant potential, anti-inflammatory actions, and alteration of signaling pathways (Basli et al., 2012; Moosavi et al., 2016). While managing neurodegenerative, novel therapeutic strategies support the application on antioxidant polyphenols as monotherapy or antioxidant cocktail formulation (Vecchia et al., 2015).

Silymarin is the polyphenolic flavonoid extracted from dried fruit of *Silybum marianum* and is most commonly used for hepatoprotective activities since ancient times (Wang et al., 2015; AbouZid et al., 2016). Among phytochemicals it is one of the most widely used flavonoid because of its extensive therapeutic properties (Mady et al., 2016). Silymarin has been indicated in pathological conditions of various origins such as prostate, lungs, CNS, pancreas, and skin. It is considered safe at therapeutic doses but improper administration of dosages may lead to cause adverse drug reactions (ADRs) where gastrointestinal effects are more common among them (Karimi et al., 2011). Neuroprotective effects of silymarin have been studied in various models of neurological disorders such as Alzheimer's disease, PD, and cerebral ischemia. Reducing oxidative stress, inflammatory cytokines, altering cellular apoptosis machinery, and estrogen receptor machinery are mechanisms that are responsible for neuroprotection by silymarin (Borah et al., 2013). Additionally because of poor aqueous solubility the bioavailability of silymarin is low and only 23–47% of silymarin reaches systemic circulation after oral administration (Yang et al., 2013). The aim of the present study is to provide comprehensive review of the recent literature exploring the effects of silymarin administration on progression of PD. Our primary focus is on the chemical basis of pharmacology of silymarin and its anti-Parkinson's mechanisms.

CHEMISTRY

Silymarin is a mixture containing isomer flavonolignans (silybin, isosilybin, and silychristin), small number of flavonoids (taxifolin), fatty acids, and other polyphenolic compounds. It is a lipophilic agent extracted from seeds of *S. marianum*. Silybin comprises 50–70% of silymarin having greatest degree of biological activity (Ghosh et al., 2010; El-Elimat et al., 2014). Seeds of *S. marianum* also contain other flavonolignans including isosilybin, dehydrosilybin, desoxysilychristin, desoxysilydianin, silandrin, silybinome, silyhermin, and neosilyhermin (Karkanis et al., 2011). Flavonolignans present in the mixture of silymarin contain flavonoid moiety links to a molecule of lignin moiety (coniferyl alcohol) (Crocenzi and Roma, 2006). The molecular formula of flavonolignan skeleton is $C_{25}H_{22}O_{10}$ and molecular weight is 482. Pelter and Hansel were first who established the structure of silybin in 1975 (Lee and Liu, 2003). It has been documented that silybin is a mixture of diastereoisomers namely silybin A and silybin B. Silybin also known as silibinin contains 1,4-dioxane ring in addition to flavonoid moiety and

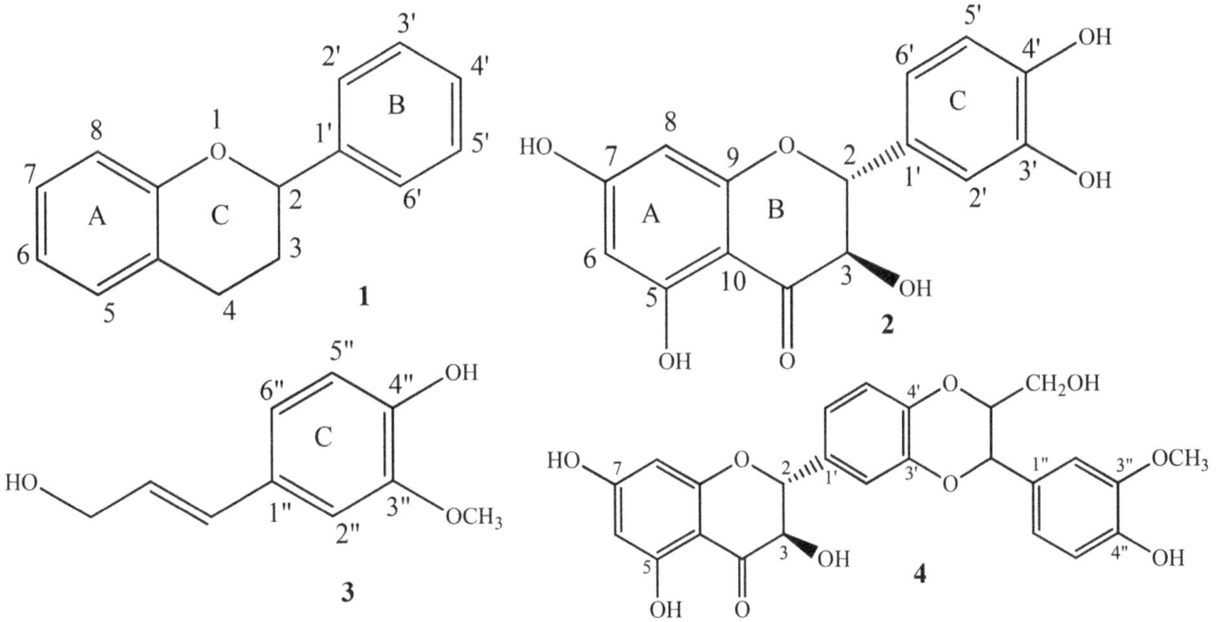

Chemical basis of Silymarin: **(1)** Basic flavonoid, **(2)** Taxifolin, **(3)** Coniferyl alcohol, **(4)** Silybin

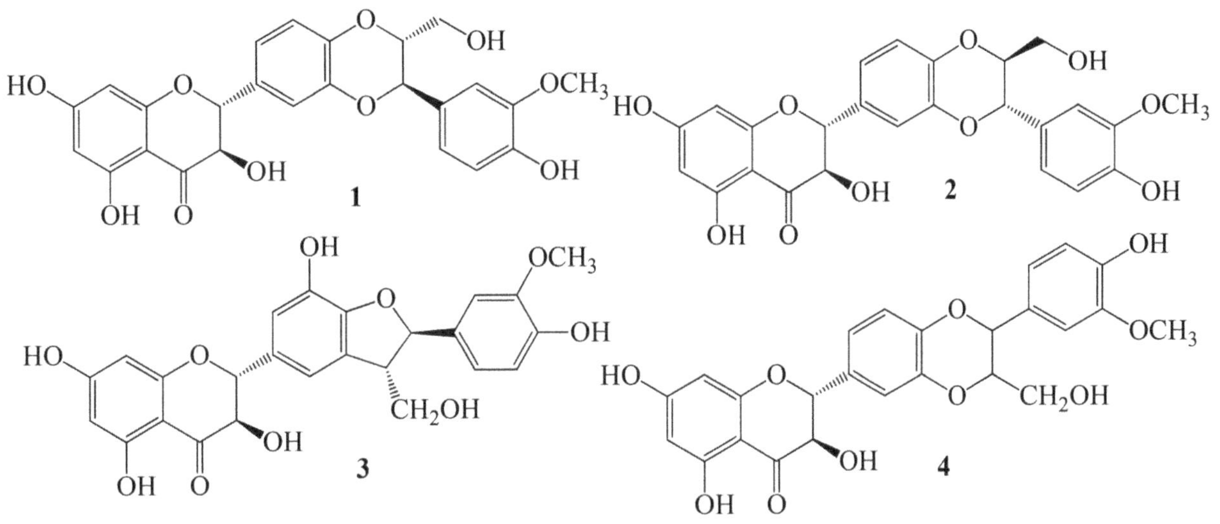

FIGURE 1 | Structures of silymarin compounds: 1, silybin A; 2, silybin B; 3, silychristin; and 4, isosilybin.

is a most active anti-hepatotoxic agent. It has been reported that the presence of 2,3-double bond in the C-ring of flavonoid structure results in increasing antioxidant activity of silybin (Ahmed et al., 2003; Ramasamy and Agarwal, 2008; Khan et al., 2011).

SOURCES

Silymarin (**Figure 1**) is a pharmacologically active phytochemical extracted from seeds and fruits of *S. marianum*, commonly known as milk thistle (Wagoner et al., 2010; Wang et al., 2015). *S. marianum* is an annual or a biennial plant and is a member of plant family Asteraceae (**Table 1**). The genus *Silybum* contains two species that are *S. marianum* and *Silybum eburneum*. Geographically this plant distributes around the globe. It is cultivated in Mediterranean region, Sinai, Afghanistan, and has been neutralized in other parts of the world (Karkanis et al., 2011; AbouZid et al., 2016). It has been used from ancient times where Theophrastus (4th century B.C.) was probably first to describe it under the name Pternix. The initial use of *S. marianum* was reported by Dioscorides for treatment of serpent bites. In 1898, the use of herb to relieve obstructions of the liver was documented by British herbalist Culpepper (Post-White

TABLE 1 | Components of silymarin mixture.

Botanical source	Local name	Constituents	Quantity (%)	Reference
Silybum marianum	Milk thistle	Silybin A	16	(Davis-Searles et al., 2005; Ross, 2008; Polyak et al., 2013)
		Silybin B	24	
		Isosilybin A	6	
		Isosilybin B	4	
		Silydianin	16	
		Silychristin	12	
		Isosilychristin	2	
		Taxifolin	2	

et al., 2007; Karkanis et al., 2011). Today, it is one of the most commonly used botanical supplement in the world. As reported in 2012, it ranked sixth in total US botanical supplement sales (Kawaguchi-Suzuki et al., 2014).

PATHOPHYSIOLOGY OF PARKINSON'S DISEASE

The neuropathological mechanisms (**Figure 2**) responsible for pathogenesis of PD include protein misfolding, disrupted protein handling, mitochondrial dysfunction, oxidative stress, impaired calcium handling, and neuroinflammation (Brundin and Melki, 2017). The substantia nigra (SN) and ventral tegmental area (VTA) are major dopaminergic nuclei located in mid-brain playing most important functions of brain. The progressive loss of dopaminergic neurons in SN pars compacta and dopaminergic denervation in forebrain areas is the main characteristic of motor symptoms of PD (Politis, 2014; Jovanovic et al., 2018). There is also non-dopaminergic neuronal loss contributing to non-motor symptoms of PD. These neurons include monoaminergic cells in the locus coeruleus and raphe nuclei, cholinergic cells in the nucleus basalis of Meynert, pedunculopontine tegmental nucleus, and hypocretin cells in the hypothalamus. Loss of cholinergic cells, pedunculopontine tegmental nucleus, and hypocretin cells are associated with cognitive dysfunction, gait problems, and sleep disorders, respectively, as seen in PD. It has been reported that the presence of 140 amino acid containing proteinaceous α-synuclein-rich inclusions called as Lewy bodies exclusively in neurons is closely related with neuronal loss in PD (Leverenz et al., 2009; Jowaed et al., 2010; Obeso et al., 2010; Surmeier et al., 2017).

Several factors either from genetic background or environmental factors play a crucial role in cellular α-synuclein misfolding. Mitochondrial dysfunction, oxidative stress, failure of liposomal autophagy, ubiquitin proteasome system, and neuroinflammation are factors responsible for α-synuclein misfolding and cell-to-cell transfer of pathogenic α-synuclein assemblies (Brundin and Melki, 2017). α-Synuclein pathology is a neurotoxic process in which the formation of oligomers occurs from soluble α-synuclein monomers, which then combines to form large insoluble α-synuclein fibrils (Kim and Lee, 2008; Melki, 2015). Liposomal autophagy and ubiquitin proteasome are both responsible for α-synuclein degradation and thus impairment of these degradation systems can contribute to α-synuclein accumulation (Xilouri et al., 2013; Kaushik and Cuervo, 2015). Like other neurodegenerative disorders, formation of reactive oxygen species (ROS) is a key mechanism in pathogenesis of PD causing degeneration of dopaminergic neurons. Metabolism of dopamine, mitochondrial dysfunction neuroinflammation, high level of iron and calcium in SN pars compacta, and aging all are contributing factors in the generation of ROS. At mitochondrial level, the electron transport chain is the major contributor in causing oxidative stress. Other sources of ROS formation are monoamine oxidase (MAO), NADPH oxidase, and other flavo-enzymes along with nitric oxide (NO). Lipid peroxidation also occurs under oxidative stress as brain contains high concentration of polyunsaturated fatty acids. Mutations in α-synuclein, parkin, PINK1, DJ-1, and LRRK2 are related to mitochondria and thus studies linked these mutations with oxidative stress (Dias et al., 2013; Yan et al., 2013).

Neuroinflammation may not be an initial trigger, but it is one of the most essential factor in pathogenesis of PD. As documented, catecholaminergic and dopaminergic neurons express MHC-I proteins which can expose them to cytotoxic T-cell-mediated death in the presence of antigens. Activation of complement system on Lewy bodies pre-exposes neurons to inflammatory processes (Loeffler et al., 2006; Poewe et al., 2017). Glial cells activation in SN pars compacta has been reported concurrently with an increased expression of pro-inflammatory mediators. CCAAT/enhancer binding protein ß (C/EBPß) is a transcription factor whose role in pathogenesis of PD has been reported. It regulates the expression of genes involved in inflammatory processes and brain injury (Morales-Garcia et al., 2017). Studies suggest important role of cyclooxygenase-2 (COX-2) enzyme in secondary activation of microglia, in the progression of the inflammatory response, and in the progressive loss of dopaminergic neurons (Vijitruth et al., 2006).

NEUROPROTECTIVE POTENTIAL OF SILYMARIN

Silymarin is a polyphenolic flavonoid with strong antioxidant activities and is in clinical practice for management of hepatic disorders. Free radicals scavenging, elevating cellular glutathione level, and improving activity of superoxide dismutase are key mechanisms attributed to antioxidant activities of silymarin. Through inhibition of oxidative stress, silymarin possesses neuroprotective effects and it can be used in the management of neurodegenerative disorders including Alzheimer's disease, PD stroke, and traumatic brain injury (Kittur et al., 2002; Chtourou et al., 2010; Muley et al., 2012; Pandima Devi et al., 2017). It has been reported that silymarin inhibits the activation of microglia as well as production of inflammatory mediators such as tumor necroses factor-alpha (TNF-α) and NO, as a result reducing damage to dopaminergic neurons (Křen and Walterova, 2005; Kaur et al., 2011). As reported, silymarin maintained striatal dopamine levels by diminishing apoptosis in the SN and preserving dopaminergic neurons. Studies linked these effects

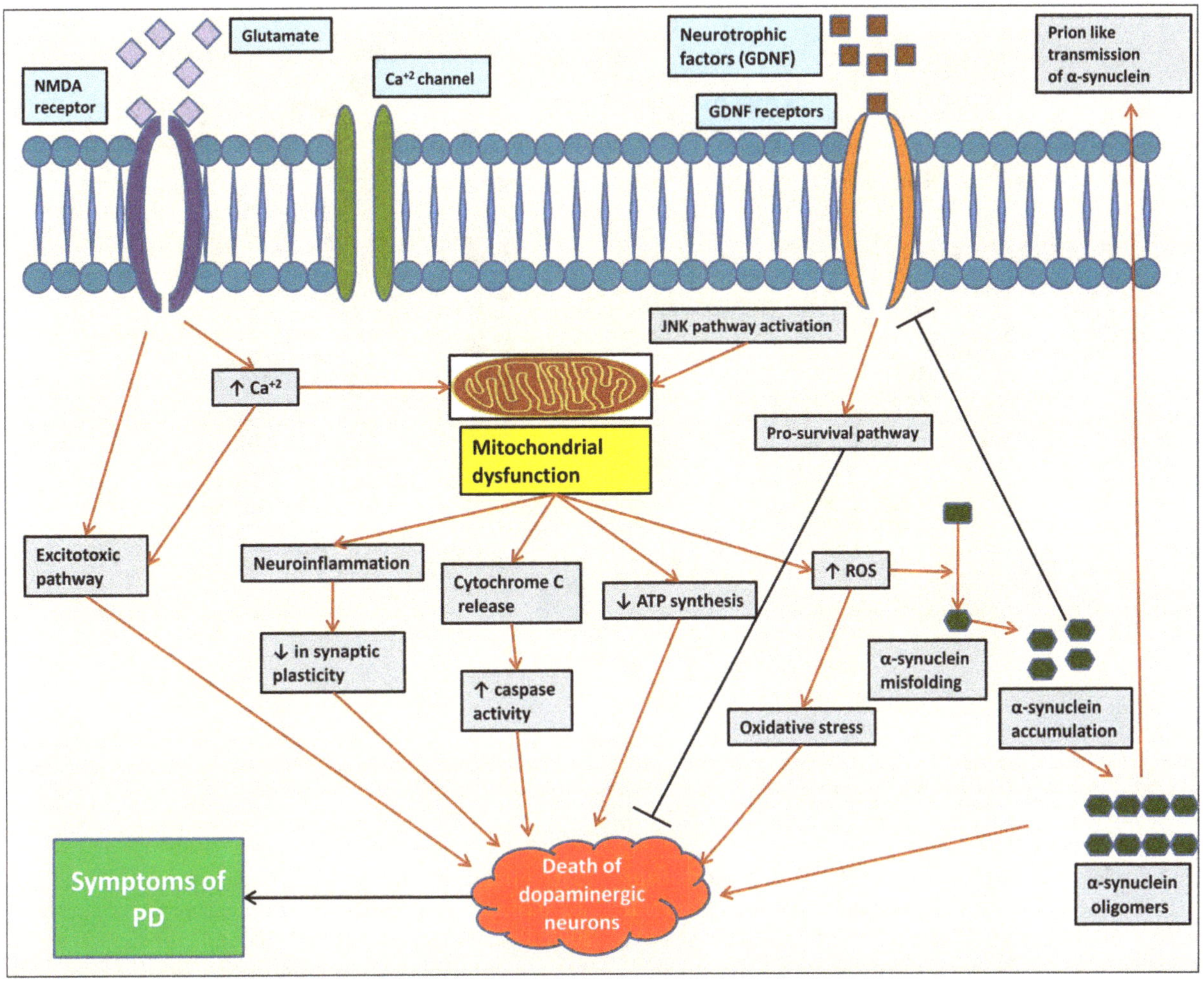

FIGURE 2 | Pathogenesis of Parkinson's disease at molecular level, showing different complex mechanistic singling pathway/events.

with antioxidant and anti-inflammatory potential of silymarin (Abushouk et al., 2017). It has been also documented from some studies that silymarin reduces level of α-synuclein protein and increasing dopamine level (Srivastava et al., 2017).

MOLECULAR MECHANISMS OF SILYMARIN

Different researchers have extensively investigated the molecular mechanisms of silymarin in various experimental models of neurological and PD (**Figure 3**).

Antioxidant Potential

Silymarin has already been reported to protect neurons against oxidative stress and nitrosative stress by elevating both enzymatic and non-enzymatic antioxidant markers. It is capable of inhibiting the formation of oxygen and peroxyl radicals along with the protein oxidation products (Galhardi et al., 2009; Borah et al., 2013). Silybin in the mixture of silymarin is mainly responsible for its antioxidant activities. However, it has been documented that a mixture of silymarin components showed higher antioxidant activities because of synergistic effects (Nabavi et al., 2012; Pérez-H et al., 2014; Pérez-Hernández et al., 2016). Silymarin treatment can reduce levels of LDH, NO, and ROS as well as oxidants/antioxidants balance (Chtourou et al., 2011). It results in elevation of glutathione levels by increasing transcriptional and translational activities of proteins used to synthesize glutathione, decreased degradation of glutathione, increased reduction of glutathione disulfide, and by increasing transport of precursors (Johnson et al., 2012). Silymarin also down regulates the expression of CYP 2E1 which induces free radical generation by mixed function oxidase activity and thus reduces oxidative stress (Singhal et al., 2011). Furthermore, it maintains mitochondrial integrity and function and inhibits mitochondrial apoptotic pathway (Fernández-Moriano et al., 2015).

Anti-inflammatory Activities

As stated earlier in this review that neuroinflammation is a consequence or a cause of nigral cell loss and thus plays one of the

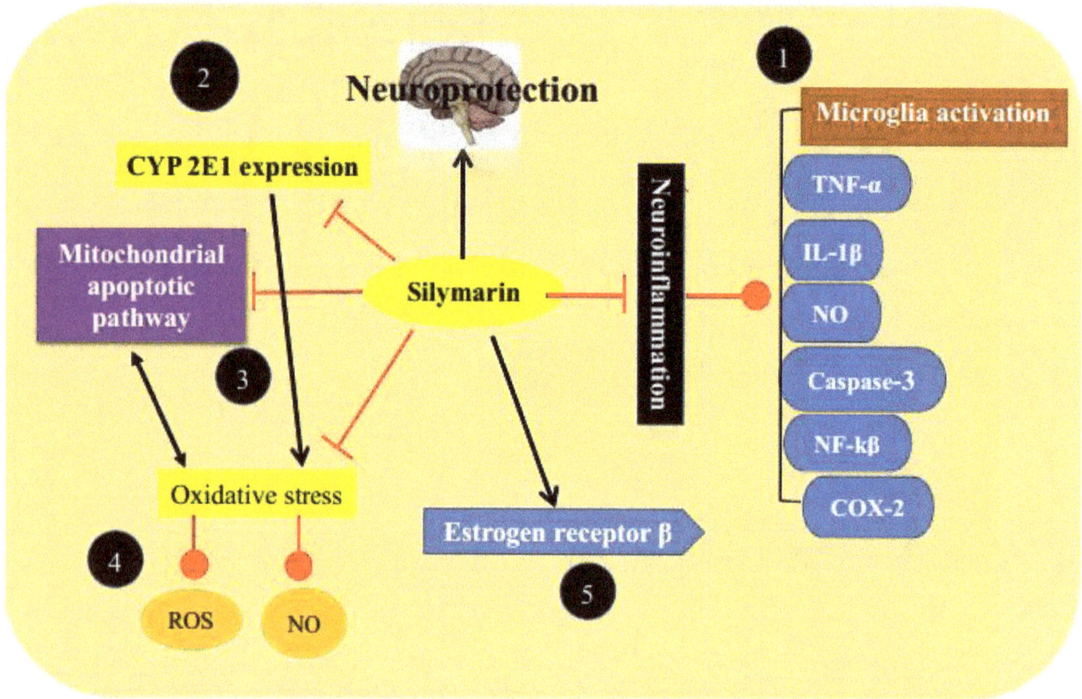

FIGURE 3 | Anti-Parkinson's targets of silymarin. (1) By acting through inhibition of neuroinflammation, (2) inhibition of CYP 2E1 expression leads to free radical formation, (3) inhibition of mitochondrial apoptotic pathway, (4) prevention of oxidative stress, and (5) modulation of estrogen receptors.

most crucial roles in pathophysiology of PD. Beside antioxidant properties silymarin also inhibits neuroinflammation by several mechanisms (Tansey and Goldberg, 2010; Machado et al., 2011). Silymarin exerts its anti-inflammatory activities mainly by inhibiting microglia activation. It reduces the production of inflammatory mediators such as TNF-α, IL-1β, and NO, and protects dopaminergic neurons against degeneration (Wang et al., 2002; Stojkovska et al., 2015). It has been documented that silymarin inhibits the production of inducible NO synthase in a dose-dependent manner. No production in neuroglial cells surrounding neurons has been correlated with neurotoxicity and pathogenesis of neurodegenerative disorders. Silymarin inhibits NO production at <300 ppm (Gazak et al., 2007; Matés et al., 2009). It decreases striatal levels of caspase-3, NF-kβ, and down regulates COX-2 reflecting its anti-apoptotic and anti-inflammatory activities (Haddadi et al., 2014; Olson and Gendelman, 2016). Activated caspase-3 is responsible for apoptosis of dopaminergic neurons and thus its reduction can protects against apoptosis (Yamada et al., 2010). It inhibits the activation of NF-κB by decreasing phosphorylation of p65 subunit which is responsible for strong transcription activating potential of NF-κB (Gu et al., 2007; Lee et al., 2014).

Anti-Parkinson's Potential: *In Vitro* Studies

Neuroprotective actions of silymarin have been reported using several *in vitro* models of PD. *In vitro* studies reported that antioxidant and anti-inflammatory activities of silymarin are basically responsible for its neuroprotection (Matkowski, 2008; Ramasamy and Agarwal, 2008). Lipopolysaccharide (LPS) is most widely used as neurotoxic agent *in vitro* models of PD. It protects dopaminergic neurons from LPS-induced neurotoxicity by inhibiting activation of microglia reflecting its anti-inflammatory actions (Kittur et al., 2002; Hald and Lotharius, 2005; Lee et al., 2014). It has been documented from *in vitro* studies that silymarin also reduces superoxide and TNF-α production while inhibiting inducible NO synthase (Wang et al., 2002). NF-κB pathway plays an important role in pathogenesis of inflammation by regulating pro-inflammatory cytokine production, leukocyte recruitment, or cell survival (Lawrence, 2009). Silymarin regulates NF-κB 100 times better than aspirin. Several kinases regulate NF-κB that belong to mitogen-activated protein kinase (MAPK) family and C-Jun N-terminal kinase (JNK). Silymarin inhibits these kinases without posing any threat to the cell (Kidd, 2009; Lawrence, 2009).

Anti-Parkinson's Potential: *In Vivo* Studies

The potential of silymarin in management on PD has been reported from several *in vivo* studies. *In vivo* models of PD show that activation of caspases in microglia leads to initiation of inflammatory cascade results in degeneration of dopaminergic neurons (Antonietta Panaro and Cianciulli, 2012). LPS exposure results in overproduction and over expression of cytokines and chemokines including IL-8, IL-1β, TNF-α, and playing a significant role in the pathogenesis of PD (Tentillier et al., 2016). *In vivo* models also suggest that MPTP treatment results in over expression of pro-inflammatory cytokine receptors (Lofrumento et al., 2011). Silymarin by diminishing apoptosis in the SN preserve dopaminergic neurons and thus maintain striatal dopaminergic levels (Pérez-H et al., 2014). It has been reported that silymarin normalizes gene expression of up-regulated NF-κB1 and caspase-9 (Raza et al., 2011; Singhal et al., 2013). However, studies also suggest that silymarin induces many features of apoptosis in *Candida albicans* such as disruption of calcium homeostasis, loss of MMP, DNA fragmentation, and caspase activation. It needs further research whether these effects have a link with neurological actions of silymarin (Lee and Lee, 2018). The binding affinity of silymarin for estrogen receptor β in CNS regions has also been reported. Estrogen attenuates toxin-induced neurotoxicity, prevents lipid peroxidation, acting synergistically with antioxidants such as glutathione (Singh et al., 2006; Baluchnejadmojarad et al., 2010).

Safety Profile of Silymarin

Being a phytochemical silymarin generally possesses favorable safety profile, although allergic reactions including anaphylactic reactions have been reported (Geier et al., 1990). Other ADRs include mild laxative effects, nausea, epigastric discomfort, arthralgia, pruritus, urticaria, and headache (Mayer et al., 2005). Silymarin also leads to inhibition of cytochrome P450 system and thus affecting the clearance of other drugs including chemotherapeutic agents (Venkataramanan et al., 2000). However, no interaction found with cisplatin, doxorubicin, vincristine, and L-asparaginase in pre-clinical studies at concentrations used. These effects may be dose related require further study at higher doses (Post-White et al., 2007).

Low Solubility of Silymarin

Low solubility of silymarin has been documented, i.e., 0.04 mg/ml and this is one of the basic reason of low oral bioavailability of silymarin from GIT. Studies also reflect that, however, silymarin has low aqueous solubility, it possess no lipophilic properties (Woo et al., 2007). Several strategies have been investigated that can improve the solubility and bioavailability of Silymarin including self-microemulsifying drug delivery systems (SMEDDS), solid dispersions, porous silica nanoparticles (PSNs), and liposomes (Yang et al., 2015). SMEDDS results in 3.6 times increase in bioavailability comparatively to reference capsule (Woo et al., 2007). A novel solid dispersion system containing silymarin, polyvinylpyrrolidone (PVP), and Tween-80 have been increased drug solubility by about 650-folds with physical and chemical stability of 6 months (Hwang et al., 2014). The PSNs are a novel approach to improve the bioavailability of drugs with poor solubility such as silymarin. The prepared PSNs consist of narrow pore size distribution of approximately 10 nm. Silymarin-loaded PSNs showed an initial burst release followed by sustained release over a period of 72 h (Cao et al., 2012). Incorporating silymarin in liposomal carrier system gave increase in AUC and Cmax and thus showed better hepatoprotective and anti-inflammatory effects when compared to silymarin suspension (Kumar et al., 2014).

CONCLUDING REMARKS

Silymarin is a polyphenolic phytochemical with promising therapeutic potential. It is extracted from dried fruit of *S. marianum* and has been used as a hepatoprotective agent since long time. Later-on, the beneficial role of silymarin in the treatment of pathological conditions of various origins including cancer has been studied and documented. It is a mixture of flavonolignans with strong antioxidant and anti-inflammatory activities. It also has binding affinity with estrogen receptor β in CNS regions which attenuates neurotoxicity and prevents lipid peroxidation. These effects make silymarin a valuable choice in therapeutics of neurodegenerative disorders such as PD. Additionally, it has shown significant neuroprotective effects in various *in vitro* and *in vivo* models. However, because of low aqueous solubility the bioavailability of silymarin is quite low i.e., 23–47%. Several techniques are available to improve the bioavailability of silymarin such as SMEDDS, solid dispersions, PSNs, and liposomes. Moreover, the bioavailability issue can be resolved via chemical derivatization. Thus, further research is required on these grounds in order to get molecule of clinical utility for the treatment of PD.

AUTHOR CONTRIBUTIONS

All authors listed have made a substantial, direct and intellectual contribution to the work, and approved it for publication.

REFERENCES

AbouZid, S. F., Chen, S.-N., McAlpine, J. B., Friesen, J. B., and Pauli, G. F. (2016). *Silybum marianum* pericarp yields enhanced silymarin products. *Fitoterapia* 112, 136–143. doi: 10.1016/j.fitote.2016.05.012

Abushouk, A. I., Negida, A., Ahmed, H., and Abdel-Daim, M. M. (2017). Neuroprotective mechanisms of plant extracts against MPTP induced neurotoxicity: future applications in Parkinson's disease. *Biomed. Pharmacother.* 85, 635–645. doi: 10.1016/j.biopha.2016.11.074

Ahmad, S., Ullah, F., Sadiq, A., Ayaz, M., Imran, M., Ali, I., et al. (2016). Chemical composition, antioxidant and anticholinesterase potentials of essential oil of *Rumex hastatus* D. Don collected from the North West of Pakistan. *BMC Complement. Altern. Med.* 16:29. doi: 10.1186/s12906-016-0998-z

Ahmed, B., Khan, S., and Alam, T. (2003). Synthesis and antihepatotoxic activity of some heterocyclic compounds containing the 1, 4-dioxane ring system. *Pharmazie* 58, 173–176.

AlDakheel, A., Kalia, L. V., and Lang, A. E. (2014). Pathogenesis-targeted, disease-modifying therapies in Parkinson disease. *Neurotherapeutics* 11, 6–23. doi: 10.1007/s13311-013-0218-1

Alves, G., Forsaa, E. B., Pedersen, K. F., Gjerstad, M. D., and Larsen, J. P. (2008). Epidemiology of Parkinson's disease. *J. Neurol.* 255, 18–32. doi: 10.1007/s00415-008-5004-3

Antonietta Panaro, M., and Cianciulli, A. (2012). Current opinions and perspectives on the role of immune system in the pathogenesis of Parkinson's disease. *Curr. Pharm. Des.* 18, 200–208. doi: 10.2174/138161212799040574

Ayaz, M., Junaid, M., Ullah, F., Sadiq, A., Khan, M. A., Ahmad, W., et al. (2015). Comparative chemical profiling, cholinesterase inhibitions and anti-radicals properties of essential oils from *Polygonum hydropiper* L: a preliminary anti-Alzheimer's study. *Lipids Health Dis.* 14, 141–147. doi: 10.1186/s12944-015-0145-8

Ayaz, M., Junaid, M., Ullah, F., Subhan, F., Sadiq, A., Ali, G., et al. (2017a). Anti-Alzheimer's Studies on β-Sitosterol Isolated from *Polygonum hydropiper* L. *Front. Pharmacol.* 8:697. doi: 10.3389/fphar.2017.00697

Ayaz, M., Sadiq, A., Junaid, M., Ullah, F., Subhan, F., and Ahmed, J. (2017b). Neuroprotective and anti-aging potentials of essential oils from aromatic and medicinal plants. *Front. Aging Neurosci.* 9:168. doi: 10.3389/fnagi.2017.00168

Băjenaru, O., Ene, A., Popescu, B., Szasz, J., Sabău, M., Mureşan, D., et al. (2016). The effect of levodopa–carbidopa intestinal gel infusion long-term therapy on motor complications in advanced Parkinson's disease: a multicenter Romanian experience. *J. Neural Transm.* 123, 407–414. doi: 10.1007/s00702-015-1496-z

Baluchnejadmojarad, T., Roghani, M., and Mafakheri, M. (2010). Neuroprotective effect of silymarin in 6-hydroxydopamine hemi-parkinsonian rat: involvement of estrogen receptors and oxidative stress. *Neurosci. Lett.* 480, 206–210. doi: 10.1016/j.neulet.2010.06.038

Basli, A., Soulet, S., Chaher, N., Mérillon, J.-M., Chibane, M., Monti, J.-P., et al. (2012). Wine polyphenols: potential agents in neuroprotection. *Oxid. Med. Cell. Longev.* 2012:805762. doi: 10.1155/2012/805762

Ben-David, E., and Tu, R. (2015). Genetics of parkinson disease. *Am. J. Neuroradiol.* 36, 445–447. doi: 10.3174/ajnr.A4092

Benvenuto, M., Fantini, M., Masuelli, L., De Smaele, E., Zazzeroni, F., Tresoldi, I., et al. (2013). Inhibition of ErbB receptors, Hedgehog and NF-kappaB signaling by polyphenols in cancer. *Front. Biosci.* 18, 1290–1310. doi: 10.2741/4180

Bhullar, K. S., and Rupasinghe, H. (2013). Polyphenols: multipotent therapeutic agents in neurodegenerative diseases. *Oxid. Med. Cell. Longev.* 2013:891748. doi: 10.1155/2013/891748

Borah, A., Paul, R., Choudhury, S., Choudhury, A., Bhuyan, B., Das Talukdar, A., et al. (2013). Neuroprotective potential of silymarin against CNS disorders: insight into the pathways and molecular mechanisms of action. *CNS Neurosci. Ther.* 19, 847–853. doi: 10.1111/cns.12175

Brundin, P., and Melki, R. (2017). Prying into the prion hypothesis for Parkinson's disease. *J. Neurosci.* 37, 9808–9818. doi: 10.1523/JNEUROSCI.1788-16.2017

Cao, X., Fu, M., Wang, L., Liu, H., Deng, W., Qu, R., et al. (2012). Oral bioavailability of silymarin formulated as a novel 3-day delivery system based on porous silica nanoparticles. *Acta Biomater.* 8, 2104–2112. doi: 10.1016/j.actbio.2012.02.011

Chtourou, Y., Fetoui, H., Sefi, M., Trabelsi, K., Barkallah, M., Boudawara, T., et al. (2010). Silymarin, a natural antioxidant, protects cerebral cortex against manganese-induced neurotoxicity in adult rats. *Biometals* 23, 985–996. doi: 10.1007/s10534-010-9345-x

Chtourou, Y., Trabelsi, K., Fetoui, H., Mkannez, G., Kallel, H., and Zeghal, N. (2011). Manganese induces oxidative stress, redox state unbalance and disrupts membrane bound ATPases on murine neuroblastoma cells in vitro: protective role of silymarin. *Neurochem. Res.* 36, 1546–1557. doi: 10.1007/s11064-011-0483-5

Connolly, B. S., and Lang, A. E. (2014). Pharmacological treatment of Parkinson disease: a review. *JAMA* 311, 1670–1683. doi: 10.1001/jama.2014.3654

Crocenzi, F. A., and Roma, M. G. (2006). Silymarin as a new hepatoprotective agent in experimental cholestasis: new possibilities for an ancient medication. *Curr. Med. Chem.* 13, 1055–1074. doi: 10.2174/092986706776360950

Davis-Searles, P. R., Nakanishi, Y., Kim, N.-C., Graf, T. N., Oberlies, N. H., Wani, M. C., et al. (2005). Milk thistle and prostate cancer: differential effects of pure flavonolignans from *Silybum marianum* on antiproliferative end points in human prostate carcinoma cells. *Cancer Res.* 65, 4448–4457. doi: 10.1158/0008-5472.CAN-04-4662

De Lau, L. M., and Breteler, M. M. (2006). Epidemiology of Parkinson's disease. *Lancet Neurol.* 5, 525–535. doi: 10.1016/S1474-4422(06)70471-9

Dias, V., Junn, E., and Mouradian, M. M. (2013). The role of oxidative stress in Parkinson's disease. *J. Parkinsons Dis.* 3, 461–491. doi: 10.3233/JPD-130230

Dorsey, E., Constantinescu, R., Thompson, J., Biglan, K., Holloway, R., Kieburtz, K., et al. (2007). Projected number of people with Parkinson disease in the most populous nations, 2005 through 2030. *Neurology* 68, 384–386. doi: 10.1212/01.wnl.0000247740.47667.03

El-Elimat, T., Raja, H. A., Graf, T. N., Faeth, S. H., Cech, N. B., and Oberlies, N. H. (2014). Flavonolignans from *Aspergillus iizukae*, a fungal endophyte of milk thistle (*Silybum marianum*). *J. Nat. Prod.* 77, 193–199. doi: 10.1021/np400955q

Fantini, M., Benvenuto, M., Masuelli, L., Frajese, G. V., Tresoldi, I., Modesti, A., et al. (2015). *In vitro* and *in vivo* antitumoral effects of combinations of polyphenols, or polyphenols and anticancer drugs: perspectives on cancer treatment. *Int. J. Mol. Sci.* 16, 9236–9282. doi: 10.3390/ijms16059236

Farooq, U., Khan, A., Naz, S., Rauf, A., Khan, H., Khan, A., et al. (2018). Sedative and antinociceptive activities of two new sesquiterpenes isolated from *Ricinus communis*. *Chin. J. Nat. Med.* 16, 225–230. doi: 10.1016/S1875-5364(18)30051-7

Fernández-Moriano, C., González-Burgos, E., and Gómez-Serranillos, M. P. (2015). Mitochondria-targeted protective compounds in Parkinson's and Alzheimer's diseases. *Oxid. Med. Cell. Longev.* 2015:408927. doi: 10.1155/2015/408927

Galhardi, F., Mesquita, K., Monserrat, J. M., and Barros, D. M. (2009). Effect of silymarin on biochemical parameters of oxidative stress in aged and young rat brain. *Food Chem. Toxicol.* 47, 2655–2660. doi: 10.1016/j.fct.2009.07.030

Gazak, R., Walterova, D., and Kren, V. (2007). Silybin and silymarin-new and emerging applications in medicine. *Curr. Med. Chem.* 14, 315–338. doi: 10.2174/092986707779941159

Geier, J., Fuchs, T., and Wahl, R. (1990). Anaphylactic shock due to an extract of *Silybum marianum* in a patient with immediate-type allergy to kiwi fruit. *Allergologie* 13, 387–388.

Ghosh, A., Ghosh, T., and Jain, S. (2010). Silymarin-a review on the pharmacodynamics and bioavailability enhancement approaches. *J. Pharm. Sci. Technol.* 2, 348–355.

Gu, M., Singh, R. P., Dhanalakshmi, S., Agarwal, C., and Agarwal, R. (2007). Silibinin inhibits inflammatory and angiogenic attributes in photocarcinogenesis in SKH-1 hairless mice. *Cancer Res.* 67, 3483–3491. doi: 10.1158/0008-5472.CAN-06-3955

Haddadi, R., Nayebi, A. M., Farajniya, S., Brooshghalan, S. E., and Sharifi, H. (2014). Silymarin improved 6-OHDA-induced motor impairment in hemi-parkisonian rats: behavioral and molecular study. *Daru* 22:38. doi: 10.1186/2008-2231-22-38

Hald, A., and Lotharius, J. (2005). Oxidative stress and inflammation in Parkinson's disease: is there a causal link? *Exp. Neurol.* 193, 279–290. doi: 10.1016/j.expneurol.2005.01.013

Hamza, T. H., Zabetian, C. P., Tenesa, A., Laederach, A., Montimurro, J., Yearout, D., et al. (2010). Common genetic variation in the HLA region is associated with late-onset sporadic Parkinson's disease. *Nat. Genet.* 42, 781–785. doi: 10.1038/ng.642

Hwang, D. H., Kim, Y.-I., Cho, K. H., Poudel, B. K., Choi, J. Y., Kim, D.-W., et al. (2014). A novel solid dispersion system for natural product-loaded medicine: silymarin-loaded solid dispersion with enhanced oral bioavailability and hepatoprotective activity. *J. Microencapsul.* 31, 619–626. doi: 10.3109/02652048.2014.911375

Jagla, F., and Pechanova, O. (2015). Age-related cognitive impairment as a sign of geriatric neurocardiovascular interactions: may polyphenols play a protective role? *Oxid. Med. Cell. Longev.* 2015:721514. doi: 10.1155/2015/721514

Johnson, W. M., Wilson-Delfosse, A. L., and Mieyal, J. J. (2012). Dysregulation of glutathione homeostasis in neurodegenerative diseases. *Nutrients* 4, 1399–1440. doi: 10.3390/nu4101399

Jovanovic, V., Salti, A., Tilleman, H., Zega, K., Jukic, M., Zou, H., et al. (2018). BMP/SMAD pathway promotes neurogenesis of midbrain dopaminergic neurons *in vivo* and in human induced pluripotent and neural stem cells. *J. Neurosci.* 38, 1662–1676. doi: 10.1523/JNEUROSCI.1540-17.2018

Jowaed, A., Schmitt, I., Kaut, O., and Wüllner, U. (2010). Methylation regulates alpha-synuclein expression and is decreased in Parkinson's disease patients' brains. *J. Neurosci.* 30, 6355–6359. doi: 10.1523/JNEUROSCI.6119-09.2010

Karimi, G., Vahabzadeh, M., Lari, P., Rashedinia, M., and Moshiri, M. (2011). "Silymarin", a promising pharmacological agent for treatment of diseases. *Iran. J. Basic Med. Sci.* 14, 308–317.

Karkanis, A., Bilalis, D., and Efthimiadou, A. (2011). Cultivation of milk thistle (*Silybum marianum* L. Gaertn.), a medicinal weed. *Ind. Crops Prod.* 34, 825–830. doi: 10.1016/j.indcrop.2011.03.027

Kaur, A. K., Wahi, A., Brijesh, K., Bhandari, A., and Prasad, N. (2011). Milk thistle (*Silybum marianum*): a review. *IJPRD* 3, 1–10.

Kaushik, S., and Cuervo, A. M. (2015). Proteostasis and aging. *Nat. Med.* 21, 1406–1415. doi: 10.1038/nm.4001

Kawaguchi-Suzuki, M., Frye, R. F., Zhu, H.-J., Brinda, B. J., Chavin, K. D., Bernstein, H. J., et al. (2014). The effects of milk thistle (*Silybum marianum*) on human cytochrome P450 activity. *Drug Metab. Dispos.* 42, 1611–1616. doi: 10.1124/dmd.114.057232

Khan, H., Amin, S., and Patel, S. (2018). Targeting BDNF modulation by plant glycosides as a novel therapeutic strategy in the treatment of depression. *Life Sci.* 196, 18–27. doi: 10.1016/j.lfs.2018.01.013

Khan, S. A., Ahmed, B., Zelalem, M., Mohammed, A.-M. I., Bekhit, A. A., Hymete, A., et al. (2011). Synthesis and antihepatotoxic activity of some new xanthones containing 1, 4-dioxane ring system. *Thai J. Pharm. Sci.* 35, 103–109.

Kidd, P. M. (2009). Bioavailability and activity of phytosome complexes from botanical polyphenols: the silymarin, curcumin, green tea, and grape seed extracts. *Altern. Med. Rev.* 14, 226–246.

Kim, C., and Lee, S. J. (2008). Controlling the mass action of α-synuclein in Parkinson's disease. *J. Neurochem.* 107, 303–316. doi: 10.1111/j.1471-4159.2008.05612.x

Kim, Y., Keogh, J. B., and Clifton, P. M. (2016). Polyphenols and glycemic control. *Nutrients* 8:E17. doi: 10.3390/nu8010017

Kittur, S., Wilasrusmee, S., Pedersen, W. A., Mattson, M. P., Straube-West, K., Wilasrusmee, C., et al. (2002). Neurotrophic and neuroprotective effects of milk thistle (*Silybum marianum*) on neurons in culture. *J. Mol. Neurosci.* 18, 265–269. doi: 10.1385/JMN:18:3:265

Křen, V., and Walterova, D. (2005). Silybin and silymarin-new effects and applications. *Biomed. Pap. Med. Fac. Univ. Palacky Olomouc Czech. Repub.* 149, 29–41. doi: 10.5507/bp.2005.002

Kumar, N., Rai, A., Reddy, N. D., Raj, P. V., Jain, P., Deshpande, P., et al. (2014). Silymarin liposomes improves oral bioavailability of silybin besides targeting hepatocytes, and immune cells. *Pharmacol. Rep.* 66, 788–798. doi: 10.1016/j.pharep.2014.04.007

Lawrence, T. (2009). The nuclear factor NF-κB pathway in inflammation. *Cold Spring Harb. Perspect. Biol.* 1:a001651. doi: 10.1101/cshperspect.a001651

Lee, A., and Gilbert, R. M. (2016). Epidemiology of Parkinson disease. *Neurol. Clin.* 34, 955–965. doi: 10.1016/j.ncl.2016.06.012

Lee, D. Y.-W., and Liu, Y. (2003). Molecular Structure and Stereochemistry of Silybin A, Silybin B, Isosilybin A, and Isosilybin B, Isolated from *Silybum marianum* (Milk Thistle). *J. Nat. Prod.* 66, 1171–1174. doi: 10.1021/np030163b

Lee, J., Jo, D.-G., Park, D., Chung, H. Y., and Mattson, M. P. (2014). Adaptive cellular stress pathways as therapeutic targets of dietary phytochemicals: focus on the nervous system. *Pharmacol. Rev.* 66, 815–868. doi: 10.1124/pr.113.007757

Lee, W., and Lee, D. G. (2018). Potential role of potassium and chloride channels in regulation of silymarin-induced apoptosis in *Candida albicans*. *IUBMB Life* 70, 197–206. doi: 10.1002/iub.1716

Leverenz, J. B., Quinn, J. F., Zabetian, C., Zhang, J., Montine, K. S., and Montine, T. J. (2009). Cognitive impairment and dementia in patients with Parkinson disease. *Curr. Top. Med. Chem.* 9, 903–912.

Li, A.-N., Li, S., Zhang, Y.-J., Xu, X.-R., Chen, Y.-M., and Li, H.-B. (2014). Resources and biological activities of natural polyphenols. *Nutrients* 6, 6020–6047. doi: 10.3390/nu6126020

Loeffler, D. A., Camp, D. M., and Conant, S. B. (2006). Complement activation in the Parkinson's disease substantia nigra: an immunocytochemical study. *J. Neuroinflammation* 3:29.

Lofrumento, D. D., Saponaro, C., Cianciulli, A., De Nuccio, F., Mitolo, V., Nicolardi, G., et al. (2011). MPTP-induced neuroinflammation increases the expression of pro-inflammatory cytokines and their receptors in mouse brain. *Neuroimmunomodulation* 18, 79–88. doi: 10.1159/000320027

Machado, A., Herrera, A., Venero, J., Santiago, M., De Pablos, R., Villarán, R., et al. (2011). Inflammatory animal model for Parkinson's disease: the intranigral injection of LPS induced the inflammatory process along with the selective degeneration of nigrostriatal dopaminergic neurons. *ISRN Neurol.* 2011:476158. doi: 10.5402/2011/476158

Mady, F. M., Essa, H., El-Ammawi, T., Abdelkader, H., and Hussein, A. K. (2016). Formulation and clinical evaluation of silymarin pluronic-lecithin organogels for treatment of atopic dermatitis. *Drug Des. Dev. Ther.* 10, 1101–1110. doi: 10.2147/DDDT.S103423

Marzocchella, L., Fantini, M., Benvenuto, M., Masuelli, L., Tresoldi, I., Modesti, A., et al. (2011). Dietary flavonoids: molecular mechanisms of action as anti-inflammatory agents. *Recent Pat. Inflamm. Allergy Drug Discov.* 5, 200–220. doi: 10.2174/187221311797264937

Matés, J., Segura, J., Alonso, F., and Márquez, J. (2009). Natural antioxidants: therapeutic prospects for cancer and neurological diseases. *Mini Rev. Med. Chem.* 9, 1202–1214. doi: 10.2174/138955709789055180

Matkowski, A. (2008). Plant in vitro culture for the production of antioxidants—a review. *Biotechnol. Adv.* 26, 548–560. doi: 10.1016/j.biotechadv.2008.07.001

Mayer, K., Myers, R., and Lee, S. (2005). Silymarin treatment of viral hepatitis: a systematic review. *J. Viral Hepat.* 12, 559–567. doi: 10.1111/j.1365-2893.2005.00636.x

Melki, R. (2015). Role of different alpha-synuclein strains in synucleinopathies, similarities with other neurodegenerative diseases. *J. Parkinsons Dis.* 5, 217–227. doi: 10.3233/JPD-150543

Moosavi, F., Hosseini, R., Saso, L., and Firuzi, O. (2016). Modulation of neurotrophic signaling pathways by polyphenols. *Drug Des. Dev. Ther.* 10, 23–42. doi: 10.2147/DDDT.S96936

Morales-Garcia, J. A., Gine, E., Hernandez-Encinas, E., Aguilar-Morante, D., Sierra-Magro, A., Sanz-SanCristobal, M., et al. (2017). CCAAT/Enhancer binding protein β silencing mitigates glial activation and neurodegeneration in a rat model of Parkinson's disease. *Sci. Rep.* 7:13526. doi: 10.1038/s41598-017-13269-4

Muley, M. M., Thakare, V. N., Patil, R. R., Kshirsagar, A. D., and Naik, S. R. (2012). Silymarin improves the behavioural, biochemical and histoarchitecture alterations in focal ischemic rats: a comparative evaluation with piracetam and protocatachuic acid. *Pharmacol. Biochem. Behav.* 102, 286–293. doi: 10.1016/j.pbb.2012.05.004

Nabavi, S. M., Nabavi, S. F., Latifi, A. M., Moghaddam, A. H., and Hellio, C. (2012). Neuroprotective effects of silymarin on sodium fluoride-induced oxidative stress. *J. Fluor. Chem.* 142, 79–82. doi: 10.1016/j.jfluchem.2012.06.029

Nakaoka, S., Ishizaki, T., Urushihara, H., Satoh, T., Ikeda, S., Yamamoto, M., et al. (2014). Prescribing pattern of anti-Parkinson drugs in Japan: a trend analysis from 2005 to 2010. *PLoS One* 9:e99021. doi: 10.1371/journal.pone.0099021

Obeso, J. A., Rodriguez-Oroz, M. C., Goetz, C. G., Marin, C., Kordower, J. H., Rodriguez, M., et al. (2010). Missing pieces in the Parkinson's disease puzzle. *Nat. Med.* 16, 653–661. doi: 10.1038/nm.2165

Olson, K. E., and Gendelman, H. E. (2016). Immunomodulation as a neuroprotective and therapeutic strategy for Parkinson's disease. *Curr. Opin. Pharmacol.* 26, 87–95. doi: 10.1016/j.coph.2015.10.006

Pagano, G., Tan, E. E., Haider, J. M., Bautista, A., and Tagliati, M. (2015). Constipation is reduced by beta-blockers and increased by dopaminergic medications in Parkinson's disease. *Parkinsonism Relat. Disord.* 21, 120–125. doi: 10.1016/j.parkreldis.2014.11.015

Pan, P.-Y., Li, X., Wang, J., Powell, J., Wang, Q., Zhang, Y., et al. (2017). Parkinson's disease-associated LRRK2 hyperactive kinase mutant disrupts synaptic vesicle trafficking in ventral midbrain neurons. *J. Neurosci.* 37, 11366–11376. doi: 10.1523/JNEUROSCI.0964-17.2017

Pandima Devi, K., Sheeja Malar, D., Braidy, N., Mohammad Nabavi, S., and Fazel Nabavi, S. (2017). A mini review on the chemistry and neuroprotective effects of silymarin. *Curr. Drug Targets* 18, 1529–1536. doi: 10.2174/1389450117666161227125121

Patel, N., Jankovic, J., and Hallett, M. (2014). Sensory aspects of movement disorders. *Lancet Neurol.* 13, 100–112. doi: 10.1016/S1474-4422(13)70213-8

Patel, S., Rauf, A., Khan, H., Khalid, S., and Mubarak, M. S. (2017). Potential health benefits of natural products derived from truffles: a review. *Trends Food Sci. Technol.* 70, 1–8. doi: 10.1016/j.tifs.2017.09.009

Pérez-H, J., Carrillo-S, C., García, E., Ruiz-Mar, G., Pérez-Tamayo, R., and Chavarría, A. (2014). Neuroprotective effect of silymarin in a MPTP mouse model of Parkinson's disease. *Toxicology* 319, 38–43. doi: 10.1016/j.tox.2014.02.009

Pérez-Hernández, J., Zaldívar-Machorro, V. J., Villanueva-Porras, D., Vega-Ávila, E., and Chavarría, A. (2016). A potential alternative against neurodegenerative diseases: phytodrugs. *Oxid. Med. Cell. Longev.* 2016:8378613. doi: 10.1155/2016/8378613

Pinto, M., Nissanka, N., and Moraes, C. T. (2018). Lack of Parkin anticipates the phenotype and affects mitochondrial morphology and mtDNA levels in a mouse model of Parkinson's Disease. *J. Neurosci.* 38, 1042–1053. doi: 10.1523/JNEUROSCI.1384-17.2017

Poewe, W., Seppi, K., Tanner, C. M., Halliday, G. M., Brundin, P., Volkmann, J., et al. (2017). Parkinson disease. *Nat. Rev. Dis. Primers* 3:17013. doi: 10.1038/nrdp.2017.13

Politis, M. (2014). Neuroimaging in Parkinson disease: from research setting to clinical practice. *Nat. Rev. Neurol.* 10, 708–722. doi: 10.1038/nrneurol.2014.205

Polyak, S. J., Ferenci, P., and Pawlotsky, J. M. (2013). Hepatoprotective and antiviral functions of silymarin components in hepatitis C virus infection. *Hepatology* 57, 1262–1271. doi: 10.1002/hep.26179

Post-White, J., Ladas, E. J., and Kelly, K. M. (2007). Advances in the use of milk thistle (*Silybum marianum*). *Integr. Cancer Ther.* 6, 104–109. doi: 10.1177/1534735407301632

Ramasamy, K., and Agarwal, R. (2008). Multitargeted therapy of cancer by silymarin. *Cancer Lett.* 269, 352–362. doi: 10.1016/j.canlet.2008.03.053

Rascol, O., Payoux, P., Ory, F., Ferreira, J. J., Brefel-Courbon, C., and Montastruc, J. L. (2003). Limitations of current Parkinson's disease therapy. *Ann. Neurol.* 53(Suppl. 3), S3–S12. doi: 10.1002/ana.10513

Rauf, A., Hadda, T. B., Uddin, G., Cerón-Carrasco, J. P., Peña-García, J., Pérez-Sánchez, H., et al. (2017a). Sedative-hypnotic-like effect and molecular docking of di-naphthodiospyrol from *Diospyros lotus* in an animal model. *Biomed. Pharmacother.* 88, 109–113. doi: 10.1016/j.biopha.2017.01.043

Rauf, A., Uysal, S., Hadda, T. B., Uddin, G., Nawaz, M. A., Khan, H., et al. (2017b). *In vivo* and *in silico* sedative-hypnotic like activity of 7-methyljuglone isolated from *Diospyros lotus* L. *Biomed. Pharmacother.* 87, 678–682. doi: 10.1016/j.biopha.2017.01.021

Raza, S. S., Khan, M. M., Ashafaq, M., Ahmad, A., Khuwaja, G., Khan, A., et al. (2011). Silymarin protects neurons from oxidative stress associated damages in focal cerebral ischemia: a behavioral, biochemical and immunohistological study in Wistar rats. *J. Neurol. Sci.* 309, 45–54. doi: 10.1016/j.jns.2011.07.035

Rizek, P., Kumar, N., and Jog, M. S. (2016). An update on the diagnosis and treatment of Parkinson disease. *Can. Med. Assoc. J.* 188, 1157–1165. doi: 10.1503/cmaj.151179

Ross, S. M. (2008). Milk thistle (*Silybum marianum*): an ancient botanical medicine for modern times. *Holist. Nurs. Pract.* 22, 299–300. doi: 10.1097/01.HNP.0000334924.77174.6d

Singh, M., Dykens, J. A., and Simpkins, J. W. (2006). Novel mechanisms for estrogen-induced neuroprotection. *Exp. Biol. Med.* 231, 514–521. doi: 10.1177/153537020623100505

Singhal, N. K., Chauhan, A. K., Jain, S. K., Shanker, R., Singh, C., and Singh, M. P. (2013). Silymarin-and melatonin-mediated changes in the expression of selected genes in pesticides-induced Parkinsonism. *Mol. Cell. Biochem.* 384, 47–58. doi: 10.1007/s11010-013-1780-x

Singhal, N. K., Srivastava, G., Patel, D. K., Jain, S. K., and Singh, M. P. (2011). Melatonin or silymarin reduces maneb-and paraquat-induced Parkinson's disease phenotype in the mouse. *J. Pineal Res.* 50, 97–109. doi: 10.1111/j.1600-079X.2010.00819.x

Srivastava, S., Sammi, S. R., Laxman, T. S., Pant, A., Nagar, A., Trivedi, S., et al. (2017). Silymarin promotes longevity and alleviates Parkinson's associated pathologies in *Caenorhabditis elegans*. *J. Funct. Foods* 31, 32–43. doi: 10.1016/j.jff.2017.01.029

Stojkovska, I., Wagner, B. M., and Morrison, B. E. (2015). Parkinson's disease and enhanced inflammatory response. *Exp. Biol. Med.* 240, 1387–1395. doi: 10.1177/1535370215576313

Surmeier, D. J., Obeso, J. A., and Halliday, G. M. (2017). Parkinson's disease is not simply a prion disorder. *J. Neurosci.* 37, 9799–9807. doi: 10.1523/JNEUROSCI.1787-16.2017

Tan, L. (2013). Epidemiology of Parkinson's disease. *Neurol. Asia* 18, 231–238.

Tansey, M. G., and Goldberg, M. S. (2010). Neuroinflammation in Parkinson's disease: its role in neuronal death and implications for therapeutic intervention. *Neurobiol. Dis.* 37, 510–518. doi: 10.1016/j.nbd.2009.11.004

Tentillier, N., Etzerodt, A., Olesen, M. N., Rizalar, F. S., Jacobsen, J., Bender, D., et al. (2016). Anti-inflammatory modulation of microglia via CD163-targeted glucocorticoids protects dopaminergic neurons in the 6-OHDA parkinson's disease model. *J. Neurosci.* 36, 9375–9390. doi: 10.1523/JNEUROSCI.1636-16.2016

Thome, A. D., Harms, A. S., Volpicelli-Daley, L. A., and Standaert, D. G. (2016). microRNA-155 regulates alpha-synuclein-induced inflammatory responses in models of Parkinson disease. *J. Neurosci.* 36, 2383–2390. doi: 10.1523/JNEUROSCI.3900-15.2016

Todorova, A., Jenner, P., and Chaudhuri, K. R. (2014). Non-motor Parkinson's: integral to motor Parkinson's, yet often neglected. *Pract. Neurol.* 14, 310–322. doi: 10.1136/practneurol-2013-000741

Vecchia, D. D., Schamne, M. G., Ferro, M. M., dos Santos, A. F. C., Latyki, C. L., de Lara, D. V., et al. (2015). Effects of *Hypericum perforatum* on turning behavior in an animal model of Parkinson's disease. *Braz. J. Pharm. Sci.* 51, 111–115. doi: 10.1590/S1984-82502015000100012

Venkataramanan, R., Ramachandran, V., Komoroski, B. J., Zhang, S., Schiff, P. L., and Strom, S. C. (2000). Milk thistle, a herbal supplement, decreases the activity of CYP3A4 and uridine diphosphoglucuronosyl transferase in human hepatocyte cultures. *Drug Metab. Dispos.* 28, 1270–1273.

Vijitruth, R., Liu, M., Choi, D.-Y., Nguyen, X. V., Hunter, R. L., and Bing, G. (2006). Cyclooxygenase-2 mediates microglial activation and secondary dopaminergic cell death in the mouse MPTP model of Parkinson's disease. *J. Neuroinflammation* 3:6.

Wagoner, J., Negash, A., Kane, O. J., Martinez, L. E., Nahmias, Y., Bourne, N., et al. (2010). Multiple effects of silymarin on the hepatitis C virus lifecycle. *Hepatology* 51, 1912–1921. doi: 10.1002/hep.23587

Wang, M., Xie, T., Chang, Z., Wang, L., Xie, X., Kou, Y., et al. (2015). A new type of liquid silymarin proliposome containing bile salts: its preparation and improved hepatoprotective effects. *PLoS One* 10:e0143625. doi: 10.1371/journal.pone.0143625

Wang, M. J., Lin, W. W., Chen, H. L., Chang, Y. H., Ou, H. C., Kuo, J. S., et al. (2002). Silymarin protects dopaminergic neurons against lipopolysaccharide-induced neurotoxicity by inhibiting microglia activation. *Eur. J. Neurosci.* 16, 2103–2112. doi: 10.1046/j.1460-9568.2002.02290.x

Weiss, H. D., and Marsh, L. (2012). Impulse control disorders and compulsive behaviors associated with dopaminergic therapies in Parkinson disease. *Neurol. Clin. Pract.* 2, 267–274. doi: 10.1212/CPJ.0b013e318278be9b

Woo, J. S., Kim, T.-S., Park, J.-H., and Chi, S.-C. (2007). Formulation and biopharmaceutical evaluation of silymarin using SMEDDS. *Arch. Pharm. Res.* 30, 82–89. doi: 10.1007/BF02977782

Xilouri, M., Brekk, O. R., and Stefanis, L. (2013). Alpha-synuclein and protein degradation systems: a reciprocal relationship. *Mol. Neurobiol.* 47, 537–551. doi: 10.1007/s12035-012-8341-2

Yamada, M., Kida, K., Amutuhaire, W., Ichinose, F., and Kaneki, M. (2010). Gene disruption of caspase-3 prevents MPTP-induced Parkinson's disease in mice. *Biochem. Biophys. Res. Commun.* 402, 312–318. doi: 10.1016/j.bbrc.2010.10.023

Yan, M. H., Wang, X., and Zhu, X. (2013). Mitochondrial defects and oxidative stress in Alzheimer disease and Parkinson disease. *Free Radic. Biol. Med.* 62, 90–101. doi: 10.1016/j.freeradbiomed.2012.11.014

Yang, G., Zhao, Y., Zhang, Y., Dang, B., Liu, Y., and Feng, N. (2015). Enhanced oral bioavailability of silymarin using liposomes containing a bile salt: preparation by supercritical fluid technology and evaluation in vitro and in vivo. *Int. J. Nanomed.* 10, 6633–6644. doi: 10.2147/IJN.S92665

Yang, K. Y., Hwang, du, H., Yousaf, A. M., Kim, D. W., Shin, Y. J., et al. (2013). Silymarin-loaded solid nanoparticles provide excellent hepatic protection: physicochemical characterization and in vivo evaluation. *Int. J. Nanomed.* 8, 3333–3343. doi: 10.2147/IJN.S50683

7

Multi-Target Protective Effects of Gintonin in 1-Methyl-4-phenyl-1,2,3,6-tetrahydropyridine-Mediated Model of Parkinson's Disease via Lysophosphatidic Acid Receptors

Jong Hee Choi[1,2], Minhee Jang[2], Seikwan Oh[3], Seung-Yeol Nah[4] and Ik-Hyun Cho[1,2,5]**

[1] Department of Science in Korean Medicine and Brain Korea 21 Plus Program, Graduate School, Kyung Hee University, Seoul, South Korea, [2] Department of Convergence Medical Science, College of Korean Medicine, Kyung Hee University, Seoul, South Korea, [3] Department of Neuroscience and Tissue Injury Defense Research Center, School of Medicine, Ewha Womans University, Seoul, South Korea, [4] Ginsentology Research Laboratory and Department of Physiology, College of Veterinary Medicine and Bio/Molecular Informatics Center, Konkuk University, Seoul, South Korea, [5] Institute of Korean Medicine, College of Korean Medicine, Kyung Hee University, Seoul, South Korea

Correspondence:
Seung-Yeol Nah
synah@konkuk.ac.kr
Ik-Hyun Cho
ihcho@khu.ac.kr;
neuropro@hanmail.net

Gintonin is a ginseng-derived lysophosphatidic acid receptor (LPAR) ligand. Although previous *in vitro* and *in vivo* studies demonstrated the therapeutic role of gintonin against Alzheimer's disease, the neuroprotective effects of gintonin in Parkinson's disease (PD) are still unknown. We investigated whether gintonin (50 and 100 mg/kg/day, p.o., daily for 12 days) had neuroprotective activities against neurotoxicity in a 1-methyl-4-phenyl-1,2,3,6-tetrahydropyridine (MPTP)-induced mouse model of PD. Pre-administration of 100 mg/kg gintonin displayed significantly ameliorating effects in neurological disorders (motor and welfare) as measuring using pole, rotarod, and nest building tests, and in the survival rate. These effects were associated to the reduction of the loss of tyrosine hydroxylase–positive neurons, microglial activation, activation of inflammatory mediators (interleukin-6, tumor necrosis factor, and cyclooxygenase-2), and alteration of blood-brain barrier (BBB) integrity in the substantia nigra pars compacta and/or striatum following MPTP injection. The benefits of gintonin treatment against MPTP also included the activation of the nuclear factor erythroid 2-related factor 2 pathways and the inhibition of phosphorylation of the mitogen-activated protein kinases and nuclear factor-kappa B signaling pathways. Interestingly, these neuroprotective effects of gintonin were blocked by LPAR1/3 antagonist, Ki16425. Overall, the present study shows that gintonin attenuates MPTP-induced neurotoxicity via multiple targets. Gintonin combats neuronal death, and acts as an anti-inflammatory and an anti-oxidant agent. It maintains BBB integrity. LPA receptors play a key role in gintonin-mediated anti-PD mechanisms. Finally, gintonin is a key agent for prevention and/or treatment of PD.

Keywords: gintonin, 1-methyl-4-phenyl-1,2,3,6-tetrahydropyridine, Parkinson's disease, lysophosphatidic acid receptor, multi-target

INTRODUCTION

Parkinson's disease (PD) is a common progressive neurodegenerative disorder characterized by profound loss of dopaminergic neurons and accumulation of α-synuclein aggregates into Lewy bodies and Lewy neuritis in the substantia nigra pars compacta (SNpc) of the midbrain, and by decreased dopamine levels in the striatum (caudate and putamen) of the basal ganglia (Shulman et al., 2011; Kalia and Lang, 2015; Poewe et al., 2017). The main symptoms of PD are movement impairments, such as slowness of movement, tremor, rigidity, and postural instability, and non-motor related disorders that include executive dysfunction, slowed cognitive speed, memory problems, genitourinary problems, and emotional changes (Shulman et al., 2011; Kalia and Lang, 2015; Poewe et al., 2017). PD has a complex, multi-factorial etiology including mitochondrial malfunction, glutamate excitotoxicity, apoptosis, oxidative stress, proteasomal dysfunction, and environmental exposures (Riess and Kruger, 1999; Shulman et al., 2011; Kalia and Lang, 2015; Poewe et al., 2017).

Although medicines for symptom relief including levodopa are the most trusted therapeutics for PD, the approach does not prevent the progressive loss of dopaminergic neurons, and does not result in cell regeneration in PD patients. In addition, they produce adverse effects including dizziness, nausea, and vomiting when therapy is prolonged (Marsden, 1994; Athauda and Foltynie, 2015). These unsatisfactory effects may be inextricably related to the targeting of only one of the multi-factorial mechanisms underlying neuronal degeneration (Riess and Kruger, 1999; Shulman et al., 2011; Kalia and Lang, 2015; Poewe et al., 2017). The recent and rapid advances in medical biology and technology have suggested a new paradigm of drug development (multi-targeted drugs) based on the multi-factorial and highly complex pathological features of various neurodegenerative disorders (Bajda et al., 2011; Dias and Viegas, 2014; Zheng et al., 2014; Calabresi and Di Filippo, 2015). The multi-targeted strategy may hopefully overcome the limitations of drugs directed at a single target. Plant-derived natural products that are proven safe, effective, and innovative, remain the best sources of drugs, encouraging continuous research, development and discovery of therapeutic approaches for a wide range of diseases and conditions (Newman and Cragg, 2012). Although increasing evidence suggests that characterizing and identifying potentially active natural products may meet the unmet demand of single-target drugs (Li et al., 2013), no approved PD protective medicines are currently available (Athauda and Foltynie, 2015).

Panax (P.) ginseng Meyer, a perennial herb of the family *Araliaceae*, has been widely used for millennia as an adaptogen, particularly in the eastern Asian countries including Korea, Chinese, and Japan (Cho, 2012; Lee et al., 2017). Beneficial effects of *P. ginseng* have been reported in various diseases including neurological disorders. The major active ingredients of *P. ginseng* are acidic polysaccharide, a carbohydrate polymer, and ginsenoside, a kind of plant saponin (Cho, 2012; Lee et al., 2017). Although the molecular mechanisms of the ingredients have been frequently studied in neurodegenerative diseases (Cho, 2012), they remain unclear. Recently, we isolated a novel ingredient from *P. ginseng*, termed gintonin. Gintonin is a non-carbohydrate polymer and a non-saponin (Choi et al., 2015b) that was identified as a novel ligand of G protein-coupled lysophosphatidic acid (Alpayci et al., 2012) receptors (LPARs). Gintonin elicits a transient increase in intracellular calcium concentration $[Ca^{2+}]_i$, which activates the calcium-dependent cellular events through the regulation of ion channels and cell surface receptors, induces anti-inflammatory activity by inhibiting mitogen-activated protein kinases (MAPKs) and nuclear factor-kappa B (NF-κB) pathways in lipopolysaccharide-induced RAW 264.7 cells, and increases the release of neurotransmitters (dopamine, catecholamine, and gliotransmitter) in cortical primary astrocytes and PC12 cells (Choi et al., 2015b; Saba et al., 2015). Intraperitoneal (i.p.) administration of gintonin to mice also increased serum dopamine concentrations (Hwang et al., 2015).

On the other hand, LPA receptors are present on most cell types and fluids within the developing and adult nervous system, and are functionally involved in many neural processes and pathways (Noguchi et al., 2009; Choi et al., 2010; Yung et al., 2014, 2015). Recent studies showed that dysregulations of brain LPA receptor pathways may lead to nervous system disorders including cognitive functions, hydrocephalus, neuropsychiatric disorders, and neuropathic pain (Noguchi et al., 2009; Choi et al., 2010; Yung et al., 2014, 2015), indicating that LPA receptors play important roles in maintenance of normal brain functions. In previous studies we demonstrated that gintonin exhibits *in vitro* and *in vivo* anti-Alzheimer's disease, one of representative neurodegenerative diseases, effects via LPA receptor signaling pathway (Hwang et al., 2012). However, little is known on the effects of gintonin on PD. In the present study we investigated whether oral gintonin administration to MPTP-induced PD animal model attenuates brain neuropathies of PD and found that the gintonin administration exhibits multiple beneficial effects on PD via LPA receptors. Presently, we demonstrated that gintonin contributes to neuroprotections against MPTP-induced neurotoxicities in mice and further discuss possible molecular mechanisms on gintonin-mediated anti-PD in animal model.

MATERIALS AND METHODS

Animals and Ethical Approval

Adult male C57BL/6 mice (Narabiotec Co., Ltd., Seoul, South Korea) that were 7–8 weeks of age and weighed 22–23 g) were housed at a constant temperature of 23 ± 2°C with a 12-h light-dark cycle (lights on from 08:00 to 20:00), and provided with food and water *ad libitum*. All experimental procedures were reviewed and approved by the Institutional Animal Care and Use Committee of Kyung Hee University [KHUASP(SE)-17-143]. In this process, proper randomization of laboratory animals and handling of data were performed in a blinded manner in accordance with recent recommendations from an NIH workshop on preclinical models of neurological diseases (Landis et al., 2012).

Preparation of Gintonin and Its Composition

Gintonin was prepared as previous described (Choi et al., 2015a). Briefly, one kilogram of 4-year-old ginseng (Korea ginseng corporation, Daejeon, South Korea) was ground into small pieces (>3 mm) and refluxed with 70% fermented ethanol eight times for 8 h each at 80°C. The extracts (340 g) were concentrated, dissolved in distilled, cold water at a ratio of 1:10, and stored at 4°C for 24–96 h. The supernatant and precipitate fractions obtained by water fractionation after ethanol extraction of ginseng were separated by centrifugation (3,000 rpm, 20 min). The precipitate was lyophilized. Gintonin consists of carbohydrates, lipids and ginseng proteins. The proportion of total carbohydrates, lipids, and proteins in gintonin was approximately 30, 20.2, and 30.3%, respectively, in addition to other minor components (Choi et al., 2015a). The lipid composition of gintonin based on LC-MS/MS analysis is as follows: fatty acids (7.53% linoleic acid, 2.82% palmitic acid, and 1.46% oleic acid); lysophospholipids and phospholipids (0.60%); and phosphatidic acids (1.75%). The total lipid content in gintonin is about 14.2%. Qualitative assays indicate that gintonin also contains diacylglycerols and triacylglycerols (Choi et al., 2015a).

Experimental Groups and Treatment With MPTP, Gintonin, and Ki16425

In order to determine the most effective dose and mechanism of pre-administration of gintonin, mice were randomly divided into sham, MPTP, MPTP + gintonin pre-administration (50 and 100 mg/kg), and gintonin groups. For MPTP injection, mice received four i.p. injections of MPTP-hydrochloride (20 mg/kg body weight; Sigma-Aldrich, St. Louis, MO, United States) dissolved in phosphate buffered saline (PBS) for 2 h intervals (Jackson-Lewis and Przedborski, 2007). Gintonin was dissolved in physiological saline and administrated orally at doses of 50 and 100 mg/kg once daily for 12 days from 5 days before the first MPTP injection. Ki16425, an antagonist against LPAR1 and LPAR3 (Tocris Bioscience, Bristol, United Kingdom), was prepared in 5% DMSO in PBS. It was administered once daily 30 min before gintonin treatment.

Behavioral Assays

To examine motor coordination, mice (n = 5 per group) were subjected to pole and rotarod tests as previous described (Choi et al., 2018). The nest building behavior was measured as an indicator of health and welfare in mice as previous described (Choi et al., 2018). The behavioral tests were performed by an experimenter who was unaware of the experimental conditions and was done under constant temperature (23 ± 2°C) and humidity (55 ± 5%) in a quiet room, 1 day before and 1, 3, 5, and 7 days after MPTP injection.

Immunohistochemical Evaluation

Seven days after the last injection of MPTP, brain (n = 5 per group) for histological evaluation were prepared as previously described (Jang et al., 2013; Lee et al., 2016). Sequential coronal sections (30 μm thickness) were acquired using a model CM3050S freezing microtome (Leica Biosystems, Wetzlar, Germany), from the level of the SNpc (bregma −2.54 to −3.40 mm) and mid-striatum (bregma +0.26 to +1.10 mm), according to the mouse brain atlas (Franklin and Paxinos, 2008). Immunohistochemical analysis of the SNpc and striatal sections was performed as previously described (Jang et al., 2013; Lee et al., 2016). Briefly, sections (n = 3 per brain) from all groups were incubated with either rabbit anti-tyrosine hydroxylase (TH; 1:1,000; Millipore, Bedford, MA, United States), rabbit anti-ionized calcium binding adapter molecule-1 (Iba-1; 1:2,000; WAKO, Osaka, Japan), rabbit anti-glial fibrillary acidic protein (GFAP; 1:5,000; DAKO, Carpinteria, CA, United States) or rat anti-platelet endothelial cell adhesion molecule-1 (PECAM-1; 1:500; Santa Cruz Biotechnology, Santa Cruz, CA, United States), followed by incubation with biotinylated rabbit IgG antibody (1:200; Vector Laboratories, Burlingame, CA, United States) and avidin–biotinylated horseradish peroxidase complex (1:200; Vector Laboratories). The sections were visualized with 3,3′-diamino-benzidine and cover-slipped with Permount.

Western Blot Analysis

Seven days after the last injection of MPTP, the brains of all groups (n = 2–3 per group) was immediately removed with lysis buffer under anesthesia. Western blot analysis was accomplished as previously described (Jang et al., 2013; Lee et al., 2016). The polyvinylidene fluoride membranes with protein were probed overnight with rabbit anti-TH (1:1,000; Millipore), rabbit anti-Iba-1 (1:500; WAKO), mouse anti-GFAP (1:1,000; Millipore), rat anti-PECAM-1 (1:500; Santa Cruz Biotechnology), rabbit anti-phospho (p)-extracellular signal-regulated kinase (ERK), rabbit anti-ERK, rabbit anti-phospho (p)-c-Jun N-terminal kinase (JNK), rabbit anti-JNK, rabbit anti-p-p38, rabbit anti-p38, rabbit anti-p-NF-κB p65, rabbit anti-NF-κB p65, rabbit anti-p-IκBα, mouse anti-IκBα (1:1,000; Cell Signaling Technology, Beverly, MA, United States), rabbit anti-nuclear factor erythroid 2-related factor 2 (Nrf2; 1:1000, Santa Cruz Biotechnology), mouse anti-heme oxygenase-1 (HO-1; 1:1,000; Enzo Life Sciences, Farmingdale, NY, United States), mouse anti-NQO1 (1:1,000; Cell Signaling Technology), rabbit anti-LPAR1 (1:1,000; Abcam, Cambridge, United Kingdom), or rabbit anti-LPAR3 (1:1,000; Abcam) at 4°C, followed by incubation with horseradish peroxidase-conjugated secondary antibody for 1 h prior to enhanced chemiluminescence analysis (Amersham Pharmacia Biotech, Piscataway, NJ, United States) and visualized using a super cooled-CCD camera system with a Davinch-K Gel imaging system (Dvinch-K, Seoul, South Korea). For normalization of the antibody signal, the membranes were stripped and reprobed with glyceraldehyde 3-phosphate dehydrogenase (GAPDH; 1:5,000; Cell Signaling Technology) or total antibody levels against each protein. After Western blot was performed three times, the density of each band was converted to a numerical value using the Photoshop CS2 program (Adobe, San Jose, CA, United States) after subtracting background values from an area of film immediately adjacent to the stained band. Data are expressed as the ratio of each expression against GAPDH or total protein in each sample. Original images of Western blots were supported in **Supplementary Figure S2**.

Real-Time Polymerase Chain Reaction (PCR) Analysis

Seven days after the MPTP injection, brain of each mouse ($n = 3$ per group) was rapidly removed under anesthesia, coronal brain slices (3 mm thickness) were prepared on ice-cold subbed slide glass using a brain matrix device (Roboz Surgical Instrument Co. Gaithersburg, MD, United States), and SNpc and striatum regions were sampled using microscissors and blade under a dissection microscope. Real-time PCR analysis was accomplished as previously described (Choi et al., 2016). The mRNA levels of each target gene were normalized to that of GAPDH mRNA. Fold-induction was calculated using the $2^{-\Delta\Delta C_T}$ method as previously described (Livak and Schmittgen, 2001). The primer sequences were as follows; interleukin (IL)-6-5′-TCC ATC CAG TTG CCT TCT TGG-3′ and 5′-CCA CGA TTT CCC AGA GAA CAT G-3′, tumor necrosis factor (TNF)-α-5′-AGC AAA CCA CCA AGT GGA GGA-3′ and 5′-GCT GGC ACC ACT AGT TGG TTG T-3′, Cyclooxygenase (COX)-2-5′-CAG TAT CAG AAC CGC ATT GCC-3′ and 5′-GAG CAA GTC CGT GTT CAA GGA-3′, endothelial intercellular adhesion molecule (ICAM)-1-5′-TGC GTT TTG GAG CTA GCG GAC CA-3′ and 5′-CGA GGA CCA TAC AGC ACG TGC AG-3′, vascular cell adhesion molecule (VCAM)-1-5′-CCT CAC TTG CAG CAC TAC GGG CT-3′ and 5′-TTT TCC AAT ATC CTC AAT GAC GGG-3′, zoula occludens (ZO)-1-5′-AAG GCA ATT CCG TAT CGT TG-3′ and 5′-CCA CAG CTG AAG GAC TCA CA-3′, claudin-3-5′-CTG GGA GGG CCT GTG GAT GAA CT-3′ and 5′-TCG CGG CGC AGA ATA GAG GAT-3′, LPAR1-5′-GAG GAA TCG GGA CAC CAT GAT-3′ and 5′-ACA TCC AGC AAT AAC AAG ACC AAT C-3′, LPAR2-5′-GAC CAC ACT CAG CCT AGT CAA GAC-3′ and 5′-CTT ACA GTC CAG GCC ATC CA-3′, LPAR3-5′-GCT CCC ATG AAG CTA ATG AAG ACA-3′ and 5′-AGG CCG TCC AGC AGC AGA-3′, LPAR4-5′-CAG TGC CTC CCT GTT TGT CTT C-3′ and 5′-GAG AGG GCC AGG TTG GTG AT-3′, LPAR5-5′-GCT CCA GTG CCC TGA CTA TC-3′ and 5′-GGG AAG TGA CAG GGT GAA GA-3′, LPAR6-5′-ACA GTG ATG GGA GGA AGT GC-3′ and 5′-CCG CTG GAA AGT TCT CAA AG-3′, and GAPDH-5′-AGG TCA TCC CAG AGC TGA ACG-3′ and 5′-CAC CCT GTT GCT GTA GCC GTA T-3′.

Statistical Analyses

All data are presented as means ± SEM. Statistical analyses were performed using the SPSS 23.0 package (SPSS Inc, Chicago, IL, United States) for Windows. Two-sample comparisons were carried out using the Student's t-test and multiple comparisons were made using two-way ANOVA with Tukey's *post hoc* test. Statistical difference was identified at the 5% level unless otherwise indicated.

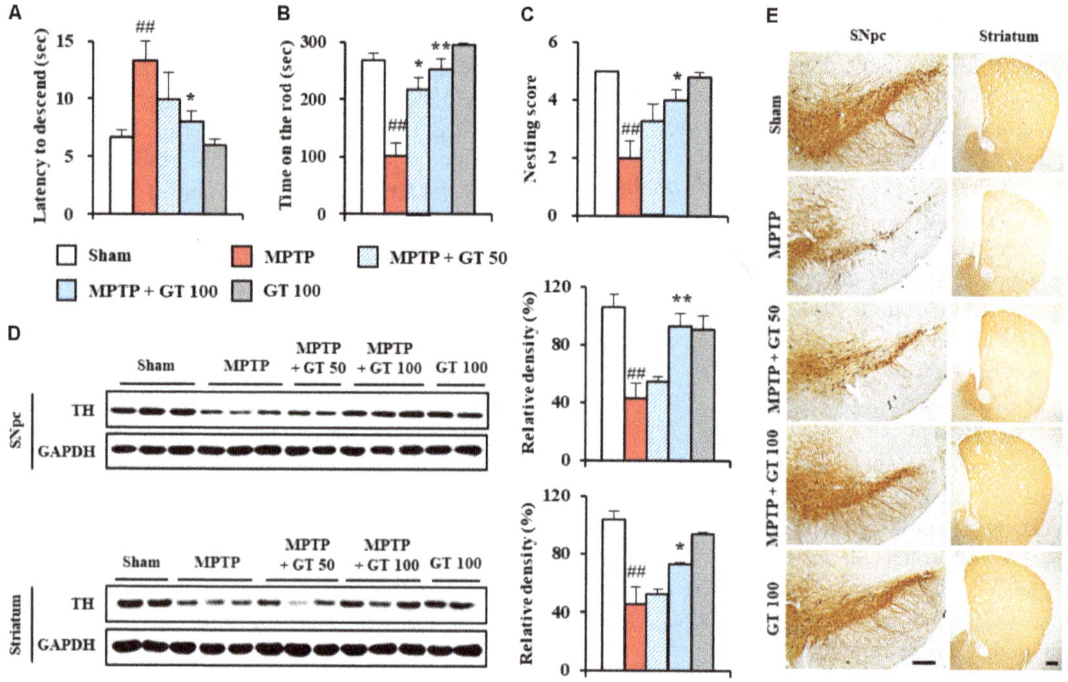

FIGURE 1 | Gintonin attenuates neurological impairment and dopaminergic cell death by MPTP neurotoxicity. **(A–C)** Mice ($n = 5$ per group) were orally administrated gintonin (50 and 100 mg/kg/day) or saline from 1 h before the first MPTP injection (20 mg/kg, every 2 h × 4 times). Pole test **(A)**, rotarod performance test **(B)**, and nest building behavior test **(C)** were performed 3, 5, and 1 days after the last MPTP-injection. **(D)** SNpc and striatum each group ($n = 2$–3 per group) were sampled 7 days after MPTP injection and quantitatively analyzed by immunoblot analysis using TH antiserum. The left panels illustrate representative Western blots. **(E)** SNpc and striatum sections ($n = 3$ per brain) from each group ($n = 5$ per group) were prepared 7 days after MPTP injection and immunostained with TH antiserum. Scale bar = 100 μm. ANOVA test; $^{\#\#}p < 0.01$ vs. Sham group; $^{*}p < 0.05$ and $^{**}p < 0.01$ vs. MPTP group.

RESULTS

Gintonin Improves Neurological Impairments and Dopaminergic Neuronal Death Following MPTP Injection

To determine the effective dose of gintonin for the treatment of MPTP-mediated neurological impairment, we investigated the motor coordination in mice. First, we performed pole test. In the MPTP group, the average descent time from the top to the bottom of the pole increased by 98.5% (13.3 ± 1.7 s) compared with the sham group (6.7 ± 0.6 s). The average descent time was decreased by 24.8–39.8% by gintonin administration (10.0 ± 2.3 and 8.0 ± 0.9 s for 50 and 100 mg/kg/day gintonin, respectively; **Figure 1A**). One hour after the pole test, rotarod performance was tested. In the MPTP group, the average latency to fall decreased by 62.0% (101.6 ± 21.7 s) compared with the sham group (267.6 ± 12.6 s), while the average latency to fall was increased by 114.5–149.0% by gintonin administration (218.0 ± 19.7 and 253.0 ± 17.9 s for 50 and 100 mg/kg/day gintonin, respectively; **Figure 1B**). As an indicator of health and welfare, nest building behavior was measured. In the MPTP group, the mean score of the quality of the resulting nest decreased by 60% (2.0 ± 0.6) compared with the sham group (5.0 ± 0.0). However, the mean score was improved by 100% following gintonin administration (4.0 ± 0.4 in the 100 mg/kg/day gintonin) compared to the MPTP group (**Figure 1C**). At the end of the experiment, the survival rate of all groups was 100% (data not shown).

Since MPTP-mediated neurological disorders results from the loss of dopaminergic neurons in the SNpc and depletion of the dopamine in the striatum (Gubellini and Kachidian, 2015), we investigated whether gintonin could prevent the loss of dopaminergic neurons/fibers by immunoblotting and immunohistochemical analyses using TH antibody 7 days after MPTP injection (**Figures 1D,E**). The expression of TH protein in the SNpc was reduced by MPTP-injection (42.7 ± 6.0%) compared to the sham group (105.7 ± 6.0%), while the reduction was significantly inhibited by gintonin administration (54.9 ± 3.8% and 92.9 ± 6.4% for 50 and 100 mg/kg/day gintonin, respectively; upper panel of **Figure 1D**). The findings agreed with the alteration in intensity of TH immunoreactivity (**Figure 1E**). Since the fibers of dopaminergic neurons in the SNpc project to the striatum (Gubellini and Kachidian, 2015; Kalinderi et al., 2016), we examined the alteration of TH immunoreactivity in the striatum. As expected, the reduction of striatal TH protein expressions by MPTP neurotoxicity (45.5 ± 3.4%) were also inhibited by gintonin (52.7 ± 3.9% and 72.8 ± 12.3% for 50 and 100 mg/kg/day gintonin, respectively; lower panel of **Figure 1D**), in agreement with the alteration of intensity of TH immunoreactiviy (**Figure 1E**). Gintonin did not induce significant alteration in TH expression in the SNpc and striatum. The findings suggest that gintonin may inhibit MPTP-mediated neurological impairments by decreasing dopaminergic degeneration in the SNpc and striatum.

Gintonin Inhibits Microglial Activation and the Expression of Inflammatory Mediators in the SNpc or Striatum Following MPTP Injection

Since microglia are activated within or around lesions of neurodegenerative disorders, such as PD, and activated microglia contribute to neurodegeneration by the producing inflammatory mediators (Liberatore et al., 1999; Lobsiger and Cleveland, 2007; Du et al., 2017), we wondered whether gintonin could have neuroprotective effects closely related with the down-regulation of the anti-inflammatory response. The level of Iba-1 (a marker for microglia) protein expression was enhanced in the SNpc (80.8 ± 3.2%) and striatum (81.5 ± 5.3%) from MPTP group compared to the sham group (35.6 ± 4.6% in the SNpc and 35.2 ± 3.7% in the striatum), whereas the enhancement was inhibited by 100 mg/kg of gintonin administration (47.0 ± 6.5% in the SNpc and 49.2 ± 7.3% in the striatum) compared to the MPTP group (**Figure 2A**). The expression trend paralleled the alteration in the intensity of Iba-1-immunoreactivity (**Figure 2B**). In the SNpc and striatum from the MPTP group, Iba-1-immunoreactive cells showed typically activated form with enlarged cell bodies and short and thick processes compared to the sham group, which generally displayed the typical forms of resting cells that included small cell bodies and thin processes (Jang et al., 2013; Jang and Cho, 2016; Lee et al., 2016). However, the morphology of Iba-1-immunoreactive cells from gintonin-administrated group was relatively similar to that of the resting cells from the sham group.

Since activated microglia may produce inflammatory mediators, which have been implicated in the degeneration of dopaminergic neurons in the SNpc and striatum from MPTP model of PD (Liberatore et al., 1999; Lobsiger and Cleveland, 2007; Du et al., 2017), we investigated whether gintonin might down-regulate the representative inflammatory mediators in the SNpc and striatum after MPTP injection. Real-time PCR analysis demonstrated that the relative mRNA expressions of IL-6, TNF-α, and COX-2 were enhanced by 3.6-, 4.2-, and 3.1-fold, respectively, in the SNpc, and by 4.0-, 2.1-, and 4.5-fold, respectively, in the striatum, 7 days following MPTP injection compared to sham group. In contrast, their enhancements were significantly prevented in the SNpc (66.7, 64.3, and 61.3%, respectively), and in the striatum (67.5, 42.9, and 71.1%, respectively) following the administration of 100 mg/kg gintonin compared with the MPTP group. Real-time PCR analysis revealed little or no mRNA expression of both genes in the SNpc and striatum from the sham groups (**Figures 2C,D**). The findings suggest that gintonin might contribute to neuroprotection against MPTP-mediated neurotoxicity by inhibiting microglial activation and the inflammatory response.

Gintonin Blocks MAPKs and NF-κB Pathways in the Striatum Following MPTP Injection

Since MAPK and NF-κB pathways have been implicated as a main signaling pathway in the neuronal death, oxidative

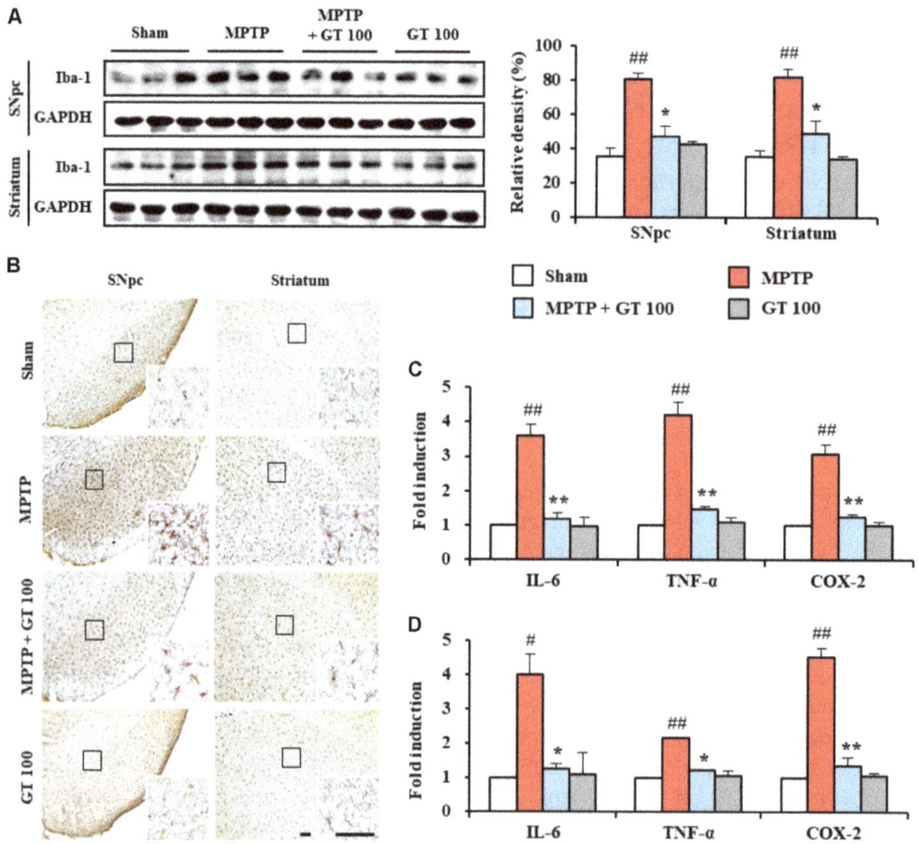

FIGURE 2 | Gintonin attenuates activation of microglia and inflammatory mediators in the SNpc and striatum after MPTP injection. **(A)** SNpc and striatum from each group (n = 3 per group) 7 days after MPTP-injection were quantified by immunoblot analysis using Iba-1 antiserum. The left panels illustrate representative Western blots. **(B)** SNpc and striatum sections (n = 3 per brain) 7 days after MPTP injection were immunostained with Iba-1 antiserum. Insets display high magnification micrographs of the areas marked with squares. **(C,D)** Real-time PCR was used to quantify mRNA expression of IL-6, TNF-α, and COX-2 in SNpc and striatum (n = 3 per group) from day 7 after MPTP injection (SNpc, **C**; striatum, **D**). Scale bar = 50 μm. ANOVA test; $^{\#}p < 0.05$ and $^{\#\#}p < 0.01$ vs. Sham group; $^{*}p < 0.05$ and $^{**}p < 0.01$ vs. MPTP group.

stress, and BBB disruption (Abbott et al., 2006; Sandoval and Witt, 2008; Zlokovic, 2008), we measured the regulation effect of gintonin on the both pathways in the SNpc and striatum after MPTP injection. The activation of ERK, JNK, and p38 proteins was significantly enhanced in the SNpc (189.8 ± 3.3%, 134.9 ± 5.9%, and 120.0 ± 17.2%, respectively) and striatum (89.5 ± 17.6%, 150.6 ± 6.7%, and 148.7 ± 9.0%, respectively) 7 days after MPTP injection compared to the sham group (68.4 ± 23.3%, 79.0 ± 18.4%, and 45.7 ± 12.5%, respectively, in the SNpc, and 19.1 ± 10.2%, 19.0 ± 8.7%, and 49.4 ± 14.0%, respectively). The enhancement of activation was blocked by pretreatment with 100 mg/kg gintonin (108.9 ± 4.1%, 102.2 ± 2.3%, and 67.5 ± 15.3%, respectively, in the SNpc, and 43.7 ± 9.0%, 49.2 ± 22.2%, and 92.6 ± 21.8%, respectively, in striatum) (**Figures 3A–D,G–J**). Subsequently, we examined whether gintonin regulates the NF-κB pathway in the SNpc and striatum following MPTP injection. Expressions of p-NF-κB and p-IκBα were significantly increased in the SNpc (283.4 ± 36.6%, and 379.6 ± 40.7%, respectively) and striatum (68.4 ± 0.1% and 114.0 ± 12.8%, respectively) 7 days after the MPTP-injection compared to the sham group (87.2 ± 17.1%, and 231.9 ± 21.1%, respectively, in the SNpc, and 21.4 ± 4.5% and 47.3 ± 13.9%, respectively, in the striatum). The expressions were significantly increased by the administration of 100 mg/kg gintonin (128.5 ± 8.7%, and 227.5 ± 5.5%, respectively, in the SNpc, and 32.5 ± 7.9% and 71.0 ± 8.5%, respectively, in the striatum) (**Figures 3A,E,F,G,K,L**). Phosphorylation of MAPKs or NF-κB pathways was not significantly affected by gintonin administration alone (**Figures 3A–L**). The results suggest that gintonin might diminish MPTP neurotoxicity by inhibiting the activation of the MAPKs and NF-κB pathways.

Gintonin Activates Nrf2 Pathway in the Striatum Following MPTP Injection

Panax ginseng extract and ginsenosides exert anti-oxidative effects through Nrf2 transcriptional activation in neural dysfunctions (Nabavi et al., 2015; Lee et al., 2017). Yet, the anti-oxidative effects of See comment in PubMed Commons below gintonin are unknown. Therefore, we examined the effect of gintonin on the Nrf2 pathway in the MPTP-mediated PD model by immunoblot blot analysis. The level of Nrf2 protein expression was slightly increased in the

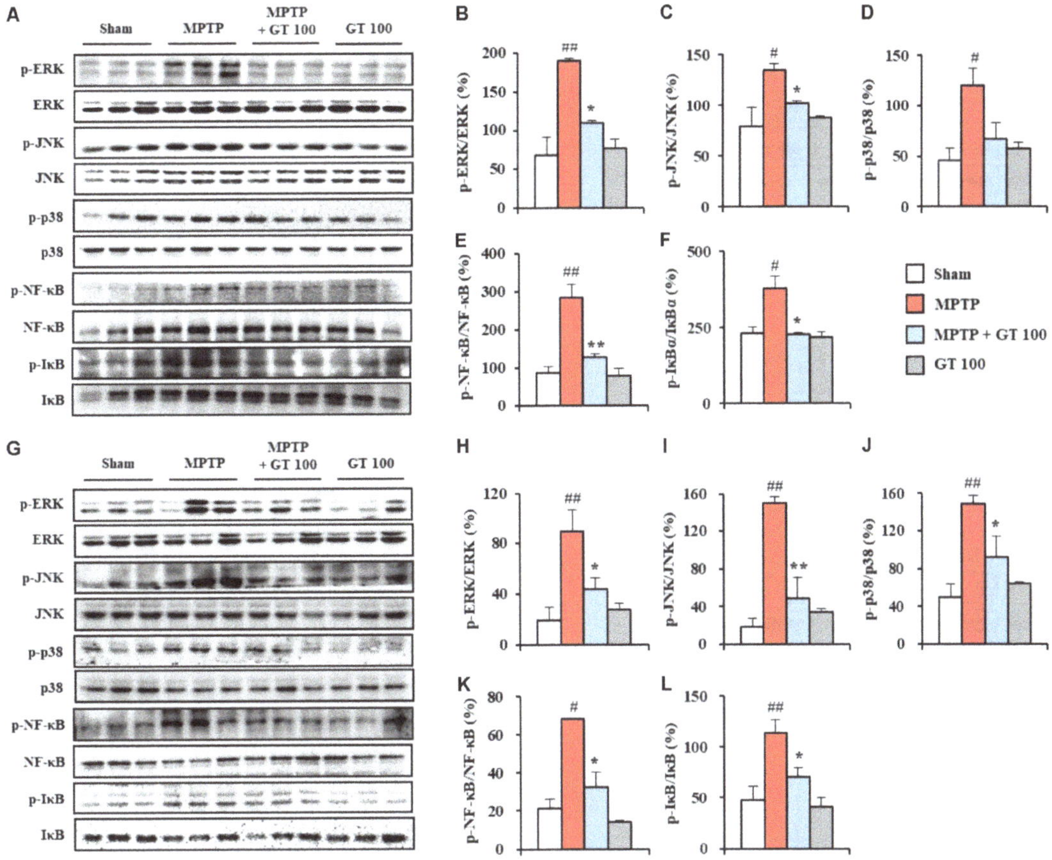

FIGURE 3 | Gintonin inhibits MAPKs and NF-κB signaling pathways in the SNpc and striatum after MPTP injection. **(A–L)** SNpc and striatum sample from each group ($n = 3$ per group) 7 days after MPTP-injection were quantified by immunoblot analysis to measure the alteration in the MAPKs **(A–D,G–J)** and NF-κB pathways **(A,E,F,G,K,L)**. SNpc **(A–F)** and striatum **(G–L)**. The left panels illustrate representative Western blots **(A,G)**. ANOVA test; $^{\#}p < 0.05$ and $^{\#\#}p < 0.01$ vs. Sham group. $^{*}p < 0.05$ and $^{**}p < 0.01$ vs. MPTP group.

SNpc (68.1 ± 18.1%) and striatum (14.7 ± 0.7%) by MPTP injection compared to the sham group (59.4 ± 6.0% in the SNpc and 8.9 ± 2.0% in the striatum), while they further increased by administration with 100 mg/kg of gintonin (113.2 ± 9.0% in the SNpc and 32.1 ± 5.1% in the striatum) (**Figures 4A,B**). Consequently, the expression of the phase II enzymes heme oxidase-1 (HO-1), and NAD(P)H:quinone oxidoreductase 1 (NQO-1) was increased by 62.3 ± 13.7% and 61.7 ± 11.4%, respectively, in the SNpc, and by 31.7 ± 0.6% and 31.4 ± 1.1%, respectively, in striatum of the gintonin-administrated group compared to that of MPTP group (114.2 ± 5.4% and 101.7 ± 5.7%, respectively, in the SNpc, and 36.7 ± 0.6% and 59.6 ± 9.2%, respectively, in striatum) (**Figures 4A,B**). The results suggest that antioxidant effect of gintonin may contribute to its neuroprotective effects in the MPTP-mediated neurotoxicity.

Gintonin Protects BBB Integrity After MPTP Injection

Since the BBB was disrupted during neurological disorders including PD (Abbott et al., 2006; Zlokovic, 2008), we examined the effect of gintonin on the level of BBB disruption and maintenance of BBB integrity 7 days after MPTP injection. Expression of PECAM-1, a marker of BBB disruption, was increased in the SNpc (107.3 ± 10.2%) and striatum (77.5 ± 3.1%) of the MPTP group compared to sham group (48.3 ± 0.9% in the SNpc and 21.2 ± 9.9% in the striatum). The increase was inhibited by the administration of 100 mg/kg gintonin (72.0 ± 4.7% and 55.4 ± 3.9%, respectively) (**Figures 5A,G**), in accordance with the alteration of PECAM-1 immunoreactivity (**Figures 5B,H**). Intensity of expression of GFAP protein, one of the main components of BBB (Abbott et al., 2006), was markedly increased in the SNpc (69.7 ± 8.1%) and striatum (155.9 ± 14.4%) of the MPTP group compared to sham group (22.4 ± 3.9% in the SNpc and 69.8 ± 31.1% in striatum). The increase was significantly inhibited by gintonin (26.6 ± 8.4% in the SNpc and 116.8 ± 1.9% in striatum) (**Figures 5A,G**), in accordance with the alteration of GFAP-immunoreactivity (**Figures 5B,H**). We tested the effect of gintonin on the changes of adhesion and junctional molecules. Real-time PCR analysis revealed increased mRNA expression of ICAM-1 and VCAM-1, representative adhesion molecules, in the SNpc (2.5 and 3.2-fold, respectively) and striatum (2.4 and 11.5-fold, respectively) following MPTP injection compared

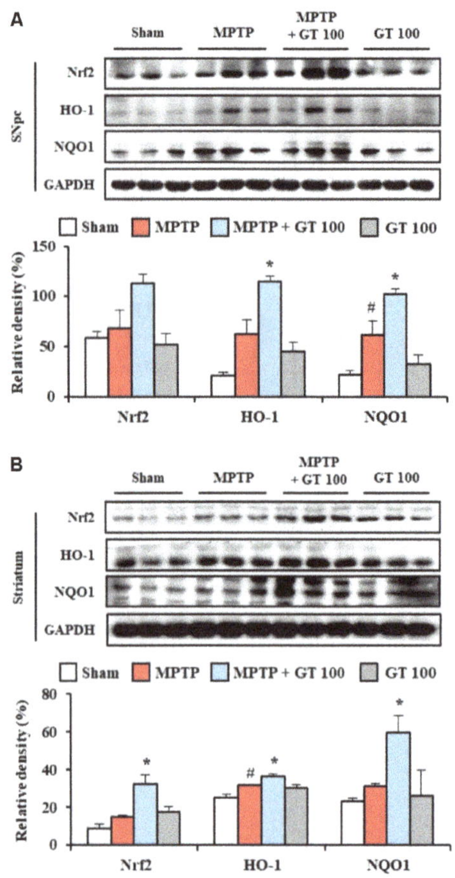

FIGURE 4 | Gintonin activates Nrf2 signaling pathway in the SNpc and striatum after MPTP injection. **(A,B)** SNpc and striatum sample (*n* = 3 per group) 7 days after MPTP-injection were quantified by immunoblot analysis. Nrf2, HO-1, and NQO1. SNpc **(A)** and striatum **(B)**. The top panels illustrate representative Western blots. ANOVA test; $^{\#}p < 0.05$ vs. Sham group. $^{*}p < 0.05$ vs. MPTP group.

to the sham group, whereas the increase was blocked by the gintonin administration (32.0 and 68.8%, respectively, in the SNpc and 45.8 and 52.2%, respectively, in the striatum) (**Figures 5C,D,I,J**). Meanwhile, mRNA expressions of ZO-1 and claudin-3, representative junctional molecules, were reduced in the SNpc (0.6 and 0.7-fold, respectively) and striatum (0.7 and 0.7-fold, respectively) following MPTP injection. The reduction was inhibited by gintonin (100.0 and 42.9%, respectively, in the SNpc and 71.4 and 42.6%, respectively, in the striatum) (**Figures 5E,F,K,L**). The collective data demonstrate that the positive activity of gintonin on the disruption and maintenance of BBB might contribute to its protective effect against MPTP toxicity.

Gintonin Activates LPARs Pathways in the SNpc and Striatum After MPTP Injection

Since gintonin as an exogenous LPA induces various cellular effects that include migration and cell proliferation through the activation of LPARs (Choi et al., 2015b), we tested the expression pattern of LPARs. Interestingly, mRNA expressions of LPAR 1 and 3 were slightly (but not significantly) increased in the SNpc and striatum by MPTP-mediated neurotoxicity. The expressions were further increased by administration of 100 mg/kg gintonin (**Figures 6A,B,F,G**), in agreement with the alteration in the mRNA expression of phospholipase C-β3 and IP_3R_3, which are representative molecules in the downstream cascade (**Figures 6C,D,H,I**) and protein expression of LPAR 1 and 3 (**Figures 6E,J**). However, mRNA expression of other types of LPAR was not significantly affected by MPTP or gintonin (**Supplementary Figure S1**). The overall results suggest a possible role of LPAR1 and LPAR3 in gintonin-mediated anti-PD effects in brain.

Multi-Target Effects of Gintonin Are Neutralized by Ki16425 Treatment

Gintonin significantly enhanced the expression of LPAR1 and 3 (**Figure 6**), resulting in multi-target effects. Gintonin combats neuronal death, exerts anti-inflammatory and anti-oxidant effects, and contributes to the maintenance of BBB integrity in the SNpc and striatum after MPTP injection (**Figures 1–6**). The results strongly suggest the possibility that interruption of the LPA pathway neutralizes the effects of gintonin on MPTP neurotoxicity. To investigate this possibility, we intraperitoneally administered Ki16425 (a LPAR1 and 3 antagonist) to mice once daily 30 min before gintonin treatment in an MPTP model. As expected, the protective effects of gintonin against neurological disorders in pole, rotarod, and nest-building tests after MPTP injection was significantly neutralized by Ki16425 (**Figures 7A–C**). Further, the increased expression of TH protein by gintonin was neutralized by Ki16425 (**Figures 7D,E**), consistent with the neutralization of gintonin expression in Iba-1, Nrf2, and PECAM-1 expression (**Figures 7D,E**). Conclusively, enhanced protein expression of LAPR1 and LPAR3 after gintonin treatment was blocked by Ki16425 (**Figures 7D,E**). The results indicate that the beneficial effects of gintonin after MPTP injection were neutralized by interrupting LPA signaling before treatment.

DISCUSSION

The pathogenesis underlying the loss of dopaminergic neurons in PD remains subject to further debate, although the cell death is multifactorial and to be associated with mitochondrial malfunction, apoptosis, oxidative stress, and inflammation (Riess and Kruger, 1999; Shulman et al., 2011; Blesa et al., 2015; Kalia and Lang, 2015; Poewe et al., 2017). Currently, most single-target therapeutics, such as levodopa, provide symptomatic relief with adverse effects when PD patients receive long-term therapy (Marsden, 1994; Guneysel et al., 2008). Therefore, to overcome these limitations, the desire to develop more effective and safer therapeutic approaches for PD is driving drug design toward multi-target compounds acting in the central nervous system designed from natural products (Bajda et al., 2011; Dias and Viegas, 2014; Zheng et al., 2014;

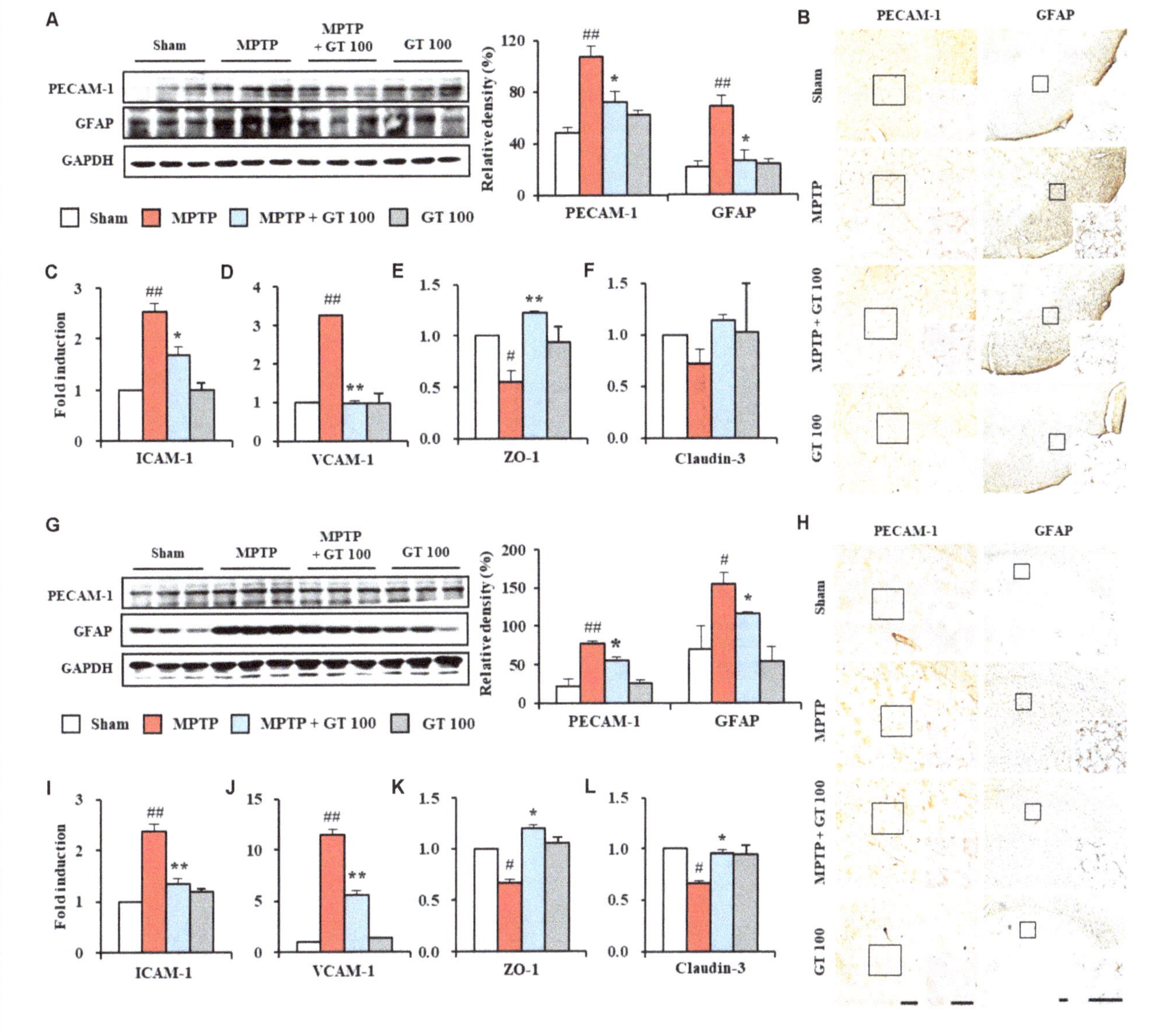

FIGURE 5 | Gintonin prevents disruption of the BBB integrity in the SNpc and striatum after MPTP injection. **(A,G)** SNpc and striatum sample (n = 3 per group) were quantified by immunoblot analysis using PECAM-1 and GFAP antisera. The left panels illustrate representative Western blots. **(B,H)** SNpc and striatum sections (n = 3 per brain) from each group (n = 5 per group) 7 days after MPTP-injection were immunostained using PECAM-1 and GFAP antisera. Insets display high magnification micrographs of the areas marked with squares. Scale bar = 50 μm. **(C–F,I–L)** Real-time PCR using primers for ICAM-1 **(C,I)**, VCAM-1 **(D,J)**, ZO-1 **(E,K)**, and claudin-3 **(F,L)** was used to quantify the expression of these molecules in SNpc **(C–F)** and striatum **(I–L)** (n = 3 per group) 7 days after MPTP-injection. ANOVA test; $^{\#}p < 0.05$ and $^{\#\#}p < 0.01$ vs. Sham group. $^{*}p < 0.05$ and $^{**}p < 0.01$ vs. MPTP group.

Calabresi and Di Filippo, 2015). Gintonin is a ligand of LPARs that was isolated from *P. ginseng*, a recognized well-known medicinal herb that has been widely used in traditional medicine to treat various diseases, including motor disabilities (Nah, 2012; Choi et al., 2015b; Hwang et al., 2015; Kim et al., 2017). The present data demonstrate the protective effects of gintonin in the MPTP-mediated SNpc and striatal toxicity through multifunctional activities including anti-neuronal death, anti-inflammation, anti-oxidant, and inhibition of BBB disruption. Thus, gintonin has potential value in functional foods and new drugs to preventive and treat PD, based on its multi-target effects.

Neuroinflammation and neuroimmune dysfunction might be closely related with the chronic features of neurodegenerative diseases, such as PD (Lobsiger and Cleveland, 2007; Du et al., 2017). Microglia are important in the development and maintenance of the brain micro-environment during inflammatory response. Activated microglia are pivotal cells in the defense against immunopathogenesis of infections and neurodegenerative disorders (Lobsiger and Cleveland, 2007; Du et al., 2017). Therefore, controlling microglial activation is considered as an attractive trial to protect dopaminergic neurons in the *in vivo* model of PD and PD patients (Du et al., 2017). *P. ginseng* extract has anti-inflammatory role in various *in vitro*

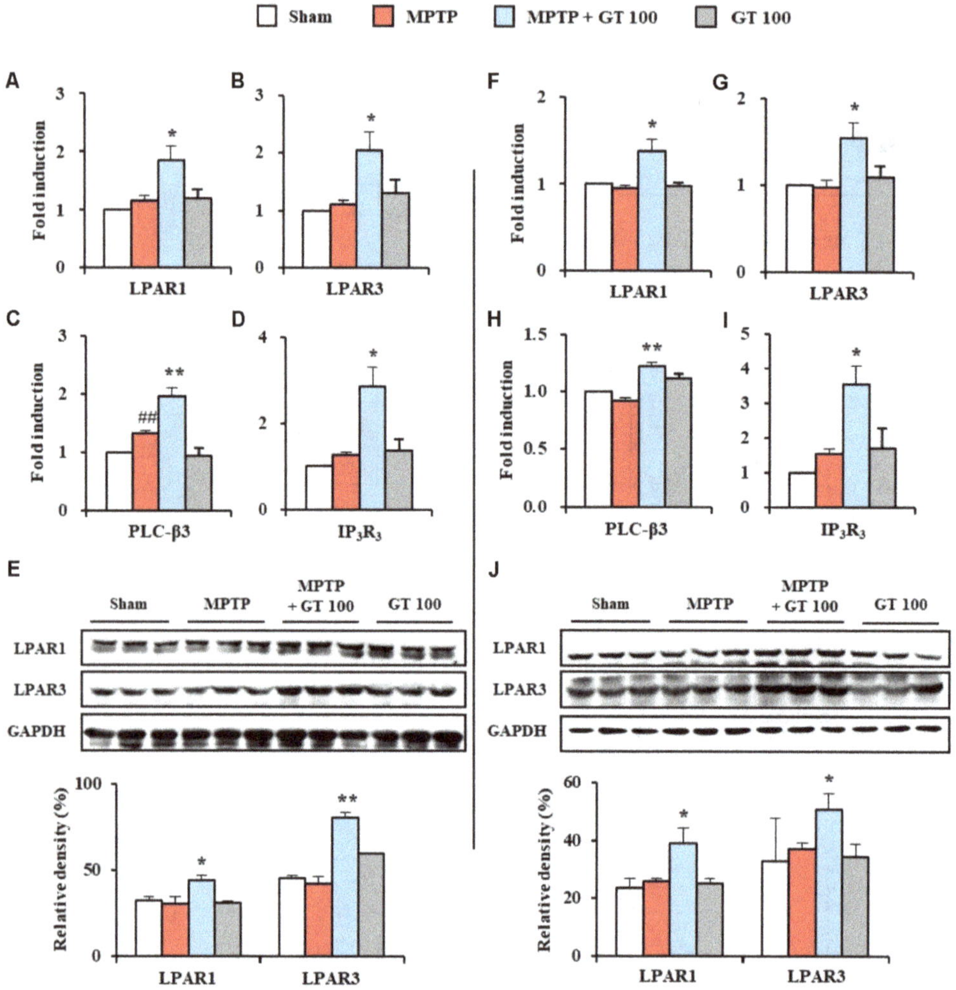

FIGURE 6 | Gintonin activates LPAR1 and 3 signaling pathways in the SNpc and striatum after MPTP injection. **(A–J)** SNpc and striatum sample from each group (n = 3 per group) 7 days after MPTP-injection were quantified by real-time PCR **(A–D,F–I)** and immunoblot analysis **(E,J)** to measure the alteration in expression of LPAR 1 and 3 or their downstream molecules. mRNA expression of LPAR1 **(A,F)**, LPAR3 **(B,G)**, PLC-β3 **(C,H)**, and IP_3R_3 **(D,I)**. Protein expression of LPAR1 and 3 **(E,J)**. The top panels illustrate representative Western blots **(E,J)**. SNpc **(A–E)** and striatum **(F–J)**. ANOVA test; $^{\#\#}p < 0.01$ vs. Sham group. $^{*}p < 0.05$ and $^{**}p < 0.01$ vs. MPTP group.

and *in vivo* studies (Cho, 2012; Choi et al., 2015b; Nabavi et al., 2015; Lee et al., 2017), and gintonin suppresses the increase in the expression of pro-inflammatory cytokines (IL-1β, IL-6, and TNF-α), COX-2, and iNOS in lipopolysaccharide-stimulated RAW 264.7 cells (Saba et al., 2015). In accordance with these reports, gintonin suppressed microglial activation and up-regulation of mRNA expressions of pro-inflammatory cytokines (IL-6, and TNF-α), and COX-2 in the SNpc and striatum following MPTP injection (**Figure 2**). Collectively, our results indicate that gintonin can exert suppressive effect dopaminergic neurodegeneration by MPTP neurotoxicity by attenuating microglial activation and its inflammatory responses.

The pathways of MAPKs and NF-κB regulate the expression of many genes involved in a variety of processes including neurodegeneration, neuroinflammation, oxidative stress, and BBB disruption (Abbott et al., 2006; Sandoval and Witt, 2008; Zlokovic, 2008). Agents to control MAPKs and NF-κB pathways may be potential medications with an ability to prevent or treat PD through various mechanisms (Kim and Choi, 2010; Flood et al., 2011). In present study, as expected, administration of gintonin inhibited phosphorylation of all three MAPKs as well as phosphorylation of NF-κB and IκBα in the SNpc and striatum following MPTP injection (**Figure 3**). Previous studies have demonstrated that gintonin inhibits inflammation by MAPKs (p-ERK, p-JNK, and p-p38) and NF-κB pathways (NF-κB and p-IκBα) in lipopolysaccharide-induced RAW 264.7 cells (Saba et al., 2015). The observations along with the present findings that gintonin activates Nrf2 and Nrf2-dependent genes and their proteins including HO-1 and NQO-1 (**Figure 4**), supports the hypothesis that triggering the Nrf2 pathway by gintonin may block activation of MAPKs and NF-κB pathways, contributing to gintonin's anti-inflammatory activity against MPTP neurotoxicity. Collectively, our findings indicate that gintonin can mitigate dopaminergic cell death by MPTP toxicity

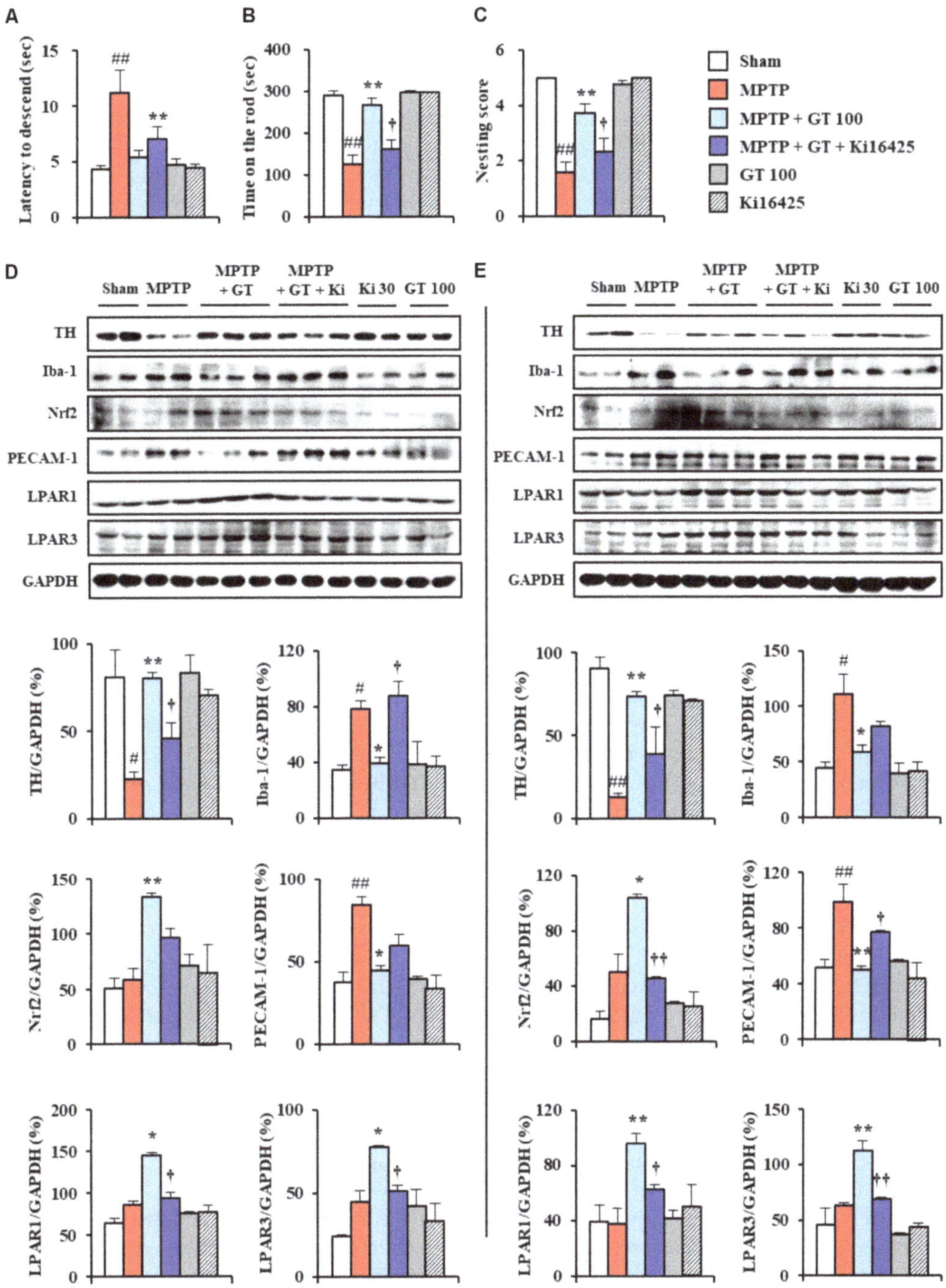

FIGURE 7 | Multi-target effects of gintonin in MPTP-induced neurotoxicity were neutralized by Ki16425, an LPAR1/3 antagonist. **(A–C)** Mice (n = 8 per group) were orally administered with gintonin or saline 1 h before the first MPTP injection. Ki16425 was used once daily 30 min before gintonin treatment. Pole test **(A)**, rotarod performance test **(B)**, and nest-building behavior test **(C)** were conducted 3, 3, and 1 days after the last MPTP-injection. **(D,E)** Immunoblot analysis of TH, Iba-1, Nrf2, PECAM-1, LPAR1, and LPAR3 was conducted in SNpc **(D)** and striatum **(E)** obtained from each group (n = 2–3 per group) 7 days after MPTP injection. The top panels illustrate representative Western blots. ANOVA test; $^{\#}p < 0.05$ and $^{\#\#}p < 0.01$ vs. Sham group. $^{*}p < 0.05$ and $^{**}p < 0.01$ vs. MPTP group. $^{\dagger}p < 0.05$ and $^{\dagger\dagger}p < 0.01$ vs. MPTP + GT 100 mg/kg/day group.

via anti-inflammatory activity by inhibiting the MAPKs and NF-κB mediated pathways by the triggered Nrf2 pathway.

The processes of oxidative stress induced by reactive oxygen species are a cause of a complex multifactorial PD (Riess and Kruger, 1999; Blesa et al., 2015). Recently, Nrf2, a phase II antioxidant 'master regulator,' was reported to demonstrably mitigate the neurotoxic actions of parkinsonian agents such as MPP^{+}, rotenone, and hydrogen peroxide *in vitro* and *in vivo* (Todorovic et al., 2016). Many natural products including sulforaphane, which is present in broccoli, and ginsenosides of *P. ginseng* protects neuronal cells by activating Nrf2-mediated signaling *in vitro* and *in vivo* (Cho, 2012; Nabavi et al., 2015; Jang and Cho, 2016). It is conceivable, therefore, that the natural product-derived pharmacological modulators of the Nrf2 pathway may be very beneficial against neural toxicity. In present study, gintonin activated Nrf2 and representative Nrf2-dependent proteins, HO-1 and NQO1, in the SNpc and striatum following MPTP injection (**Figure 4**). The results may be supported by anti-oxidant effect of *P. ginseng* extract, fractions, and ginsenosides by activation of Nrf2 pathway *in vitro* and *in vivo* (Ong et al., 2015). Taken together, the data indicate that gintonin contributes to anti-dopaminergic cell death via anti-oxidant activity.

The blood-brain barrier (BBB) is a multicellular vascular structure that consists of the foot processes of astrocytes, pericytes, and endothelial cells. Inter-endothelial connections contain a variety of junctional molecule species, such as adherens, tight, and gap junctions (Abbott et al., 2006; Zlokovic, 2008). The BBB restricts the passage of various biological or chemical entities to brain tissue and maintains a constant micro-environment of the central nervous system (CNS). Disruption of the BBB by disease or drugs can compromise the CNS. Thus, agents that maintain BBB integrity may be powerful preventive and therapeutic approaches for neurological diseases including PD (Abbott et al., 2006; Sandoval and Witt, 2008; Zlokovic, 2008). BBB disruption is associated with astroglial activation, and the alteration of endothelial adhesive and tight junctional molecules (Abbott et al., 2006; Sandoval and Witt, 2008; Zlokovic, 2008). Many synthetic or natural agents, such as resveratrol and shikonin, block BBB disruption by reducing astroglial activation and the alteration of expression of junctional molecules (Lee et al., 2016; Zhao et al., 2017). In the present study, gintonin inhibited astroglial activation and blocked increase in the mRNA expression of endothelial adherens junctional molecules (ICAM-1 and VCAM-1) and in the SNpc and striatum following MPTP injection, while it prevented the decrease in that of tight junctional molecules (ZO-1 and claudin-3) (**Figure 5**). Taken together, that data indicate that gintonin could attenuate the degeneration of dopaminergic neurons caused by MPTP neurotoxicity, directly or indirectly mitigating BBB disruption. The cellular mechanism remains unclear.

Whether activation of LPA pathway protects dopaminergic neurons that are normally damaged in PD and whether gintonin could be critical role in the LPA pathway in PD are unclear. Here, although expression of LPARs was not investigated in all neural cell types in the SNpc and striatum following MPTP injection, the level of mRNA and protein expression of LPAR 1 and 3 was not significantly changed in the both tissues following MPTP injection, but their expressions were significantly increased by co-administration of gintonin with MPTP (**Figure 6**). Other types of LPAR did not show significant alteration. Currently, we failed to elucidate why gintonin administration enhanced the expression of only LPAR1 and 3 subtypes. It is possible that the gintonin-mediated anti-PD effects were mediated via LPAR1 and 3 in the brain rather than other subtypes in SNpc and striatum, based on the observation that gintonin-mediated anti-PD activity was blocked by Ki16425, an LPAR1/3 antagonist (**Figure 7**). Thus, the enhanced expression of LPAR 1 and 3 by gintonin in the presence of MPTP contributed to the protective effect against MPTP-induced neurotoxicity. However, further studies are needed to elucidate the precise molecular mechanisms underlying differential increases in brain LPAR1 and 3 levels following gintonin treatment in MPTP-induced PD animal model. Taken together, the present study showed that gintonin-mediated regulation of LPAR1 and 3 plays a key role in the amelioration of MPTP-induced SNpc and striatal toxicity.

Interestingly, multi-target effects of gintonin on MPTP neurotoxicity were neutralized by pre-treatment with Ki16425 (**Figure 7**). The results suggest that increased LPAR1 and 3 by gintonin directly or indirectly contributed to the protective effect against MPTP neurotoxicity via multiple targets, which was supported biologically. LPARs are widely expressed in neurons, microglia, astrocytes, and endothelial cells at a higher level in pathological conditions such as traumatic brain injury, neuropsychiatric disorders, and neuropathic pain (Crack et al., 2014; Yung et al., 2015; Velasco et al., 2017). LPA signaling stabilizes Nrf2 and increases the expression of genes (NQO1 and HMOX1) involved in oxidative stress response through LPAR1 (Venkatraman et al., 2015). Nrf2 modulation in response to NF-κB activation acts as a protective mechanism against inflammation (Wardyn et al., 2015). Taken together, the data support the suggestion that gintonin might contribute to anti-dopaminergic neuronal death via multi-target effects including anti-inflammation, anti-oxidant, and maintenance of BBB integrity through direct or indirect regulation of LPAR signaling pathway. Therefore gintonin may be exploited natural product-derived medication to prevent or treat PD via multi-target effects. The precise roles of gintonin on LPA pathway in the intact and diseased nervous system remain to be determined in the future.

CONCLUSION

Most medications are available to control symptoms, because no innovative neuroprotective agents are yet available to treat multifactoral PD. Discovery of a multifunctional therapy targeting both symptomatic treatment and neuroprotection is a very attractive challenge to treat PD. Here, gintonin significantly inhibited the degeneration of dopaminergic neurons from MPTP-mediated neurotoxicity, possibly by multi-functional mechanisms including anti-dopaminergic cell death activity, anti-oxidative activity by stimulation of the Nrf2 pathway, anti-inflammatory activity by inhibition of the MAPKs and NF-κB pathways, and maintenance of BBB integrity, through the regulation of the LPA-LPARs signal pathway. Therefore, gintonin may be applied as natural product-derived multi-target drug to prevent and treat multifactoral PD.

AUTHOR CONTRIBUTIONS

JC performed the behavioral experiments, immunohistochemistry and Western blots, and prepared all figures. MJ carried out real-time PCR analysis and contributed to data interpretation. SO and S-YN contributed to draft of article and critical revision for important intellectual content. I-HC conceived all experiments, analyzed the results, and wrote the manuscript. All authors have read and approved the final manuscript.

FUNDING

This research was supported by the Brain Research Program and the Basic Science Research Program through the National Research Foundation of Korea (NRF) funded by the Ministry of Science and ICT (NRF-2017R1A2A2A05069493 and NRF-2016M3C7A1905074 for I-HC and NRF-2016M3C7A1913845 for S-YN).

SUPPLEMENTARY MATERIAL

FIGURE S1 | Gintonin do not significantly affect LPAR2 and 4–6 signaling pathways in the SNpc and striatum after MPTP injection. **(A–H)** SNpc and striatum sample (n = 3 per group) from 7 days after MPTP-injection were quantified by real-time PCR to measure the alteration in expression of LPARs. mRNA expression of LPAR2 **(A,E)**, 4 **(B,F)**, 5 **(C,G)**, and 6 **(D,H)**. SNpc **(A–D)** and striatum **(E–H)**.

FIGURE S2 | Original images of Western blots: Western blot analysis was performed using membrane strips containing specific proteins.

REFERENCES

Abbott, N. J., Ronnback, L., and Hansson, E. (2006). Astrocyte-endothelial interactions at the blood-brain barrier. *Nat. Rev. Neurosci.* 7, 41–53. doi: 10.1038/nrn1824

Alpayci, M., Bozan, N., Erdem, S., Gunes, M., and Erden, M. (2012). The possible underlying pathophysiological mechanisms for development of multiple sclerosis in familial Mediterranean fever. *Med. Hypotheses* 78, 717–720. doi: 10.1016/j.mehy.2012.02.017

Athauda, D., and Foltynie, T. (2015). The ongoing pursuit of neuroprotective therapies in Parkinson disease. *Nat. Rev. Neurol.* 11, 25–40. doi: 10.1038/nrneurol.2014.226

Bajda, M., Guzior, N., Ignasik, M., and Malawska, B. (2011). Multi-target-directed ligands in Alzheimer's disease treatment. *Curr. Med. Chem.* 18, 4949–4975. doi: 10.2174/092986711797535245

Blesa, J., Trigo-Damas, I., Quiroga-Varela, A., and Jackson-Lewis, V. R. (2015). Oxidative stress and Parkinson's disease. *Front. Neuroanat.* 9:91. doi: 10.3389/fnana.2015.00091

Calabresi, P., and Di Filippo, M. (2015). Multitarget disease-modifying therapy in Parkinson's disease? *Lancet Neurol.* 14, 975–976. doi: 10.1016/S1474-4422(15)00227-6

Cho, I. H. (2012). Effects of *Panax ginseng* in neurodegenerative diseases. *J. Ginseng Res.* 36, 342–353. doi: 10.5142/jgr.2012.36.4.342

Choi, J. H., Jang, M., Kim, E. J., Kim, H., Ye, S. K., and Cho, I. H. (2016). Oriental medicine Woohwangchungsimwon attenuates Kainic acid-induced seizures and neuronal cell death in the hippocampus. *Rejuvenation Res.* 19, 394–405. doi: 10.1089/rej.2015.1779

Choi, J. H., Jang, M., Nah, S. Y., Oh, S., and Cho, I. H. (2018). Multitarget effects of Korean red ginseng in animal model of Parkinson's disease: antiapoptosis, antioxidant, antiinflammation, and maintenance of blood–brain barrier integrity. *J. Ginseng Res.* (in press). doi: 10.1016/j.jgr.2018.01.002

Choi, J. W., Herr, D. R., Noguchi, K., Yung, Y. C., Lee, C. W., Mutoh, T., et al. (2010). LPA receptors: subtypes and biological actions. *Annu. Rev. Pharmacol. Toxicol.* 50, 157–186. doi: 10.1146/annurev.pharmtox.010909.105753

Choi, S. H., Jung, S. W., Kim, H. S., Kim, H. J., Lee, B. H., Kim, J. Y., et al. (2015a). A brief method for preparation of gintonin-enriched fraction from ginseng. *J. Ginseng Res.* 39, 398–405. doi: 10.1016/j.jgr.2015.05.002

Choi, S. H., Jung, S. W., Lee, B. H., Kim, H. J., Hwang, S. H., Kim, H. K., et al. (2015b). Ginseng pharmacology: a new paradigm based on gintonin-lysophosphatidic acid receptor interactions. *Front. Pharmacol.* 6:245. doi: 10.3389/fphar.2015.00245

Crack, P. J., Zhang, M., Morganti-Kossmann, M. C., Morris, A. J., Wojciak, J. M., Fleming, J. K., et al. (2014). Anti-lysophosphatidic acid antibodies improve traumatic brain injury outcomes. *J Neuroinflammation* 11:37. doi: 10.1186/1742-2094-11-37

Dias, K. S., and Viegas, C. Jr. (2014). Multi-target directed drugs: a modern approach for design of new drugs for the treatment of Alzheimer's disease. *Curr. Neuropharmacol.* 12, 239–255. doi: 10.2174/1570159X1203140511153200

Du, L., Zhang, Y., Chen, Y., Zhu, J., Yang, Y., and Zhang, H. L. (2017). Role of microglia in neurological disorders and their potentials as a therapeutic target. *Mol. Neurobiol.* 54, 7567–7584. doi: 10.1007/s12035-016-0245-0

Flood, P. M., Qian, L., Peterson, L. J., Zhang, F., Shi, J. S., Gao, H. M., et al. (2011). Transcriptional factor NF-kappaB as a target for therapy in Parkinson's disease. *Parkinsons Dis.* 2011:216298. doi: 10.4061/2011/216298

Franklin, K. B. J., and Paxinos, G. (2008). *The Mouse Brain in Stereotaxic Coordinates*. San Diego, CA: Elsevier.

Gubellini, P., and Kachidian, P. (2015). Animal models of Parkinson's disease: an updated overview. *Rev. Neurol.* 171, 750–761. doi: 10.1016/j.neurol.2015.07.011

Guneysel, O., Onultan, O., and Onur, O. (2008). Parkinson's disease and the frequent reasons for emergency admission. *Neuropsychiatr. Dis. Treat.* 4, 711–714. doi: 10.2147/NDT.S3007

Hwang, S. H., Lee, B. H., Choi, S. H., Kim, H. J., Jung, S. W., Kim, H. S., et al. (2015). Gintonin, a novel ginseng-derived lysophosphatidic acid receptor ligand, stimulates neurotransmitter release. *Neurosci. Lett.* 584, 356–361. doi: 10.1016/j.neulet.2014.11.007

Hwang, S. H., Shin, E. J., Shin, T. J., Lee, B. H., Choi, S. H., Kang, J., et al. (2012). Gintonin, a ginseng-derived lysophosphatidic acid receptor ligand, attenuates Alzheimer's disease-related neuropathies: involvement of non-amyloidogenic processing. *J. Alzheimers Dis.* 31, 207–223. doi: 10.3233/JAD-2012-120439

Jackson-Lewis, V., and Przedborski, S. (2007). Protocol for the MPTP mouse model of Parkinson's disease. *Nat. Protoc.* 2, 141–151. doi: 10.1038/nprot.2006.342

Jang, M., and Cho, I. H. (2016). Sulforaphane ameliorates 3-nitropropionic acid-induced striatal toxicity by activating the Keap1-Nrf2-ARE pathway and inhibiting the MAPKs and NF-kappaB pathways. *Mol. Neurobiol.* 53, 2619–2635. doi: 10.1007/s12035-015-9230-2

Jang, M., Lee, M. J., Kim, C. S., and Cho, I. H. (2013). Korean red ginseng extract attenuates 3-nitropropionic acid-induced Huntington's-like symptoms. *Evid. Based Complement. Alternat. Med.* 2013:237207. doi: 10.1155/2013/237207

Kalia, L. V., and Lang, A. E. (2015). Parkinson's disease. *Lancet* 386, 896–912. doi: 10.1016/S0140-6736(14)61393-3

Kalinderi, K., Bostantjopoulou, S., and Fidani, L. (2016). The genetic background of Parkinson's disease: current progress and future prospects. *Acta Neurol. Scand.* 134, 314–326. doi: 10.1111/ane.12563

Kim, E. K., and Choi, E. J. (2010). Pathological roles of MAPK signaling pathways in human diseases. *Biochim. Biophys. Acta* 1802, 396–405. doi: 10.1016/j.bbadis.2009.12.009

Kim, H. J., Kim, J. Y., Lee, B. H., Choi, S. H., Rhim, H., Kim, H. C., et al. (2017). Gintonin, an exogenous ginseng-derived LPA receptor ligand, promotes corneal wound healing. *J. Vet. Sci.* 18, 387–397. doi: 10.4142/jvs.2017.18.3.387

Landis, S. C., Amara, S. G., Asadullah, K., Austin, C. P., Blumenstein, R., Bradley, E. W., et al. (2012). A call for transparent reporting to optimize the predictive value of preclinical research. *Nature* 490, 187–191. doi: 10.1038/nature 11556

Lee, M. J., Jang, M., Choi, J., Chang, B. S., Kim, D. Y., Kim, S. H., et al. (2016). Korean red ginseng and ginsenoside-Rb1/-Rg1 alleviate experimental autoimmune encephalomyelitis by suppressing Th1 and Th17 cells and upregulating regulatory T cells. *Mol. Neurobiol.* 53, 1977–2002. doi: 10.1007/s12035-015-9131-4

Lee, Y. M., Yoon, H., Park, H. M., Song, B. C., and Yeum, K. J. (2017). Implications of red *Panax ginseng* in oxidative stress associated chronic diseases. *J. Ginseng Res.* 41, 113–119. doi: 10.1016/j.jgr.2016.03.003

Li, X. Z., Zhang, S. N., Liu, S. M., and Lu, F. (2013). Recent advances in herbal medicines treating Parkinson's disease. *Fitoterapia* 84, 273–285. doi: 10.1016/j.fitote.2012.12.009

Liberatore, G. T., Jackson-Lewis, V., Vukosavic, S., Mandir, A. S., Vila, M., McAuliffe, W. G., et al. (1999). Inducible nitric oxide synthase stimulates dopaminergic neurodegeneration in the MPTP model of Parkinson disease. *Nat. Med.* 5, 1403–1409. doi: 10.1038/70978

Livak, K. J., and Schmittgen, T. D. (2001). Analysis of relative gene expression data using real-time quantitative PCR and the 2(-Delta Delta C(T)) Method. *Methods* 25, 402–408. doi: 10.1006/meth.2001.1262

Lobsiger, C. S., and Cleveland, D. W. (2007). Glial cells as intrinsic components of non-cell-autonomous neurodegenerative disease. *Nat. Neurosci.* 10, 1355–1360. doi: 10.1038/nn1988

Marsden, C. D. (1994). Problems with long-term levodopa therapy for Parkinson's disease. *Clin. Neuropharmacol.* 17(Suppl. 2), S32–S44.

Nabavi, S. F., Sureda, A., Habtemariam, S., and Nabavi, S. M. (2015). Ginsenoside Rd and ischemic stroke; a short review of literatures. *J. Ginseng Res.* 39, 299–303. doi: 10.1016/j.jgr.2015.02.002

Nah, S. Y. (2012). Gintonin: a novel ginseng-derived ligand that targets G protein-coupled lysophosphatidic acid receptors. *Curr. Drug Targets* 13, 1659–1664. doi: 10.2174/138945012803529947

Newman, D. J., and Cragg, G. M. (2012). Natural products as sources of new drugs over the 30 years from 1981 to 2010. *J. Nat. Prod.* 75, 311–335. doi: 10.1021/np200906s

Noguchi, K., Herr, D., Mutoh, T., and Chun, J. (2009). Lysophosphatidic acid (LPA) and its receptors. *Curr. Opin. Pharmacol.* 9, 15–23. doi: 10.1016/j.coph.2008.11.010

Ong, W. Y., Farooqui, T., Koh, H. L., Farooqui, A. A., and Ling, E. A. (2015). Protective effects of ginseng on neurological disorders. *Front. Aging Neurosci.* 7:129. doi: 10.3389/fnagi.2015.00129

Poewe, W., Seppi, K., Tanner, C. M., Halliday, G. M., Brundin, P., Volkmann, J., et al. (2017). Parkinson disease. *Nat. Rev. Dis. Primers* 3:17013. doi: 10.1038/nrdp.2017.13

Riess, O., and Kruger, R. (1999). Parkinson's disease–a multifactorial neurodegenerative disorder. *J. Neural Transm. Suppl.* 56, 113–125. doi: 10.1007/978-3-7091-6360-3_6

Saba, E., Jeon, B. R., Jeong, D. H., Lee, K., Goo, Y. K., Kwak, D., et al. (2015). A novel Korean red ginseng compound gintonin inhibited inflammation by MAPK and NF-kappaB pathways and recovered the levels of mir-34a and mir-93 in RAW 264.7 Cells. *Evid. Based Complement. Alternat. Med.* 2015, 624132. doi: 10.1155/2015/624132

Sandoval, K. E., and Witt, K. A. (2008). Blood-brain barrier tight junction permeability and ischemic stroke. *Neurobiol. Dis.* 32, 200–219. doi: 10.1016/j.nbd.2008.08.005

Shulman, J. M., De Jager, P. L., and Feany, M. B. (2011). Parkinson's disease: genetics and pathogenesis. *Annu. Rev. Pathol.* 6, 193–222. doi: 10.1146/annurev-pathol-011110-130242

Todorovic, M., Wood, S. A., and Mellick, G. D. (2016). Nrf2: a modulator of Parkinson's disease? *J. Neural Transm.* 123, 611–619. doi: 10.1007/s00702-016-1563-0

Velasco, M., O'Sullivan, C., and Sheridan, G. K. (2017). Lysophosphatidic acid receptors (LPARs): potential targets for the treatment of neuropathic pain. *Neuropharmacology* 113(Pt B), 608–617. doi: 10.1016/j.neuropharm.2016.04.002

Venkatraman, G., Benesch, M. G., Tang, X., Dewald, J., McMullen, T. P., and Brindley, D. N. (2015). Lysophosphatidate signaling stabilizes Nrf2 and increases the expression of genes involved in drug resistance and oxidative stress responses: implications for cancer treatment. *FASEB J.* 29, 772–785. doi: 10.1096/fj.14-262659

Wardyn, J. D., Ponsford, A. H., and Sanderson, C. M. (2015). Dissecting molecular cross-talk between Nrf2 and NF-kappaB response pathways. *Biochem. Soc. Trans.* 43, 621–626. doi: 10.1042/BST20150014

Yung, Y. C., Stoddard, N. C., and Chun, J. (2014). LPA receptor signaling: pharmacology, physiology, and pathophysiology. *J. Lipid Res.* 55, 1192–1214. doi: 10.1194/jlr.R046458

Yung, Y. C., Stoddard, N. C., Mirendil, H., and Chun, J. (2015). Lysophosphatidic Acid signaling in the nervous system. *Neuron* 85, 669–682. doi: 10.1016/j.neuron.2015.01.009

Zhao, X., Chen, R., Liu, M., Feng, J., Chen, J., and Hu, K. (2017). Remodeling the blood-brain barrier microenvironment by natural products for brain tumor therapy. *Acta Pharm. Sin. B* 7, 541–553. doi: 10.1016/j.apsb.2017.07.002

Zheng, H., Fridkin, M., and Youdim, M. (2014). From single target to multitarget/network therapeutics in Alzheimer's therapy. *Pharmaceuticals* 7, 113–135. doi: 10.3390/ph7020113

Zlokovic, B. V. (2008). The blood-brain barrier in health and chronic neurodegenerative disorders. *Neuron* 57, 178–201. doi: 10.1016/j.neuron.2008.01.003

8

Lavandula stoechas (L) a Very Potent Antioxidant Attenuates Dementia in Scopolamine Induced Memory Deficit Mice

Aamir Mushtaq[1,2]*, *Rukhsana Anwar*[1] *and Mobasher Ahmad*[1,2]

[1] *Department of Pharmacology, Punjab University College of Pharmacy, University of the Punjab, Lahore, Pakistan,* [2] *Gulab Devi Institute of Pharmacy, Gulab Devi Educational Complex, Lahore, Pakistan*

Correspondence:
Aamir Mushtaq
aamir_mushtaq@hotmail.com

The objective of the current project was to explore the pharmacotherapeutic role of *Lavandula stoechas* (L) for the management of dementia. Dementia is considered a global challenge of current century seeking special attention of pharmacologists to explore its best remedies. Methanolic extract of aerial parts of *L. stoechas* was tested for phytochemical analysis along with free radical scavenging activity. Behavioral studies were performed on scopolamine induced amnesic mice by using elevated plus maze (EPM), light and dark test and hole board paradigms. Biochemical investigations were made after decapitating the mice. Their brains were isolated for biochemical estimation of acetylcholinesterase (AChE), malondialdehyde (MDA), superoxide dismutase (SOD), catalase (CAT), and glutathione (GSH). Phytochemical study ensured the presence of total phenolic contents (285.91 $\pm$ 0.75 mg of GAE/g of extract), total flavonoids (134.06 $\pm$ 0.63 mg of RE/g of extract), total tannins (149.60 $\pm$ 0.93 mg of TAE/g of extract) and free radical scavenging activity (IC_{50} value = 76.73 μg/ml found by DPPH method). Behavioral studies indicated that animals of GVII showed higher inflexion ratio (0.40 $\pm$ 0.03) for EPM, spent most of time (227.17 $\pm$ 2.13 s) in dark area of light dark test and had many hole pockings (39.83 $\pm$ 1.88) for hole board paradigm. Moreover, biochemical studies revealed that methanolic extract of *L. stoechas* (800 mg/kg/p.o.) significantly ($P < 0.001$) reduced brain AChE and MDA levels while improved SOD, CAT, and GSH levels. Thus the findings suggest that *L. stoechas* stabilizes memory by enhancing cholinergic neurotransmission and by providing defense against oxidative stress in mice brain.

Keywords: dementia, neurodegeneration, AChE, *L. stoechas*, elevated plus maze

INTRODUCTION

Dementia results from neurodegenerative insult in brain neurons. Neurodegeneration not only leads to the impairment of memory but also alters the social and behavioral compliance. Cholinergic hypothesis (Francis et al., 1999) describes the pathogenesis of dementia, according to which severity of the disease is coupled with neuronal damages in septohippocampal cholinergic system (Giovannini et al., 1997) associated with learning and cognitions (Ballard et al., 2005). Acetyl cholinesterase inhibitors like donepezil, galantamine, rivastigmine (Bejar et al., 1999) and tacrine can be used for the symptomatic management of mild dementia but they have little therapeutic success because they do not prevent neurodegeneration and are associated with serious adverse effects (Hake, 2001). Herbal remedies are considered more safe, gentle and reliable in enhancing memory and cognitive functions (Bhattacharjee et al., 2015). Roughly, 150 traditional plants and herbs have been used so for, either singly or in combined preparations to stop neurodegeneration in brain (Adams et al., 2007). This is of great worth to identify the active constituent for the management of dementia and cognitive disorders which will definitely enhance the practice of customary herbs in the field of neuropharmacology (Kumar et al., 2012).

Lavandula stoechas L. (Lamiaceae) has been extensively used by traditional healers for the management of CNS disorders including epilepsy, dementia, and migraine (Hakeem et al., 1991). This is also known as the broom of the brain. Its aerial parts have been extensively studied for phytochemical work (Gilani et al., 2000). The present research work was aimed to explore the pharmacological basis of enhancement of memory to strengthen the folk and traditional use of *L. stoechas* as a memory enhancer.

MATERIALS AND METHODS

Drugs and Chemicals

Acetic acid (71251), 2,2-diphenyl-1-picrylhydrazyl (DPPH) (D9132), acetyl thiocholine iodide (A22300), carboxy methyl cellulose (CMC) (419273), 5,5′-dithiobis-2-nitrobenzoic acid (DTNB) (D218200), aluminum chloride (563919), ascorbic acid (A0278), chloroform (C2432), ethanol (E7023), Folin-Ciocalteu reagent (FCR) (F9252), gallic acid (G7384), methanol (34860), *n*-butanol, nitro blue tetrazolium (NBT) (N5514), phenyl methanesulfonate (PMS) (495085), superoxide dismutase (SOD) (S9697), hydrogen peroxide (H_2O_2) (16911), potassium acetate (P1190), potassium dichromate (P5271), reduced nicotinamide adenine dinucleotide (NADH) (N8129), rutin (R5143), sodium carbonate (S7795), sodium dodecyl sulfate (436143), tannic acid (403040), trichloracetic acid (TCA) (T6399) and thiobarbituric acid (TBA) (T5500) all were procured from Sigma-Aldrich, Ms Traders, Lahore Pakistan. Piracetam and scopolamine was donated by Jiangxi Yuehua Pharmaceutical, China and Merck Pharmaceutical Pvt. Ltd. Pakistan, respectively, upon special request. All chemicals of analytical grades were used in this research.

Preparation of Plant Extract

Dried aerial parts of *L. stoechas* were purchased from local market of Lahore, Pakistan and were identified by Department of Botany GC-University, Lahore. Plant specimen was preserved in herbarium with voucher number GC.Herb.Bot.3386. For extraction, dried aerial parts were ground into coarse size powder and 1 kg of it was soaked into 5 L methanol (99.5%) in glass jar for 3 days. It was then filtered first by muslin cloth and then through Whatman No. 1 filter paper. Filtrate was concentrated in buchi rotavapor and residue was again macerated in recovered methanol for another 3 days. In this way, after three consecutive soakings concentrated filtrates were mixed up and dried in dry heat oven at 37°C. Finally dark green colored thick extract was obtained which was labeled after sealing in glass jar and put into refrigerator at 4°C temperature. Percentage yield was calculated as;

$$\% \text{ Age yield} = \text{Weight of extract (g)/Weight of plant material (g)} \times 100$$

Phytochemical Analysis of Plant Extract

Preliminary phytochemical testing of *L. stoechas* methanolic extract was performed to explore the major phytochemical classes actually responsible for anti-oxidant and anti-amnesic activities. Proteins, carbohydrates, alkaloids, glycosides, flavonoids, steroids, terpenoids, saponins, tannins, phenols, quinones, phytosterol, terpenes, and fixed oil were tested qualitatively (Mushtaq et al., 2013).

Estimation of Phenolic Contents

Total phenolic contents of plant extract were determined by using FCR as described by Kumaran and Karunakaran (2007). For determination of total phenols sample solution was prepared by mixing 100 μl of *L. stoechas* methanolic extract (100 μg/ml), 500 μl of FCR and 1.5 ml of 20% sodium carbonate. Solution was shaken vigorously in vortex mixer after making the volume of solution 10 ml by adding distilled water and mixture was incubated for 2 h. Similarly, standard solution was prepared by adding 100 μl of different dilutions of gallic acid (50, 100, 150, 200, 250, 300, 350, and 400 μg/ml) separately in reaction mixture instead of *L. stoechas* extract. Then absorbance of both sample and standard solutions were determined at 765 nm against blank. All readings were taken in triplicates and total phenolic contents in plant extract were expressed as gallic acid equivalent (GAE) by drawing gallic acid calibration curve. Following formula was used to find total phenol contents in plant extract; $C = Ci \times V/W$

C = total phenolic content in mg/g, Ci = concentration of gallic acid established from calibration curve in mg/ml, V = volume of extract in ml, and W = weight of plant extract in gram.

Estimation of Total Flavonoids

Flavonoid contents were found by using aluminum chloride method as proposed by Kumaran and Karunakaran (2007). Stock solutions were prepared separately by taking 0.5 ml of plant extract (1 mg/ml) and standard rutin (10–100 μg/ml). To each test tube, 1.5 ml of methanol, 0.10 ml potassium acetate, 0.10 ml aluminum chloride and 2.8 ml distilled water was added with constant shaking. All solutions were filtered and absorbance was taken at 510 nm. A calibration curve was drawn for rutin and total flavonoid contents were found as mg rutin equivalents (RE)/g dry extract.

Estimation of Total Tannins

Tannins in plant extract were determined by modified Folin-Ciocalteu's method by preparing 0.1 ml standard tannic acid solutions of different dilutions (50, 100, 150, 200, 250, 300, 400, and 500 μg/ml). Sample solution was prepared by taking 0.1 ml of *L. stoechas* methanotic extract (200 μg/ml). To each test tube,

FCR (0.5 ml) and 35% sodium carbonate (1 ml) were mixed and final volume was made 10 ml by adding distilled water. All the test tubes were shaken and kept at room temperature for half an hour and absorbance was read at 725 nm against a blank. Tannic acid calibration curve was drawn and total tannin contents of extract were expressed as mg tannic acid equivalent/g of extract (Polshettiwar et al., 2007).

In vitro Antioxidant Activity

DPPH Free Radical Scavenging Assay

Antioxidant activity of *L. stoechas* methanolic extract was determined by using DPPH free radical scavenging assay developed by Blois (1958). Methanolic solution of DPPH (1.0 mmol/L) was prepared in volumetric flask, covered with aluminum foil and put into dark place after marking as reagent stock solution. Different solutions of plant extract and standard ascorbic acid (1 ml each) having concentrations (20, 40, 60, 80, 100, and 200 μg/ml) were prepared separately in test tubes. Then, 2 ml of reagent stock solution was put into each test tube, mixed on vortex and incubated for 30 min, at 37°C in dark place. Blank solution was prepared in the same way having all the ingredients except test substances. The absorbance of blank and all test solutions was measured at 517 nm by using UV-Vis spectrophotometer. Percentage scavenging activity was determined by applying following formula:

$$\text{Radical scavenging (\%)} = \text{Absorbance of Blank} - \text{Absorbance of Sample} \times 100/\text{Absorbance of Blank}$$

Experimental Animals

Male Swiss albino mice (20–25 g) were used in this study. They were housed in polycarbonate cages in animal house of Punjab University College of Pharmacy, University of the Punjab, Lahore. Special permission regarding animal ethics was obtained from research ethics committee of the institute with diary number AEC/PUCP/1072. The animals were provided with standard living conditions (temperature; 25 ± 2°C, humidity; 50 ± 5% and 12:12 light/dark span) and had free access of standard pellet diet and water *ad libitum.* Animals were acclimatized in lab and were trained for all three paradigms for 1 week before the start of behavioral experiments.

Study Design

Mice were divided into seven groups (n = 6) and were treated accordingly as shown in **Table 1**.

Behavioral Studies

All behavioral experiments were performed in sound proof room in dim day light and mice were put apart to avoid acoustic and visual disturbances. Observations were recorded by using digital camera connected with computer monitor.

Elevated Plus Maze

Elevated plus maze (EPM) is considered the most reliable paradigm for evaluation of memory (Pahaye et al., 2017), which was made up of two poly acrylic sheets joined together in shape of plus sign in such a way that it had two open arms (16 cm × 5 cm), two closed arms (16 cm × 5 cm × 12 cm) and a central platform (5 cm × 5 cm). Apparatus was put on a wooden stand elevated 25 cm from floor (Kulkarni et al., 2011). Mouse was put on open arm by facing it away from central platform and time taken (s) by it to move in any of closed arm with all its four legs was recorded and then returned into its home cage. Each animal was given maximum 90 s to explore the apparatus. If it failed to find closed arms for given time then it was pushed into closed arm with its tale and latency time was marked as 90 s for that animal. Initial transfer latency was observed after 45 min of administration of scopolamine and retention of latency was recorded after 24 h of administration of scopolamine and inflexion ratio (IR) (Kasture et al., 2007) was calculated by following formula; $IR = (L_0 - L_1)/L_0$ where, IR = inflexion ratio, L_0 is initial transfer latency (s) and L_1 is retention transfer latency in seconds.

Light and Dark Test Apparatus

This paradigm is used for the evaluation of learning tasks as proposed by Barry et al. (1987), which is based upon the principle that rodents prefer to live in dark compartment. Apparatus was made up of poly acrylic sheets and had two compartments; larger (30 cm × 30 cm × 35 cm) transparent chamber separated from smaller chamber (20 cm × 30 cm × 35 cm) which was colored black to make it dark. Both chambers had small opening (5 cm × 5 cm) in the middle bottom of separating wall for entrance. The floor of both chambers was marked by lines each 1 mm apart. Mouse was put in the light chamber and was observed carefully for 5 min to record the time spent in each chamber. According to study designs, the animals were given doses and observations were recorded by using light and dark test apparatus for 2 days after the completion of last dose.

Hole Board Test

For assessment of learning behavior, hole board test paradigm (Durcan and Lister, 1988) was used with minor modification (Hossain and Uma Devi, 2001) which was composed of rectangular shaped, poly acrylic box (35 cm × 45 cm × 45 cm). Black colored sheet contained sixteen holes (2 cm diameter and at equal distance) was supported on corners, 5 cm above the bottom of box. The animal was put in the middle of box and observed for 5 min to record number of hole pokings. Animals were given doses according to the protocols of study design and then observations were recorded for two consecutive days.

Biochemical Assessment

After performance of behavioral tests the animals were given anesthesia by using chloroform and were decapitated to isolate brains. Each brain was rinsed with ice cold normal saline after weighing it and 20 mg of it was homogenized in 1 ml ice cold phosphate buffer (pH 7.4.) by using tissue homogenizer. To separate out the nuclear debris, the homogenized mixture was then centrifuged for 5 min at 69.40 × g by keeping the temperature 4°C. Supernatant was again centrifuged for 20 min at 1,0845 × g at the same temperature and supernatant thus obtained was used for biochemical tests (Rajesh et al., 2017).

TABLE 1 | Study design.

No.	Treatment from day 1 to day 7	Treatment on day 7th, 45 min after administration of the last dose
G-I (Normal Control)	Normal saline 10 ml/kg/p.o.	–
G-II (Amnesic Control)	5% CMC 10 ml/kg/p.o.	Scopolamine (10 mg/kg/p.o.)
G-III (Standard Control-A)	Piracetam 200 mg/kg/p.o.	–
G-IV (Standard Control-B)	Piracetam 200 mg/kg/p.o.	Scopolamine (10 mg/kg/p.o.)
G-V (Experimental Control-I)	meL.s 200 mg/kg/p.o.	Scopolamine (10 mg/kg/p.o.)
G-VI (Experimental Control-II)	meL.s 400 mg/kg/p.o.	Scopolamine (10 mg/kg/p.o.)
G-VII (Experimental Control-III)	meL.s 800 mg/kg/p.o.	Scopolamine (10 mg/kg/p.o.)

Scopolamine and piracetam were dissolved in normal saline while L. stoechas was suspended in 5% CMC for dose preparation. Then animals were subjected to elevated plus maze (EPM), light and dark test apparatus and hole board test apparatus for behavioral assessment.

Acetylcholinesterase (AChE) Activity

Ellman's method was used for estimation of AChE level for which 0.4 ml of supernatant was taken in cuvette already contained 2.6 ml of phosphate buffer (0.1 M/L, pH; 8) and 100 μL of 5,5′-dithiobis-2-nitrobenzoic acid. The reaction mixture was thoroughly mixed and absorbance was recorded several times by using UV-Vis spectrophotometer at 412 nm. Then 20 μL of acetyl thiocholine iodide was added as substrate in the reaction mixture and variations in absorbance were recorded five times at 2 min interval and finally change in absorbance per min was found (Ellman et al., 1961). Then following formula was applied to find level of AChE;

$$R = 5.74 \times 10^{-4} \times A/CO$$

R is the rate (moles) of substrate hydrolyzed/min/g of brain tissue, A is change in absorbance per min, and CO is original concentration (20 mg/ml) of tissue.

Assessment of Malondialdehyde (MDA) Level in Brain

The level of malondialdehyde (MDA) was determined by mixing 100 μL of brain homogenates with 1.5 ml of TBA (0.8% w/v), 1.5 ml of acetic acid (20% v/v) and 200 μL of sodium dodecyl sulfate (8% w/v). The reaction mixture was heated at 95°C for 1 h and then 5 mL of *n*-butanol was added to mixture after cooling it at room temperature. Mixture was centrifuged at 976 × *g* for 10 min and organic layer formed at top was collected for which the absorbance was measured at 532 nm (Xian et al., 2011). The following formula was used to find the concentration of MDA in brain.

$$\text{MDA } (\mu\text{M}) = A \text{ (sample)} \times DF/I \times \varepsilon$$

I = light path = 1 cm, ε = molar absorptivity = 1.56×10^5 $M^{-10}cm^{-1}$ and DF = dilution factor = 21.

Measurement of Superoxide Dismutase (SOD) Level

The level of SOD was found by diluting brain homogenate (0.5 ml) with distilled water (1 ml) which was then added chilled ethanol (2.5 ml) and chloroform (1.5 ml). Mixture was well shaken and centrifuged for 1 min at 4°C. The supernatant was mixed with 1.2 ml of (0.025 M, pH 8.4) sodium pyrophosphate buffer, 0.3 ml of 30 μM NBT, 0.1 ml of 186 μM PMS, 0.2 ml of 780 μM of reduced nicotinamide adenine dinucleotide (NADH) and 3 ml of distilled water. The reaction mixture was incubated for 90 s at 30°C and the reaction which was initiated by addition of NADH was stopped by subsequent addition of glacial acetic acid (1 ml). Reaction mixture was vigorously stirred and then mixed with *n*-butanol by gentle shaking. Butanol layer was separated out and absorbance was measured at 560 nm against butanol blank. Amount of SOD was expressed as unit/mg of protein (Kakkar et al., 1984).

Measurement of Catalase (CAT) Activity

Catalase (CAT) activity was found by mixing tissue homogenate (0.1 ml) with 1.0 ml of 0.01 M phosphate buffer (pH 7.0) and 0.4 ml of 2 M H_2O_2. Then 2 ml of dichromate acetic acid reagent composed of 5% potassium dichromate and glacial acetic acid in ratio 1:3 was added in reaction mixture to stop the reaction and absorbance was taken at 620 nm. CAT activity was expressed as μM of H_2O_2 decomposed/min/mg of protein (Sinha, 1972).

Determination of Glutathione (GSH) Activity

Brain homogenate (0.4 ml) was mixed with 0.4 ml of 20% TCA and mixture was centrifuged at 10,000 × *g* for 20 min at 4°C. The supernatant (0.25 ml) was then added 0.6 M DTNB (2 ml) and phosphate buffer (0.2 M, pH 8.0) was used to make final volume of 3 ml. Then absorbance was read at 412 nm against blank. Standard calibration curve was made by using different concentrations of glutathione (GSH) (10–50 μM) by dissolving in TCA (0.4 ml) and concentration of GSH in brain was expressed as μM/mg of tissue protein (Moron et al., 1979).

Statistical Analysis

The data were expressed as mean ± SEM. Student's *t*-test analysis was applied on data with paired comparisons and multiple comparisons were made by ANOVA followed by Dunnett's test by using GraphPad Prism software version 7. Value of $P < 0.05$ was marked as significant.

RESULTS

Percentage Yield of Plant Extract

Simple methanolic extraction of *L. stoechas* gave 220 g semi solid extract per 1,000 g of dried powdered plant material and hence % age yield was 22% w/w.

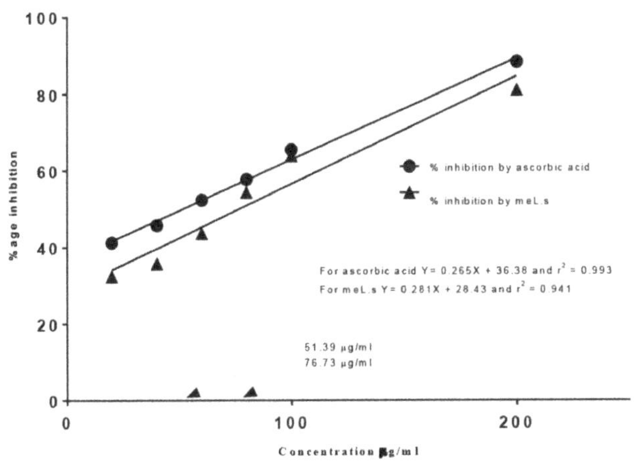

FIGURE 1 | Free radical scavenging activity of meL.s and standard (ascorbic acid) along with their IC_{50} values.

Phytochemical Constituents

Qualitative phytochemical analysis of methanolic extract of *L. stoechas* (meL.s) showed the presence of following constituents as expressed in **Table 2**.

Quantitative Analysis of Bioactive Constituents of Methanolic Extract of *L. stoechas* (meL.s)

Total phenolic, flavonoid, and tannin contents in methanolic extract of *L. stoechas* (meL.s) were found to be 285.91 ± 0.75 mg of GAE/g of extract, 134.06 ± 0.63 mg of RE/g of extract and 149.60 ± 0.93 mg of TAE/g of dried plant extract, respectively.

TABLE 2 | Phytochemical analysis of methanolic extract of *Lavandula stoechas* (meL.s).

No.	Phytochemical constituents	Tests	Presence
1	Proteins	Ninhydrin test	++
2	Carbohydrates	Molish test	+
3	Alkaloids	Hagers's test	++
		Wagner's test	++
		Dragendroff's test	+
		Mayer's test	++
4	Glycosides	Killer-Kiliani test	+
5	Flavonoids	Alkaline reagent test	+
6	Steroids	Ring test	+
7	Terpenoids		+
8	Saponins	Foam test	+
9	Tannins	Ferric chloride test	+
10	Phenols	FC method	++
11	Quinones		–
12	Phytosterol	Liebermann–Burchard test	++
13	Terpenes	Salkowski test	+
14	Fixed oils	Spot test	–

+, present; ++, highly present; and –, absent.

Free Radical Scavenging Activity

Free radical scavenging activity found by DPPH assay indicated that IC_{50} value for methanolic extract of *L. stoechas* (meL.s) was 76.73 µg/ml and that of standard ascorbic acid it was 51.39 µg/ml as shown in **Figure 1**. Moreover, considering yield of extract, it was calculated that 1 mg of crude plant powder was equal to 220 µg of meL.s.

Effect of Methanolic Extract of *L. stoechas* (meL.s) on Transfer Latency (TL) in EPM Paradigm

Initial transfer latency (ITL) was recorded on day 7th of treatment (45 min after administration of scopolamine) which reflected the learning behavior of animal while, retention transfer latency (RTL) was noted after 24 h of administration of last dose which exhibited retention of learning tasks. Inflexion ratio was calculated from transfer latencies which indicated the improvement of memories in mice. It was observed that ITL and RTL values of Group-II (amnesic control) were significantly ($P < 0.001$) high from values of Group-I (normal control) which clearly indicated the loss of memory in amnesic group. Standard control, meL.s 400 mg/kg/p.o. and meL.s 800 mg/kg/p.o. significantly ($P < 0.001$) reduced the time spent by animal in open arms as compared to Group-II which indicated improvement of memory as shown in **Figure 2A**. Similarly, RTL values of Groups-III to VII were significantly less ($P < 0.001$) than values of Group-II which indicated the retention of memory by animals as shown in **Figure 2B**. Inflexion ratios of Group-IV and VII were 0.44 ± 0.04 and 0.40 ± 0.03, respectively, which were significantly ($p < 0.001$) higher than amnesic group having IR = −0.20 ± 0.03. While Group V and VI have IR = 0.11 ± 0.05 and 0.17 ± 0.03, respectively, as shown in **Figure 2C**.

Effect of Methanolic Extract of *L. stoechas* (meL.s) on Time Spent in Light and Dark Compartment

Effect of meL.s on time spent in both compartments of light and dark paradigm is shown in **Figure 3**. Animals in Group-I spent less time in light compartment and remained most of time in dark compartment. Time spent by animals in light compartment was significantly increased ($P < 0.001$) in Group-II as compared to Group-I animals. Similarly, animals in Groups III-VII spent most of the time in dark arena both on first and second day which indicated that they significantly ($P < 0.001$) improved memory as compared to amnesic group.

Effect of Methanolic Extract of *L. stoechas* (meL.s) on Number of Hole Pokings in Hole Board Paradigm

It has been observed that no of hole pokings by mice in amnesic group was significantly ($P < 0.001$) reduced as compared to normal control group which indicated induction of amnesia. However, Groups-IV and VII significantly ($P < 0.001$) increased

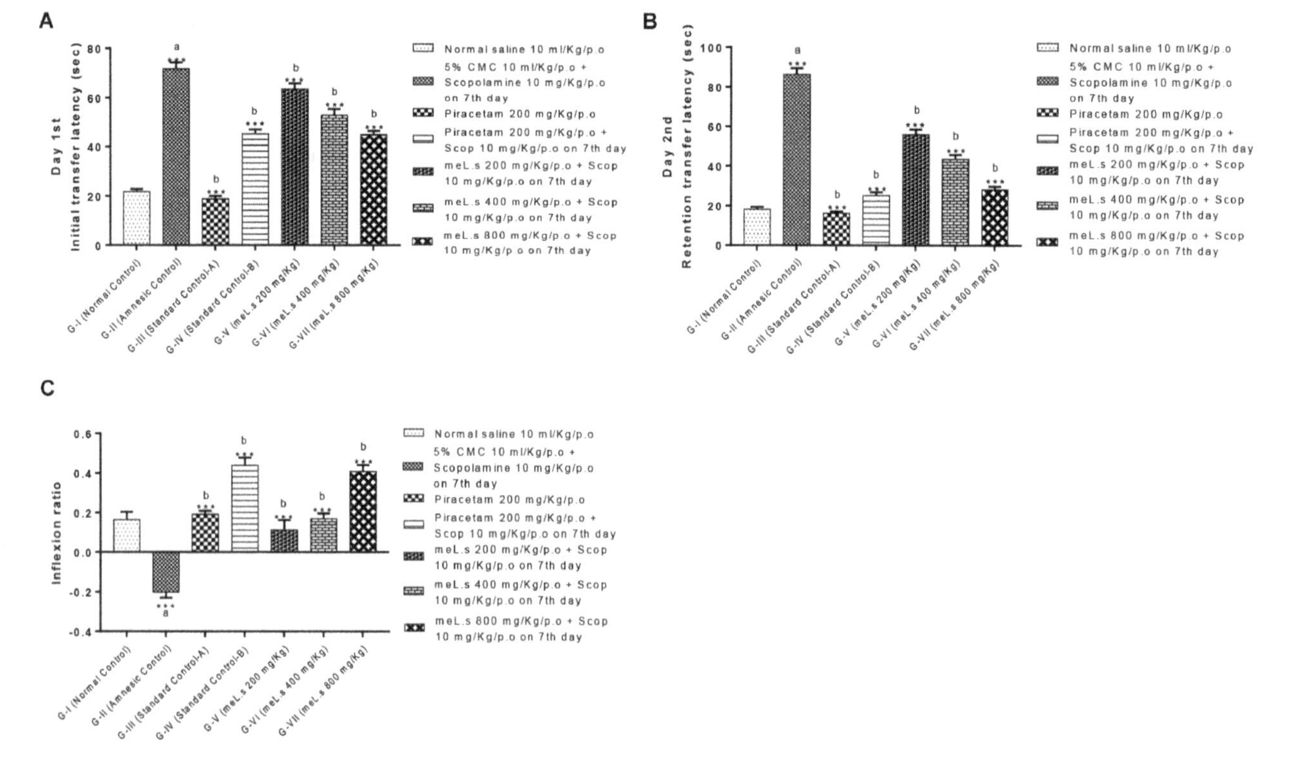

FIGURE 2 | Effect of meL.s on **(A)** initial transfer latency, **(B)** retention transfer latency, and **(C)** Inflexion ratio in elevated plus maze paradigm. All values were expressed as mean ± SEM with $n = 6$ per group. One-way ANOVA followed by Dunnett's test was applied on data set and G-II was compared with G-I (presented by sign "a" on bar) while other groups (G-III to G-VII) were compared with G-II (presented by sign "b" on bars). Value of $P \geq 0.05$ was shown by marking "ns" while P-values ≤0.05, ≤0.01, and ≤0.001 were expressed as *, **, and ***, respectively.

no of hole pokings as compared to Group-II. Groups V–VI produced non-significant changes in hole pokings both at day 1st and 2nd. All details are shown in **Figure 4** which indicated that meL.s 800 mg/kg/p.o. was more effective than both of its lower doses.

Effect of Methanolic Extract of *L. stoechas* (meL.s) on Concentration of Acetylcholinesterase (AChE) in Mice Brain

Group-II animals significantly ($P < 0.001$) increased the level of AChE as compared to normal control animals. However, pretreatment of animals with standard drug piracetam and plant extract in different doses showed marked reduction in level of AChE. Among treatment groups meL.s 800 mg/kg/p.o. caused maximum reduction in the level of AChE which was significantly ($P < 0.001$) less than the amnesic group. The details are given in **Figure 5A**.

Effect of Methanolic Extract of *L. stoechas* (meL.s) on MDA, SOD, CAT, and GSH Levels in Mice Brain

It was observed that administration of scopolamine to Group-II animals significantly ($P < 0.001$) increased the level of MDA in brain while SOD, CAT, and GSH levels were declined in comparison to normal control group. A significant ($P < 0.001$) reduction in MDA and elevation in SOD, CAT, and GSH level was observed in animals treated with standard drug piracetam in comparison to Group-II animals. Pretreatment of animals with meL.s 800 mg/kg/p.o. significantly decreased the MDA contents of mice brain while SOD and GSH were significantly ($P < 0.001$) improved as compared to groups treated with same extract in low doses but CAT level was non-significantly improved by it. From **Figure 5** it is clear that meL.s 200 mg/kg/p.o. did not increase the level of SOD, GSH, and CAT while meL.s 400 mg/kg/p.o. produced less significant ($P < 0.05$) results as compared to amnesic group. Similarly, 800 mg/kg/p.o. non-significantly improved the CAT level. The detailed results of biochemical markers are shown in **Figures 5B–E**.

DISCUSSION

Neurodegeneration in the brain, initially results into loss of short term memory (Burns and Iliffe, 2009) which progresses toward disorientation speech, mood swing, social withdrawals, altered behavioral patterns and ultimately death (Todd et al., 2013) due to loss of cognition over a time span of a decade or more (Alzheimer's Association Report, 2017). Cholinergic hypothesis best narrates the pathogenesis of dementia by loss of

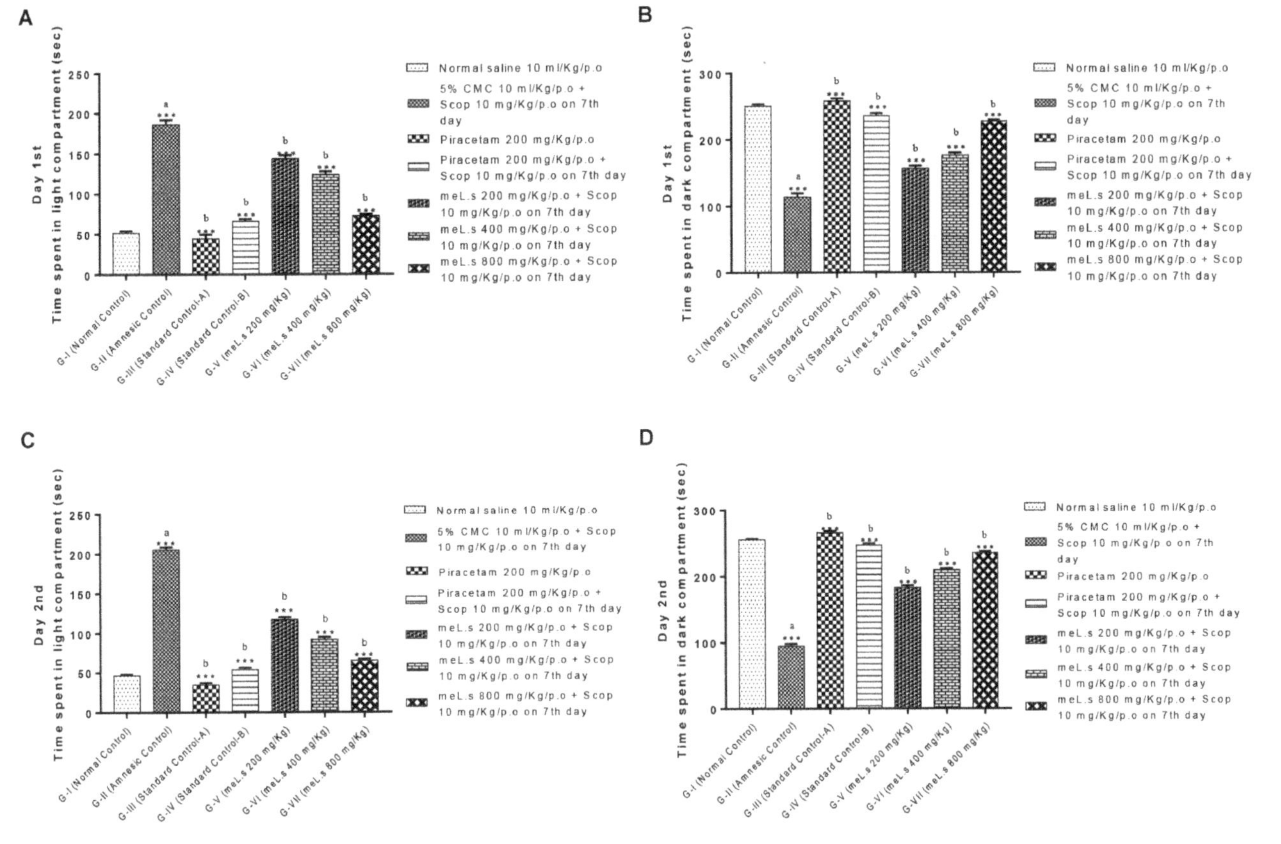

FIGURE 3 | Effect of meL.s on **(A)** time spent (s) in light compartment on day 1st, **(B)** time spent (s) in dark compartment on day 1st, **(C)** time spent (s) in light compartment on day 2nd, and **(D)** time spent (s) in dark compartment on day 2nd. All values were expressed as mean ± SEM with $n = 6$ per group. One-way ANOVA followed by Dunnett's test was applied on data set and G-II was compared with G-I (presented by sign "a" on bar) while other groups (G-III to G-VII) were compared with G-II (presented by sign "b" on bars). Value of $P \geq 0.05$ was shown by marking "ns" while P-values ≤ 0.05, ≤ 0.01, and ≤ 0.001 were expressed as *, **, and ***, respectively.

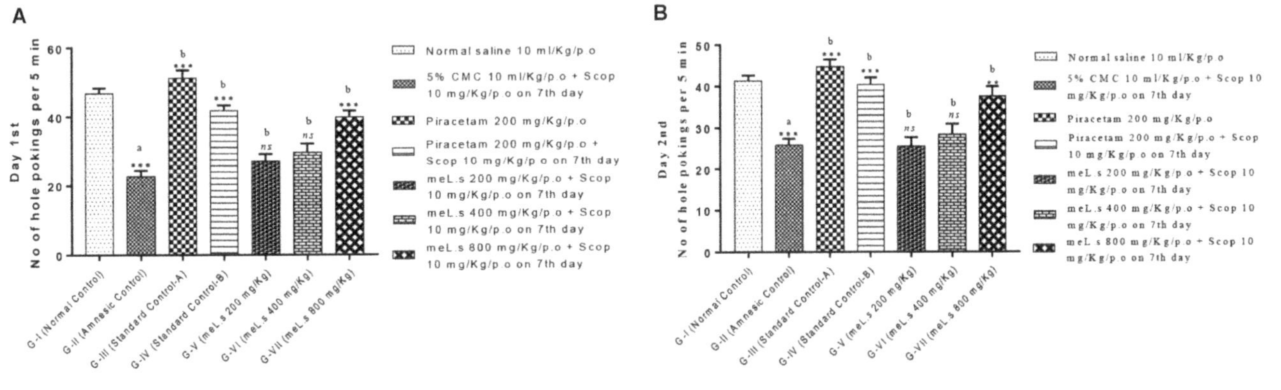

FIGURE 4 | Effect of meL.s on **(A)** no of hole pokings by mice on day 1st and **(B)** no of hole pokings by mice on day 2nd. All values were expressed as mean ± SEM with $n = 6$ per group. One-way ANOVA followed by Dunnett's test was applied on data set and G-II was compared with G-I (presented by sign "a" on bar) while other groups (G-III to G-VII) were compared with G-II (presented by sign "b" on bars). Value of $P \geq 0.05$ was shown by marking "ns" while P-values ≤ 0.05, ≤ 0.01, and ≤ 0.001 were expressed as *, **, and ***, respectively.

cholinergic innervations in frontal cortex, cingulated gyrus and hippocampus of the brain (Wenk, 2003). Similarly, accumulation of β-amyloid protein and extra neuronal plaque formation due to severe oxidative damage (Da Silva Filho et al., 2017; Omar et al., 2017) are main causes of memory loss (Hardy and Higgins, 1992; Wilson and Binder, 1997; Da Silva Filho et al., 2017). It has been roughly estimated that oxidative stress is responsible for pathogenesis of more than hundred

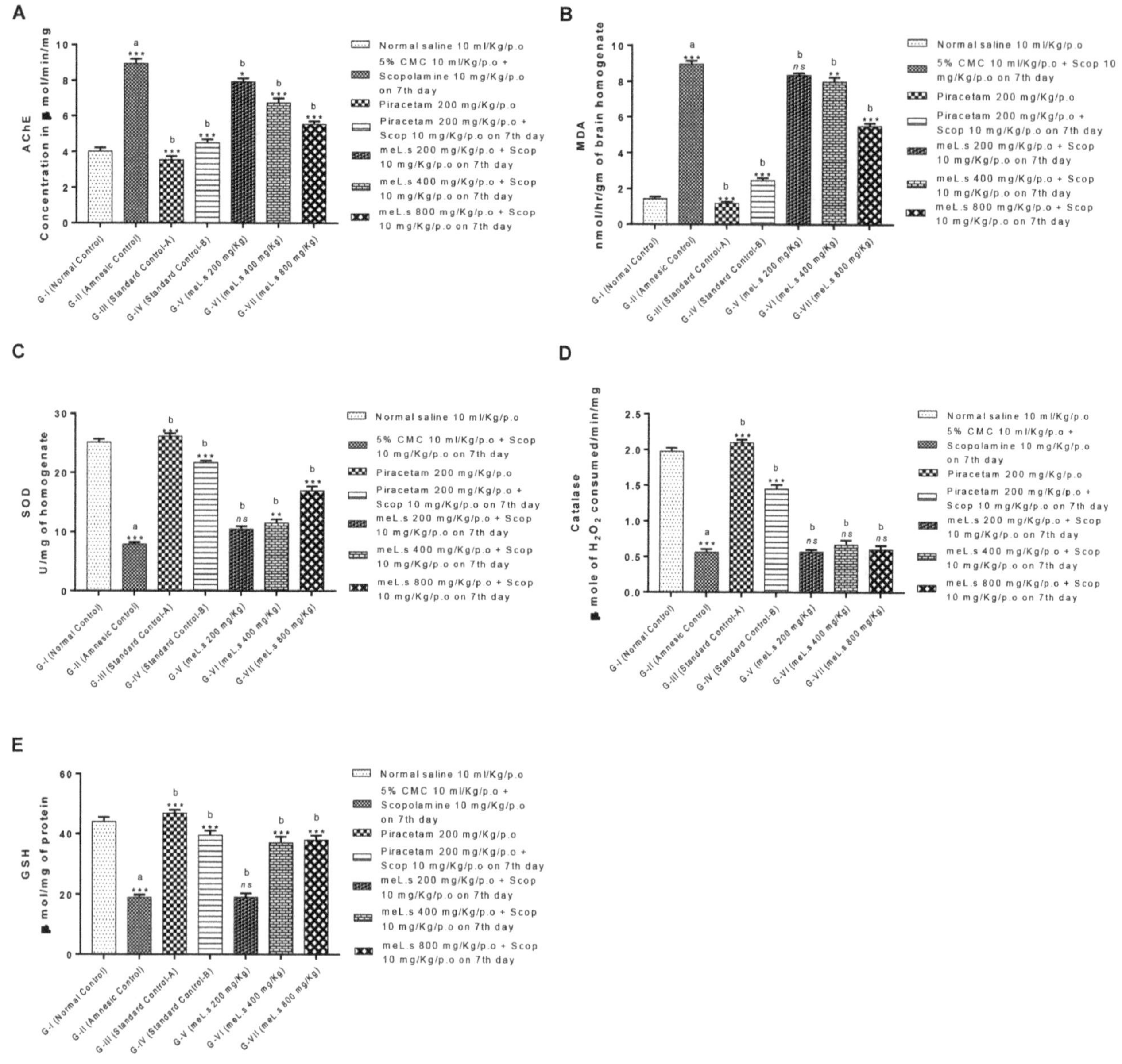

FIGURE 5 | Effect of meL.s on concentration of **(A)** acetylcholinesterase (AChE), **(B)** MDA, **(C)** SOD, **(D)** CAT, and **(E)** GSH in brain homogenate. All values were expressed as mean ± SEM with $n = 6$ per group. One-way ANOVA followed by Dunnett's test was applied on data set and G-II was compared with G-I (presented by sign "a" on bar) while other groups (G-III to G-VII) were compared with G-II (presented by sign "b" on bars). Value of $P \geq 0.05$ was shown by marking "ns" while P-values ≤ 0.05, ≤ 0.01, and ≤ 0.001 were expressed as *, **, and ***, respectively.

diseases (McCord, 2000) including dementia (Pratico, 2008). Anticholinergic drugs especially scopolamine disrupt both short term and working memory by muscarinic blockade of neurons and hence can be employed for induction of amnesia in rodents to evaluate antiamnesic activity of an agent (Baxter et al., 2013). In contrary, agents enhancing cholinergic neuronal activity in brain and those preventing oxidative stress in brain can be used to prevent progression of dementia (Rabiei et al., 2014; Rajesh et al., 2017). Currently, very few drugs are available for the management of dementia including piracetam, galantamine, donepezil, memantine and rivastigmine which only provide symptomatic relief and are associated of severe toxicity. They do not prevent the progression of underlying pathophysiological aspects of dementia (Salomone et al., 2012). Bioactive herbal constituents (Howes et al., 2003) demonstrating anti-amnesic properties are of great interest of researchers in current era to explore successful remedy of dementia (Houghton and Howes, 2005). A toxicity free profile and sustained long lasting neuroprotective benefits of herbal remedies are empirical evidence for the best therapeutic applications of natural plants in the management of memory related disorders (Omar et al., 2017). Considering potential beneficial effects of *Lavandula stoechas* (L) in management of dementia in traditional medicinal practice (Nadkarni, 1996), this study was planned to explore its active constituents responsible for anti amnesic activity. The current research paper is initial finding of this series. In this investigation EPM, light and dark test and hole board paradigms were used for behavioral observations to reach the conclusion as proposed by Hossain and Uma Devi (2001).

Behavioral studies using EPM paradigm indicated that methanolic extract of *L. stoechas* showed dose dependent decrease in transfer latencies (decrease latency means improvement of learning tasks) and increased the inflexion ratio (a hallmark of improvement in retaining learned tasks) in comparison to amnesic group. Currently, EMP is widely employed paradigm in assessment of memory and learning tasks in rodents (Barez-Lopez et al., 2017) and considered reliable method of assessment of memory (Chauhan and Chaudhary, 2012). Pre treatment of animals with plant extract prior to administration of scopolamine prevented the impairment of learning and retaining capabilities which indicates the effectiveness of *L. stoechas* in memory build up. Similarly, findings of light dark paradigm illustrate that extract treated animals retained their learned ability of spending most of time in dark area while G-II animals (scopolamine treated) lost their memory to go into dark compartment and hence lived most of the time in light area. This supported the effectiveness of memory enhancing effect of plant along with efficiency of this paradigm in evaluation of memory tasks (Barry et al., 1987). Hole board paradigm used for behavioral analysis was based upon concept that increased no of hole pokings by mice retained their exploration behavior while scopolamine impaired their memory of exploration (Durcan and Lister, 1988). Thus it was observed that standard drug piracetam and plant extract in high doses increased the no of hole pokings by mice as compared to scopolamine treated mice. Investigation of memory enhancing effect of *L. stoechas* through behavioral analysis was further supported by evaluation of biochemical markers in brain homogenates of mice.

Acetylcholine is degraded by AChE at the level of synaptic cleft which diminishes cholinergic transmission (Ballard et al., 2005). An agent enhancing the level of AChE will impair memory by reducing acetylcholine levels as scopolamine did in amnesic group. In contrary, standard drug piracetam and methanolic plant extract (800 mg/kg/p.o.) retained the memory of mice as observed by behavioral studies by significantly ($P < 0.001$) lowering the level of AChE in brain (**Figure 5A**). Presence of alkaloids and flavonoids (134.06 ± 0.63 mg/g) in *L. stoechas* supported the acetyl cholinesterase activity of plant extract (Ma and Gang, 2008). Moreover, anti-oxidant studies suggested that plant extract also prevented the brain from oxidative stress (Pratico, 2008) by raising the level of SOD, GSH and CAT as shown in **Figures 5B–E**. Brain is highly susceptible to be damaged by oxidizing agents because high oxygen consumption, low GSH levels and polyunsaturated fat deposition in brain damage the neurons in brain (Mamelak, 2007; Sonnen et al., 2008). Exposure of brain with hydrogen peroxide results into production of several enzymes like β-secretase and γ-secretase which cleave amyloid precursor protein into amyloid β-peptide. Accumulation of amyloid β-peptide in brain is hallmark of loss of memory (Butterfield, 2002; Tong et al., 2005). Similarly, lipid peroxidation in brain elevates the level of MDA in brain which suggested loss of memory due to oxidative stress (Sultana et al., 2013). Thus, anti-oxidants protect the brain from this damage by scavenging free radicals (Omar et al., 2017). *In vitro* antioxidant activity of plant extract as observed by DPPH method ensured that it exhibited free radical scavenging activity (**Figure 1**). Total phenols were estimated to be 85.91 mg/g plant extract which were supposed to scavenge free oxygen, hydrogen peroxide, superoxide, and hydroxyl radicals (Pereira et al., 2009) and prevented the brain from oxidative stress. Scopolamine damaged the memory by depleting natural antioxidants present in brain, i.e., SOD, GSH, and CAT (El-Sherbiny et al., 2003) but current findings clearly declared *L. stoechas* a strong anti oxidant which reduced the level of MDA and increased SOD, GSH, and CAT levels in mice brain. Elevation of SOD and CAT prevented the damage caused by superoxide radicals and H_2O_2 respectively (Bhattacharjee et al., 2015) while GSH scavenged free radicals in brain proteins (Farombi et al., 2000). Based upon concluding results of current study, it is increasingly evidenced that antioxidant supplementation improves cognition on one hand and slows down the progression of dementia on other side.

CONCLUSION

It is concluded that dementia is linked with oxidative stress and loss of cholinergic innervations in brain neurons. *L. stoechas* could prove helpful in attenuation of dementia as it reduces oxidative burden of neurons and decreases neuro-degradation of cholinergic transmission in mice brain. This research is first finding of the series and further studies are in progress in our lab to reach a bio molecule of *L. stoechas* actually responsible for anti amnesic activity along with an appropriate mechanism of action.

AUTHOR CONTRIBUTIONS

AM conducted the experimental work. MA and RA proposed the study design, supervised the experimental work, and guided in writing manuscript.

ACKNOWLEDGMENTS

Special vote of thanks to Prof. Dr. Mobasher Ahmad Butt who not only supervised the work but provided the full technical and scientific support also to conduct the study smoothly. A bundle of gratitude to the management of Gulab Devi Institute of Pharmacy, Gulab Devi Educational Complex, Lahore and Punjab University College of Pharmacy, University of the Punjab, Lahore to facilitate the project.

REFERENCES

Adams, M., Gmünder, F., and Hamburger, M. (2007). Plants traditionally used in age related brain disorders—a survey of ethnobotanical literature. *J. Ethnopharmacol.* 113, 363–381. doi: 10.1016/j.jep.2007.07.016

Alzheimer's Association Report. (2017). 2017 Alzheimer's disease facts and ures. *Alzheimers Dement.* 13, 325–373. doi: 10.1016/j.jalz.2017.02.001

Ballard, C. G., Greig, N. H., Guillozet-Bongaarts, A. L., Enz, A., and Darvesh, S. (2005). Cholinesterases: roles in the brain during health and disease. *Curr. Alzheimer Res.* 2, 307–318. doi: 10.2174/1567205054367838

Barez-Lopez, S., Montero-Pedrazuela, A., Bosch-García, D., Venero, C., and Guadaño-Ferraz, A. (2017). Increased anxiety and fear memory in adult mice lacking type 2 deiodinase. *Psychoneuroendocrinology* 84, 51–60. doi: 10.1016/j.psyneuen.2017.06.013

Barry, J. M., Costall, B., Kelly, M. E., and Naylor, R. J. (1987). Withdrawal syndrome following subchronic treatment with anxiolytic agents. *Pharmacol. Biochem. Behav.* 27, 239–245. doi: 10.1016/0091-3057(87)90565-X

Baxter, M. G., Bucci, D. J., Gorman, L. K., Wiley, R. G., and Gallagher, M. (2013). Selective immunotoxic lesions of basal forebrain cholinergic cells: effects on learning and memory in rats. *Behav. Neurosci.* 127, 619–627. doi: 10.1037/a0033939

Bejar, C., Wang, R.-H., and Weinstock, M. (1999). Effect of rivastigmine on scopolamine-induced memory impairment in rats. *Eur. J. Pharmacol.* 383, 231–240. doi: 10.1016/S0014-2999(99)00643-3

Bhattacharjee, A., Shashidhara, S. C., and Saha, S. (2015). Nootropic activity of crataeva nurvala buch-ham against scopolamine induced cognitive impairment. *EXCLI J.* 14:335. doi: 10.17179/excli2014-541

Blois, M. S. (1958). Antioxidant determinations by the use of a stable free radical. *Nature* 181, 1199–1200. doi: 10.1038/1811199a0

Burns, A., and Iliffe, S. (2009). Alzheimer's disease. *BMJ* 338:b158. doi: 10.1136/bmj.b158

Butterfield, D. (2002). Amyloid β-peptide (1-42)-induced oxidative stress and neurotoxicity: implications for neurodegeneration in Alzheimer's disease brain. a review. *Free Radic. Res.* 36, 1307–1313. doi: 10.1080/1071576021000049890

Chauhan, B., and Chaudhary, A. K. (2012). Memory enhancing activity of methanolic extract of pterocarpus marsupium roxb. *Phytopharmacology* 2, 72–80.

Da Silva Filho, S. R. B., Barbosa, J. H. O., Rondinoni, C., dos Santos, A. C., Salmon, C. E. G., et al. (2017). Neuro-degeneration profile of Alzheimer's patients: a brain morphometry study. *NeuroImage Clin.* 15, 15–24. doi: 10.1016/j.nicl.2017.04.001

Durcan, M. J., and Lister, R. G. (1988). Time course of ethanol's effects on locomotor activity, exploration and anxiety in mice. *Psychopharmacology* 96, 67–72. doi: 10.1007/BF02431535

Ellman, G. L., Courtney, K. D., Andres, V., and Featherstone, R. M. (1961). A new and rapid colorimetric determination of acetylcholinesterase activity. *Biochem. Pharmacol.* 7, 88–95. doi: 10.1016/0006-2952(61)90145-9

El-Sherbiny, D. A., Khalifa, A. E., Attia, A. S., and Eldenshary Eel, D. (2003). Hypericum perforatum extract demonstrates antioxidant properties against elevated rat brain oxidative status induced by amnestic dose of scopolamine. *Pharmacol. Biochem. Behav.* 76, 525–533. doi: 10.1016/j.pbb.2003.09.014

Farombi, E. O., Olowu, B. I., and Emerole, G. O. (2000). Effect of three structurally related antimalarial drugs on liver microsomal components and lipid peroxidation in rats. *Comp. Biochem. Physiol. C Pharmacol. Toxicol. Endocrinol.* 126, 217–224.

Francis, P. T., Palmer, A. M., Snape, M., and Wilcock, G. K. (1999). The cholinergic hypothesis of Alzheimer's disease: a review of progress. *J. Neurol. Neurosurg. Psychiatry* 66, 137–147. doi: 10.1136/jnnp.66.2.137

Gilani, A., Aziz, N., Khan, M., Shaheen, F., Jabeen, Q., Siddiqui, B., et al. (2000). Ethnopharmacological evaluation of the anticonvulsant, sedative and antispasmodic activities of *Lavandula stoechas* L. *J. Ethnopharmacol.* 71, 161–167. doi: 10.1016/S0378-8741(99)00198-1

Giovannini, M., Casamenti, F., Bartolini, L., and Pepeu, G. (1997). The brain cholinergic system as a target of cognition enhancers. *Behav. Brain Res.* 83, 1–5. doi: 10.1016/S0166-4328(97)86038-X

Hake, A. M. (2001). Use of cholinesterase inhibitors for treatment of Alzheimer disease. *Cleve. Clin. J. Med.* 68, 608–609, 613–604, 616. doi: 10.3949/ccjm.68.7.608

Hakeem, M., Siddiqui, M., and Khan, A. (1991). Antiepileptic activity of ustu khudoos in secondary epilepsy—a case report. *Hamdard Med.* 34, 33–39.

Hardy, J. A., and Higgins, G. A. (1992). Alzheimer's disease: the amyloid cascade hypothesis. *Science* 256:184. doi: 10.1126/science.1566067

Hossain, M., and Uma Devi, P. (2001). Effect of irradiation at the early foetal stage on adult brain function of mouse: learning and memory. *Int. J. Radiat. Biol.* 77, 581–585. doi: 10.1080/09553000110037394

Houghton, P. J., and Howes, M.-J. (2005). Natural products and derivatives affecting neurotransmission relevant to Alzheimer's and Parkinson's disease. *Neurosignals* 14, 6–22. doi: 10.1159/000085382

Howes, M. J. R., Perry, N. S., and Houghton, P. J. (2003). Plants with traditional uses and activities, relevant to the management of Alzheimer's disease and other cognitive disorders. *Phytother. Res.* 17, 1–18. doi: 10.1002/ptr.1280

Kakkar, P., Das, B., and Viswanathan, P. (1984). A modified spectrophotometric assay of superoxide dismutase. *Indian J. Biochem. Biophys.* 21, 130–132.

Kasture, S., Kasture, V., Joshua, A., Damodaran, A., and Amit, A. (2007). Nootropic activity of bacomind tm, an enriched phytochemical composition from *Bacopa monnieri*. *J. Nat. Remedies* 7, 166–173.

Kulkarni, P. D., Ghaisas, M. M., Chivatbe, N., and Sankpal, P. S. (2011). Memory enhancing activity of *Cissampelos pariera* in mice. *Int. J. Pharm. Pharm. Sci.* 3, 206–211.

Kumar, H., More, S. V., Han, S.-D., Choi, J.-Y., and Choi, D.-K. (2012). Promising therapeutics with natural bioactive compounds for improving learning and memory—a review of randomized trials. *Molecules* 17, 10503–10539. doi: 10.3390/molecules170910503

Kumaran, A., and Karunakaran, R. J. (2007). In vitro antioxidant activities of methanol extracts of five *Phyllanthus* species from India. *LWT Food Sci. Technol.* 40, 344–352. doi: 10.1016/j.lwt.2005.09.011

Ma, X., and Gang, D. R. (2008). In vitro production of huperzine A, a promising drug candidate for Alzheimer's disease. *Phytochemistry* 69, 2022–2028. doi: 10.1016/j.phytochem.2008.04.017

Mamelak, M. (2007). Alzheimer's disease, oxidative stress and gammahydroxybutyrate. *Neurobiol. Aging* 28, 1340–1360. doi: 10.1016/j.neurobiolaging.2006.06.008

McCord, J. M. (2000). The evolution of free radicals and oxidative stress. *Am. J. Med.* 108, 652–659. doi: 10.1016/S0002-9343(00)00412-5

Moron, M. S., Depierre, J. W., and Mannervik, B. (1979). Levels of glutathione, glutathione reductase and glutathione S-transferase activities in rat lung and liver. *Biochim. Biophys. Acta Gen. Sub.* 582, 67–78. doi: 10.1016/0304-4165(79)90289-7

Mushtaq, A., Mahmood, A., and Jabeen, Q. (2013). Hepatoprotective action of a polyherbal aqueous ethanolic extract against nimesulide intoxicated albino rats. *IJPRBS* 2, 332–347.

Nadkarni, K. M. (1996). *Indian Materia Medica; Dr. KM Nadkarni's Indian Materia Medica: with Ayurvedic, Unani-Tibbi, Siddha, Allopathic, Homeopathic, Naturopathic & Home Remedies, Appendices & Indexes. 1*, Vol. 1 Mumbai: Popular Prakashan.

Omar, S. H., Scott, C. J., Hamlin, A. S., and Obied, H. K. (2017). The protective role of plant biophenols in mechanisms of Alzheimer's disease. *J. Nutr. Biochem.* 47, 1–20. doi: 10.1016/j.jnutbio.2017.02.016

Pahaye, D. B., Bum, E. N., Taïwé, G. S., Ngoupaye, G. T., Sidiki, N., Moto, F. C. O., et al. (2017). Neuroprotective and antiamnesic effects of *Mitragyna inermis* willd (*Rubiaceae*) on scopolamine-induced memory impairment in mice. *Behav. Neurol.* 2017, 1–11. doi: 10.1155/2017/5952897

Pereira, D. M., Valentão, P., Pereira, J. A., and Andrade, P. B. (2009). Phenolics: from chemistry to biology. *Molecules* 14, 2201–2211. doi: 10.3390/molecules14062202

Polshettiwar, S., Ganjiwale, R., Wadher, S., and Yeole, P. (2007). Spectrophotometric estimation of total tannins in some ayurvedic eye drops. *Indian J. Pharm. sci.* 69, 574–576. doi: 10.4103/0250-474X.36949

Pratico, D. (2008). Oxidative stress hypothesis in Alzheimer's disease: a reappraisal. *Trends Pharmacol. sci.* 29, 609–615. doi: 10.1016/j.tips.2008.09.001

Rabiei, Z., Rafieian-kopaei, M., Heidarian, E., Saghaei, E., and Mokhtari, S. (2014). Effects of *Zizyphus jujube* extract on memory and learning impairment induced by bilateral electric lesions of the nucleus basalis of meynert in rat. *Neurochem. Res.* 39, 353–360. doi: 10.1007/s11064-013-1232-8

Rajesh, V., Riju, T., Venkatesh, S., and Babu, G. (2017). Memory enhancing activity of *Lawsonia inermis* linn. leaves against scopolamine induced memory impairment in Swiss albino mice. *Orient. Pharm. Exp. Med.* 17, 127–142. doi: 10.1007/s13596-017-0268-8

Salomone, S., Caraci, F., Leggio, G. M., Fedotova, J., and Drago, F. (2012). New pharmacological strategies for treatment of Alzheimer's disease: focus on disease modifying drugs. *Br. J. Clin. Pharmacol.* 73, 504–517. doi: 10.1111/j.1365-2125.2011.04134.x

Sinha, A. K. (1972). Colorimetric assay of catalase. *Anal. Biochem.* 47, 389–394. doi: 10.1016/0003-2697(72)90132-7

Sonnen, J. A., Breitner, J. C., Lovell, M. A., Markesbery, W. R., Quinn, J. F., and Montine, T. J. (2008). Free radical-mediated damage to brain in Alzheimer's disease and its transgenic mouse models. *Free Radic. Biol. Med.* 45, 219–230. doi: 10.1016/j.freeradbiomed.2008.04.022

Sultana, R., Perluigi, M., and Butterfield, D. A. (2013). Lipid peroxidation triggers neurodegeneration: a redox proteomics view into the Alzheimer disease brain. *Free Radic. Biol. Med.* 62, 157–169. doi: 10.1016/j.freeradbiomed.2012.09.027

Todd, S., Barr, S., Roberts, M., and Passmore, A. P. (2013). Survival in dementia and predictors of mortality: a review. *Int. J. Geriatr. Psychiatry* 28, 1109–1124. doi: 10.1002/gps.3946

Tong, Y., Zhou, W., Fung, V., Christensen, M., Qing, H., Sun, X., et al. (2005). Oxidative stress potentiates BACE1 gene expression and Aβ generation. *J. Neural. Transm.* 112, 455–469. doi: 10.1007/s00702-004-0255-3

Wenk, G. L. (2003). Neuropathologic changes in Alzheimer's disease. *J. Clin. Psychiatry* 64, 7–10.

Wilson, D. M., and Binder, L. I. (1997). Free fatty acids stimulate the polymerization of tau and amyloid beta peptides. in vitro evidence for a common effector of pathogenesis in Alzheimer's disease. *Am. J. pathol.* 150:2181–2195.

Xian, Y.-F., Lin, Z.-X., Zhao, M., Mao, Q.-Q., Ip, S.-P., and Che, C.-T. (2011). Uncaria rhynchophylla ameliorates cognitive deficits induced by D-galactose in mice. *Planta Med.* 77, 1977–1983. doi: 10.1055/s-0031-128 0125

9

Target Proteins in the Dorsal Hippocampal Formation Sustain the Memory-Enhancing and Neuroprotective Effects of *Ginkgo biloba*

Renan Barretta Gaiardo*[1]*, Thiago Ferreira Abreu*[2]*, Alexandre Keiji Tashima*[2]*,
Monica Marques Telles*[3] *and Suzete Maria Cerutti*[1]*

[1] Departamento de Ciências Biológicas, Laboratório de Farmacologia Celular e Comportamental, Universidade Federal de São Paulo, Diadema, Brazil, [2] Departamento de Bioquímica, Escola Paulista de Medicina, Universidade Federal de São Paulo, São Paulo, Brazil, [3] Departamento de Ciências Biológicas, Laboratório de Fisiologia Metabólica, Universidade Federal de São Paulo, Diadema, Brazil

***Correspondence:**
Suzete Maria Cerutti
smcerutti@unifesp.br;
smcerutti@gmail.com

We have previously shown that standardized extracts of *Ginkgo biloba* (EGb) modulate fear memory formation, which is associated with CREB-1 (mRNA and protein) upregulation in the dorsal hippocampal formation (dHF), in a dose-dependent manner. Here, we employed proteomic analysis to investigate EGb effects on different protein expression patterns in the dHF, which might be involved in the regulation of CREB activity and the synaptic plasticity required for long-term memory (LTM) formation. Adult male Wistar rats were randomly assigned to four groups (n = 6/group) and were submitted to conditioned lick suppression 30 min after vehicle (12% Tween 80) or EGb (0.25, 0.50, and 1.00 $g{\cdot}kg^{-1}$) administration (p.o). All rats underwent a retention test session 48 h after conditioning. Twenty-four hours after the test session, the rats were euthanized *via* decapitation, and dHF samples were removed for proteome analysis using two-dimensional polyacrylamide gel electrophoresis, followed by peptide mass fingerprinting. In agreement with our previous data, no differences in the suppression ratios (SRs) were identified among the groups during first trial of CS (conditioned stimulus) presentation ($P > 0.05$). Acute treatment with 0.25 $g{\cdot}kg^{-1}$ EGb significantly resulted in retention of original memory, without prevent acquisition of extinction within-session. In addition, our results showed, for the first time, that 32 proteins were affected in the dHF following treatment with 0.25, 0.50, and 1.00 $g{\cdot}kg^{-1}$ doses of EGb, which upregulated seven, 19, and five proteins, respectively. Additionally, EGb downregulated two proteins at each dose. These proteins are correlated with remodeling of the cytoskeleton; the stability, size, and shape of dendritic spines; myelin sheath formation; and composition proteins of structures found in the membrane of the somatodendritic and axonal compartments. Our findings suggested that EGb modulates conditioned suppression LTM through differential protein expression profiles, which may be a target for cognitive enhancers and for the prevention or treatment of neurocognitive impairments.

Keywords: conditioned suppression, proteomic, *Ginkgo biloba*, long-term memory, protein–protein interaction

INTRODUCTION

The ability to extract meaning from sensory input, i.e., acquiring new knowledge about the world, and storing this information as past experiences for subsequent retrieval is part of the normal development of living beings and has been well studied in invertebrates animals (Carew and Sahley, 1986; Kandel et al., 2014). These events are largely coordinated and are crucial to memory formation, being characterized by specific cellular and/or molecular modifications that might last from seconds or minutes to hours. If these modifications persist over time, they guarantee that long-lasting changes, which are essential to long-term memory (LTM) formation, will occur (Stork, 1999; Won and Silva, 2008; Mayford et al., 2012). In vertebrates, LTM seems to occur in parallel on the day of training within the specific neural circuitry for each memory type and may involve the hippocampus, prefrontal cortex, and amygdaloid complex (Izquierdo et al., 1997; Cammarota et al., 2008).

The early phase of LTM occurs as a result of transient modifications to the activity of already existing proteins that are present on the membrane or in the cytosol of a neural cell, which act by regulating ionic conductivity as NMDA receptors or by phosphorylation of proteins as alpha calcium/calmodulin-dependent kinase II and the mitogen-activated protein kinases family as ERK1/2 (Fendt and Fanselow, 1999; Giese and Mizuno, 2013). The maintenance of these signals, in parallel with other downstream activation targets, is necessary for long-lasting neuronal plasticity and cellular consolidation of memory, a protein synthesis-dependent stage of memory formation that may last for hours, weeks, or months.

Subsequent evidence has demonstrated that *de novo* proteins have multiple functions in cells and are essential for dendritic spicule growth, functional synaptic area increase, and synaptic cleft narrowing, which are involved in new synaptic formation and/or in the strength of existing synapses over time. Furthermore, changes may occur through underutilized synapses that weaken or eliminate some inputs. Both mechanisms provide a cellular substrate for the formation of learned associations (McGaugh, 1966; Frey et al., 1993; Hotulainen and Hoogenraad, 2010).

In addition to the neuronal adaptations, the cross-talk between neurons and glial cells is crucial to the maintenance of the appropriate environment for neural functioning, electrochemical homeostasis, transmitter release, memory formation, or the effects of drug therapy (Lynch, 2002; Barco et al., 2003; Cerutti et al., 2009). Hence, beyond the synaptic and extrasynaptic changes that underlie memory formation, alterations in the intrinsic cell functions, such as redox balance regulation and hypoxia tolerance, may guarantee better conditions and, consequently, better cell functioning, which promote memory maintenance (Kandel, 2001).

In recent decades, popular and institutional interest in the use of herbal medicines as a therapeutic resource in the prevention, promotion, and recovery of health has grown in many countries. Currently, the standardized extract of *Ginkgo biloba* (EGb) is the plant product that has been most frequently indicated for the treatment and prevention of the loss of function related to ageing of the nervous system, in particular for treatment of diseases associated with cognitive and memory dysfunctions (Itil et al., 1996; DeFeudis, 2002; Ahlemeyer and Krieglstein, 2003b).

Studies from our laboratory have characterized the protective and preventive effects of EGb treatment on the dorsal hippocampal formation (dHF) of middle-aged rats, which is associated with short-term memory (Ribeiro et al., 2016), or of adult rats during LTM enhancement (Oliveira et al., 2009, 2013; Zamberlam et al., 2016). Our group showed that upregulation of CREB-1 in the dHF is essential for conditioned suppression memory and that short or long-term treatment with EGb upregulated the expression of CREB-1 (mRNA and protein) and of glial fibrillary acidic protein in the dHF in a dose-dependent manner (Oliveira et al., 2009, 2013). Conversely, EGb treatment downregulated the product of the gene expression (mRNA and protein) of growth associated protein 43 (also called neuromodulin), a neural-specific protein kinase C substrate, in the dHF of rats subjected to the suppression of licking response test in parallel with cellular and molecular changes in the prefrontal cortex and the amygdaloid complex. Recently, we suggested that treatment with EGb prior to conditioned suppression modulates molecular mechanisms that are associated with acquisition or consolidation, resulting in the retention of fear memory over time (Zamberlam et al., 2016). These pieces of evidence were recently corroborated since we found that the effects of EGb treatment on the modulation of fear memory retrieval over time were correlated with differential expression patterns of serotoninergic, GABAergic, and glutamatergic receptors in the dHF (Zamberlam et al., unpublished). Altogether, these findings established the proprieties of EGb on memory and raised questions about the role of the dHF as a key structure in the acquisition of conditioned lick suppression. However, intrahippocampal downstream proteins that may be involved in the regulation of CREB activity, as well as in the synaptic plasticity required for LTM formation, have not been characterized.

To address these questions, we employed quantitative proteomic analysis to investigate the effects of treatment with EGb before conditioning on differential protein expression.

MATERIALS AND METHODS

Animals

Twenty-four male adult *Wistar* rats, 12 weeks old (250–300 g) were obtained from the Center for the Development of Experimental Medicine and Biology, Universidade Federal de São Paulo (São Paulo, Brazil). All animals were experimentally naive and were housed three per cage with food and water freely available. They were kept under a controlled temperature of 21 ± 2°C, a relative humidity of 53 ± 2%, and a 12:12 h light cycle with lights on at 06:00 hours throughout the experimental period. The experiments were performed in the light phase of the cycle. All procedures were approved by the Ethics Committee on Animal Use of the Federal University of Sao Paulo (CEUA 0043/12) and in accordance with the rules issued by the National Council for the Control of Animal Experimentation (CONCEA). The rats were randomly assigned to the control (vehicle) or EGb (0.25, 0.50, and 1.00 g·kg^{-1}) group (n = 6 per group).

Drug

A standardized EGb, containing 24% flavonol glycosides, 5–7% terpene trilactones (2.8–3.4% ginkgolides A, B, C, J, M and 2.6–3.2% bilobalide), and <5 ppm ginkgolic acids provided by Galena Pharmaceutical, Campinas, Brazil) was used. EGb was re-suspended in water containing 12% Tween 80®. Single doses of EGb or vehicle solution were administered orally *via* a gastric tube 30 min prior to the acquisition session. The dose rational of choice in this work was based on previous work in our lab (Oliveira et al., 2009, 2013; Zamberlam et al., 2016) and published studies; several clinical studies have demonstrated that higher dosages (up to 600 mg day^{-1}) appear to be necessary to enhance memory when an acute dosage is used (Allain et al., 1993; Le Bars and Kastelan, 2000). However, pre-clinical studies have demonstrated conflicting findings; however, a dose lower than 240–300 mg·kg^{-1} did not have an effect on cognitive performance when an acute dose (p.o) was administered. This finding is inconsistent with the findings reported for chronic treatment, in which a dose of 100 mg·kg^{-1} appears to be effective (Tchantchou et al., 2007; Blecharz-Klin et al., 2009; Yoshitake et al., 2010; Kehr et al., 2012).

Behavioral Procedure

Conditioned suppression of licking responses was assessed as previously described (Oliveira et al., 2016; Zamberlam et al., 2016), and the assessments were conducted for 8 days. Briefly, prior to each experimental session, the rats were deprived of water for 12–16 h. On days 1–5, the rats were subjected to the acquisition of the lick response for 20 min during each session to obtain a stable baseline of drinking behavior. On day 6, each rat was returned to the experimental chamber, and the animals were subjected to four tone-shock (tone: 85 dB, 30 s; shock: 0.4 mA, 1.0 s) pairings; with the shock immediately following tone termination and a 5-min interval separating each successive pairing. On day 7, the animals were exposed to the experimental chamber, without stimuli presentation, to minimize the influence of context on this process and for the reacquisition of the licking response. On day 8, each rat was subjected to a retention test session, whereby the fear memory was retrieved *via* 10 successive conditioned stimulus (CS, tone) presentations (trials). The latencies to complete 10 licks prior to and during the tone were recorded and were used to calculate the suppression ratio (SR).

Protein Sample Preparation

Twenty-four hours after the retention test ended, the animals were euthanized *via* decapitation, in the absence of anesthesia, and the dHF was rapidly removed, frozen in liquid nitrogen, and stored at −80°C until it was analyzed. Sample preparation was performed as previously described (Pedroso et al., 2012), with minor modifications. The entire dHF was homogenized in 1 mL of extraction buffer (7 M urea, 2 M thiourea, 4% CHAPS, 0.5% Triton X-100) containing cOmplete™, Mini Protease Inhibitor Cocktail Tablets (Roche Diagnostics, Basel, Switzerland). Sample lysates were centrifuged at 4°C (14,000 rpm/30 min), and the supernatants were stored at −80°C until analysis. Protein concentrations of the supernatants were determined using a 2-D Quant Kit (GE Healthcare, Chicago, IL, United States) according to the manufacturer's recommendations, using bovine albumin as a standard. The method applied to analysis of protein profile in this study was bottom-up proteomics file to aliquots of 750 μg of protein were precipitated with a solution of 35% chlorate potassium, 43% chloroform, and 22% methanol (v/v). The mixture was homogenized and centrifuged at 15,000 rpm and at 4°C for 15 min. The pellet was recovered and air-dried at room temperature.

Two-Dimensional Gel Electrophoresis and Image Analysis

For isoelectric focusing (IEF), the pellet was dissolved in 500 μL of rehydration buffer [7 M urea, 2 M thiourea, 4% CHAPS, 0.5% Triton X-100, 100 mM DTT, 0.2% IPG buffer, pH 3–10 (GE Healthcare, United States), and traces of bromophenol blue]. IEF was carried out on a Protean® IEF Cell (Bio-Rad, Hercules, CA, United States), using an Immobiline™ DryStrip, with a pH of 3–10, an 18-cm linear gradient (GE Healthcare, United States), and having been previously rehydrated for 12–14 h. IEF was performed with the current limit set at 50 mA per IPG strip at 18°C with the following conditions: 250 V for 30 min, 500 V for 1 h, 1000 V for 1 h, 2000 V for 1 h, 4000 V for 1 h, and 8000 V for 1 h followed by 8000 V until 40,000 Vh. After focusing, the strips were equilibrated for 15 min in buffer containing 6 M urea, 2% SDS, 1.5 M Tris pH 8.8, 30% glycerol, and 1% DDT, followed by an additional 15 min in the same buffer containing 2.5% iodoacetamide instead of DTT. Strips were then loaded onto 12% SDS-polyacrylamide gels. After running in Protean® II XL Multi-Cell (Bio-Rad, United States) at 60 mA per gel for 5 h, the gels were stained for 48 h with Coomassie Brilliant Blue G-250 (Bio-Rad, United States). The stained gels were scanned (GS-800™ Calibrated Densitometer) and analyzed using the PDQuest™ 2-D Analysis Software Version 8.0.1 (Bio-Rad, United States).

Protein Identification

Protein Digestion

The protein spots that were quantitatively altered in response to treatment with EGb were manually excised from the gels, distained in 50% methanol and 2.5% acetic acid for 3 h, dehydrated with 100% acetonitrile, and dried in a vacuum concentrator. To the dried spots, 10 mM DTT was added, and the mixture was incubated for 30 min at room temperature, followed by a 50 mM iodoacetamide addition under the same conditions. The spots were washed and dehydrated with 100 mM ammonium bicarbonate and 100% acetonitrile, respectively, and were dried in vacuum concentrator. Digestion was performed overnight at 37°C with 20 ng/μL of trypsin (Promega, Fitchburg, WI, United States) in 50 mM ammonium bicarbonate. The digested samples were dried and re-suspended in 0.1% formic acid and were stored at −20°C until analysis (Shevchenko et al., 1996).

Mass Spectrometry Analysis

For the liquid chromatography–mass spectrometry analysis (LC–MS), peptides from the digested samples were injected onto a trap column (C18 trap column symmetry 180 μm × 20 mm, Waters, Milford, MA, United States) and were separated in the analytical column (C18 BEH 75 μm × 200 mm, 1.7 mm, Waters, United States) using a capillary UPLC system (nanoAcquity, Waters, United States). The elution gradient of 7–35% phase B (phase A: 0.1% formic acid in water, phase B: 0.1% formic acid in acetonitrile) was performed in 45 min at 275 nL/min. Multiple charged protonated peptides were generated by electrospray ionization and analyzed in a quadrupole time-of-flight mass spectrometer (Synapt HDMS G2, Waters, United States). Data were acquired in the MSE mode, switching from low (4 eV) to high (ramped from 19 to 45 eV) collision energy with scan times of 1.25 s. An external calibration was performed every 60 s using Glu-fibrinopeptide B (Waters, United States).

Data Analysis

Liquid chromatography–mass spectrometry analysis data were processed in the ProteinLynx Global SERVER^{TM} version 3.0.3 (Waters, United States) using low energy threshold of 750 counts and high-energy threshold of 50 counts. The MS/MS spectra were exported as mascot generic format (.mgf) files to MASCOT Server version 2.4 (Matrix Science, United Kingdom) for database search. Searches were performed in the UniprotKB[1] (92,378 sequences) and NCBI-nr[2] (92,378 sequences) protein databases. The following parameters were used in the searches: no restrictions on protein molecular weight; trypsin digest with up to one missing cleavage; monoisotopic mass; taxonomy limited to *Rattus*; carbamidomethylation of cysteine as a fixed modification; oxidation of methionine and tryptophan as variable modifications; a peptide mass tolerance of 10 ppm; and a fragment mass tolerance of 0.05 Da. The false discovery rate was estimated by the decoy database approach, and set to a maximum of 1%.

Protein matching probabilities were determined using the MASCOT protein scores, with the identification confidence indicated by the number of matches and by the coverage of the protein sequence by the matching peptides. The presence of at least one peptide with a significant ion score was required for positive protein identification. Only statistically significant MASCOT score results ($P < 0.05$) were included in the analysis.

Statistical Analysis

The behavioral data were evaluated according to the mean SR of each trial for each rat daily. A two-way analysis of variance for repeated measures, followed by Tukey's multiple comparisons test, was used to test for the presence of group and trial effects, as well as for the interaction between these variables. The optic densities of the spots were expressed as the percentage of change relative to the basal levels (vehicle) and were compared using one-way analysis of variance, followed by Tukey's multiple comparisons test. The data were analyzed using GraphPad Prism version 7.00 (GraphPad Software, San Diego, CA, United States), and the significance level was 5%. All data are shown as the means ± standard error of the mean (see **Supplementary Material**).

Interaction Network Analysis

Pathway analysis of the significantly altered optical density spots was performed using STRING[3]. Three protein–protein interaction networks (one for each EGb dose) of different spots were constructed with the confidence score set at 0.7 (high confidence).

RESULTS

Behavioral Analysis

Data regarding the first SR (SR_1) means during the retention test demonstrated that all groups experienced the acquisition of conditioned suppression, namely, the EGb 0.25 g·kg^{-1} (SR_1 = 0.77), 0.50 g·kg^{-1} (SR_1 = 0.78), and 1.0 g·kg^{-1} (SR_1 = 0.82) groups and the vehicle (SR_1 = 0.89) group. **Figure 1** shows SR means recorded across the ten trials of the memory retention sessions for the EGb-treated and vehicle groups, and all SRs are available in **Supplementary Table S1**. The first trial is presented independently because it represents the first presentation of the CS after conditioning and can characterize the level of fear of the animal in each situation. A two-way ANOVA analysis revealed no interaction between group × trial [$F_{(9,60)}$ = 1.355; P = 0.2290] and a main effect of trial [$F_{(3,60)}$ = 26.74; P < 0.0001] and no effect of group [$F_{(3,20)}$ = 0.2604; P = 0.8531]. The comparisons between trials showed a significant decrease in the mean SR of the first trial compared with those of the three-trial blocks across all groups, except to group treated with 0.25 g·kg^{-1} dose during second three-trial block. Comparisons of the results for the first trial in the retention test sessions between groups revealed elevated SR in the subgroups treated with EGb and vehicle. The analysis of SR in the first three-trial block (second to fourth trials) showed a significant decrease in mean SR relative to the first trial in the vehicle and EGb groups. These results indicated the acquisition of extinction of fear memory within the session (**Figure 1A**). Furthermore, comparing the three-trial blocks revealed differences within sessions (P < 0.05). Rats treated with 0.25 g·kg^{-1} had return of fear during fifth to seventh trials of CS presentation. Furthermore, a reliable decrease in suppression and a reduction of fear to control and EGb at dose 0.5 g·kg^{-1}. In summary, our data show that EGb did not prevent acquisition of lick suppression as well as within-session extinction (**Figure 1B**).

Proteomics Analysis

The 2DE gels of the dHF (n = 5 per group) showed 344.0 ± 10.1 spots in the vehicle group and 355.6 ± 5.3 (0.25 g·kg^{-1}), 361.6 ± 6.6 (0.50 g·kg^{-1}), and 363.0 ± 4.7 (1.00 g·kg^{-1}) spots in the EGb-treated groups. To analyze memory formation and the EGb treatment effect on protein expression, we analyzed the

[1]www.uniprot.org

[2]www.ncbi.nlm.nih.gov/protein

[3]http://string-db.org/

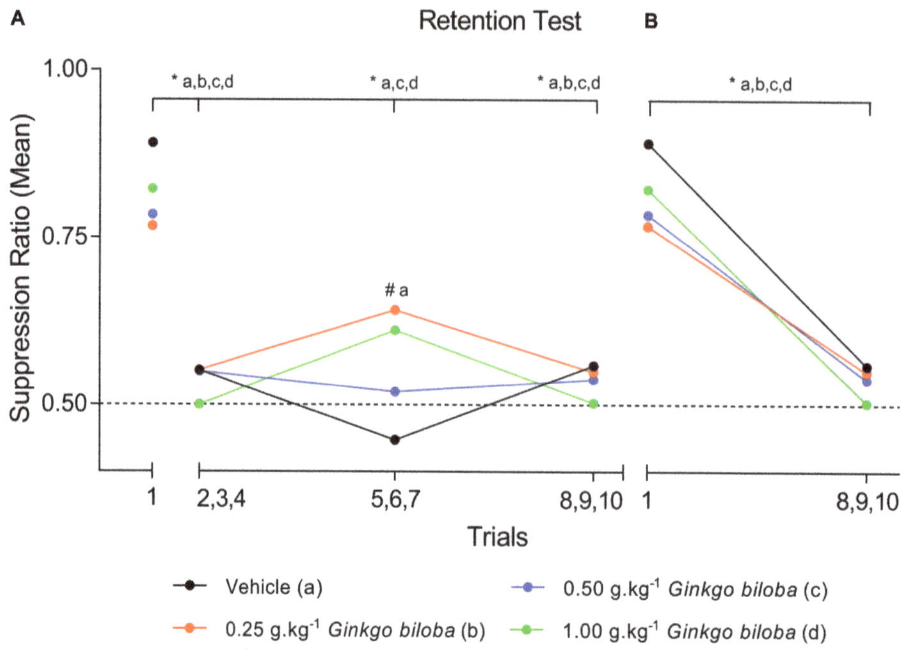

FIGURE 1 | SR means of conditioned lick suppression during the retention test session (day 8). The points indicate the SR means of the first trial and the three-trial blocks for the control (vehicle) and EGb-treated (0.25, 0.50, and 1.00 g·kg^{-1}) groups (n = 6 per group) **(A)** and first trial *versus* last three trial block **(B)**. Data represent mean. *P < 0.05 (two-way repeated measures ANOVA–Tukey *post hoc* test). #Comparison among groups; *comparison intragroup.

fold changes in protein expression between the control and EGb-treated groups. We identified 32 spots with significant changes in their optical density values (**Table 1** and **Supplementary Table S2**). EGb treatment at all doses resulted in altered protein expression. Herein, six (0.25 g·kg^{-1}), 12 (0.50 g·kg^{-1}), and four (1.00 g·kg^{-1}) proteins were upregulated, while six proteins and two proteins at each dose were downregulated in the EGb-treated groups in comparison to the vehicle group. The comparisons among the EGb-treated groups revealed that the intermediary dose (0.50 g·kg^{-1}) positively affected protein expression in relation to the other doses. Ten proteins were found to be upregulated following treatment with 0.5 g·kg^{-1} EGb in relation to the lower dose (0.25 g·kg^{-1}). Additionally, 13 proteins were upregulated, and two other proteins were downregulated in comparison to the group treated with 1.00 g·kg^{-1} EGb. Moreover, three proteins were significantly upregulated at the 1.00 g·kg^{-1} dosage, and three other proteins were downregulated in relation to the 0.25 g·kg^{-1} dose (**Table 1**).

Figure 2 shows a representative image of a 2DE gel of the vehicle group, with the indication of spots significantly affected by EGb treatment and submitted to conditioned lick suppression. The spots with significant optical density differences were analyzed using mass spectrometry for protein identification (**Supplementary Table S3**).

The analysis of protein–protein interactions showed significant enrichments among the 21 proteins affected by EGb treatment at a dose of 0.50 g·kg^{-1} (P = 0.000335). On the other hand, treatment with EGb at doses of 0.25 g·kg^{-1} (nine nodes; P = 0.127) and 1.00 g·kg^{-1} (seven nodes; P = 0.592) indicated no significant interaction enrichments (**Figure 3**). The pathway analysis indicated that membrane-bound vesicles, cellular component morphogenesis, and cell projections were significantly modified following EGb treatment at a dose of 0.25 g·kg^{-1}. Furthermore, treatment with EGb at a dose of 0.50 g·kg^{-1} modified pathways involved in processes related to heterocyclic compound binding, organic cyclic compound binding, and cell projection, as well as to the somatodendritic compartment, myelin sheath, neuronal cell body, tight junctions, and neurons. In addition, the group treated with EGb at the higher dose of 1.00 g·kg^{-1} exhibited modifications to the ribosomal small subunit assembly pathway (**Table 2**).

DISCUSSION

The present data provided evidence of the modulatory effects of EGb on the acquisition of conditioned lick suppression by differential protein expression profiles in the dHF, corroborating our previous data (Oliveira et al., 2009; Zamberlam et al., 2016) and expanding our current knowledge about EGb effects on memory formation. Rats treated with EGb at all doses acquired suppression of the licking response and within-session extinction. However, our data revealed elevated SR in the subgroups treated with EGb at dose 0.25 g·kg^{-1} in relation to control group during second three-trial block (fifth to seventh), but in the subsequent trial, they had a reliable decrease in suppression and a reduction of fear, similar to all groups by the end of the session. Furthermore, comparisons between the first trial and the three-trial blocks showed reduced suppression of the licking response in the EGb at doses 0.5 and 1.0 g·kg^{-1}, similar to the vehicle group.

TABLE 1 | Proteins differentially expressed in the dorsal hippocampal formation of the rats treated with *Ginkgo biloba* (0.25, 0.50, and 1.0 g·kg^{-1}) or vehicle groups and submitted to conditioned lick suppression.

Fold change (*P*-value)[1]						**Protein description**
0.25/vehicle[2]	**0.50/vehicle[2]**	**1.00/vehicle[2]**	**0.50/0.25[2]**	**1.00/0.25[2]**	**1.00/0.50[2]**	
3.27 (0.0247)						Dual specificity mitogen-activated protein kinase kinase 1
3.24 (0.0219)						Phosphoglycerate mutase 1
2.85 (0.0374)						Dihydropyrimidinase-related protein 5
4.30 (0.0120)						T-complex protein 1 subunit delta
	2.52 (0.0110)					Dihydropyrimidinase-related protein 2
	4.09 (0.0125)					Myosin-8
	1.95 (0.0098)	1.86 (0.0286)				Septin-6
			4.26 (0.0490)			Proteasome subunit alpha type-1
			4.09 (0.0126)			Vesicle-fusing ATPase
		6.11 (0.0020)		2.14 (0.0496)		Chain A, tetra-(5-fluorotryptophanyl)-glutathione transferase
		42.0 (0.0322)		12.4 (0.0336)	8.41 (0.0428)	Hypoxanthine-guanine phosphoribosyltransferase
					3.43 (0.0342)	40S ribosomal protein S14
0.56 (0.0255)	0.43 (0.0016)					Proteasome subunit alpha type-7
0.40 (0.0301)		0.47 (0.0458)				Endophilin-A1
	0.46 (0.0340)	0.51 (0.0464)				40S ribosomal protein SA
				0.35 (0.0333)		Synapsin-2
					0.32 (0.0488)	Beta-synuclein
					0.41 (0.0365)	Creatine kinase M-type
					0.46 (0.0378)	Transcriptional activator protein Pur-alpha
					0.46 (0.0032)	Myosin-6
2.61 (0.0225)				0.40 (0.0277)		WD repeat-containing protein 1
2.14 (0.0115)				0.35 (0.0039)		Dihydropyrimidinase-related protein 1
	2.16 (0.0411)				0.37 (0.0153)	MICOS complex subunit Mic60
	2.55 (0.0114)				0.41 (0.0213)	Myosin heavy chain IIa
	2.09 (0.0469)		2.72 (0.0210)		0.26 (0.0043)	14-3-3 protein eta
	2.38 (0.0250)		2.43 (0.0227)		0.36 (0.0130)	Heat shock protein HSP 90-alpha
	2.09 (0.0132)		1.89 (0.0262)		0.31 (0.0014)	Protein disulfide-isomerase A3
	2.06 (0.0082)		1.91 (0.0210)		0.58 (0.0301)	Hexokinase 1
	1.89 (0.0435)		2.69 (0.0098)		0.43 (0.0134)	Dynamin-1
	3.66 (0.0158)		2.50 (0.0362)		0.33 (0.0276)	Tubulin polymerization-promoting protein
			2.04 (0.0305)		0.47 (0.0235)	Myosin-4
	5.67 (0.0136)	6.77 (0.0044)	3.57 (0.0445)	4.27 (0.0142)		Proteasome subunit alpha type-6

[1]*A fold change value > 1.0 indicates upregulation and a value of < 1.0 indicates downregulation. P-value for Tukey post hoc test.* [2]*The fold change was calculated as ratio of A/B where A is mean of group in the numerator and B mean of group in denominator.*

Our current findings corroborate with previous data from our lab about modulatory effects of EGb treatment on original memory, which was somewhat enhanced, i.e., better preserved, similar to found to the flavones from *Erythrina falcata* (Oliveira et al., 2016). These findings aligned with our hypothesis that EGb is able to modulate in a dose-dependent manner molecular mechanisms

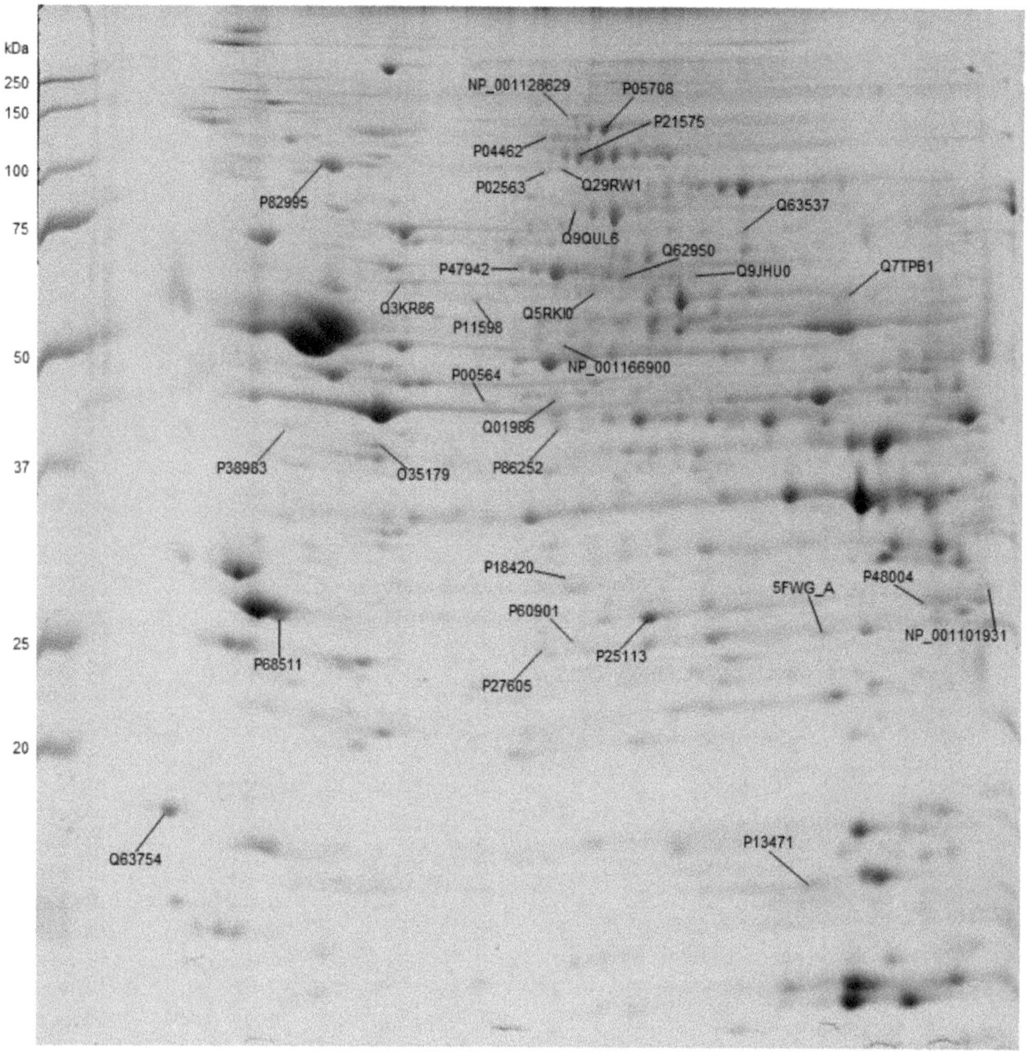

FIGURE 2 | Representative image of a 2DE gel of a control (vehicle) dorsal hippocampal formation depicting the proteins that were significantly affected by EGb treatment. The numbers indicate the protein accession number.

that underlie the acquisition/consolidation of fear memories and anxiety.

Acute doses of EGb have been demonstrated to enhance attention and memory in young healthy volunteers. A significant improvement in short-term memory has been demonstrated following *G. biloba* extract administration at a dose of 600 mg in volunteers with cognitive impairment (Allain et al., 1993; Le Bars and Kastelan, 2000) and healthy volunteers (Subhan and Hindmarch, 1984). Higher dosages (up to 600 mg·day^{-1}) appear to be necessary to enhance memory when an acute dosage is used (Allain et al., 1993; Le Bars and Kastelan, 2000). One study demonstrated the efficacy of an acute treatment of EGb with 240 and 360 mg in young volunteers (Kennedy et al., 2000). Furthermore, EGb at a daily dose of 240 mg (chronic treatment) has been considered necessary to successfully ameliorate clinical symptoms, such as apathy, depression, motor alterations, and cognitive deficits (Gavrilova et al., 2014). Additionally, effects of EGb on mitochondrial function might substantiate their function on cognition and ameliorate the age-associated cognitive disorders (Müller et al., 2017).

In rats, several studies have showed that a lower than 240–300 mg·kg^{-1} did not have effect on cognitive performance when acute dose is administered, different than observed to chronic treatment (Tchantchou et al., 2007; Blecharz-Klin et al., 2009; Yoshitake et al., 2010; Kehr et al., 2012). Subacute treatment with EGb, at dose 300 mg·kg^{-1} was a significant increase in extracellular monoamines in pre-frontal cortex was related (5HT, Ach, and DOPA), which was considered relevant to clinical doses (Yoshitake et al., 2010; Kehr et al., 2012). Nevertheless, studies that evaluated the effects of chronic treatment of EGb in mice AD model showed that plasma concentration of EGb metabolites after chronic administration (5 months) of diet supplementary with EGb in dose around 69 mg·kg^{-1}·day^{-1}), was similar to secondary metabolites found in plasma human after with chronic treatment with 240 mg·day^{-1} EGb. Further chronic treatment with EGb 761 at dose 240–480 mg was effective in reduces

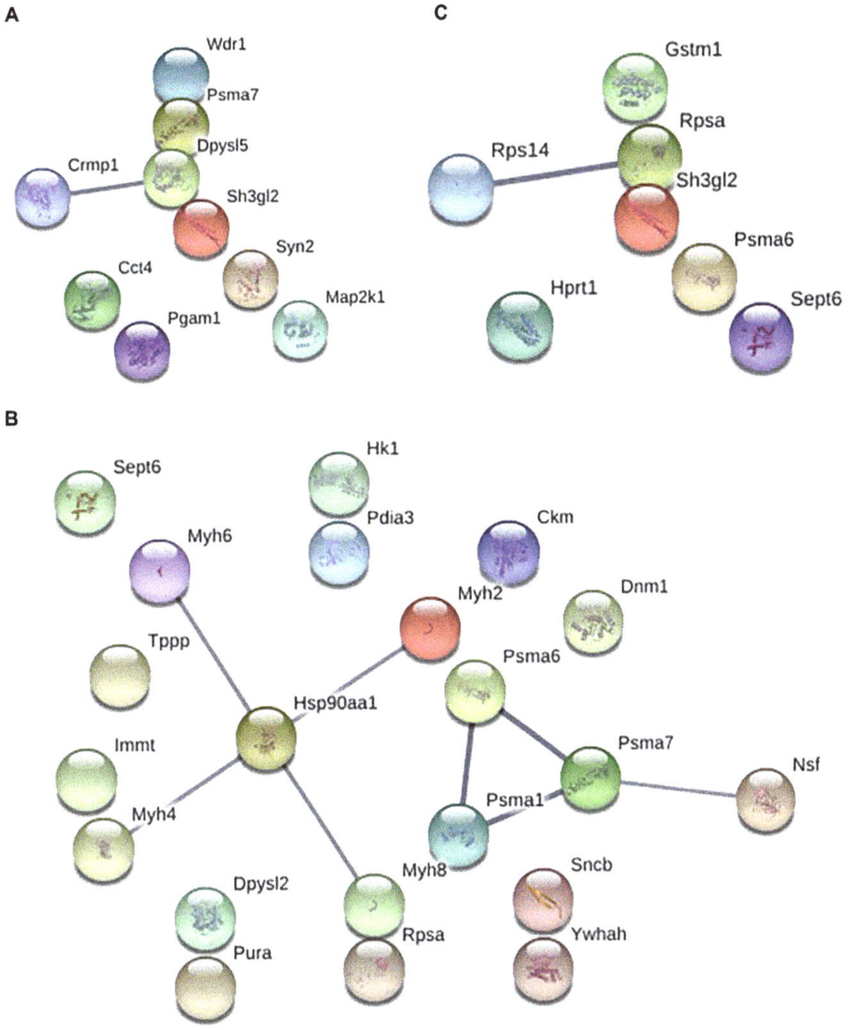

FIGURE 3 | Graphic representation of the protein–protein interaction networks with significant differences between the groups in dorsal hippocampal formation. EGb 0.25 g·kg^{-1} (nine nodes), enrichment *P*-value = 0.127 **(A)**. EGb 0.50 g·kg^{-1} (21 proteins), enrichment *P*-value = 0.000335 **(B)**. EGb 1.00 g·kg^{-1} (seven proteins), enrichment *P*-value = 0.592 **(C)**.

anxiety in middle-age patients with anxiety disorders, but in higher dose, the effects were more pronounced (Woelk et al., 2007). In this study, a dose of 500 mg·kg^{-1} was effective in reduce a conditioned suppression (anxiety-like effects) without impair fear memory. A comparative analysis between specific effects of EGb *in vivo* from pre clinical studies and equivalent dosage for humans was showed for Serrano-García et al. (2013), but all studies evaluate was for subacute or chronic treatment. In recent study, Tan et al. (2015) showed that treatment chronic with EGb was a be able to stabilize or slow decline in cognition function, global function, and behavior symptoms in patients with neuropsychiatric symptoms. Conversely, Birks and Colleagues (Birks and Evans, 2009; Yuan et al., 2017) showed in a meta-analysis study, that treatments of EGb seems no correlated with dose only. Furthermore, in attempt to evaluate drugs safety and efficacy, our group evaluate the suppression of licking behavior in rats submitted to acute, subacute, and chronic treatment with EGb (Oliveira et al., 2009, 2013), that results was compared with another anti-anxiety drugs. Acute (one dose), subacute (14 days), or chronic (30 days) treatment with EGb at dose of 500 and 1000 mg·kg^{-1} did not impair acquisition of fear memory. Furthermore, although the dose and regime of treatments were different, we found similar effects on gene expression in prefrontal cortex, amygdala, and hippocampus. However, in higher dose the effects were more pronounced.

We depicted for the first time that EGb modulates 32 proteins through both upregulation and downregulation in the dHF in a dose-dependent manner. We also found that treatment with EGb at a dose of 0.50 g·kg^{-1} affected the expression of a greater number of regulatory proteins when compared with the other doses. Furthermore, our results suggested that EGb modulates proteins, which might have therapeutic relevance since that they may be modulated for new pharmacological agents that can be used to enhance memory formation and to prevent or

TABLE 2 | Pathway significantly affected in the dorsal hippocampal formation of rats following treatment with standardized extract of *Ginkgo biloba* and acquisition of conditioned lick suppression.

	Pathway description	Protein	False discovery rate
0.25 g·kg^{-1} *Ginkgo biloba*	Membrane-bounded vesicle	T-complex protein 1 subunit delta ↑	0.0206
		Dual specificity mitogen-activated protein kinase kinase 1 ↑	
		Endophilin-A1 ↓	
		Synapsin-2 ↑	
		WD repeat-containing protein 1 ↑	
	Cellular component morphogenesis	Dihydropyrimidinase-related protein 1 ↑	0.0396
		Dihydropyrimidinase-related protein 5 ↑	
		Dual specificity mitogen-activated protein kinase kinase 1 ↑	
		WD repeat-containing protein 1 ↑	
	Cell projection	Dihydropyrimidinase-related protein 1 ↑	0.0429
		Dual specificity mitogen-activated protein kinase kinase 1 ↑	
		Synapsin-2 ↑	
		WD repeat-containing protein 1 ↑	
0.50 g·kg^{-1} *Ginkgo biloba*	Heterocyclic and organic cyclic compound binding	Creatine kinase M-type ↑	0.00615
		Dynamin-1 ↑	
		Hexokinase 1 ↑	
		Heat shock protein HSP 90-alpha ↑	
		Myosin-4 ↑	
		Myosin-6 ↑	
		Vesicle-fusing ATPase ↑	
		Protein disulfide-isomerase A3 ↑	
		Proteasome subunit alpha type-6 ↑	
	Cell projection part	Dynamin-1 ↑	0.00992
		Dihydropyrimidinase-related protein 2 ↑	
		Heat shock protein HSP 90-alpha ↑	
		Vesicle-fusing ATPase ↑	
		Beta-synuclein ↑	
	Somatodendritic compartment	Dihydropyrimidinase-related protein 2 ↑	0.0110
		Heat shock protein HSP 90-alpha ↑	
		Vesicle-fusing ATPase ↑	
		40S ribosomal protein SA ↓	
		Beta-synuclein ↑	
	Myelin sheath	Dihydropyrimidinase-related protein 2 ↑	0.0110
		Heat shock protein HSP 90-alpha ↑	
		Protein disulfide-isomerase A3 ↑	
	Neuronal cell body	Dihydropyrimidinase-related protein 2 ↑	0.0280
		Heat shock protein HSP 90-alpha ↑	
		40S ribosomal protein SA ↓	
		Beta-synuclein ↑	
	Tight junction	Myosin heavy chain IIa ↑	0.0305
		Myosin-4 ↑	
		Myosin-6 ↑	
	Neuron part	Dynamin-1 ↑	0.0499
		Heat shock protein HSP 90-alpha ↑	
		Vesicle-fusing ATPase ↑	
		40S ribosomal protein SA ↓	
		Beta-synuclein ↑	
1.00 g·kg^{-1} *Ginkgo biloba*	Ribosomal small subunit assembly	40S ribosomal protein S14 ↑	0.0300
		40S ribosomal protein SA ↓	

Up ↑ and down ↓ arrows indicate upregulation and downregulation, respectively. False discovery rate (corrected P-values for multiple testing using the method of Benjamini and Hochberg, 1995).

treat memory decline or anxiety disorders. To understand the differential effects of EGb, we investigated the protein–protein interactions at each dose.

Memory formation and its maintenance might involve distinct processes that occur over time and both *de novo* protein synthesis and post-translational modification of existing proteins (Jarome and Helmstetter, 2014; Yau et al., 2015). In this context, our present findings corroborated those of a large number of studies showing that molecular changes underlie memory acquisition and consolidation and have since shown that acquisition of conditioned lick suppression and treatment with EGb are correlated with multiple biological processes and signaling pathways that are crucial to the formation and maintenance of LTM. The differential protein expression patterns recognized in our studies have been found to be correlated with dendritic spine expansion or projection, the composition of structures in the somatodendritic compartment of neurons, the proteins involved in myelin sheath formation, and tight-junction composition.

The upregulated expression of dynamin-1, vesicle-fusing ATPase, and dihydropyrimidinase-related protein 2 in the dHF after treatment with EGb at a dose of 0.5 $g{\cdot}kg^{-1}$ suggested that EGb modulates events correlated to remodeling of the cytoskeleton and those involved in the control of the distinct pathways involved in neurotransmission events since they are also involved in dendritic spine development and maintenance, synaptic vesicle recycling, and insertion of glutamatergic receptors at synaptic sites, which are events that are described as essential to LTM formation and neurogenesis. Still, changes in these protein expression levels have been found to be correlated with hippocampal-dependent memory formation (Beretta et al., 2005; Guo et al., 2010; Fà et al., 2014; Migues et al., 2014; Jin et al., 2016; Yoo et al., 2016; Zhang et al., 2016). Corroborating with previous study, our data showed that EGb treatment modulate proteins whose activity are essential for normal mitochondrial function and synaptic plasticity in hippocampus as Dynanin-1 (Shields et al., 2015) and proteins, as Hexokinase 1 (HKI), which is associated with the outer mitochondrial membrane. HKI activity in neurons has been associated with cell survival and neuroprotection by suppressing apoptosis and oxidative stress (Saraiva et al., 2010).

Our results showed that the 0.50 $g{\cdot}kg^{-1}$ dose of EGb upregulated heat shock protein 90 alpha, disulfide-isomerase A3, and beta-synuclein, which are important in cellular homeostasis since they are involved in the transient changes in the activity of specific proteins that participate in the intracellular cascades that regulate gene transcription and *de novo* protein synthesis in the brain, cell stress responses, synaptic transmission, and autophagy (Stetler et al., 2010; Jarome and Helmstetter, 2014; Yau et al., 2015).

Several studies have noted that the heat shock protein 90 family facilitates cell signaling; assists in the efficient folding of newly translated proteins intracellular transport, maintenance and degradation of proteins; and the protection of mesenchymal stem cells from apoptosis and stimulates their migration. Furthermore, their roles in calcium homeostasis, neuron survival, axonal regeneration, and neuroprotection of the central and peripheral nervous systems have been shown (Loones et al., 2000; Gao et al., 2015; Ousman et al., 2017). The pharmacological inhibition of HSP 90 has been associated with neurodegenerative disease, suggesting the protective role of these proteins (Luo et al., 2010). Recent evidence has suggested their role in the enhancement of memory formation (Gyurko et al., 2014). Another chaperone protein that is important in the quality control of protein folding is disulfide-isomerase A3, which is an enzyme in the endoplasmic reticulum of eukaryotic cells that acts as a binding partner for other proteins and has a role in myelin sheath preservation. Their therapeutic roles as neuroprotective/anti-apoptotic and prosurvival proteins in several neurological disorders, including Alzheimer's disease, have been investigated (Hoffstrom et al., 2010; Imaoka, 2011; Gonzalez-Perez et al., 2015). Regarding beta-synuclein, its role in the central nervous system remains unclear. Beta-synuclein has been found to be associated with membrane stability and/or turnover of membrane components, and it also might act as a chaperone and might be found in pre-synaptic nerve terminals that are presently thought to be important for neural plasticity (George, 2001; Mori et al., 2002; Fujita et al., 2006). Their role in neurodegenerative diseases, such as Alzheimer's, Parkinson's, or ischemic disease, has been evaluated (Tanaka et al., 2000; Hashimoto et al., 2004; Hoffstrom et al., 2010; Leak, 2014).

Therefore, the upregulation of these proteins following treatment with EGb at a dose of 0.50 $g{\cdot}kg^{-1}$ aligned with the antioxidant and neuroprotective effects that have been proposed for EGb (DeFeudis, 2002; Ahlemeyer and Krieglstein, 2003a; Ribeiro et al., 2016) and indicated a possible therapeutic use of this extract in the prevention of neural diseases. Furthermore, previous data from our group showed that conditioned lick suppression downregulated alpha-synuclein (Gaiardo et al., unpublished) and that EGb upregulated beta-synuclein, which has been recognized as playing a role in chaperone activity more efficiently than alpha-synuclein (Lee et al., 2004). The correlation between the presence of beta-synuclein and the significant reduction in the rate of alpha-synuclein aggregation was shown by Brown et al. (2016), suggests a neuroprotective effect.

Myosin IIA is less predominant in the central nervous system, is required in the maintenance of tensile adhesion and neurite retraction, and is regulated during the induction of long-term potentiation. Their actions combine to generate the vectorial forces that are required for neurite extension (Wylie and Chantler, 2003; Liu and Cheney, 2012; Luissint et al., 2012). Myosin IIA was found to have a stronger association with actin filaments under oxidative stress, and the inhibition of the myosin IIA–actin interaction was found to be correlated with attenuated apoptosis and enhanced survival of PC12 neural cells in culture (Wang et al., 2017) and modulates synaptic plasticity in the lateral amygdaloid complex, which is involved in fear memory formation, seemingly preventing irrelevant memories (Lamprecht et al., 2006). Myosin VI is found in Golgi complexes and has a higher affinity for ADP. It is involved in the endocytosis and phagocytosis of AMPA receptors and serves as a target for other proteins involved in neurodegenerative disorders, such as Huntington's disease (Osterweil et al., 2005). Similarly, we observed upregulation of myosin IV following treatment with

EGb at a dose of 0.5 g·kg^{-1}. Both myosin IIA and VI play roles in calcium binding and protein phosphorylation (Buss and Kendrick-Jones, 2008).

Regarding the role of myosin, the present data allowed us to suggest that EGb might act by enabling the neural network to become more stable since it was found to promote changes in the cellular morphology and physiology of neural cells *via* changes in the activity of the different isoforms of myosin.

Concerning the effects on rats treated with EGb at a dose 0.25 g·kg^{-1}, we found that EGb modulates different pathways and proteins, and it may have the same effects *via* other pathways, for example, upregulation of proteins such as dual specificity mitogen-activated protein kinase 1, synapsin-2, dihydropyrimidinase-related protein 5, dihydropyrimidinase-related protein 1, and T-complex protein 1 subunit delta (molecular chaperone). These proteins have a crucial role in the control of signaling in long-lasting forms of synaptic plasticity and memory, modulating neurotransmitter release at the pre-synaptic cell, and playing a role in the generation and survival of newly generated neurons in the areas of the adult brain with a high level of activity-dependent neuronal plasticity (Kelleher et al., 2004; Bretin et al., 2005; Cesca et al., 2010).

The analysis of protein expression in the dHFs of rats treated with EGb at a dose of 1.0 g·kg^{-1} revealed an upregulation of septin-6, a member of a protein family that is highly expressed in the brain and takes part in processes such as regulation of the formation, growth and stability of axons and dendrites, synaptic plasticity, and vesicular trafficking, which are essential for memory formation (Cho et al., 2011; Hall and Russell, 2012). In addition, EGb treatment in higher doses may promote protective and preventive effects since proteasome 6 and tetra-(5-fluorotryptophanyl)-glutathione-S-transferase (all four tryptophan residues are replaced by the synthetic amino acid 5-fluorotryptophan, which causes a modest increase in catalytic activity) were upregulated. Further analyses are necessary, but these proteins might result in the improvement of fear memory consolidation and in the spontaneous recovery of fear memory established at this dose in previous studies by our group Zamberlam et al., 2016).
(

Protein degradation is a stage in protein turnover regulation. Studies over the last decade have demonstrates strong links between the maintenance of long-term potentiation and protein degradation (Dong et al., 2008; Hegde, 2010). Several behavioral studies have also confirmed the crucial role of the ubiquitin-proteasome system (UPS) in memory consolidation in the hippocampal formation (Lopez-Salon et al., 2001; Artinian et al., 2008). The effects of dysregulation of the UPS on neurons and glial cells may contribute to several neural diseases because large insoluble aggregates of misfolded proteins can form and then result in neurotoxicity (Lehman, 2009; Jansen et al., 2014). These proteins are essential for the disposal of exogenous toxic compounds and for antioxidant responses to reactive oxygen species (Strange et al., 2001). Our findings showed upregulation of the alpha type subunits (1 and 6) of the UPS, corroborating the findings of previous studies, which showed upregulation of the UPS following EGb treatment (Liu et al., 2009; Stark and Behl, 2014).

Furthermore, proteasome subunit alpha type-7, endophilin-A1, and 40S ribosomal protein SA were downregulated following EGb treatment in comparison with the vehicle group. Despite the reduction observed in these proteins, other proteins with the same effects were upregulated. For example, proteasome subunit alpha type-7 was downregulated by the 0.25 and 0.50 g·kg^{-1} doses; conversely, these doses upregulated other proteins with similar functions, such as T-complex protein 1 subunit delta, proteasome subunit alpha type-1, and heat shock protein HSP 90-alpha. In this context, EGb modulates, in a dose-dependent manner, different pathways, which may correlate with the behavioral effects that were previously described by our group in relation to fear memory and anxiety.

In summary, the comparative dHF proteome analysis allowed us to identify proteins whose altered expression may underlie the effects of EGb on conditioned suppression. We identified 32 different protein expression patterns that correlated with dendritic spine expansion or projection, the composition of structures in the somatodendritic compartment, and with proteins involved in myelin sheath formation and preservation, as well as those involved in tight-junction composition, which are mechanisms that are involved in the long-term changes that are crucial for LTM formation. The present data might explain, at least in part, the beneficial effects of EGb on memory formation.

PROTEOME PROFILING DATA

The mass spectrometry proteomics data have been deposited to the PRIDE Archive (http://www.ebi.ac.uk/pride/archive/) *via* the PRIDE partner repository with the data set identifier PXD009894.

AUTHOR CONTRIBUTIONS

RG performed all the experiments and was responsible for the writing of the manuscript in its entirety. TA performed the mass spectrometry analysis. SC was responsible for conceptualizing and revising the manuscript. AT and MT were involved in conceptualizing and proofreading. All authors gave their final approval for the submission of the manuscript.

FUNDING

This study was financed in part by the Coordenação de Aperfeiçoamento de Pessoal de Nível Superior – Brasil (CAPES) – Finance Code 001, the Studies and Projects Financier (FINEP), and the São Paulo State Research Foundation (FAPESP) grant 2013/20378-8 and 2016/18039-9 (to SC) and 2016/03839-0 (to AT).

REFERENCES

Ahlemeyer, B., and Krieglstein, J. (2003a). Neuroprotective effects of *Ginkgo biloba* extract. *Cell Mol. Life Sci. C* 60, 1779–1792. doi: 10.1007/s00018-003-3080-1

Ahlemeyer, B., and Krieglstein, J. (2003b). Pharmacological studies supporting the therapeutic use of *Ginkgo biloba* extract for Alzheimer's disease. *Pharmacopsychiatry* 36, 8–14. doi: 10.1055/s-2003-40454

Allain, H., Raoul, P., Lieury, A., LeCoz, F., Gandon, J. M., and d'Arbigny, P. (1993). Effect of two doses of *Ginkgo biloba* extract (EGb 761) on the dual-coding test in elderly subjects. *Clin. Ther.* 15, 549–558.

Artinian, J., McGauran, A.-M. T., De Jaeger, X., Mouledous, L., Frances, B., and Roullet, P. (2008). Protein degradation, as with protein synthesis, is required during not only long-term spatial memory consolidation but also reconsolidation. *Eur. J. Neurosci.* 27, 3009–3019. doi: 10.1111/j.1460-9568.2008.06262.x

Barco, A., Pittenger, C., and Kandel, E. R. (2003). CREB, memory enhancement and the treatment of memory disorders: promises, pitfalls and prospects. *Expert Opin. Ther. Targets* 7, 101–114. doi: 10.1517/14728222.7.1.101

Benjamini, Y., and Hochberg, Y. (1995). Controlling the false discovery rate: a practical and powerful approach to multiple testing. *J. R. Stat. Soc.* 57, 289–300. doi: 10.1111/j.2517-6161.1995.tb02031.x

Beretta, F., Sala, C., Saglietti, L., Hirling, H., Sheng, M., and Passafaro, M. (2005). NSF interaction is important for direct insertion of GluR2 at synaptic sites. *Mol. Cell. Neurosci.* 28, 650–660. doi: 10.1016/j.mcn.2004.11.008

Birks, J., and Evans, J. G. (2009). *Ginkgo biloba* for cognitive impairment and dementia. *Cochr. Database Syst. Rev.* 18:CD003120. doi: 10.1002/14651858.CD003120.pub3

Blecharz-Klin, K., Piechal, A., Joniec, I., Pyrzanowska, J., and Widy-Tyszkiewicz, E. (2009). Pharmacological and biochemical effects of *Ginkgo biloba* extract on learning, memory consolidation and motor activity in old rats. *Acta Neurobiol. Exp. (Wars)* 69, 217–231.

Bretin, S., Reibel, S., Charrier, E., Maus-Moatti, M., Auvergnon, N., Thevenoux, A., et al. (2005). Differential expression of CRMP1, CRMP2A, CRMP2B, and CRMP5 in axons or dendrites of distinct neurons in the mouse brain. *J. Comp. Neurol.* 486, 1–17. doi: 10.1002/cne.20465

Brown, J. W. P., Buell, A. K., Michaels, T. C. T., Meisl, G., Carozza, J., Flagmeier, P., et al. (2016). β-Synuclein suppresses both the initiation and amplification steps of α-synuclein aggregation via competitive binding to surfaces. *Sci. Rep.* 6:36010. doi: 10.1038/srep36010

Buss, F., and Kendrick-Jones, J. (2008). How are the cellular functions of myosin VI regulated within the cell? *Biochem. Biophys. Res. Commun.* 369, 165–175. doi: 10.1016/j.bbrc.2007.11.150

Cammarota, M., Bevilaqua, L. R., Rossato, J. I., Lima, R. H., Medina, J. H., and Izquierdo, I. (2008). Parallel memory processing by the CA1 region of the dorsal hippocampus and the basolateral amygdala. *Proc. Natl. Acad. Sci. U.S.A.* 105, 10279–10284. doi: 10.1073/pnas.0805284105

Carew, T. J., and Sahley, C. L. (1986). Invertebrate learning and memory: from behavior to molecules. *Annu. Rev. Neurosci.* 9, 435–487. doi: 10.1146/annurev.ne.09.030186.002251

Cerutti, S. M., Gomide, V. C., de Moraes Ferrari, E. A., and Chadi, G. (2009). Long-term astroglial reaction and neuronal plasticity in the subcortical visual pathways after a complete ablation of telencephalon in pigeons (*Columba livia*). *Int. J. Neurosci.* 119, 384–403. doi: 10.1080/00207450802480291

Cesca, F., Baldelli, P., Valtorta, F., and Benfenati, F. (2010). The synapsins: key actors of synapse function and plasticity. *Prog. Neurobiol.* 91, 313–348. doi: 10.1016/j.pneurobio.2010.04.006

Cho, S.-J., Lee, H., Dutta, S., Song, J., Walikonis, R., and Moon, I. S. (2011). Septin 6 regulates the cytoarchitecture of neurons through localization at dendritic branch points and bases of protrusions. *Mol. Cells* 32, 89–98. doi: 10.1007/s10059-011-1048-9

DeFeudis, F. V. (2002). Effects of *Ginkgo biloba* extract (EGb 761) on gene expression: possible relevance to neurological disorders and age-associated cognitive impairment. *Drug Dev. Res.* 57, 214–235. doi: 10.1002/ddr.10151

Dong, C., Upadhya, S. C., Ding, L., Smith, T. K., and Hegde, A. N. (2008). Proteasome inhibition enhances the induction and impairs the maintenance of late-phase long-term potentiation. *Learn. Mem.* 15, 335–347. doi: 10.1101/lm.984508

Fà, M., Staniszewski, A., Saeed, F., Francis, Y. I., and Arancio, O. (2014). Dynamin 1 is required for memory formation. *PLoS One* 9:e91954. doi: 10.1371/journal.pone.0091954

Fendt, M., and Fanselow, M. S. (1999). The neuroanatomical and neurochemical basis of conditioned fear. *Neurosci. Biobehav. Rev.* 23, 743–760. doi: 10.1016/S0149-7634(99)00016-0

Frey, U., Huang, Y., and Kandel, E. (1993). Effects of cAMP simulate a late stage of LTP in hippocampal CA1 neurons. *Science (80-)* 260, 1661–1664. doi: 10.1126/science.8389057

Fujita, M., Wei, J., Nakai, M., Masliah, E., and Hashimoto, M. (2006). Chaperone and anti-chaperone: two-faced synuclein as stimulator of synaptic evolution. *Neuropathology* 26, 383–392. doi: 10.1111/j.1440-1789.2006.00732.x

Gao, F., Hu, X., Xie, X., Liu, X., and Wang, J. (2015). Heat shock protein 90 stimulates rat mesenchymal stem cell migration via PI3K/Akt and ERK1/2 pathways. *Cell Biochem. Biophys.* 71, 481–489. doi: 10.1007/s12013-014-0228-6

Gavrilova, S. I., Preuss, U. W., Wong, J. W. M., Hoerr, R., Kaschel, R., and Bachinskaya, N. (2014). Efficacy and safety of *Ginkgo biloba* extract EGb 761? in mild cognitive impairment with neuropsychiatric symptoms: a randomized, placebo-controlled, double-blind, multicenter trial. *Int. J. Geriatr. Psychiatry* 29, 1087–1095. doi: 10.1002/gps.4103

George, J. M. (2001). The synucleins. *Genome Biol.* 3:reviews3002.1.

Giese, K. P., and Mizuno, K. (2013). The roles of protein kinases in learning and memory. *Learn. Mem.* 20, 540–552. doi: 10.1101/lm.028449.112

Gonzalez-Perez, P., Woehlbier, U., Chian, R.-J., Sapp, P., Rouleau, G. A., Leblond, C. S., et al. (2015). Identification of rare protein disulfide isomerase gene variants in amyotrophic lateral sclerosis patients. *Gene* 566, 158–165. doi: 10.1016/j.gene.2015.04.035

Guo, C.-H., Senzel, A., Li, K., and Feng, Z.-P. (2010). De novo protein synthesis of syntaxin-1 and dynamin-1 in long-term memory formation requires CREB1 gene transcription in *Lymnaea stagnalis*. *Behav. Genet.* 40, 680–693. doi: 10.1007/s10519-010-9374-9

Gyurko, D. M., Soti, C., Stetak, A., and Csermely, P. (2014). System level mechanisms of adaptation, learning, memory formation and evolvability: the role of chaperone and other networks. *Curr. Protein Pept. Sci.* 15, 171–188. doi: 10.2174/1389203715666140331110522

Hall, P. A., and Russell, S. H. (2012). Mammalian septins: dynamic heteromers with roles in cellular morphogenesis and compartmentalization. *J. Pathol.* 226, 287–299. doi: 10.1002/path.3024

Hashimoto, M., Bar-on, P., Ho, G., Takenouchi, T., Rockenstein, E., Crews, L., et al. (2004). β-synuclein regulates Akt activity in neuronal cells. *J. Biol. Chem.* 279, 23622–23629. doi: 10.1074/jbc.M313784200

Hegde, A. N. (2010). The ubiquitin-proteasome pathway and synaptic plasticity. *Learn. Mem.* 17, 314–327. doi: 10.1101/lm.1504010

Hoffstrom, B. G., Kaplan, A., Letso, R., Schmid, R. S., Turmel, G. J., Lo, D. C., et al. (2010). Inhibitors of protein disulfide isomerase suppress apoptosis induced by misfolded proteins. *Nat. Chem. Biol.* 6, 900–906. doi: 10.1038/nchembio.467

Hotulainen, P., and Hoogenraad, C. C. (2010). Actin in dendritic spines: connecting dynamics to function. *J. Cell Biol.* 189, 619–629. doi: 10.1083/jcb.201003008

Imaoka, S. (2011). "Chemical stress on protein disulfide isomerases and inhibition of their functions," in *International Review of Cell and Molecular Biology*, ed. K. W. Jeon (Amsterdam: Elsevier Inc.), 121–166.

Itil, T. M., Eralp, E., Tsambis, E., Itil, K. Z., and Stein, U. (1996). Central nervous system effects of *Ginkgo biloba*, a plant extract. *Am. J. Ther.* 3, 63–73. doi: 10.1097/00045391-199601000-00009

Izquierdo, I., Quillfeldt, J. A., Zanatta, M. S., Quevedo, J., Schaeffer, E., Schmitz, P. K., et al. (1997). Sequential role of hippocampus and amygdala, entorhinal cortex and parietal cortex in formation and retrieval of memory for inhibitory avoidance in rats. *Eur. J. Neurosci.* 9, 786–793. doi: 10.1111/j.1460-9568.1997.tb01427.x

Jansen, A. H. P., Reits, E. A. J., and Hol, E. M. (2014). The ubiquitin proteasome system in glia and its role in neurodegenerative diseases. *Front. Mol. Neurosci.* 7:73. doi: 10.3389/fnmol.2014.00073

Jarome, T. J., and Helmstetter, F. J. (2014). Protein degradation and protein synthesis in long-term memory formation. *Front. Mol. Neurosci.* 7:61. doi: 10.3389/fnmol.2014.00061

Jin, X., Sasamoto, K., Nagai, J., Yamazaki, Y., Saito, K., Goshima, Y., et al. (2016). Phosphorylation of CRMP2 by Cdk5 regulates dendritic spine development of cortical neuron in the mouse hippocampus. *Neural Plast.* 2016, 1–7. doi: 10.1155/2016/6790743

Kandel, E. R. (2001). The molecular biology of memory storage: a dialogue between genes and synapses. *Science (80-)* 294, 1030–1038. doi: 10.1126/science.1067020

Kandel, E. R., Dudai, Y., and Mayford, M. R. (2014). The molecular and systems biology of memory. *Cell* 157, 163–186. doi: 10.1016/j.cell.2014.03.001

Kehr, J., Yoshitake, S., Ijiri, S., Koch, E., Nöldner, M., and Yoshitake, T. (2012). *Ginkgo biloba* leaf extract (EGb 761®) and its specific acylated flavonol constituents increase dopamine and acetylcholine levels in the rat medial prefrontal cortex: possible implications for the cognitive enhancing properties of EGb 761®. *Int. Psychogeriatr.* 24(Suppl. 1), S25–S34. doi: 10.1017/S1041610212000567

Kelleher, R. J., Govindarajan, A., Jung, H.-Y., Kang, H., and Tonegawa, S. (2004). Translational control by MAPK signaling in long-term synaptic plasticity and memory. *Cell* 116, 467–479. doi: 10.1016/S0092-8674(04)00115-1

Kennedy, D. O., Scholey, A. B., and Wesnes, K. A. (2000). The dose-dependent cognitive effects of acute administration of *Ginkgo biloba* to healthy young volunteers. *Psychopharmacology (Berl)* 151, 416–423. doi: 10.1007/s002130000501

Lamprecht, R., Margulies, D. S., Farb, C. R., Hou, M., Johnson, L. R., and LeDoux, J. E. (2006). Myosin light chain kinase regulates synaptic plasticity and fear learning in the lateral amygdala. *Neuroscience* 139, 821–829. doi: 10.1016/j.neuroscience.2005.12.055

Le Bars, P. L., and Kastelan, J. (2000). Efficacy and safety of a *Ginkgo biloba* extract. *Public Heal Nutr.* 3, 495–499. doi: 10.1017/S1368980000000574

Leak, R. K. (2014). Heat shock proteins in neurodegenerative disorders and aging. *J. Cell Commun. Signal.* 8, 293–310. doi: 10.1007/s12079-014-0243-9

Lee, D., Paik, S. R., and Choi, K. Y. (2004). β-Synuclein exhibits chaperone activity more efficiently than α-synuclein. *FEBS Lett.* 576, 256–260. doi: 10.1016/j.febslet.2004.08.075

Lehman, N. L. (2009). The ubiquitin proteasome system in neuropathology. *Acta Neuropathol.* 118, 329–347. doi: 10.1007/s00401-009-0560-x

Liu, K. C., and Cheney, R. E. (2012). Myosins in cell junctions. *Bioarchitecture* 2, 158–170. doi: 10.4161/bioa.21791

Liu, X.-P., Goldring, C. E. P., Wang, H.-Y., Copple, I. M., Kitteringham, N. R., and Park, B. K. (2009). Extract of *Ginkgo biloba* induces glutathione-S-transferase subunit-P1 in vitro. *Phytomedicine* 16, 451–455. doi: 10.1016/j.phymed.2008.11.001

Loones, M.-T., Chang, Y., and Morange, M. (2000). The distribution of heat shock proteins in the nervous system of the unstressed mouse embryo suggests a role in neuronal and non-neuronal differentiation. *Cell Stress Chaper.* 5:291. doi: 10.1379/1466-1268(2000)005<0291:TDOHSP>2.0.CO;2

Lopez-Salon, M., Alonso, M., Vianna, M. R. M., Viola, H. E., Souza, T. M., Izquierdo, I., et al. (2001). The ubiquitin-proteasome cascade is required for mammalian long-term memory formation. *Eur. J. Neurosci.* 14, 1820–1826. doi: 10.1046/j.0953-816x.2001.01806.x

Luissint, A.-C., Artus, C., Glacial, F., Ganeshamoorthy, K., and Couraud, P.-O. (2012). Tight junctions at the blood brain barrier: physiological architecture and disease-associated dysregulation. *Fluids Barriers CNS* 9:23. doi: 10.1186/2045-8118-9-23

Luo, W., Sun, W., Taldone, T., Rodina, A., and Chiosis, G. (2010). Heat shock protein 90 in neurodegenerative diseases. *Mol. Neurodegener.* 5:24. doi: 10.1186/1750-1326-5-24

Lynch, G. (2002). Memory enhancement: the search for mechanism-based drugs. *Nat. Neurosci.* 5(Suppl.), 1035–1038. doi: 10.1038/nn935

Mayford, M., Siegelbaum, S. A., and Kandel, E. R. (2012). Synapses and memory storage. *Cold Spring Harb. Perspect. Biol.* 4, 1–18. doi: 10.1101/cshperspect.a005751

McGaugh, J. L. (1966). Time-dependent processes in memory storage. *Science (80-)* 153, 1351–1358. doi: 10.1126/science.153.3742.1351

Migues, P. V., Hardt, O., Finnie, P., Wang, Y. W., and Nader, K. (2014). The maintenance of long-term memory in the hippocampus depends on the interaction between N -ethylmaleimide-sensitive factor and GluA2. *Hippocampus* 24, 1112–1119. doi: 10.1002/hipo.22295

Mori, F., Tanji, K., Yoshimoto, M., Takahashi, H., and Wakabayashi, K. (2002). Immunohistochemical comparison of α- and β-synuclein in adult rat central nervous system. *Brain Res.* 941, 118–126. doi: 10.1016/S0006-8993(02)02643-4

Müller, W. E., Eckert, A., Eckert, G. P., Fink, H., Friedland, K., Gauthier, S., et al. (2017). Therapeutic efficacy of the Ginkgo special extract EGb761® within the framework of the mitochondrial cascade hypothesis of Alzheimer's disease. *World J. Biol. Psychiatry* [Epub ahead of print]. doi: 10.1080/15622975.2017.1308552

Oliveira, D. R., de Zamberlam, C. R., Rêgo, G. M., Cavalheiro, A. J., Cerutti, J. M., and Cerutti, S. M. (2016). Effects of the a flavonoid-rich fraction on the acquisition and extinction of fear memory: pharmacological and molecular approaches. *Front. Behav. Neurosci.* 9:345. doi: 10.3389/fnbeh.2015.00345

Oliveira, D. R., Sanada, P. F., Filho, A. C. S., Conceição, G. M. S., Cerutti, J. M., and Cerutti, S. M. (2013). Long-term treatment with standardized extract of *Ginkgo biloba* L. enhances the conditioned suppression of licking in rats by the modulation of neuronal and glial cell function in the dorsal hippocampus and central amygdala. *Neuroscience* 235, 70–86. doi: 10.1016/j.neuroscience.2013.01.009

Oliveira, D. R., Sanada, P. F., Saragossa, F. A. C., Innocenti, L. R., Oler, G., Cerutti, J. M., et al. (2009). Neuromodulatory property of standardized extract *Ginkgo biloba* L. (*EGb* 761) on memory: behavioral and molecular evidence. *Brain Res.* 1269, 68–89. doi: 10.1016/j.brainres.2008.11.105

Osterweil, E., Wells, D. G., and Mooseker, M. S. (2005). A role for myosin VI in postsynaptic structure and glutamate receptor endocytosis. *J. Cell Biol.* 168, 329–338. doi: 10.1083/jcb.200410091

Ousman, S. S., Frederick, A., and Lim, E. M. F. (2017). Chaperone proteins in the central nervous system and peripheral nervous system after nerve injury. *Front. Neurosci.* 11:79. doi: 10.3389/fnins.2017.00079

Pedroso, A. P., Watanabe, R. L. H., Albuquerque, K. T., Telles, M. M., Andrade, M. C. C., Perez, J. D., et al. (2012). Proteomic profiling of the rat hypothalamus. *Proteome Sci.* 10, 26–40. doi: 10.1186/1477-5956-10-26

Ribeiro, M. L., Moreira, L. M., Arçari, D. P., dos Santos, L. F., Marques, A. C., Pedrazzoli, J., et al. (2016). Protective effects of chronic treatment with a standardized extract of *Ginkgo biloba* L. in the prefrontal cortex and dorsal hippocampus of middle-aged rats. *Behav. Brain Res.* 313, 144–150. doi: 10.1016/j.bbr.2016.06.029

Saraiva, L. M., Seixas da Silva, G. S., Galina, A., da-Silva, W. S., Klein, W. L., Ferreira, S. T., et al. (2010). Amyloid-β triggers the release of neuronal Hexokinase 1 from mitochondria. *PLoS One* 5:e15230. doi: 10.1371/journal.pone.0015230

Serrano-García, N., Pedraza-Chaverri, J., Mares-Sámano, J. J., Orozco-Ibarra, M., Cruz-Salgado, A., Jiménez-Anguiano, A., et al. (2013). Antiapoptotic effects of EGb 761. *Evid. Based Complement. Alternat. Med.* 2013:495703. doi: 10.1155/2013/495703

Shevchenko, A., Wilm, M., Vorm, O., and Mann, M. (1996). Mass spectrometric sequencing of proteins from silver-stained polyacrylamide gels. *Anal. Chem.* 68, 850–858. doi: 10.1021/ac950914h

Shields, L. Y., Kim, H., Zhu, L., Haddad, D., Berthet, A., Pathak, D., et al. (2015). Dynamin-related protein 1 is required for normal mitochondrial bioenergetic and synaptic function in CA1 hippocampal neurons. *Cell Death Dis.* 6:e1725. doi: 10.1038/cddis.2015.94

Stark, M., and Behl, C. (2014). The *Ginkgo biloba* extract EGb 761 modulates proteasome activity and polyglutamine protein aggregation. *Evid. Based Complement. Altern. Med.* 2014, 1–14. doi: 10.1155/2014/940186

Stetler, R. A., Gan, Y., Zhang, W., Liou, A. K., Gao, Y., Cao, G., et al. (2010). Heat shock proteins: cellular and molecular mechanisms in the central nervous system. *Prog. Neurobiol.* 92, 184–211. doi: 10.1016/j.pneurobio.2010.05.002

Stork, O. (1999). Memory formation and the regulation of gene expression. *Cell Mol. Life Sci.* 55, 575–592. doi: 10.1007/s000180050316

Strange, R. C., Spiteri, M. A., Ramachandran, S., and Fryer, A. A. (2001). Glutathione-S-transferase family of enzymes. *Mutat. Res. Mol. Mech. Mutagen.* 482, 21–26. doi: 10.1016/S0027-5107(01)00206-8

Subhan, Z., and Hindmarch, I. (1984). The psychopharmacological effects of *Ginkgo biloba* in normal healthy volunteers. *Int. J. Clin. Pharmacol. Res.* 4, 89–93.

Tan, M. S., Yu, J. T., Tan, C. C., Wang, H. F., Meng, X. F., Wang, C., et al. (2015). Efficacy and adverse effects of *Ginkgo biloba* for cognitive impairment and dementia: a systematic review and meta-analysis. *J. Alzheimer's Dis.* 43, 589–603. doi: 10.3233/JAD-140837

Tanaka, S., Uehara, T., and Nomura, Y. (2000). Up-regulation of protein-disulfide isomerase in response to hypoxia/brain ischemia and its protective effect against apoptotic cell death. *J. Biol. Chem.* 275, 10388–10393. doi: 10.1074/jbc.275.14.10388

Tchantchou, F., Xu, Y., Wu, Y., Christen, Y., and Luo, Y. (2007). EGb 761 enhances adult hippocampal neurogenesis and phosphorylation of CREB in transgenic mouse model of Alzheimer's disease. *FASEB J.* 21, 2400–2408. doi: 10.1096/fj.06-7649com

Wang, Y., Xu, Y., Liu, Q., Zhang, Y., Gao, Z., Yin, M., et al. (2017). Myosin IIA-related actomyosin contractility mediates oxidative stress-induced neuronal apoptosis. *Front. Mol. Neurosci.* 10:75. doi: 10.3389/fnmol.2017.00075

Woelk, H., Arnoldt, K. H., Kieser, M., and Hoerr, R. (2007). *Ginkgo biloba* special extract EGb 761 in generalized anxiety disorder and adjustment disorder with anxious mood: a randomized, double-blind, placebo-controlled trial. *J. Psychiatr. Res.* 41, 472–480. doi: 10.1016/j.jpsychires.2006.05.004

Won, J., and Silva, A. J. (2008). Molecular and cellular mechanisms of memory allocation in neuronetworks. *Neurobiol. Learn. Mem.* 89, 285–292. doi: 10.1016/j.nlm.2007.08.017

Wylie, S. R., and Chantler, P. D. (2003). Myosin {IIA} drives neurite retraction. *Mol. Biol. Cell* 14, 4654–4666. doi: 10.1091/mbc.e03-03-0187

Yau, S., Li, A., and So, K.-F. (2015). Involvement of adult hippocampal neurogenesis in learning and forgetting. *Neural Plast.* 2015, 1–13. doi: 10.1155/2015/717958

Yoo, D. Y., Jung, H. Y., Kim, J. W., Yim, H. S., Kim, D. W., Nam, H., et al. (2016). Reduction of dynamin 1 in the hippocampus of aged mice is associated with the decline in hippocampal-dependent memory. *Mol. Med. Rep.* 14, 4755–4760. doi: 10.3892/mmr.2016.5804

Yoshitake, T., Yoshitake, S., and Kehr, J. (2010). The *Ginkgo biloba* extract EGb 761(R) and its main constituent flavonoids and ginkgolides increase extracellular dopamine levels in the rat prefrontal cortex. *Br. J. Pharmacol.* 159, 659–668. doi: 10.1111/j.1476-5381.2009.00580.x

Yuan, Q., Wang, C., Shi, J., and Lin, Z. (2017). Effects of *Ginkgo biloba* on dementia: an overview of systematic reviews. *J. Ethnopharmacol.* 195, 1–9. doi: 10.1016/j.jep.2016.12.005

Zamberlam, C. R., Vendrasco, N. C., Oliveira, D. R., Gaiardo, R. B., and Cerutti, S. M. (2016). Effects of standardized *Ginkgo biloba* extract on the acquisition, retrieval and extinction of conditioned suppression: evidence that short-term memory and long-term memory are differentially modulated. *Physiol. Behav.* 165, 55–68. doi: 10.1016/j.physbeh.2016.06.036

Zhang, H., Kang, E., Wang, Y., Yang, C., Yu, H., Wang, Q., et al. (2016). Brain-specific Crmp2 deletion leads to neuronal development deficits and behavioural impairments in mice. *Nat. Commun.* 7, 1–11. doi: 10.1038/ncomms11773

10

Anti-Neuroinflammatory Potential of Natural Products in Attenuation of Alzheimer's Disease

Bushra Shal[1†], Wei Ding[2†], Hussain Ali[1], Yeong S. Kim[3*] and Salman Khan[1*]

[1] Department of Pharmacy, Faculty of Biological Sciences, Quaid-i-Azam University, Islamabad, Pakistan, [2] Department of Neurosurgery, Rizhao Hospital of Traditional Chinese Medicine, Rizhao, China, [3] College of Pharmacy, Seoul National University, Seoul, South Korea

***Correspondence:**
Salman Khan
skhan@qau.edu.pk
Yeong S. Kim
kims@snu.ac.kr

† These authors have contributed equally to this work.

Alzheimer's disease (AD) is a chronic progressive neurodegenerative disorder associated with dementia and cognitive impairment most common in elderly population. Various pathophysiological mechanisms have been proposed by numerous researcher, although, exact mechanism is not yet elucidated. Several studies have been indicated that neuroinflammation associated with deposition of amyloid- beta (Aβ) in brain is a major hallmark toward the pathology of neurodegenerative diseases. So, there is a need to unravel the link of inflammatory process in neurodegeneration. Increased microglial activation, expression of cytokines, reactive oxygen species (ROS), and nuclear factor kappa B (NF-κB) participate in inflammatory process of AD. This review mainly concentrates on involvement of neuroinflammation and the molecular mechanisms adapted by various natural compounds, phytochemicals and herbal formulations in various signaling pathways involved in neuroprotection. Currently, pharmacologically active natural products, having anti-neuroinflammatory potential are being focused which makes them potential candidate to cure AD. A number of preclinical and clinical trials have been done on nutritional and botanical agents. Analysis of anti-inflammatory and neuroprotective phytochemicals such as terpenoids, phenolic derivatives, alkaloids, glycosides, and steroidal saponins displays therapeutic potential toward amelioration and prevention of devastating neurodegeneration observed in AD.

Keywords: Alzheimer's disease, neuroinflammation, natural products, herbal formulation, phytochemicals, neuroprotection

INTRODUCTION

Alzheimer's disease (AD) is a neurodegenerative disorder that accounts for age-related dementia in more than 80% cases worldwide (Anand et al., 2013). It is a progressive disease leading to disturbances of memory and cognitive function. It is estimated that ~5 million people with age 65 years or older and 200,000 people younger than 65 years are affected by AD. However, the total estimated prevalence by 2050 is expected to be 13.8 million (Alzheimer's Association, 2015). Limitation of existing preventive methods has increased the importance of intervention therapies using natural products rich in antioxidant and flavonoid content. The neuroprotective effect of natural compounds has been explored through preclinical and clinical studies using *in vitro* and *in vivo* models (Essa et al., 2012). Currently, approved treatments by US Food and Drug Administration (FDA), includes acetylcholinesterase inhibitors (AChEIs) and N-Methyl-D-Aspartate (NMDA) receptor antagonists that are involved in the symptomatic treatment of AD (Auld et al., 2002). However, due to serious side effects and limitations these drugs are rarely prescribed (Kumar and Singh, 2015). These are forms of palliative care, which slows the progression of cognitive symptoms and prevents any worsening of the patient's symptoms (Farlow et al., 2008). There is no proper treatment leading to cure AD till now (Ramirez-Bermudez, 2012). Immense efforts are directed toward identification of various disease-modifying therapies and discovering drugs targeting molecular pathways and blocking progression of AD (Kurz and Perneczky, 2011).

Multiple biological processes such as cognitive decline, abnormal deposition of amyloid β peptide (Aβ), accumulation of neurofibrillary tangles (NFTs), neuroinflammation, depletion or insufficient synthesis of neurotransmitters, oxidative stress, and abnormal ubiquitination linked to neurodegenerative diseases such as AD (Korolev, 2014). Genetic and environmental factors both contribute to the pathogenesis of the AD. On the basis of a number of causative factors several hypotheses have been presented to explain this multifactorial disorder, this includes the Aβ hypothesis, tau hypothesis, cholinergic hypothesis, and inflammation hypothesis (Rashid and Ansari, 2014). Recently inflammation hypothesis has gained considerable importance, innate immunity and neuroinflammation is involved in pathogenesis of neurodegenerative processes such as Alzheimer's disease (AD) due to the production of pro-inflammatory cytokines influencing the surrounding brain tissue, shown in **Figure 1** (Tan et al., 2013). Immune cells such as microglia activate resulting in production and release of proinflammatory cytokines, such as IFN-γ, IL-1β, and TNF-α (Tan et al., 2013). These cytokines stimulate the nearby astrocyte–neuron to produce further amounts of Aβ42 oligomers, thus, activating more Aβ42 production and dispersal (Dal Prà et al., 2015). Increase in the level of pro-inflammatory cytokines has been observed in the brain, serum, and cerebrospinal fluid (CSF) of AD patients in previous reports (Dursun et al., 2015). In AD Aβ form insoluble and extracellular pathological aggregates which attract microglial cells, forming clusters of microglia at sites of Aβ deposition (Streit et al., 2004). Experimental studies in animals supported the idea of involvement of microglia in phagocytosis and degradation of amyloid, such phagocytosis is ineffective in AD (Weldon et al., 1998). Activation of microglial cells and neuronal loss have been reported by direct injection of Aβ into the brain (Weldon et al., 1998). TNF-α and IL-1β affects the function of blood-brain barrier, as well as also leads to the activation of astrocytes as a secondary response, long-term effect of these cytokines can be detrimental to the astrocyte survival (Lim et al., 2013). However, it reveals a potential new target cell explaining negative effects of cytokines on brain tissue during neuroinflammation (Lim et al., 2013). Many studies have also directly associated cognitive decline with the levels of cytokines in AD patients at all stages, however, there are no drugs approved for neuroinflammation in AD (Garcez et al., 2017).

Natural polyphenolic phytochemicals have recently gained greater attention as alternative therapeutic agents against AD (Essa et al., 2012). They are considered less toxic and more effective than novel synthetic drugs (Kim et al., 2010). However, commonly herbal medicines are prepared from the crude materials, which raise questions regarding their mechanism of action and medicinal effects. Recently, research has been focused on specific active components rather than on an entire herb (Morales et al., 2014). Therefore, there is a need to identify a number of active constituents and to characterize them according to their therapeutic potentials, focusing on their effects toward neurodegenerative diseases such as AD (Kim et al., 2010). This review focuses on the natural products and their derivatives that are involved in regulation of inflammatory pathways to treat AD. Sufficient evidence suggests the role of phytochemicals in prevention and treatment of AD by targeting neuroinflammatory pathway.

NEUROINFLAMMATION AND SIGNALING CASCADES IN ALZHEIMER'S DISEASE

NF-κB Pathway in Alzheimer's Disease

The nuclear factor-kappa B (NF-κB) is a best-characterized transcription factor, expressed ubiquitously and regulating the expression of many genes, responsible for encoding proteins involved in the processes of inflammation and immunity as shown in **Figure 2** (Li and Verma, 2002). Apart of these roles NF-κB is shown to be involved in brain function, particularly in neurodegenerative diseases like AD (O'neill and Kaltschmidt, 1997). Aβ induced neurotoxicity has been linked to NF-κB activation (Longpré et al., 2006). Neuronal and microglial cells when treated with Aβ results in activation of NF-κB signaling (Longpré et al., 2006). In brains of AD patients, NF-κB activation has been detected (Boissière et al., 1997). Use of long-term anti-inflammatory drugs has shown to suppress the progression and onset of AD indicating a close relation between NF-κB and pathogenesis of AD (Hong, 2017). Therefore, potential therapeutic approach against AD can involve the modulation of Aβ-induced activation of NF-κB signaling.

Akt/PI3K Pathway in Alzheimer's Disease

The Akt/PI3K pathway is involved in survival, proliferation, growth, and migration of cells (Yu and Koh, 2017). Akt is an important and direct effectors of PI3K/Akt pathway; reportedly involved in many different substrates activation in cellular signaling as shown in **Figure 2** (Yu and Koh, 2017). Among them glycogen synthase kinase (GSK)-3β is important and well-known involved in direct induction of tau phosphorylation. GSK-3β at serine 9 when phosphorylated by activated Akt, results in inhibition of GSK-3β (Plyte et al., 1992). In AD GSK-3β phosphorylates tau protein thus inducing detachment of tau proteins from microtubules, which aggregates with each other. This causes the loss of function of microtubule, thus increasing vulnerability of cells and inducing cell death (Yu and Koh, 2017). In addition Akt also activates mTOR, whose signaling is closely related to the presence of soluble amyloid beta (Aβ) and tau protein. Injecting Aβ oligomers into the hippocampus of normal mice has shown mTOR hyperactivation (Caccamo et al., 2011). In AD mTOR signaling pathway is considered to be one of the mechanisms involved in Aβ-induced toxicity (Lafay-Chebassier et al., 2005). Increased Aβ concentration increases

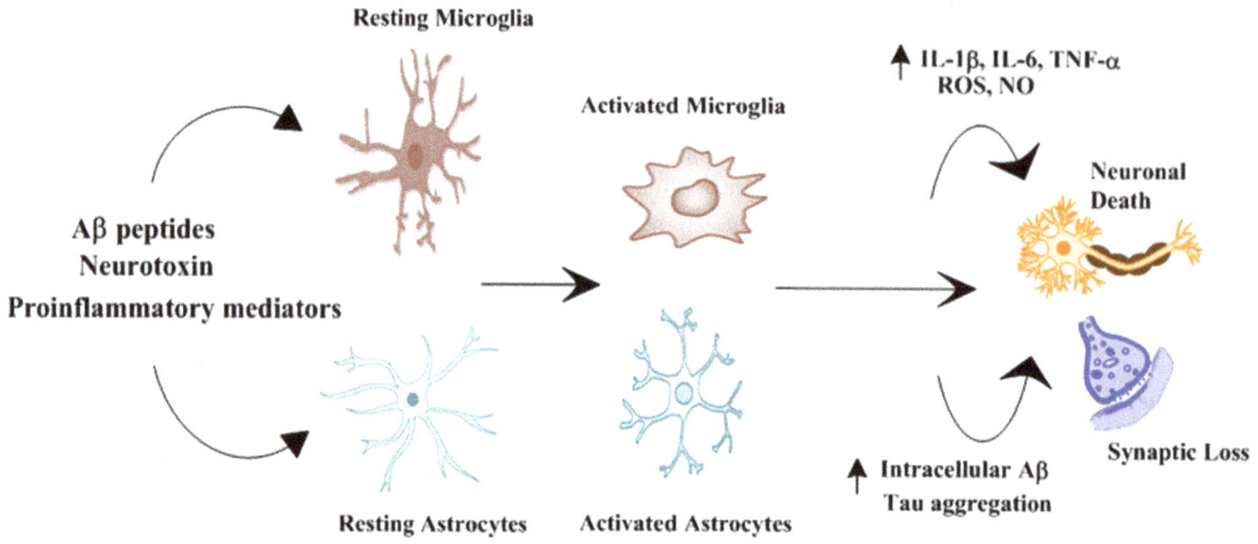

FIGURE 1 | Schematic representation of role of glial cells in pathophysiology of Alzheimer's disease. Numerous stimuli such as Aβ peptides, neurotoxin and proinflammatory mediators activates microglial cells and astrocytes. Activated microglial cells and astrocytes results in increased production of proinflammatory cytokines and intracellular Aβ and Tau aggregation resulting in synaptic loss and neuronal death (Morales et al., 2014).

mTOR signaling, however, large concentration of cytotoxic Aβ decreases mTOR signaling (Lafay-Chebassier et al., 2005). This role of mTOR signaling is controversial in amyloid hypothesis.

MAPK Pathways in Alzheimer's Disease

MAPK plays an important role in neuronal survival and death *in vitro* and in brain by signaling oxidative stress and cell cycle control as shown in **Figure 2** (Zhu et al., 2000). Various studies have shown the increased level of active ERK in AD (Zhu et al., 2001a). Thus, resulting in impaired hippocampus function and contribute toward memory impairment (Zhu et al., 2001a). JNK has shown to have role in AD pathogenesis; it co-localizes with DNA damage and is associated with neurofibrillary pathology (Smith et al., 2000). Since the oxidative stress has a well-documented role in AD, so it is suspected that JNK pathway is activated as a response to cellular stress in AD (Smith et al., 2000). Increased level associated with the pathology of NFTs and senile plaque in AD brain (Zhu et al., 2000). Further evidence has been provided convincing the abnormally activated p38 pathway in AD because of the increased activation of MKK6 as an immediate upstream activator of p38 (Zhu et al., 2001b). The activated MKK6-p38 is more prominent in neurons than in microglia, suggesting direct contribution toward degeneration of neurons in AD (Zhu et al., 2001b).However, simultaneous activation of ERK and JNK has a high tendency to develop AD representing one of the initial events in disease pathogenesis likely precipitating further alterations (Zhu et al., 2001a).

Nrf2 Pathway in Alzheimer's Disease

Nuclear factor E2-related factor 2 (Nrf2) is the transcription factor which activates expression of the genes with antioxidant activity translocating in response to oxidative stress from the cytoplasm into the nucleus as indicated in **Figure 2** (Itoh et al., 1997). It is an attractive therapeutic target for the prevention of AD (Kerr et al., 2017). Antioxidant response element (ARE) is a common response element of the genes involved in the reduction of oxidative stress, inflammation and accumulation of toxic metabolites. As a result of oxidative damage in AD, there is an upregulation of Nrf2 expressions in the neuron. In AD, there is a reduction in the levels of some ARE-containing gene products, suggesting disruption of the pathway (Itoh et al., 1997). Moreover, the *in-vivo* evidence also suggests that inhibition of Keap 1, prevents the neuronal toxicity caused by Aβ42 peptides initiating AD, correlating with activation of Nrf2 (Kerr et al., 2017).

CREB Signaling in Alzheimer's Disease

Cyclic-AMP response element binding protein (CREB) has been known to be important in memory formation (Kandel, 2012). Studies propose dysfunctions in the CREB signaling in various mouse models of AD (Bartolotti et al., 2016). It has been shown that CREB and pCREB its activated form, along with CREB-binding protein (CBP) the transcription cofactors and p300 are reduced in prefrontal cortex of AD, indicating dysfunctional CREB signaling in AD (Bartolotti et al., 2016).

Potential Role of Natural Products in Treatment of Alzheimer's Disease

Despite the accumulation of valuable knowledge and incredible innovation of modern medicine there is no effective cure of world's most problematic diseases such as Alzheimer Disease (Rasool et al., 2014). Synthetic drugs are useful for managing these diseases, however, they still possesses severe side effects (Rasool et al., 2014). Due to the increase need of novel and effective treatment, natural products have gained attention as promising therapeutic agents recently

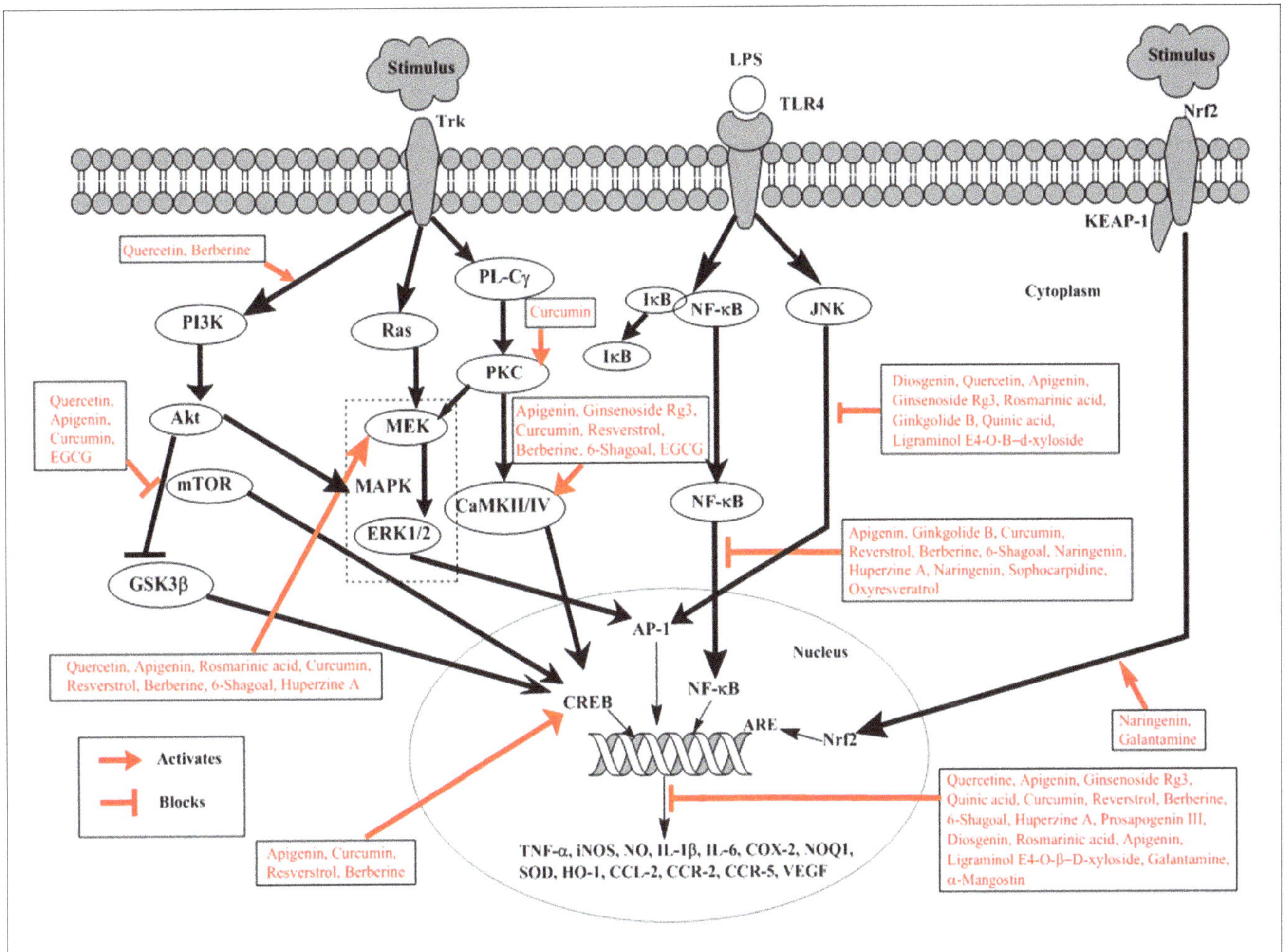

FIGURE 2 | Schematic representation of natural products involved in neuroprotection against Alzheimer's disease. External stimulus binds to Trk receptor activating PI3K/AKT, Ras/MAPK, and PL-Cγ pathways. LPS binds to TLRs activating NF-κB and JNK signaling. External stimulus releases Nrf2 from Nrf2-KEAP-1 complex and activates ARE. Trk, tyrosine kinase receptor; LPS, lipopolysaccharide; TLRs, toll-like receptors; PI3K, phosphatidylinsoitol-3-kinase; MAPK, mitogen-activated protein kinase; mTOR, mammalian target of rapamycin; ERK, extracellular signal-regulated kinases; Nrf2, nuclear factor e2-related factor 2; KEAP-1, Kelch-like ECH-associated protein-1; MEK, mitogen-activated protein kinase; PL-Cγ, phospholipase Cγ; NF-κB, nuclear factor-kappa B; PKC, protein kinase C; JNK, c-Jun N-terminal kinase; ARE, Antioxidant response element; CREB, cyclic adenosine monophosphate response element binding protein; IκB, inhibitory kappa B; CaMKII/IV, Ca2+-calmodulin kinase II/IV; GSK3β, glucose synthase kinase-3β. Diosgenin, Prosapogenin III, Quercetin, Apigenin, Ginsenoside Rg3, Rosmarinic acid, Ginkgolide B, Limonoid, Quinic acid, Curcumin, Resverstrol, Berberine, 6- Shagoal, Ligraminol E4-*O*-β-d-xyloside, Huperzine A, Sophocarpidine, Naringenin, Epigallocatechin-3-galate (EGCG), Oxyresveratrol, α-Mangostin, Galantamine.

neuroprotective treatments have demonstrated that animal based products such as omega-3, fatty acids, and plant based compounds inhibit cellular toxicity and shows anti-inflammatory effects (Wollen, 2010). Due to the potential of anti-inflammatory, antioxidant and neuroprotective properties of phytochemicals with minimal side effects have revealed the potential to improve and prevent neurodegeneration in AD (Cooper and Ma, 2017). It is speculated that onset and progression of AD might be lowered by traditional herbs and phytochemicals by targeting multiple pathological targets (Venkatesan et al., 2015). Herbs are found to be involved in regulation of mitochondrial stress; free radical scavenging systems, apoptotic factors, and neurotrophic factors (Starkov and Beal, 2008). Progression of AD is also accelerated by inflammation contributing to neurodegeneration (Cooper and Ma, 2017). Therefore, early prevention and management of inflammation might serve as a potential treatment or reducing symptoms of AD (Cooper and Ma, 2017).

Phytochemicals having anti-inflammatory, antioxidant and anti-amyloid activity can interact with neuroinflammatory mediators. The evidence of blood brain permeability of various natural products is still not conclusive. However, history of their traditional use and abundant data from animal studies demonstrates their ability to penetrate the blood brain barrier (BBB) (Kam et al., 2012). After an oral administration, principle metabolites of (−)-epicatechin have been detected in rodent brain (Van Praag et al., 2007). Similar results were also observed with epigallocatechin-3-galate (EGCG) (Lin et al., 2007) and *Ginko biloba* extract (Rangel-Ordóñez et al., 2010). It was observed that the flavonoids from *G. biloba* extract were distributed in the hippocampus, striatum, prefrontal cortex and cerebellum

TABLE 1 | Steroid phytochemicals that affect Alzheimer's disease.

Plant source	Phytochemicals	Pharmacological effects	Medicinal use	References
STEROID PHYTOCHEMICALS				
Dioscorea nipponica	Diosgenin	Inhibits IκB/ NF-κB pathway and MAPK pathways; ERK, p38, and JNK	Neuroinflammation, and neuroprotection	Hirai et al., 2010
Liriope platyphylla	Prosapogenin III	Blocks MAPK/NF-κB pathway, inhibiting release of inflammatory mediators	Anti-inflammation, antioxidant, and neuriotogenic properties	Han et al., 2013

(Rangel-Ordóñez et al., 2010). The ability of metabolites to penetrate the BBB depends upon the degree of lipophilicity, polarity, and molecular weight of each compound (Rajadhyaksha et al., 2011). Less polar lipophylic compounds with molecular weight < 500 daltons are easily permeable (Rajadhyaksha et al., 2011). The brain entry also depends on the ability to interact with specific efflux transporters expressed in BBB which includes P-glycoprotein, as observed in quercetin and naringenin flux into the brain (Youdim et al., 2004). Furthermore, the time-dependent transport studies across cerebral capillary endothelial cells of quercetin and catechin suggest the capability of BBB transfer (Faria et al., 2010). These studies demonstrate the ability of natural products to reach the areas of brain involved in neurodegenerative disease. Despite this, further investigation regarding extent of brain bioavailability of natural compounds can be performed before any firm conclusion.

Neuroprotective Effect of Steroid Phytochemicals in Alzheimer's Disease

Diosgenin

Diosgenin is a saponin aglycon a chemical constituent of *Dioscorea nipponica* (**Table 1**), chemical structure in **Figure 3**. It is also found in numerous other plants such as *Dioscorea villosa, Trigonella foenum graecum, Solanum xanthocarpum, S. incanum Lloydia,* and *Costus speciosus.* It has a wide variety of reported functions, which includes its anticancer, antifungal, and anti-inflammatory properties (Chiu and Lin, 2008). A previous report has shown anti-inflammatory effect of saponin aglycons, including diosgenin on LPS-stimulated RAW 264.7 macrophages (Chiu and Lin, 2008). Furthermore, it regulates the activity of NF-kB (Shishodia and Aggarwal, 2006), lipoxygenase (Nappez et al., 1995), and cyclooxygenase-2 (Moalic et al., 2001), also antagonizes the CXCR3 chemokine receptor involved in mediation of inflammatory responses (Ondeyka et al., 2005). Diosgenin dose dependently suppresses the production of inflammatory factors like nitric oxide (NO), monocyte chemoattractant protein-1 (MCP-1), and tumor necrosis factor-α (TNF-α) in the case of coculture of macrophages and adipocytes (Hirai et al., 2010). The nitrogen analog of diosgenin, tomatidine a steroid saponin has been reported to inhibit NF-kB and JNK signaling acting as an anti-inflammatory agent (Chiu and Lin, 2008). Consistent with these reports, it is suggested that in macrophages FFA-induced inflammation is inhibited by diosgenin through suppression of both JNK/AP-1 and IkB/NF-kB signaling pathways (Hirai et al., 2010). Therefore, through various studies it has been suggested that diosgenin has anti-neuroinflammatory potential against neurodegenerative diseases such as AD.

Prosapogenin III

Prosapogenin III (**Table 1**), a steroidal saponin extracted from roots of *Liriope platyphylla* (Liriopis Tuber). It is a medicinal plant reported to possess anti-diabetes, anti-asthma, neuriotogenic and anti-inflammatory properties (Han et al., 2013). Effect of prosapogenin III (**Figure 3**) was evaluated in LPS-induced RAW264.7 cells expressing inflammatory mediators such as anti-inflammatory cytokines, inducible nitric oxide (iNOS), nitric oxide (NO), and cyclooxygenase-2 (COX-2), also interleukin-1β (IL-1β), and IL-6. Results obtained from the study indicated its anti-inflammatory effects in activated macrophages by blocking MAPK/NF-κB signaling inhibiting production of inflammatory mediators (Han et al., 2013). For investigation of neuroprotective effect of *Liriope platyphylla* extract (LPE), its effect was evaluated in SH-SY5Y human neuroblastoma cells having hydrogen peroxide (H_2O_2)-induced injury (Park et al., 2015). The results demonstrated that LPE has neuroprotective effects by protecting cell growth through inhibition of p38 phosphorylation in a H_2O_2-induced stressful background (Park et al., 2015). Therefore, prosapogenin III might be a potential candidate for the amelioration of AD.

Neuroprotective Effect of Phenolic Phytochemicals in Alzheimer's Disease

Quercetin

Quercetin, a flavonoid is derived from mulberry fruit *Morus alba* (**Table 2**) from family Moraceae (Dajas, 2012). This fruit contains palmitic acid, linoleic acid, vitamin C, phenolics, oleic acid, gallic acid, anthocyanins, and quercetin having anti-inflammatory, anti-carcinogenic, and antioxidant properties (Dajas, 2012). Due to its anti-inflammatory property, it has been studied as a lead compound showing neuroprotective effect in the animal model of neurodegeneration (Bahar et al., 2017). Quercetin (**Figure 3**) is a strong inhibitor of both 5-lipoxygenase (5-LOX) and cyclooxygenase-2 (COX-2) enzymes involved in production of eicosanoids from arachidonic acid and also has inhibitory action on prostaglandins (PG) production and NF- κB activation (Pany et al., 2014). Quercetin enhance neuroprotection through their antioxidant property by scavenging of free radicals (Kim et al., 1999). It easily crosses the blood brain barrier (Chen et al., 2009). It has also been shown that in the

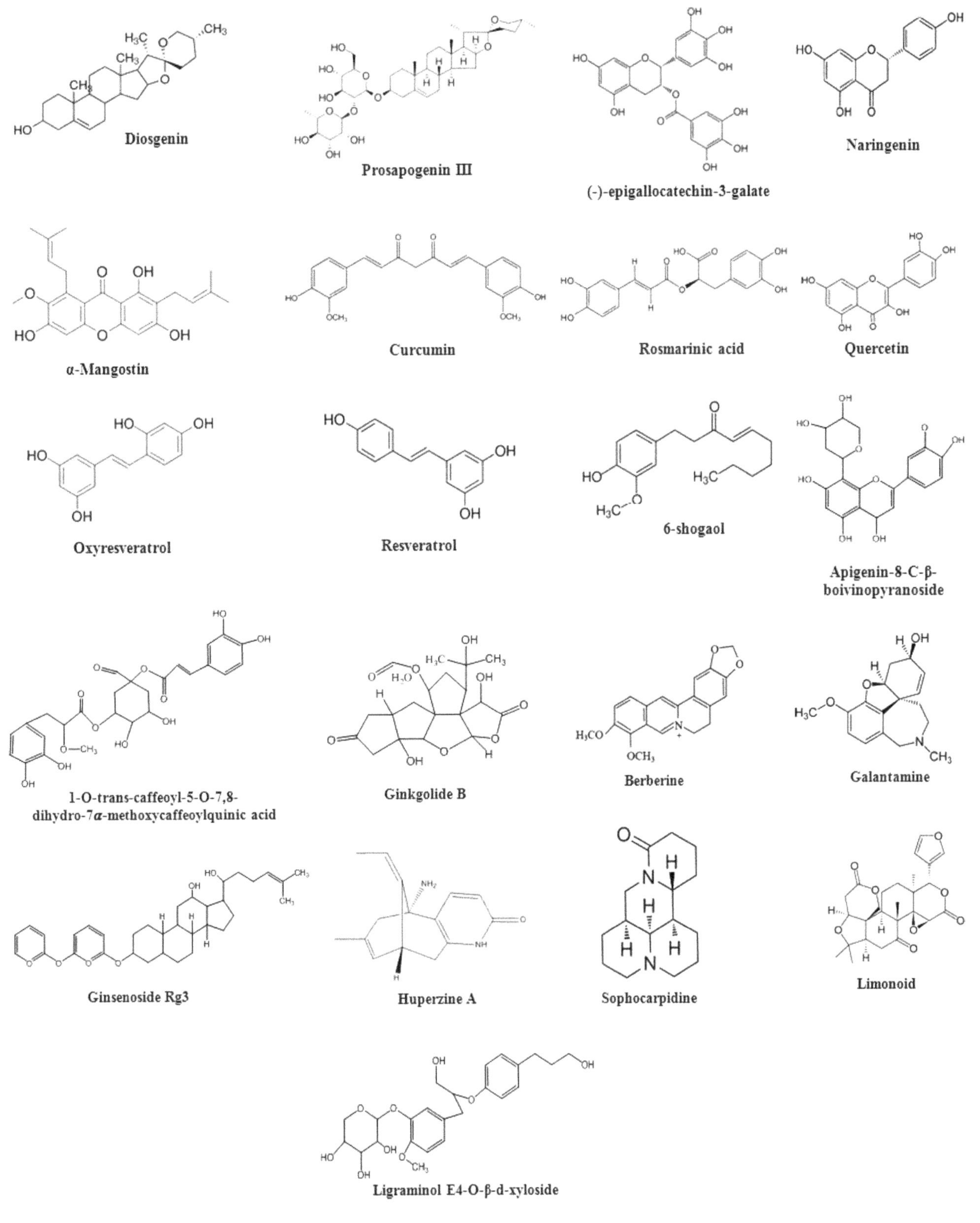

FIGURE 3 | Chemical Structures of natural compounds.

TABLE 2 | Phenolic phytochemicals that affect Alzheimer's disease.

Plant source	Phytochemicals	Pharmacological effects	Medicinal use	References
PHENOLIC PHYTOCHEMICALS				
Camellia sinensis	Epigallocatechin-3-galate (EGCG)	Inhibits MAPK and NF-κB activation, attenuates IL-1, IL-6, IL-8, COX-2 and PGE_2 production. Also induces BDNF, NGF secretion, and inhibits cas3 and ROS level	Neuroinflammation, neuroprotection, and cognitive deficit	Kim et al., 2007; Liu et al., 2014
Cirus paradise and Citrus sinensis	Naringenin	Activating Nrf2/ARE signaling, upregulates antioxidant enzymes, decreases NO, cytokines and NF-κB signaling	Anti-inflammatory, antioxidant and neuroprotective	Raza et al., 2013; Lou et al., 2014
Curcuma longa	Curcumin	Activates PKC/ERK-mediated CREB regulation and Akt/GSK-3β mediated regulation, induces BDNF secretion, and inhibits Cas3, TNF-α, and NF-κB levels	Neuritogenesis, neuroinflammation, and anti-oxidant properties	Hoppe et al., 2013; Nam et al., 2014
Garcinia mangostana	α-Mangostin	Suppresses inflammation, increases BDNF level and decreasing phospho-tau (p-tau)	Alzheimer's Disease	Huang et al., 2014
Melissa officinalis	Rosmarinic acid	Suppresses the expression of HIF-α, IL-1β, TNF-α and caspase 3	Neuroprotective, antioxidant properties	Bayat et al., 2012
Morus alba	Quercetin	Inhibits COX-2, 5-LOX enzymes and GSK-3β in PI3K pathway and inhibits NF-κB activation, also is involved in free radical scavenging	Anti-inflammatory and antioxidant properties	Kimata et al., 2000; Pany et al., 2014
Morus alba L.	Oxyresveratrol	Decreases TNF-α, IL-6 and inhibits activation of NALP3, caspase-1, NF-κB and inhibits phosphorylation of ERK, c-JNK and p38	Anti-inflammatory and anti-apoptotic effects	Chung et al., 2003; Wang et al., 2014
Passiflora edulis and P. alata	Apigenin-8-C-β-digitoxopyranoside, luteolin-8-C-β-boivinopyranoside, and apigenin-8-C-β-boivinopyranoside	Inhibits NO and PGE2 production, suppresses expression of ERK 1/2, p38, MAPK, JNK and COX-2	Anti-AD, and anti-inflammatory properties	Choi et al., 2014
Pimpinella brachycarpa	3,5-O-trans-dicaffeoylquinic acid methyl ester, 1-O-trans-caffeoyl-5-O-7,8-dihydro-7α-methoxycaffeoylquinic acid	Inhibits NO, iNOS production, and boost antioxidant system	Antioxidant, anti-inflammatory, and neuroinflammation	Soh et al., 2003; Lee et al., 2013
Vitis vinifera	Resveratrol	Inhibits synthesis and release of pro-inflammatory mediators, inhibits iNOS, COX-2, NF-κB, AP-1 and promotes anti-inflammatory molecules IL-10	Antioxidant, anti-inflammatory, and neurodegenerative disorders	Song et al., 2014
Zingiber officinale	6-shogaol	Induces NGF, BDNF, and GDNF secretion, inhibiting NO, TNF-α, IL-1β, p38, Bax, NF-κB, iNOS, PGE2, and ROS level and increases Bcl-2, and SOD levels.	Anti-inflammatory, and antioxidant	Ha et al., 2012

brains of Sprague-Dawley (SD) rats and SK-N-MC cell lines of human neuroblastoma quercetin could inhibit apoptosis and inflammatory response induced by manganese (Mn) by activating HO-1/Nrf2 and inhibiting NF-κB signaling (Bahar et al., 2017). These studies suggest the neuroprotective property of quercetin and various other extracts of *M. alba* against the AD.

Oxyresveratrol

Oxyresveratrol, a major stilbene of white mulberry *M. alba* (**Table 2**), family Moraceae showed interesting anti-inflammatory effects (Chung et al., 2003). It has shown to inhibit NO production by reducing iNOS protein expression in lipopolysaccharide-activated macrophages (Chung et al., 2003). In addition, oxyreveratrol (**Figure 3**) has a neuroprotective effects against neurotoxicity in cortical neurons induced by Aβ peptides (Niidome et al., 2007). Furthermore, decrease of NO and TNF-α in macrophages was demonstrated by a crude methanolic extract of mulberry leaves via reduction of activation of transcription factor NF-κB (Shibata et al., 2007). Another study has been proposed to elicit anti-inflammatory and neuroprotective effects useful in the treatment of brain ischemic injury (Wang et al., 2014). The mechanistic study showed that Mulberroside A exhibits anti-inflammatory and anti-apoptotic effects by decreasing the IL-6, IL-1β and TNF-α expression and inhibiting activation of LRR, NACHT, and PYD domains-containing protein 3 (NALP3), caspase-1, and NF-κB activation. All these findings indicate that oxyreveratrol is a potential candidate as a multifactorial neuroprotectant in AD (Wang et al., 2014).

Resveratrol

Resveratrol is a polyphenol derivative from *Vitis vinifera* (**Table 2**) belonging to the family of Vitaceae. It is reported to possess cardioprotective, anticarcinogenic, antioxidant, and anti-inflammatory activities in context to neurodegenerative disorders (Ma et al., 2014). Previous studies have revealed neuroprotective effect of resveratrol in rats having chronic unpredictable mild stress induced cognitive and emotional deficiencies (Yazir et al., 2015). Resveratrol (**Figure 3**) inhibits proinflammatory mediator's synthesis and release by modifying synthesis of eicosanoids, COX-2 and iNOS *via* inhibition of NF-κB (Alarcon De La Lastra and Villegas, 2005). Furthermore, in microglial cells resveratrol suppresses the level of expression of proinflammatory mediators TNF-α and NF-κB while promotes the IL-10 anti-inflammatory molecule (Song et al., 2014). These studies suggest its role against neurodegenerative diseases specially AD.

Apigenin Derivatives

Passiflora edulis and *P. alata* (**Table 2**) produces flavonoids that improve behavioral performances in rats (Xu et al., 2013). *Passiflora* has been used as a sedative, tranquilizer and natural anxiolytic agent (Barbosa et al., 2008). Flavonoids such as apigenin-8-*C*-β-digitoxopyranoside, luteolin-8-*C*-β-boivinopyranoside, and apigenin-8-*C*-β-boivinopyranoside (**Figure 3**) are the major phytochemicals contributing toward the effect of *Passiflora* (Xu et al., 2013). Recently apigenin has shown to reduce inflammation in case of LPS-induced microglial activation by inhibiting PGE_2 and NO production by free radical scavenging (Xu et al., 2013). Furthermore, apigenin also decreases MAPK, JNK, p38, and ERK1/2 and also modulate neurite outgrowth induced by nerve growth factor (NGF) in PC12 cells (Xu et al., 2013). Additionally due to its BBB permeability, it serves as an effective phytochemical involved in the treatment of neurodegenerative diseases such as AD (Yang et al., 2014). Furthermore, apigenin and its *C*-glycosylated derivatives such as isovitexin and Vitexin possess activities against diabetes, Alzheimer's disease, and inflammatory activities (Choi et al., 2014).Due to its low intrinsic toxicity, apigenin has gained interest as a beneficial and health promoting agent. In LPS-induced macrophages the potential of apigenin and its derivatives were investigated against diabetes, Alzheimer's disease, and inflammation (Choi et al., 2014). The results showed relatively weak anti-AD and anti-diabetic potentials of apigenin as compared to anti-inflammatory properties that are shown by inhibiting iNOS, COX-2, and NO production as compared to its *C*-glycosylated derivatives (Choi et al., 2014). It can be assumed through these studies that apigenin might be useful against AD.

α-Mangostin

Garcinia mangostana (**Table 2**), commonly called mangosteen is the fruit of a tropical evergreen tree native to Southeast Asia. Mangosteen possesses beneficial neuroprotective, anti-inflammatory and antioxidant effects. It consists of various polyphenolic xanthone derivatives such as α-mangostin. α-Mangostin (**Figure 3**) has shown to concentration-dependently attenuate Aβ-(1-40) or Aβ-(1-42) oligomers induced neurotoxocity, as observed in primary rat cortical neurons showing decrease in cell viability and impaired neurite outgrowth (Wang et al., 2012). Promising treatment and improved inflammation has been shown by mice fed with mangosteen supplemented diet (Huang et al., 2014). These studies suggest role of mangosteen in attenuation of AD.

Rosmarinic Acid

Melissa officinalis (**Table 2**), commonly named as lemon balm, is used traditionally for its neuroprotective and antioxidant actions. It prevents neuronal cell death by scavenging free radicals (Pereira et al., 2009). Rosmarinic acid (**Figure 3**) from *Rosmarinus officinalis* enhances cholinergic activity in cell differentiation mediated by ERK1/2 suggesting neurotrophic effect in PC 12 cells (El Omri et al., 2010). Rosmarinic acid has show protection against neuronal damage induced by hypoxia resulting in proinflammatory cytokines such as TNF-α, IL-1β, and caspase 3 through suppression of hypoxia inducible factor-1α (HIF-1α) expression (Bayat et al., 2012). All these studies shows the rosmarinic acid and other derivatives from *M. officinalis* play an important role in improving cholinergic activity by the mechanisms underlying memory enhancing function. These studies suggest rosmarinic acid as a potential therapeutic agent against AD.

Quinic Acid Derivatives

Pimpinella brachycarpa (**Table 2**), belongs to family Umbelliferea. It is distributed in Asia, Europe, and Africa (Lee, 2003). Quinic acid derivatives were isolated from the MeOH extract of *P. brachycarpa* (Lee et al., 2013). Beneficial effects of quinic acid derivatives include antioxidant, anti-hepatitis B virus, carcinogenesis and anti-inflammatory effects (Wang et al., 2009). *Aster scaber*, from the family Asteraceae is another source of quinic acid derivatives containing (–)-3,5-dicaffeoylmucoquinic acid and (–)-4,5-dicaffeoylquinic acid (Hur et al., 2004). In a previous study, the anti-inflammatory activities of potential components of MeOH extract isolated from *P. brachycarpa* were evaluated on LPS-activated BV-2 microglial cells (Lee et al., 2013). MeOH extract obtained from aerial parts of *P. brachycarpa* were separated through column chromatography, which furnished fifteen quinic acid derivatives. Among these derivatives 1-**O**-trans-caffeoyl-5-**O**-7,3,5-**O**-trans-dicaffeoylquinic acid and 8-dihydro-7**α**-methoxycaffeoylquinic acid methyl ester (**Figure 3**) significantly inhibited inflammatory mediators in cell lines activated by LPS (Lee et al., 2013). Furthermore, *A. scaber* isolated quinic acid has been found to increase survival of C6 glioma cell upon tetrahydropalmatine (THP) induced toxicity because of free radical scavenging malondialdehyde (MDA) and superoxide dismutase (SOD) (Soh et al., 2003). It is also shown that (-)-3,5-dicaffeoylmucoquinic acid an extract from *A. scaber* affects neurite outgrowth by affecting PI3K and ERK1/2 *via* activation of TrkA signaling (Xiao et al., 2011). Thus, quinic acid extracted from *A. scaber* alleviate neurodegenerative diseases by protecting neurons from free radicals by enhancing the free radical scavenging system and attenuating pro-inflammatory responses by inhibiting iNOS expression (Soh et al., 2003). Therefore, this herb might be a potential candidate for AD due to significant anti-inflammatory activities.

Epigallocatechin-3-Galate

Epigallocatechin-3-galate (EGCG) is a member of Theaceae family. This polyphenol is extracted from *Camellia sinensis* (**Table 2**) which is a natural green tea (Gramza-Michalowska and Regula, 2007). This herb is reported as beverage worldwide and is abundant in hilly areas of Asia (Gramza-Michalowska and Regula, 2007). Green tea catechins are brain permeable and in recent studies it has been ascribed to have neuroprotective actions as well (Singh et al., 2008). Several molecular biological roles are served by green tea catechins which include activation of antioxidant enzymes, protein survival genes, and kinase C, and APP processing (Levites et al., 2002). Green tea may also be involved in protection of neurons from Aβ-induced damages evidenced from several *in-vitro* studies (Bastianetto et al., 2006). Catechins have well documented anti-inflammatory properties. EGCG (**Figure 3**) inhibits NF-κB and MAPK in activation. It also inhibits the production of vascular endothelial growth factor IL-6, and IL-8 in U373MG cells of human astrocytoma (Kim et al., 2007). Anti-inflammatory activities of various cytokines are suppressed by EGCG, through inhibition of IL-1β and Aβ-induced COX-2 expression (Kim et al., 2007). Reportedly EGCG inhibits LPS-induced microglial activation, protection against neuronal injury mediated by inflammation (Li et al., 2004). EGCG increases NGF and CREB expression levels in APP/PS1 providing neuroprotection through ameliorating cognitive impairment in mice model, neuroprotection is also mediated by ERK1/2/ C-Raf by phosphorylating TrkA (Li et al., 2004). It also reduces activation of JNK2 and p75/CD reducing the expression levels of caspase 3 leading to reduction in levels of Aβ (1-40) and hippocampal APP expression (Liu et al., 2014). Prolonged consumption of green tea positively effects age-related neurodegeneration by increasing glutathione, potentiating, scavenging system, activating Bcl-2 protein and CREB levels and also boosting BDNF levels (Paulo Andrade and Assuncao, 2012). Chronic treatment has shown to improve spatial learning and memory due to the presence of catechins in green tea as shown in SAMP8 mice having impairment in memory and learning. Catechins through PKA/CREB signaling suppresses Aβ (1-42) level in the hippocampus and increases CaMKII and BDNF levels (Li et al., 2009).

Several animal models have been reported regarding the effects of green tea catechins on memory function. For instance, in Tg2576 mice reduction in cognitive impairment is shown by EGCG (Rezai-Zadeh et al., 2005). Intracerebroventricular injection of $A\beta_{1-40}$ in rats showed less memory impairment when provided with high levels of green tea catechins especially EGCG with drinking water (Haque et al., 2008). Injecting tea catechins also ameliorates hippocampal neuronal damage and memory impairment in mouse model of cerebral ischemia (Lee et al., 2003). Thus, it is a better therapeutic approach to use green catechins, especially EGCG for the treatment of cognitive decline as in AD.

Curcumin

Curcuma longa (**Table 2**) from the family Zingiberaceae is commonly known as turmeric. It contains phenolic constituents which includes curcumin, bisdemethoxycurcumin, and demethoxycurcumin (Akbik et al., 2014). It is used in flavoring food preparations commonly, also due to its good medicinal properties it is used for the treatment of coughs, biliary disorders, hepatic disorder, diabetic ulcer, rheumatism and sinusitis (Akbik et al., 2014). Curcumin (**Figure 3**) exhibits anti-inflammatory and anti-oxidant properties (Aggarwal and Harikumar, 2009). In rat model of olfactory-bulb-ablation, curcumin has been found to suppress the levels of TNF-α and caspase 3, the neuroinflammatory mediators by increasing the BDNF levels (Rinwa et al., 2013). Studies have revealed the involvement of curcumin in regulation of CREB and BDNF levels in D-galactose-induced memory and learning deficits in mouse models (Nam et al., 2014). Curcumin also treated chronic unpredictable stress induced cognitive deficiency in rats by recovering the ERK1/2 and BDNF levels in hippocampus (Liu et al., 2014). In cisplatin-treated PC12 cells curcumin affected expression level of p53 and inhibition of neurodifferentiation was reduced (Mendonça et al., 2013). Apoptosis induced by β-amyloid was attenuated by curcumin *via* inhibition of NF-κB activation (Kuner et al., 1998). Moreover cognitive decline induced by Aβ (1-42) in rats was treated by nanoencapsulated curcumin by increasing the levels of BDNF and regulating signaling of Akt/GSK-3 β in microglial cells and astrocytes leading to modulation of tau hyperphosphorylation along with an increase in synaptophysin levels in hippocampus (Hoppe et al., 2013). Furthermore, lead acetate-induced oxidative stress in rats can be regulated by curcumin has shown to increase the levels of antioxidants (Hosseinzadeh et al., 2013). Through various models of neurodegeneration, curcumin has shown to be involved in neuroprotection and recovery of memory and learning by increasing the BDNF levels and exerting anti-neuroinflammatory and anti-oxidant properties, which speculates the beneficial role of curcumin in the treatment of AD.

6-Shogaol

Zingiber officinale (**Table 2**) from the family Zingiberaceae is commonly known as ginger. It contains a phenolic phytochemical, 6-shogaol, a compound used as a culinary spice and traditionally used for centuries in Siddha, Indian, Unani, Chinese, Tibetan, and Arabic medicinal practices (Haniadka et al., 2012). A wide variety of phytochemicals are derived from ginger which includes 6-shogaol, 6-gingerol, 8-gingerol, and 10-gingerol, showing positive effects in motion sickness, vomiting, and nausea (Palatty et al., 2013). It also has reported anti-inflammatory, antioxidant, and anti-cancer activity (Shim et al., 2011). Many studies have shown potent activity of 6-Shogaol (Figure 3) against AD, enhancing memory, inhibiting inflammation and boosting antioxidant system (Moon et al., 2014). In scopolamine–and Aβ (1-42)-induced dementia mice models, it improved cognitive impairment by inhibiting inflammatory mediators and increasing NGF levels, and postsynaptic proteins in hippocampus (Moon et al., 2014).

On LPS-treated BV2 and primary microglial cells, 6-shagaol has a beneficial effect by inhibiting COX-2, PGE_2, NO, iNOS, P38 MAPK, IL-1β, TNF-α, and NF-κB (Ha et al., 2012). Additionally 6-shagaol exhibits neuroprotective effect by increasing the choline acetyltransferase, BDNF expression, and reducing ROS release through TrkB-mediated signaling in H_2O_2-treated HT22 hippocampal neuronal cells (Shim and Kwon, 2012). Further studies also assessed the neuroprotective role of 6-shagaol against LPS-induced inflammation (Shim et al., 2011). It suppressed the pro-inflammatory cytokines release and decreases the level of iNOS, NF-κB, and COX-2 in astrocytes treated with LPS (Shim et al., 2011). These studies revealed the valuable phytotherapeutic property of 6-shagaol for the treatment of neurodegenerative diseases like AD.

Naringenin

Naringenin a potent flavonoid is found to be abundant in citrus fruits such as grapefruit (*Cirus paradise*) and oranges (*Citrus sinensis*) (**Table 2**). In male SD rats, naringenin (**Figure 3**) showed protection against focal cerebral ischemia by downregulating NF-κB, nucleotide oligomerization domain protein 2 (NOD2), mitochondrial membrane potential (MMP), receptor-interacting protein 2 (RIP2) and upregulating claudin-5 (Bai et al., 2014). Recent studies have shown the protective ability of naringenin in rat models of focal cerebral I/R injury by prevention of inflammatory damage mediated by NF-κB and oxidative stress (Raza et al., 2013). It upregulates antioxidant status, decreases myeloperoxidases, nitric oxide, and cytokines, also downregulates the expression level of NF-κB (Raza et al., 2013). Naringenin also prevented 6-hydroxydopamine (6-OHDA)-induced neurotoxicity by activating Nrf2/ARE signaling (Lou et al., 2014). Through these studies naringenin can be speculated as a potential agent against AD.

Neuroprotective Effect of Terpenoid-Derived Phytochemicals in Alzheimer's Disease

Ligraminol E4-*O*-*β*-d-Xyloside

Abies holophylla is a member of the family Pinaceae, commonly named as the Needle Fir or Manchurian Fir. *A. holophylla* (**Table 3**) is present in evergreen forests of Korea, Russia and China, and (Kim et al., 2013). Seventeen different lignans were found in the ethanol extract of *A. holophylla*. In murine microglial cells, LPS-induced production of NO was potently inhibited by lignans and were also found to increase NGF levels in C6 glial cell cultures (Kim et al., 2013). Two novel sesquiterpenes, such as (8R,9S,7′S,8′R)-4,4′,7′-trihydroxy-3,3′,9-trimethoxy-9,9′-epoxylignan and ligraminol E4-***O***-***β***-D-xyloside (**Figure 3**) were found in *A. holophylla* exhibited significant inhibition of NO expression in activated microglial cells (Xia et al., 2012). Abies spp. has shown to have protective effect due to potently reducing inflammation in brain cells (Xia et al., 2012). Therefore, this herb due to its significant anti-inflammatory properties in brain can be used as a potential therapeutic agent in AD.

Ginsenoside Rg3

Panax ginseng (**Table 3**) is a member of family the Araliaceae. It is a perennial plant mostly found in Korea, Vietnam China, Russia, and Japan (Chung et al., 2011). Triterpenoid saponin, ginsenoside Rg3 and steroidal saponins are the main constituents of *P. ginseng* (Chung et al., 2011). Ginsenoside Rg3 (**Figure 3**) and other derivatives crosses BBB to a sufficient degree (Wang et al., 2006b). Previous studies have shown that extract of red ginseng is therapeutically effective against neurodegenerative diseases through control of apoptotic-and inflammatory-related events (Joo et al., 2008). It also reduces Aβ42-induced toxicity in BV-2 cells by inhibiting TNF-α, NF-κB, IL-1β, and iNOS (Joo et al., 2008). In addition, ginsenoside Rg3 potently increases neuritogenesis and cholinergic markers through targeting NGF-TrkA signaling (Kim et al., 2014). Therefore, *P.ginseng* strongly reduces neuroinflammatory cytokines and also induces immune cells to ingest the oligomeric plaques formed in AD.

Ginkgolide

Ginkgo biloba, a member of family Ginkgoaceae, traditionally used in Chinese medicine. For thousands of years it has been used for the treatment of neurological diseases such as neurosensory disorders and dementia associated with neurodegeneration (Fang et al., 2010). Extensive studies have revealed that *G. biloba* (**Table 3**) has promising effects against AD, PD, ischemic stroke (Fang et al., 2010). Ginkogolide B (**Figure 3**) is a potent neuroprotective compound used in treatment of neurodegenerative diseases is extracted from *G.biloba*. it is reported to have the ability to cross BBB, more particularly in ischemic conditions (Fang et al., 2010). Numerous studies have reported the protective effect of ginkgolide B against ischemic stroke by increasing sirt1 (silent mating type information regulation 2 homolog-1) expression, suppresses NF-κB, inhibits PI3K/Akt pathway and TLR-4/ NF-κB, up-regulates heme oxygenase 1, anti-apoptotic protein expression, and erythropoietin secretion (Nabavi et al., 2015). It also inhibited pro-apoptotic protein expression, and improves endothelial NO synthesis (Nabavi et al., 2015). It has also been shown that *G. biloba* possesses antioxidant activity by attenuating endoplasmic reticulum (ER) and mitochondrial dysfunctions induced by bupivacaine and ROS (Li et al., 2013). This activity attained through reduction in mitochondrial toxicity *via* reduction in the protein levels of Htra2, caspase 3, caspase 12 and the mRNA in cell lines of human neuroblastoma (Li et al., 2013). In Aβ25-35-treated neuron cultures of primary hippocampus, ginkogolide B was shown to increase BDNF expression levels exerting neuroprotection by reducing caspase 3, the K^+ ion level and lactate dehydrogenase (LDH) (Xiao et al., 2010). Extracts of *G.biloba* have shown to exhibit neuronal protection by inducing Trk-mediated axonal growth and suppressing apoptotic factors and ROS production (Xiao et al., 2010). On the basis of these studies it can be assumed that ginkolide can be used in amelioration of AD.

Limonoids

Melia toosendan, belongs to the family Meliaceae containing triterpenoids. Limonoids (**Figure 3**) have shown to have

TABLE 3 | Terpenoid-derived phytochemicals that affect Alzheimer's disease.

Plant source	Phytochemicals	Pharmacological effects	Medicinal use	References
TERPENOID-DERIVED PHYTOCHEMICALS				
Abies holophylla	Ligraminol E4-O-β-d-xyloside	Inhibits NO production	Neurodegenerative disease, and neuroinflammatory	Xia et al., 2012
Ginkgo biloba	Ginkgolide B	Suppresses NF-κB, PI3K/Akt pathway, upregulates anti-apoptotic proteins expression, induces BDNF secretion and reduces ROS, LDH and caspase3	Dementia, neuroprotective, antioxidant and neuroinflammation	Xiao et al., 2010; Nabavi et al., 2015
Melia toosendan	Limonoid, 1α,3α-dihydroxyl-7α-tigloyloxy-12α-ethoxylnimbolinin & 12-O-ethyl-1-deacetyl-nimbolinin B	Activates PKA/ERK1/2-mediated neurite outgrowth, induces NGF secretion, and decreases LDH activity	Neurodegenerative disease, neuroprotective, and neuroinflammatory.	Roy and Saraf, 2006
Panax ginseng	Ginsenoside Rg3	Activates cAMP/MAPK & Trk-mediated Neuritogenesis and inhibits TNF-α, NF-κB, IL-1β, and iNOS	Neuroinflammation, neurodegenerative disease, and neuroprotection	Joo et al., 2008

TABLE 4 | Alkaloidal phytochemicals that affect Alzheimer's disease.

Plant source	Phytochemicals	Pharmacological effects	Medicinal use	References
ALKALOIDAL PHYTOCHEMICALS				
Coptis chinensis	Berberine	Activates AKT/GSK-3β/Nrf2-mediated regulation, induces NGF and BDNF secretion, and inhibits COX-2, TNF-α, NF-κB, IL-1β, and iNOS levels	neuroinflammation, and neuroprotection	Jia et al., 2012; Lee et al., 2012
Galanthus Sp.	Galantamine	AChE inhibitor, inhibits IL-1β generation and microglial accumulation, increases antioxidant enzymes	Neurodegenerative diseases, neuroprotection, anti-inflammatory and anti-oxidant	Furukawa et al., 2014
Huperzia serrata	Huperzine A	Increases secretion of BDNF, SOD, GST and catalase, inhibits AChE, NF-κB, TNF-α, and caspase-3	Antioxidant, anti-inflammatory, and neuroprotection	Mao et al., 2014
Sophora flavescens	Sophocarpidine	Decreases expression of interleukin-1β	Antineuroinflammatory, Anti Alzheimer's disease	Ni et al., 2006

antibacterial, neuroprotective effects, and anti-carcinogenic properties (Roy and Saraf, 2006). *M. toosendan* contains 12-O-ethyl-1-deacetyl-nimbolinin B and 1α, 3α-dihydroxyl-7α-tigloyloxy-12α-ethoxylnimbolinin fruit extracts, which dose-dependently induce the neuronal differentiation by causing increase in neurite outgrowth in macrophages in rats along with the increase in secretion of NGF (Zhang et al., 2013). *M. toosendan* contains many neuroactive compounds involved in induction of neurite outgrowth in PC12 cells exposed to PKA inhibitors (Jowie and Ip, 2004). These studies suggest a significant potential of limonoids extracted from *M. toosendan* aganist neurodegenerative diseases like AD (**Table 3**).

Neuroprotective Effect of Alkaloidal Phytochemicals in Alzheimer's Disease

Berberine

Coptis chinensis, belongs to the Ranunculaceae family. The major component of the plant is berberine (**Figure 3**) is an isoquinoline alkaloid (Asai et al., 2007). In China it is widely used as a herbal medicine for treatment of liver disease, microbial infection and skin inflammation since decades (Asai et al., 2007). Various studies have reported the neuroprotective effects of berberine using neurodegenerative disease models (Jia et al., 2012). In scopolamine-induced memory impairments berberine reduces production of the proinflammatory cytokines TNF-α, COX-2, and IL-1β and restores levels of CREB and BDNF as well as reduces the latency of escape in rats (Lee et al., 2012). In Aβ-induced neuroinflammation in murine primary microglia and cultured BV2 cells, pretreatment with berberine prevented MCP-1 and IL-6 productions and also downregulated the expression of COX-2 and iNOS expression (Jia et al., 2012). This anti-neuroinflammatory potential of berberine suggests its role in attenuation of AD (**Table 4**).

Huperzine A

Huperzia serrata contains a sesquiterpene alkaloid i.e., huperzine A (**Table 4**). For decades it has been used in Chinese medicines as a reversible acetylcholinesterase (AChE) inhibitor (Zu Zhu et al., 2004). It exerted neuroprotective effect toward AD by promoting anti-apoptotic protein expression, inhibiting AChE, and NGF, resulting in alteration of Aβ peptide processing and reduction of oxidative stress (Zhang and Tang, 2006). Huperzine A (**Figure 3**) reduced the D-galactose-induced inflammatory loss in rat hippocampus through NF-κB and inhibiting neurovascular damage and BBB impairment (Ruan et al., 2014). (Ruan et al., 2014). In mouse models of reperfusion injury and transient cerebral ischemia, memory impairment was recovered by increasing the levels of BDNF, TGF-β and NGF *via* MAPK/ERK-mediated neuroprotection (Wang et al., 2006a). In SHSY5Y neuroblastoma cells, treatment with huperzine A caused activation of $p75_{NTR}$ and TrkA receptors that resulted increase in MAP/ERK signaling reversing the reduction in NGF level in H_2O_2-induced oxidative stress model (Tang et al., 2005). In streptozotocin-induced diabetic rats, huperzine A has shown to attenuate cognitive defects by increasing the levels of glutathione peroxidase, BDNF, catalase, and SOD while simultaneously inhibiting, CAT, MDA, TNF-α, NF-κB, AChE IL-6, and caspase-3 (Mao et al., 2014). Huperzine A also prevented cognitive decline and brain damage in neonatal rats having hypoxia-ischemia induced brain injury (Wang et al., 2008). In rats with transient focal cerebral ischemia huperzine A is involved in protection through cholinergic anti-inflammatory pathway (Wang et al., 2008). This anti-inflammatory potential of huperzine A suggests that this herb can be used in the treatment and prevention of AD.

Galantamine

Galantamine is an alkaloid derivative of *Galanthus* species (**Table 4**), belonging to the family of Amaryllis. It displays therapeutic benefits against AD (Furukawa et al., 2014). However, it was reported therapy against mild AD, due to reversible antagonism of acetylcholinesterase (AChE) by degrading acetylcholine (Jackisch et al., 2009). Due to its hydrophobic nature, galantamine crosses blood brain barrier, similar to AChE inhibitor i.e., physostigmine (Jackisch et al., 2009). Galantamine (**Figure 3**) has also been reported to decrease brain injury in rats induced by hypoxia-ischemia via inhibition of IL-1β generation and microglial accumulation (Furukawa et al., 2014). In preclinical studies, galantamine has also been shown to increase antioxidant enzymes offering neuroprotection reducing neurodegeneration caused by ROS induced by Aβ in AD (Jackisch et al., 2009).

Sophocarpidine

Sohocarpidine is isolated from roots of *Sophora flavescens*. Evidences suggests sophocarpidine (**Figure 3**) decreases expression of interleukin-1β in cerebral cortex and hippocampus and in AD rat model it also alleviates injury in mitochondria of neuronal cells, established by ibotenic acid injection into the hippocampus (Ni et al., 2006). The anti-AD effect of sophocarpidine is due to the mitigation of inflammation by suppressed release of inflammatory cytokines in the brain (**Table 4**) and thus improving the status of neuronal cells injury and reduction in apoptosis of neuron (Ni et al., 2006).

CONCLUSION

Despite the increasing prevalence of AD worldwide, there is still no cure of this disease. Extensive efforts have been made by researchers to find its solution, however, currently available therapeutic agents unfortunately target only the symptoms not the exact cause of this disease. Various hypotheses have been put forward to explain the etiology and pathology of AD in order to deal with the devastating cognitive decline observed in patients with AD. The multi target approach provides more therapeutic value. In order to extend these observations, anti-inflammatory and antioxidant targets have been focused to evaluate the protective effects against Aβ-induced neurotoxicity. Early trail with NSAIDs such as indometacin and other drugs from this group suggested reduced cognitive decline but could not replicate the results on large scale trails which seemed to be unsuccessful (Aisen et al., 2003; de Jong et al., 2008). Likewise, randomized trials with other anti-inflammatory drugs such as simvastatin (Simons et al., 2002), hydroxychloroquine (Van Gool et al., 2001), prednisone (Aisen et al., 2000), aspirin (Bentham et al., 2008), atorvastatin (Sparks et al., 2005), and rosiglitazone (Harrington et al., 2011) failed to show significant clinical changes in patients with primary cognitive decline. However, NSAIDs like naproxen and celecoxib initially showed a detrimental effect, a longer-term follow up of these patients suggested that naproxen provided protection in patients who had been asymptomatic at baseline (Breitner et al., 2011). This indicates that timing and choice of specific anti-inflammatory will provide better results (Breitner et al., 2011). There is an empirical evidence of prevention and treatment of AD by natural products (Howes et al., 2003). Plant rich diet like fruits, grains, and vegetables are correlated with healthy aging and well-being with reduced risk of AD (Howes et al., 2003). Their potential application in cure and prevention is supported by various experimental studies (Essa et al., 2012). Pharmacological basis for the use of natural products is due to their safety and efficacy as compared to other investigational drugs. Therefore, they might be used as an alternative to conventional treatments. Evidence from the previous literature suggests that phytochemicals that affect anti-inflammatory and downstream signaling targets have shown promising results in *in-vivo* and *in-vitro* studies, and therefore could be used to prevent the AD progression. The review comprehensively discussed the protective role of phytochemicals and their mechanism of action and demonstrated a safer approach toward the protection of neuronal damage caused by inflammation and oxidative stress in AD. Phytochemicals are promising therapeutic agents against neurodegenerative diseases due to their anti-inflammatory, antioxidant as well as anticholinesterase properties. This review focused on the neuroinflammation driven neurodegeneration particularly in AD and the importance of phytochemicals in its prevention and cure by targeting various molecular pathways involved in regulating neurodegenerative diseases.

FUTURE PERSPECTIVE

The numbers of neurodegenerative cases are increasing with the increase in aging in population. This might be due to the increase in chronic inflammatory diseases. Understanding the mechanism of neuroinflammation and neurodegeneration relating to systemic inflammation would be an interesting area for future research. There is still an underrepresentation of phytochemicals that regulate neurodegenerative diseases in preclinical *in vivo* studies. The possible preclinical stages could provide the best window for therapeutic or preventive approaches toward the systemic and central role of inflammation in neurodegenerative diseases.

AUTHOR CONTRIBUTIONS

BS and WD equally to this work in study design and writing of the manuscript. HA perform interpretation and critical review and drafting of the manuscript. SK and YK substantial contribution to the concept and designing of study and revision of manuscript thoroughly. All authors listed have made a substantial, direct, and intellectual contribution to the work. They also read and approved the final manuscript.

ACKNOWLEDGMENTS

This work was supported by the Higher Education Commission (HEC), Pakistan under the SRGP funding (No. 357 SRGP/HEC/2014) and under the indigenous fellowship (No.17-5(Ph-II)/2MD4-051/HEC/IS/2017). The authors are grateful to the National Research Foundation of Korea (NRF), Seoul National University, grant funded by the Korean Government (MSIP) (No. 2009-0083533).

REFERENCES

Aggarwal, B. B., and Harikumar, K. B. (2009). Potential therapeutic effects of curcumin, the anti-inflammatory agent, against neurodegenerative, cardiovascular, pulmonary, metabolic, autoimmune and neoplastic diseases. *Int. J. Biochem. Cell Biol.* 41, 40–59. doi: 10.1016/j.biocel.2008.06.010

Aisen, P. S., Davis, K. L., Berg, J. D., Schafer, K., Campbell, K., Thomas, R., et al. (2000). A randomized controlled trial of prednisone in Alzheimer's disease. *Neurology* 54, 588–588. doi: 10.1212/WNL.54.3.588

Aisen, P. S., Schafer, K. A., Grundman, M., Pfeiffer, E., Sano, M., Davis, K. L., et al. (2003). Effects of rofecoxib or naproxen vs placebo on Alzheimer disease progression: a randomized controlled trial. *JAMA* 289, 2819–2826. doi: 10.1001/jama.289.21.2819

Akbik, D., Ghadiri, M., Chrzanowski, W., and Rohanizadeh, R. (2014). Curcumin as a wound healing agent. *Life Sci.* 116, 1–7. doi: 10.1016/j.lfs.2014.08.016

Alarcon De La Lastra, C., and Villegas, I. (2005). Resveratrol as an anti-inflammatory and anti-aging agent: mechanisms and clinical implications. *Mol. Nutr. Food Res.* 49, 405–430. doi: 10.1002/mnfr.200500022

Alzheimer's Association (2015). 2015 Alzheimer's disease facts and figures. *Alzheimers Dement.* 11, 332–384. doi: 10.1016/j.jalz.2015.02.003

Anand, R., Gill, K. D., and Mahdi, A. A. (2013). Therapeutics of Alzheimer's disease: Past, present and future. *Neuropharmacology* 76(Pt A), 27–50. doi: 10.1016/j.neuropharm.2013.07.004

Asai, M., Iwata, N., Yoshikawa, A., Aizaki, Y., Ishiura, S., Saido, T. C., et al. (2007). Berberine alters the processing of Alzheimer's amyloid precursor protein to decrease Aβ secretion. *Biochem. Biophys. Res. Commun.* 352, 498–502. doi: 10.1016/j.bbrc.2006.11.043

Auld, D. S., Kornecook, T. J., Bastianetto, S., and Quirion, R. (2002). Alzheimer's disease and the basal forebrain cholinergic system: relations to β-amyloid peptides, cognition, and treatment strategies. *Prog. Neurobiol.* 68, 209–245. doi: 10.1016/S0301-0082(02)00079-5

Bahar, E., Kim, J. Y., and Yoon, H. (2017). Quercetin attenuates manganese-induced neuroinflammation by alleviating oxidative stress through regulation of apoptosis, iNOS/NF-κB and HO-1/Nrf2 pathways. *Int. J. Mol. Sci.* 18:1989. doi: 10.3390/ijms18091989

Bai, X., Zhang, X., Chen, L., Zhang, J., Zhang, L., Zhao, X., et al. (2014). Protective effect of naringenin in experimental ischemic stroke: down-regulated NOD2, RIP2, NF-κB, MMP-9 and up-regulated claudin-5 expression. *Neurochem. Res.* 39, 1405–1415. doi: 10.1007/s11064-014-1326-y

Barbosa, P. R., Valvassori, S. S., Bordignon, C. L. Jr., Kappel, V. D., Martins, M. R., Gavioli, E. C., et al. (2008). The aqueous extracts of *Passiflora alata* and *Passiflora edulis* reduce anxiety-related behaviors without affecting memory process in rats. *J. Med. Food* 11, 282–288. doi: 10.1089/jmf.2007.722

Bartolotti, N., Bennett, D. A., and Lazarov, O. (2016). Reduced pCREB in Alzheimer's disease prefrontal cortex is reflected in peripheral blood mononuclear cells. *Mol. Psychiatry* 21:1158. doi: 10.1038/mp.2016.111

Bastianetto, S., Yao, Z. X., Papadopoulos, V., and Quirion, R. (2006). Neuroprotective effects of green and black teas and their catechin gallate esters against β-amyloid-induced toxicity. *Eur. J. Neurosci.* 23, 55–64. doi: 10.1111/j.1460-9568.2005.04532.x

Bayat, M., Azami Tameh, A., Ghahremani, M. H., Akbari, M., Mehr, S. E., Khanavi, M., et al. (2012). Neuroprotective properties of *Melissa officinalis* after hypoxic-ischemic injury both *in vitro* and *in vivo*. *J. Pharm. Sci.* 20:42. doi: 10.1186/2008-2231-20-42

Bentham, P., Gray, R., Sellwood, E., Hills, R., Crome, P., and Raftery, J. (2008). Aspirin in Alzheimer's disease (AD2000): a randomised open-label trial. *Lancet Neurol.* 7, 41–49. doi: 10.1016/S1474-4422(07)70293-4

Boissière, F., Hunot, S., Faucheux, B., Duyckaerts, C., Hauw, J. J., Agid, Y., et al. (1997). Nuclear translocation of NF-κB in cholinergic neurons of patients with Alzheimer's disease. *Neuroreport* 8, 2849–2852. doi: 10.1097/00001756-199709080-00009

Breitner, J. C., Baker, L. D., Montine, T. J., Meinert, C. L., Lyketsos, C. G., Ashe, K. H., et al. (2011). Extended results of the Alzheimer's disease anti-inflammatory prevention trial. *Alzheimers. Dement.* 7, 402–411. doi: 10.1016/j.jalz.2010.12.014

Caccamo, A., Maldonado, M. A., Majumder, S., Medina, D. X., Holbein, W., Magrí, A., et al. (2011). Naturally secreted amyloid-β increases mammalian target of rapamycin (mTOR) activity via a PRAS40-mediated mechanism. *J. Biol. Chem.* 286, 8924–8932. doi: 10.1074/jbc.M110.180638

Chen, G., Bower, K. A., Xu, M., Ding, M., Shi, X., Ke, Z. J., et al. (2009). Cyanidin-3-glucoside reverses ethanol-induced inhibition of neurite outgrowth: role of glycogen synthase kinase 3 beta. *Neurotox. Res.* 15, 321–331. doi: 10.1007/s12640-009-9036-y

Chiu, F. L., and Lin, J. K. (2008). Tomatidine inhibits iNOS and COX-2 through suppression of NF-κB and JNK pathways in LPS-stimulated mouse macrophages. *FEBS Lett.* 582, 2407–2412. doi: 10.1016/j.febslet.2008.05.049

Choi, J. S., Nurul Islam, M., Yousof Ali, M., Kim, E. J., Kim, Y. M., and Jung, H. A. (2014). Effects of C-glycosylation on anti-diabetic, anti-Alzheimer's disease and anti-inflammatory potential of apigenin. *Food Chem. Toxicol.* 64, 27–33. doi: 10.1016/j.fct.2013.11.020

Chung, H. S., Lee, Y. C., Rhee, Y. K., and Lee, S. Y. (2011). Consumer acceptance of ginseng food products. *J. Food Sci.* 76, S516–S521. doi: 10.1111/j.1750-3841.2011.02399.x

Chung, K. O., Kim, B. Y., Lee, M. H., Kim, Y. R., Chung, H. Y., Park, J. H., et al. (2003). *In-vitro* and *in-vivo* anti-inflammatory effect of oxyresveratrol from *Morus alba* L. *J. Pharm. Pharmacol.* 55, 1695–1700. doi: 10.1211/0022357022313

Cooper, E. L., and Ma, M. J. (2017). Alzheimer Disease: clues from traditional and complementary medicine. *J. Tradit. Complement. Med.* 7, 380–385. doi: 10.1016/j.jtcme.2016.12.003

Dajas, F. (2012). Life or death: neuroprotective and anticancer effects of quercetin. *J. Ethnopharmacol.* 143, 383–396. doi: 10.1016/j.jep.2012.07.005

Dal Prà, I., Chiarini, A., Gui, L., Chakravarthy, B., Pacchiana, R., Gardenal, E., et al. (2015). Do astrocytes collaborate with neurons in spreading the "infectious" Aβ and Tau drivers of Alzheimer's disease? *Neuroscientist* 21, 9–29. doi: 10.1177/1073858414529828

de Jong, D., Jansen, R., Hoefnagels, W., Jellesma-Eggenkamp, M., Verbeek, M., Borm, G., et al. (2008). No effect of one-year treatment with indomethacin on Alzheimer's disease progression: a randomized controlled trial. *PLoS ONE* 3:e1475. doi: 10.1371/journal.pone.0001475

Dursun, E., Gezen-Ak, D., Hanagasi, H., Bilgiç, B., Lohmann, E., Ertan, S., et al. (2015). The interleukin 1 alpha, interleukin 1 beta, interleukin 6 and α-2-macroglobulin serum levels in patients with early or late onset Alzheimer's disease, mild cognitive impairment or Parkinson's disease. *J. Neuroimmunol.* 283, 50–57. doi: 10.1016/j.jneuroim.2015.04.014

El Omri, A., Han, J., Yamada, P., Kawada, K., Abdrabbah, M. B., and Isoda, H. (2010). *Rosmarinus officinalis* polyphenols activate cholinergic activities in PC12 cells through phosphorylation of ERK1/2. *J. Ethnopharmacol.* 131, 451–458. doi: 10.1016/j.jep.2010.07.006

Essa, M. M., Vijayan, R. K., Castellano-Gonzalez, G., Memon, M. A., Braidy, N., and Guillemin, G. J. (2012). Neuroprotective effect of natural products against Alzheimer's disease. *Neurochem. Res.* 37, 1829–1842. doi: 10.1007/s11064-012-0799-9

Fang, W., Deng, Y., Li, Y., Shang, E., Fang, F., Lv, P., et al. (2010). Blood brain barrier permeability and therapeutic time window of Ginkgolide B in ischemia–reperfusion injury. *Eur. J. Pharm. Sci.* 39, 8–14. doi: 10.1016/j.ejps.2009.10.002

Faria, A., Pestana, D., Teixeira, D., Azevedo, J., De Freitas, V., Mateus, N., et al. (2010). Flavonoid transport across RBE4 cells: a blood-brain barrier model. *Cell. Mol. Biol. Lett.* 15, 234–241. doi: 10.2478/s11658-010-0006-4

Farlow, M., Miller, M., and Pejovic, V. (2008). Treatment Options in Alzheimer's Disease: maximizing benefit, managing expectations. 25, 408–422. doi: 10.1159/000122962

Furukawa, S., Yang, L., and Sameshima, H. (2014). Galantamine, an acetylcholinesterase inhibitor, reduces brain damage induced by hypoxia-ischemia in newborn rats. *Int. J. Dev. Neurosci.* 37, 52–57. doi: 10.1016/j.ijdevneu.2014.06.011

Garcez, M. L., Mina, F., Bellettini-Santos, T., Carneiro, F. G., Luz, A. P., Schiavo, G. L., et al. (2017). Minocycline reduces inflammatory parameters in the brain structures and serum and reverses memory impairment caused by the administration of amyloid β (1-42) in mice. *Progr. Neuro Psychopharmacol. Biol. Psychiatry* 77, 23–31. doi: 10.1016/j.pnpbp.2017.03.010

Gramza-Michalowska, A., and Regula, J. (2007). Use of tea extracts (*Camelia sinensis*) in jelly candies as polyphenols sources in human diet. *Asia Pac. J. Clin. Nutr.* 16, 43–46. doi: 10.6133/apjcn.2007.16.s1.09

Ha, S. K., Moon, E., Ju, M. S., Kim, D. H., Ryu, J. H., Oh, M. S., et al. (2012). 6-Shogaol, a ginger product, modulates neuroinflammation: a new approach to neuroprotection. *Neuropharmacology* 63, 211–223. doi: 10.1016/j.neuropharm.2012.03.016

Han, Y., Jung, H. W., Lee, D. H., Kwon, S. Y., Son, K. H., and Park, Y. K. (2013). Anti-inflammatory effects of prosapogenin III from the dried roots of *Liriope platyphylla* in LPS-stimulated RAW264.7 cells. *J. Asian Nat. Prod. Res.* 15, 1038–1049. doi: 10.1080/10286020.2013.825253

Haniadka, R., Rajeev, A. G., Palatty, P. L., Arora, R., and Baliga, M. S. (2012). *Zingiber officinale* (ginger) as an anti-emetic in cancer chemotherapy: a review. *J. Altern. Complem. Med.* 18, 440–444. doi: 10.1089/acm.2010.0737

Haque, A. M., Hashimoto, M., Katakura, M., Hara, Y., and Shido, O. (2008). Green tea catechins prevent cognitive deficits caused by Aβ1–40 in rats. *J. Nutr. Biochem.* 19, 619–626. doi: 10.1016/j.jnutbio.2007.08.008

Harrington, C., Sawchak, S., Chiang, C., Davies, J., Donovan, C. M., Van Dyck, C., et al. (2011). Rosiglitazone does not improve cognition or global function when used as adjunctive therapy to AChE inhibitors in mild-to-moderate Alzheimer's disease: two phase 3 studies. *Curr. Alzheimer Res.* 8, 592–606. doi: 10.2174/156720511796391935

Hirai, S., Uemura, T., Mizoguchi, N., Lee, J. Y., Taketani, K., Nakano, Y., et al. (2010). Diosgenin attenuates inflammatory changes in the interaction between adipocytes and macrophages. *Mol. Nutr. Food Res.* 54, 797–804. doi: 10.1002/mnfr.200900208

Hong, J. T. (2017). NF-kB as a mediator of brain inflammation in AD. *CNS Neurol. Disord. Drug Targets.* doi: 10.2174/1871527316666170807130011. [Epub ahead of print].

Hoppe, J. B., Coradini, K., Frozza, R. L., Oliveira, C. M., Meneghetti, A. B., Bernardi, A., et al. (2013). Free and nanoencapsulated curcumin suppress β-amyloid-induced cognitive impairments in rats: involvement of BDNF and Akt/GSK-3β signaling pathway. *Neurobiol. Learn. Mem.* 106, 134–144. doi: 10.1016/j.nlm.2013.08.001

Hosseinzadeh, S., Roshan, V. D., and Mahjoub, S. (2013). Continuous exercise training and curcumin attenuate changes in brain-derived neurotrophic factor and oxidative stress induced by lead acetate in the hippocampus of male rats. *Pharm. Biol.* 51, 240–245. doi: 10.3109/13880209.2012.717230

Howes, M. J., Perry, N. S., and Houghton, P. J. (2003). Plants with traditional uses and activities, relevant to the management of Alzheimer's disease and other cognitive disorders. *Phytother. Res.* 17, 1–18. doi: 10.1002/ptr.1280

Huang, H.-J., Chen, W.-L., Hsieh, R.-H., and Hsieh-Li, H. M. (2014). Multifunctional effects of mangosteen pericarp on cognition in C57BL/6J and triple transgenic Alzheimer’s mice. *Evid. Based Complement. Altern. Med.* 2014:18. doi: 10.1155/2014/813672

Hur, J. Y., Lee, P., Kim, H., Kang, I., Lee, K. R., and Kim, S. Y. (2004). (-)-3,5-Dicaffeoyl-muco-quinic acid isolated from *Aster scaber* contributes to the differentiation of PC12 cells: through tyrosine kinase cascade signaling. *Biochem. Biophys. Res. Commun.* 313, 948–953. doi: 10.1016/j.bbrc.2003.11.178

Itoh, K., Chiba, T., Takahashi, S., Ishii, T., Igarashi, K., Katoh, Y., et al. (1997). An Nrf2/small Maf heterodimer mediates the induction of phase II detoxifying enzyme genes through antioxidant response elements. *Biochem. Biophys. Res. Commun.* 236, 313–322. doi: 10.1006/bbrc.1997.6943

Jackisch, R., Förster, S., Kammerer, M., Rothmaier, A. K., Ehret, A., Zentner, J., et al. (2009). Inhibitory potency of choline esterase inhibitors on acetylcholine release and choline esterase activity in fresh specimens of human and rat neocortex. *J. Alzheimer's Dis.* 16, 635–647. doi: 10.3233/JAD-2009-1008

Jia, L., Liu, J., Song, Z., Pan, X., Chen, L., Cui, X., et al. (2012). Berberine suppresses amyloid-β-induced inflammatory response in microglia by inhibiting nuclear factor-kappaB and mitogen-activated protein kinase signalling pathways. *J. Pharm. Pharmacol.* 64, 1510–1521. doi: 10.1111/j.2042-7158.2012.01529.x

Joo, S. S., Yoo, Y. M., Ahn, B. W., Nam, S. Y., Kim, Y. B., Hwang, K. W., et al. (2008). Prevention of inflammation-mediated neurotoxicity by Rg3 and its role in microglial activation. *Biological and Pharmaceutical Bulletin* 31, 1392–1396. doi: 10.1248/bpb.31.1392

Jowie, C., and Ip, N. Y. (2004). *Melia toosendan* regulates PC12 cell differentiation via the activation of protein kinase A and extracellular signal-regulated kinases. *Neurosignals* 13, 248–257. doi: 10.1159/000079339

Kam, A., Li, K. M., Razmovski-Naumovski, V., Nammi, S., Chan, K., Li, Y., et al. (2012). The protective effects of natural products on blood-brain barrier breakdown. *Curr. Med. Chem.* 19, 1830–1845. doi: 10.2174/092986712800099794

Kandel, E. R. (2012). The molecular biology of memory: cAMP, PKA, CRE, CREB-1, CREB-2, and CPEB. *Mol. Brain* 5:14. doi: 10.1186/1756-6606-5-14

Kerr, F., Sofola-Adesakin, O., Ivanov, D. K., Gatliff, J., Gomez Perez-Nievas, B., Bertrand, H. C., et al. (2017). Direct Keap1-Nrf2 disruption as a potential therapeutic target for Alzheimer's disease. *PLoS Genet.* 13:e1006593. doi: 10.1371/journal.pgen.1006593

Kim, C. S., Kwon, O. W., Kim, S. Y., and Lee, K. R. (2013). Bioactive lignans from the trunk of Abies holophylla. *J. Nat. Prod.* 76, 2131–2135. doi: 10.1021/np4005322

Kim, J., Lee, H. J., and Lee, K. W. (2010). Naturally occurring phytochemicals for the prevention of Alzheimer's disease. *J. Neurochem.* 112, 1415–1430. doi: 10.1111/j.1471-4159.2009.06562.x

Kim, M. S., Yu, J. M., Kim, H. J., Kim, H. B., Kim, S. T., Jang, S. K., et al. (2014). Ginsenoside Re and Rd enhance the expression of cholinergic markers and neuronal differentiation in Neuro-2a cells. *Biol. Pharm. Bull.* 37, 826–833. doi: 10.1248/bpb.b14-00011

Kim, S. Y., Gao, J. J., Lee, W. C., Ryu, K. S., Lee, K. R., and Kim, Y. C. (1999). Antioxidative flavonoids from the leaves of *Morus alba*. *Arch. Pharm. Res.* 22, 81–85. doi: 10.1007/BF02976442

Kim, S. J., Jeong, H. J., Lee, K. M., Myung, N. Y., An, N. H., Yang, W. M., et al. (2007). Epigallocatechin-3-gallate suppresses NF-κB activation and phosphorylation of p38 MAPK and JNK in human astrocytoma U373MG cells. *J. Nutr. Biochem.* 18, 587–596. doi: 10.1016/j.jnutbio.2006.11.001

Kimata, M., Shichijo, M., Miura, T., Serizawa, I., Inagaki, N., and Nagai, H. (2000). Effects of luteolin, quercetin and baicalein on immunoglobulin E-mediated mediator release from human cultured mast cells. *Clin. Exp. Allergy* 30, 501–508. doi: 10.1046/j.1365-2222.2000.00768.x

Korolev, I. O. (2014). Alzheimer's disease: a clinical and basic science review. *Med. Stud. Res. J.* 4, 24–33.

Kumar, A., and Singh, A. (2015). A review on Alzheimer's disease pathophysiology and its management: an update. *Pharmacol. Rep.* 67, 195–203. doi: 10.1016/j.pharep.2014.09.004

Kuner, P., Schubenel, R., and Hertel, C. (1998). β-amyloid binds to p75NTR and activates NFκB in human neuroblastoma cells. *J. Neurosci. Res.* 54, 798–804. doi: 10.1002/(SICI)1097-4547(19981215)54:6<798::AID-JNR7>3.0.CO;2-T

Kurz, A., and Perneczky, R. (2011). Novel insights for the treatment of Alzheimer's disease. *Prog. Neuropsychopharmacol. Biol. Psychiatry* 35, 373–379. doi: 10.1016/j.pnpbp.2010.07.018

Lafay-Chebassier, C., Paccalin, M., Page, G., Barc-Pain, S., Perault-Pochat, M. C., Gil, R., et al. (2005). mTOR/p70S6k signalling alteration by Aβ exposure as well as in APP-PS1 transgenic models and in patients with Alzheimer's disease. *J. Neurochem.* 94, 215–225. doi: 10.1111/j.1471-4159.2005.03187.x

Lee, B., Sur, B., Shim, I., Lee, H., and Hahm, D.-H. (2012). *Phellodendron amurense* and its major alkaloid compound, berberine ameliorates scopolamine-induced neuronal impairment and memory dysfunction in rats. *Korean J./ Physiol. Pharmacol.* 16, 79–89. doi: 10.4196/kjpp.2012.16.2.79

Lee, S. Y., Moon, E., Kim, S. Y., and Lee, K. R. (2013). Quinic acid derivatives from *Pimpinella brachycarpa* exert anti-neuroinflammatory activity in lipopolysaccharide-induced microglia. *Bioorg. Med. Chem. Lett.* 23, 2140–2144. doi: 10.1016/j.bmcl.2013.01.115

Lee, S. Y., Kim, C. Y., Lee, J. J., Jung, J. G., and Lee, S. R. (2003). Effects of delayed administration of (-)-epigallocatechin gallate, a green tea polyphenol on the changes in polyamine levels and neuronal damage after transient forebrain ischemia in gerbils. *Brain Res. Bull.* 61, 399–406. doi: 10.1016/S0361-9230(03)00139-4

Lee, T. (2003). *Coloured Flora of Korea, Vol I, II.* Seoul: Hayangmunsa.

Levites, Y., Amit, T., Youdim, M. B., and Mandel, S. (2002). Involvement of protein kinase C activation and cell survival/cell cycle genes in green tea polyphenol (-)-epigallocatechin 3-gallate neuroprotective action. *J. Biol. Chem.* 277, 30574–30580. doi: 10.1074/jbc.M202832200

Li, L., Zhang, Q. G., Lai, L. Y., Wen, X. J., Zheng, T., Cheung, C. W., et al. (2013). Neuroprotective effect of ginkgolide B on bupivacaine-induced apoptosis in SH-SY5Y cells. *Oxid. Med. Cell. Longev.* 2013:159864. doi: 10.1155/2013/159864

Li, Q., and Verma, I. M. (2002). NF-κB regulation in the immune system. *Nat. Rev. Immunol.* 2:725. doi: 10.1038/nri968

Li, Q., Zhao, H., Zhang, Z., Liu, Z., Pei, X., Wang, J., et al. (2009). Long-term green tea catechin administration prevents spatial learning and memory impairment in senescence-accelerated mouse prone-8 mice by decreasing Aβ1-42 oligomers and upregulating synaptic plasticity-related proteins in the hippocampus. *Neuroscience* 163, 741–749. doi: 10.1016/j.neuroscience.2009.07.014

Li, R., Huang, Y. G., Fang, D., and Le, W. D. (2004). (-)-Epigallocatechin gallate inhibits lipopolysaccharide-induced microglial activation and protects against inflammation-mediated dopaminergic neuronal injury. *J. Neurosci. Res.* 78, 723–731. doi: 10.1002/jnr.20315

Lim, D., Iyer, A., Ronco, V., Grolla, A. A., Canonico, P. L., Aronica, E., et al. (2013). Amyloid β deregulates astroglial mGluR5-mediated calcium signaling via calcineurin and Nf-kB. *Glia* 61, 1134–1145. doi: 10.1002/glia.22502

Lin, L. C., Wang, M. N., Tseng, T. Y., Sung, J. S., and Tsai, T. H. (2007). Pharmacokinetics of (-)-epigallocatechin-3-gallate in conscious and freely moving rats and its brain regional distribution. *J. Agric. Food Chem.* 55, 1517–1524. doi: 10.1021/jf062816a

Liu, D., Wang, Z., Gao, Z., Xie, K., Zhang, Q., Jiang, H., et al. (2014). Effects of curcumin on learning and memory deficits, BDNF, and ERK protein expression in rats exposed to chronic unpredictable stress. *Behav. Brain Res.* 271, 116–121. doi: 10.1016/j.bbr.2014.05.068

Liu, M., Chen, F., Sha, L., Wang, S., Tao, L., Yao, L., et al. (2014). (-)-Epigallocatechin-3-gallate ameliorates learning and memory deficits by adjusting the balance of TrkA/p75NTR signaling in APP/PS1 transgenic mice. *Mol. Neurobiol.* 49, 1350–1363. doi: 10.1007/s12035-013-8608-2

Longpré, F., Garneau, P., and Ramassamy, C. (2006). Protection by EGb 761 against β-amyloid-induced neurotoxicity: involvement of NF-κB, SIRT1, and MAPKs pathways and inhibition of amyloid fibril formation. *Free Radical Biol. Med.* 41, 1781–1794. doi: 10.1016/j.freeradbiomed.2006.08.015

Lou, H., Jing, X., Wei, X., Shi, H., Ren, D., and Zhang, X. (2014). Naringenin protects against 6-OHDA-induced neurotoxicity via activation of the Nrf2/ARE signaling pathway. *Neuropharmacology* 79, 380–388. doi: 10.1016/j.neuropharm.2013.11.026

Ma, T., Tan, M. S., Yu, J. T., and Tan, L. (2014). Resveratrol as a therapeutic agent for Alzheimer's disease. *Biomed Res. Int.* 2014:350516. doi: 10.1155/2014/350516

Mao, X.-Y., Cao, D.-F., Li, X., Yin, J.-Y., Wang, Z.-B., Zhang, Y., et al. (2014). Huperzine A ameliorates cognitive deficits in streptozotocin-induced diabetic rats. *Int. J. Mol. Sci.* 15, 7667–7683. doi: 10.3390/ijms15057667

Mendonça, L. M., Da Silva Machado, C., Teixeira, C. C., De Freitas, L. P., Bianchi, M. D. L. P., and Antunes, L.M.G. (2013). Curcumin reduces cisplatin-induced neurotoxicity in NGF-differentiated PC12 cells. *Neurotoxicology* 34, 205–211. doi: 10.1016/j.neuro.2012.09.011

Moalic, S., Liagre, B., Corbière, C., Bianchi, A., Dauça, M., Bordji, K., et al. (2001). A plant steroid, diosgenin, induces apoptosis, cell cycle arrest and COX activity in osteosarcoma cells. *FEBS Lett.* 506, 225–230. doi: 10.1016/S0014-5793(01)02924-6

Moon, M., Kim, H. G., Choi, J. G., Oh, H., Lee, P. K., Ha, S. K., et al. (2014). 6-Shogaol, an active constituent of ginger, attenuates neuroinflammation and cognitive deficits in animal models of dementia. *Biochem. Biophys. Res. Commun.* 449, 8–13. doi: 10.1016/j.bbrc.2014.04.121

Morales, I., Guzman-Martinez, L., Cerda-Troncoso, C., Farias, G. A., and Maccioni, R. B. (2014). Neuroinflammation in the pathogenesis of Alzheimer's disease. A rational framework for the search of novel therapeutic approaches. *Front. Cell. Neurosci.* 8:112. doi: 10.3389/fncel.2014.00112

Nabavi, S. M., Habtemariam, S., Daglia, M., Braidy, N., Loizzo, M. R., Tundis, R., et al. (2015). Neuroprotective effects of Ginkgolide B against ischemic stroke: a review of current literature. *Curr. Top. Med. Chem.* 15, 2222–2232. doi: 10.2174/1568026615666150610142647

Nam, S. M., Choi, J. H., Yoo, D. Y., Kim, W., Jung, H. Y., Kim, J. W., et al. (2014). Effects of curcumin (*Curcuma longa*) on learning and spatial memory as well as cell proliferation and neuroblast differentiation in adult and aged mice by upregulating brain-derived neurotrophic factor and CREB signaling. *J. Med. Food* 17, 641–649. doi: 10.1089/jmf.2013.2965

Nappez, C., Liagre, B., and Beneytout, J. (1995). Changes in lipoxygenase activities in human erythroleukemia (HEL) cells during diosgenin-induced differentiation. *Cancer Lett.* 96, 133–140. doi: 10.1016/0304-3835(95)03923-K

Ni, J., Wu, Z., Ling, S., Zhu, X., and Lu, P. (2006). Effect of Matrine injection on IL−1beta level and ultrastructural changes of hippocampal neuron in Alzheimer's disease rat. *Chin. J. Anat.* 29, 608–611.

Niidome, T., Takahashi, K., Goto, Y., Goh, S., Tanaka, N., Kamei, K., et al. (2007). Mulberry leaf extract prevents amyloid beta-peptide fibril formation and neurotoxicity. *Neuroreport* 18, 813–816. doi: 10.1097/WNR.0b013e3280dce5af

Ondeyka, J. G., Jayasuriya, H., Polishook, J. D., Bills, G. F., Dombrowski, A. W., Mojena, M., et al. (2005). Discovery of structurally diverse natural product antagonists of chemokine receptor CXCR3. *Mol. Divers.* 9, 123–129. doi: 10.1007/s11030-005-1296-8

O'neill, L. A., and Kaltschmidt, C. (1997). NF-kB: a crucial transcription factor for glial and neuronal cell function. *Trends Neurosci.* 20, 252–258. doi: 10.1016/S0166-2236(96)01035-1

Palatty, P. L., Haniadka, R., Valder, B., Arora, R., and Baliga, M. S. (2013). Ginger in the prevention of nausea and vomiting: a review. *Crit. Rev. Food Sci. Nutr.* 53, 659–669. doi: 10.1080/10408398.2011.553751

Pany, S., Pal, A., and Sahu, P. K. (2014). Neuroprotective effect of quercetin in neurotoxicity induced rats: role of neuroinflammation in neurodegeneration. *Asian J. Pharm. Clin. Res.* 7, 152–156.

Park, H. R., Lee, H., Park, H., Jeon, J. W., Cho, W. K., and Ma, J. Y. (2015). Neuroprotective effects of *Liriope platyphylla* extract against hydrogen peroxide-induced cytotoxicity in human neuroblastoma SH-SY5Y cells. *BMC Complement. Altern. Med.* 15:171. doi: 10.1186/s12906-015-0679-3y

Paulo Andrade, J., and Assuncao, M. (2012). Protective effects of chronic green tea consumption on age-related neurodegeneration. *Curr. Pharm. Des.* 18, 4–14. doi: 10.2174/138161212798918986

Pereira, R. P., Fachinetto, R., de Souza Prestes, A., Puntel, R. L., Da Silva, G. N. S., Heinzmann, B. M., et al. (2009). Antioxidant effects of different extracts from *Melissa officinalis, Matricaria recutita* and *Cymbopogon citratus. Neurochem. Res.* 34, 973–983. doi: 10.1007/s11064-008-9861-z

Plyte, S. E., Hughes, K., Nikolakaki, E., Pulverer, B. J., and Woodgett, J. R. (1992). Glycogen synthase kinase-3: functions in oncogenesis and development. *Biochim. Biophys. Acta Rev. Cancer* 1114, 147–162. doi: 10.1016/0304-419X.(92)90012-N.

Rajadhyaksha, M., Boyden, T., Liras, J., El-Kattan, A., and Brodfuehrer, J. (2011). Current advances in delivery of biotherapeutics across the blood-brain barrier. *Curr. Drug Discov. Technol.* 8, 87–101. doi: 10.2174/157016311795563866

Ramirez-Bermudez, J. (2012). Alzheimer's disease: critical notes on the history of a medical concept. *Arch. Med. Res.* 43, 595–599. doi: 10.1016/j.arcmed.2012.11.008

Rangel-Ordóñez, L., Noldner, M., Schubert-Zsilavecz, M., and Wurglics, M. (2010). Plasma levels and distribution of flavonoids in rat brain after single and repeated doses of standardized *Ginkgo biloba* extract EGb 761(R). *Planta Med.* 76, 1683–1690. doi: 10.1055/s-0030-1249962

Rashid, U., and Ansari, F. L. (2014). "Challenges in designing therapeutic agents for treating alzheimer's disease-from serendipity to rationality," in *Drug Design and Discovery in Alzheimer's Disease*, eds Atta-ur-Rahman and M. I. Choudhary (Karachi: Elsevier), 40–141.

Rasool, M., Malik, A., Qureshi, M. S., Manan, A., Pushparaj, P. N., Asif, M., et al. (2014). Recent updates in the treatment of neurodegenerative disorders using natural compounds. *Evid. Based Complem. Altern. Med.* 2014:7. doi: 10.1155/2014/979730

Raza, S. S., Khan, M. M., Ahmad, A., Ashafaq, M., Islam, F., Wagner, A. P., et al. (2013). Neuroprotective effect of naringenin is mediated through suppression of NF-κB signaling pathway in experimental stroke. *Neuroscience* 230, 157–171. doi: 10.1016/j.neuroscience.2012.10.041

Rezai-Zadeh, K., Shytle, D., Sun, N., Mori, T., Hou, H., Jeanniton, D., et al. (2005). Green tea epigallocatechin-3-gallate (EGCG) modulates amyloid precursor protein cleavage and reduces cerebral amyloidosis in Alzheimer transgenic mice. *J. Neurosci.* 25, 8807–8814. doi: 10.1523/JNEUROSCI.1521-05.2005

Rinwa, P., Kumar, A., and Garg, S. (2013). Suppression of neuroinflammatory and apoptotic signaling cascade by curcumin alone and in combination with piperine in rat model of olfactory bulbectomy induced depression. *PLoS ONE* 8:e61052. doi: 10.1371/journal.pone.0061052

Roy, A., and Saraf, S. (2006). Limonoids: overview of significant bioactive triterpenes distributed in plants kingdom. *Biol. Pharm. Bull.* 29, 191–201. doi: 10.1248/bpb.29.191

Ruan, Q., Hu, X., Ao, H., Ma, H., Gao, Z., Liu, F., et al. (2014). The neurovascular protective effects of huperzine A on D-galactose-induced inflammatory damage in the rat hippocampus. *Gerontology* 60, 424–439. doi: 10.1159/000358235

Shibata, Y., Kume, N., Arai, H., Hayashida, K., Inui-Hayashida, A., Minami, M., et al. (2007). Mulberry leaf aqueous fractions inhibit TNF-α-induced nuclear factor κB (NF-κB) activation and lectin-like oxidized LDL receptor-1 (LOX-1) expression in vascular endothelial cells. *Atherosclerosis* 193, 20–27. doi: 10.1016/j.atherosclerosis.2006.08.011

Shim, S., and Kwon, J. (2012). Effects of [6]-shogaol on cholinergic signaling in HT22 cells following neuronal damage induced by hydrogen peroxide. *Food Chem. Toxicol.* 50, 1454–1459. doi: 10.1016/j.fct.2012.02.014

Shim, S., Kim, S., Choi, D. S., Kwon, Y. B., and Kwon, J. (2011). Anti-inflammatory effects of [6]-shogaol: potential roles of HDAC inhibition and HSP70 induction. *Food Chem. Toxicol.* 49, 2734–2740. doi: 10.1016/j.fct.2011.08.012

Shishodia, S., and Aggarwal, B. (2006). Diosgenin inhibits osteoclastogenesis, invasion, and proliferation through the downregulation of Akt, IκB kinase activation and NF-κB-regulated gene expression. *Oncogene* 25:1463. doi: 10.1038/sj.onc.1209194

Simons, M., Schwärzler, F., Lütjohann, D., Von Bergmann, K., Beyreuther, K., Dichgans, J., et al. (2002). Treatment with simvastatin in normocholesterolemic patients with Alzheimer's disease: a 26-week randomized, placebo-controlled, double-blind trial. *Ann. Neurol.* 52, 346–350. doi: 10.1002/ana.10292

Singh, M., Arseneault, M., Sanderson, T., Murthy, V., and Ramassamy, C. (2008). Challenges for research on polyphenols from foods in Alzheimer's disease: bioavailability, metabolism, and cellular and molecular mechanisms. *J. Agric. Food Chem.* 56, 4855–4873. doi: 10.1021/jf0735073

Smith, M. A., Nunomura, A., Zhu, X., Takeda, A., and Perry, G. (2000). Metabolic, metallic, and mitotic sources of oxidative stress in Alzheimer disease. *Antioxidants Redox Signal.* 2, 413–420. doi: 10.1089/15230860050192198

Soh, Y., Kim, J. A., Sohn, N. W., Lee, K. R., and Kim, S. Y. (2003). Protective effects of quinic acid derivatives on tetrahydropapaveroline-induced cell death in C6 glioma cells. *Biol. Pharm. Bull.* 26, 803–807. doi: 10.1248/bpb.26.803

Song, J., Cheon, S. Y., Jung, W., Lee, W. T., and Lee, J. E. (2014). Resveratrol induces the expression of interleukin-10 and brain-derived neurotrophic factor in BV2 microglia under hypoxia. *Int. J. Mol. Sci.* 15, 15512–15529. doi: 10.3390/ijms150915512

Sparks, D. L., Sabbagh, M. N., Connor, D. J., Lopez, J., Launer, L. J., Browne, P., et al. (2005). Atorvastatin for the treatment of mild to moderate Alzheimer disease: preliminary results. *Arch. Neurol.* 62, 753–757. doi: 10.1001/archneur.62.5.753

Starkov, A. A., and Beal, F. M. (2008). Portal to Alzheimer's disease. *Nat. Med.* 14, 1020–1021. doi: 10.1038/nm1008-1020

Streit, W. J., Mrak, R. E., and Griffin, W. S. T. (2004). Microglia and neuroinflammation: a pathological perspective. *J. Neuroinflammation* 1:14. doi: 10.1186/1742-2094-1-14

Tan, M. S., Yu, J. T., Jiang, T., Zhu, X. C., and Tan, L. (2013). The NLRP3 inflammasome in Alzheimer's disease. *Mol. Neurobiol.* 48, 875–882. doi: 10.1007/s12035-013-8475-x

Tang, L.-L., Wang, R., and Tang, X.-C. (2005). Huperzine A protects SHSY5Y neuroblastoma cells against oxidative stress damage via nerve growth factor production. *Eur. J. Pharmacol.* 519, 9–15. doi: 10.1016/j.ejphar.2005.06.026

Van Gool, W. A., Weinstein, H. C., Scheltens, P. K., and Walstra, G. J. (2001). Effect of hydroxychloroquine on progression of dementia in early Alzheimer's disease: an 18-month randomised, double-blind, placebo-controlled study. *Lancet* 358, 455–460. doi: 10.1016/S0140-6736(01)05623-9

Van Praag, H., Lucero, M. J., Yeo, G. W., Stecker, K., Heivand, N., Zhao, C., et al. (2007). Plant-derived flavanol (-)epicatechin enhances angiogenesis and retention of spatial memory in mice. *J. Neurosci.* 27, 5869–5878. doi: 10.1523/JNEUROSCI.0914-07.2007

Venkatesan, R., Ji, E., and Kim, S. Y. (2015). Phytochemicals that regulate neurodegenerative disease by targeting neurotrophins: a comprehensive review. *Biomed Res. Int.* 2015:814068. doi: 10.1155/2015/814068

Wang, C. P., Zhang, L. Z., Li, G. C., Shi, Y. W., Li, J. L., Zhang, X. C., et al. (2014). Mulberroside A protects against ischemic impairment in primary culture of rat cortical neurons after oxygen-glucose deprivation followed by reperfusion. *J. Neurosci. Res.* 92, 944–954. doi: 10.1002/jnr.23374

Wang, G. F., Shi, L. P., Ren, Y. D., Liu, Q. F., Liu, H. F., Zhang, R. J., et al. (2009). Anti-hepatitis B virus activity of chlorogenic acid, quinic acid and caffeic acid *in vivo* and *in vitro*. *Antiviral Res.* 83, 186–190. doi: 10.1016/j.antiviral.2009.05.002

Wang, Y., Xia, Z., Xu, J.-R., Wang, Y.-X., Hou, L.-N., Qiu, Y., et al. (2012). α-Mangostin, a polyphenolic xanthone derivative from mangosteen, attenuates β-amyloid oligomers-induced neurotoxicity by inhibiting amyloid aggregation. *Neuropharmacology* 62, 871–881. doi: 10.1016/j.neuropharm.2011.09.016

Wang, Z. F., Wang, J., Zhang, H. Y., and Tang, X. C. (2008). Huperzine a exhibits anti-inflammatory and neuroprotective effects in a rat model of transient focal cerebral ischemia. *J. Neurochem.* 106, 1594–1603. doi: 10.1111/j.1471-4159.2008.05504.x

Wang, Z. F., Tang, L. L., Yan, H., Wang, Y. J., and Tang, X. C. (2006a). Effects of huperzine A on memory deficits and neurotrophic factors production after transient cerebral ischemia and reperfusion in mice. *Pharmacol. Biochem. Behav.* 83, 603–611. doi: 10.1016/j.pbb.2006.03.027

Wang, Z. J., Nie, B. M., Chen, H. Z., and Lu, Y. (2006b). Panaxynol induces neurite outgrowth in PC12D cells via cAMP-and MAP kinase-dependent mechanisms. *Chem. Biol. Interact.* 159, 58–64. doi: 10.1016/j.cbi.2005.09.003

Weldon, D. T., Rogers, S. D., Ghilardi, J. R., Finke, M. P., Cleary, J. P., O'hare, E., et al. (1998). Fibrillar β-amyloid induces microglial phagocytosis, expression of inducible nitric oxide synthase, and loss of a select population of neurons in the rat CNS *in vivo*. *J. Neurosci.* 18, 2161–2173. doi: 10.1523/JNEUROSCI.18-06-02161.1998

Wollen, K. A. (2010). Alzheimer's disease: the pros and cons of pharmaceutical, nutritional, botanical, and stimulatory therapies, with a discussion of treatment strategies from the perspective of patients and practitioners. *Altern. Med. Rev.* 15, 223–244.

Xia, J.-H., Zhang, S.-D., Li, Y.-L., Wu, L., Zhu, Z.-J., Yang, X.-W., et al. (2012). Sesquiterpenoids and triterpenoids from *Abies holophylla* and their bioactivities. *Phytochemistry* 74, 178–184. doi: 10.1016/j.phytochem.2011.11.011

Xiao, H., Cao, X., Wang, L., Run, X., Su, Y., Tian, C., et al. (2011). 1, 5-dicaffeoylquinic acid protects primary neurons from amyloid β 1-42-induced apoptosis via PI3K/Akt signaling pathway. *Chin. Med. J.* 124, 2628–2635. doi: 10.3760/cma.j.issn.0366-6999.2011.17.012

Xiao, Q., Wang, C., Li, J., Hou, Q., Li, J., Ma, J., et al. (2010). Ginkgolide B protects hippocampal neurons from apoptosis induced by beta-amyloid 25–35 partly via up-regulation of brain-derived neurotrophic factor. *Eur. J. Pharmacol.* 647, 48–54. doi: 10.1016/j.ejphar.2010.08.002

Xu, F., Wang, C., Yang, L., Luo, H., Fan, W., Zi, C., et al. (2013). C-dideoxyhexosyl flavones from the stems and leaves of *Passiflora edulis* sims. *Food Chem.* 136, 94–99. doi: 10.1016/j.foodchem.2012.07.101

Yang, Y., Bai, L., Li, X., Xiong, J., Xu, P., Guo, C., et al. (2014). Transport of active flavonoids, based on cytotoxicity and lipophilicity: an evaluation using the blood–brain barrier cell and Caco-2 cell models. *Toxicology In Vitro* 28, 388–396. doi: 10.1016/j.tiv.2013.12.002

Yazir, Y., Utkan, T., Gacar, N., and Aricioglu, F. (2015). Resveratrol exerts anti-inflammatory and neuroprotective effects to prevent memory deficits in rats exposed to chronic unpredictable mild stress. *Physiol. Behav.* 138, 297–304. doi: 10.1016/j.physbeh.2014.10.010

Youdim, K. A., Qaiser, M. Z., Begley, D. J., Rice-Evans, C. A., and Abbott, N. J. (2004). Flavonoid permeability across an in situ model of the blood-brain barrier. *Free Radic. Biol. Med.* 36, 592–604. doi: 10.1016/j.freeradbiomed.2003.1break1.023

Yu, H.-J., and Koh, S.-H. (2017). The role of PI3K/AKT pathway and its therapeutic possibility in Alzheimer's disease. *Hanyang Med. Rev.* 37, 18–24. doi: 10.7599/hmr.2017.37.1.18

Zhang, H. Y., and Tang, X. C. (2006). Neuroprotective effects of huperzine A: new therapeutic targets for neurodegenerative disease. *Trends Pharmacol. Sci.* 27, 619–625. doi: 10.1016/j.tips.2006.10.004

Zhang, Q., Li, J.-K., Ge, R., Liang, J.-Y., Li, Q.-S., and Min, Z.-D. (2013). Novel NGF-potentiating limonoids from the fruits of *Melia toosendan*. *Fitoterapia* 90, 192–198. doi: 10.1016/j.fitote.2013.07.019

Zhu, X., Castellani, R. J., Takeda, A., Nunomura, A., Atwood, C. S., Perry, G., et al. (2001a). Differential activation of neuronal ERK, JNK/SAPK and p38 in Alzheimer disease: the 'two hit'hypothesis. *Mech. Ageing Dev.* 123, 39–46. doi: 10.1016/S0047-6374(01)00342-6

Zhu, X., Rottkamp, C. A., Boux, H., Takeda, A., Perry, G., and Smith, M. A. (2000). Activation of p38 kinase links tau phosphorylation, oxidative stress, and cell cycle-related events in Alzheimer disease. *J. Neuropathol. Exp. Neurol.* 59, 880–888. doi: 10.1093/jnen/59.10.880

Zhu, X., Rottkamp, C. A., Hartzler, A., Sun, Z., Takeda, A., Boux, H., et al. (2001b). Activation of MKK6, an upstream activator of p38, in Alzheimer's disease. *J. Neurochem.* 79, 311–318. doi: 10.1046/j.1471-4159.2001.00597.x

Zu Zhu, X., Li, X.-Y., and Liu, J. (2004). Recent pharmacological studies on natural products in China. *Eur. J. Pharmacol.* 500, 221–230. doi: 10.1016/j.ejphar.2004.07.027

11

Taraxasterol Inhibits LPS-Induced Inflammatory Response in BV2 Microglia Cells by Activating LXRα

*Bin Liu[1], Zhaoqi He[2], Jingjing Wang[2], Zhuoyuan Xin[3], Jiaxin Wang[2], Fan Li[3] and Yunhe Fu[2,3]**

[1] *Cardiovascular Disease Center, First Hospital of Jilin University, Changchun, China,* [2] *Department of Clinical Veterinary Medicine, College of Veterinary Medicine, Jilin University, Changchun, China,* [3] *Department of Pathogenobiology, The Key Laboratory of Zoonosis, Chinese Ministry of Education, College of Basic Medicine, Jilin University, Changchun, China*

Correspondence:
Yunhe Fu
fuyunhesky@sina.com

Neuroinflammation plays a critical role in the development of neurodegenerative diseases. Taraxasterol, a pentacyclic-triterpene isolated from *Taraxacum officinale*, has been reported to have anti-inflammatory effect. The aim of this study was to investigate the anti-inflammatory effects and mechanism of taraxasterol in LPS-stimulated BV2 microglia cells. BV2 microglia cells were treated with taraxasterol 12 h before LPS stimulation. The effects of taraxasterol on LPS-induced TNF-α and IL-1β production were detected by ELISA. The effects of taraxasterol on LXRα, ABCA1, TLR4, and NF-κB expression were detected by western blot analysis. The results showed that taraxasterol dose-dependently inhibited LPS-induced TNF-α and IL-1β production and NF-κB activation. Taraxasterol also disrupted the formation of lipid rafts and inhibited translocation of TLR4 into lipid rafts. Furthermore, taraxasterol was found to activate LXRα-ABCA1 signaling pathway which induces cholesterol efflux from cells. In addition, our results showed that the anti-inflammatory effect of taraxasterol was attenuated by transfection with LXRα siRNA. In conclusion, these results suggested that taraxasterol inhibits LPS-induced inflammatory response in BV2 microglia cells by activating LXRα-ABCA1 signaling pathway.

Keywords: taraxasterol, LPS, ABCA1, LXRα, lipid rafts

INTRODUCTION

Neuroinflammation, a chronic inflammation in the brain, has been reported to play critical roles in the development of neurodegenerative diseases, such as Alzheimer's disease and Parkinson's disease (Sun et al., 2010). Microglia, a type of primary immune cells in the brain, play critical roles in host defense and tissue repair in brain (Cameron and Landreth, 2010). Stimulation of microglia by LPS leads to the activation of TLR4 signaling pathway (Qin et al., 2005). The activation of TLR4 signaling pathway leads to the activation of NF-κB and release of inflammatory cytokines such as TNF-α and IL-1β (Kawai and Akira, 2007). TLR4 is the major receptor of LPS and inhibition of TLR4 signaling pathway could attenuate neurodegenerative diseases. Overproduction of these inflammatory cytokines leads to cell death and brain injury (Ziebell and Morganti-Kossmann, 2010). Therefore, the control of microglial activation could be a therapeutic approach for the treatment of neurodegenerative diseases.

Taraxasterol, a pentacyclic-triterpene isolated from *Taraxacum officinale*, has been reported to have anti-inflammatory effects (Xiong et al., 2014). Taraxasterol has been reported to inhibited iNOS and COX-2 expression in LPS-stimulated RAW264.7 cells (Xiong et al., 2014). Taraxasterol also inhibited IL-1β-induced NO and PGE2 production in human osteoarthritic chondrocytes (Piao et al., 2015). *In vivo*, taraxasterol was found to protect LPS-induced acute lung injury and endotoxic shock in mice (San et al., 2014; Zhang et al., 2014). Furthermore, taraxasterol has been reported to protect against OVA-induced allergic asthma in mice (Liu et al., 2013). However, the anti-inflammatory effects of taraxasterol on LPS-induced inflammatory response in BV2 microglia cells have not been reported. In addition, the anti-inflammatory mechanism of taraxasterol has not been fully clarified. In the present study, we detected the anti-inflammatory effects and mechanism of taraxasterol in LPS-stimulated BV2 microglia cells. Our results showed that taraxasterol inhibited LPS-induced inflammatory response in BV2 microglia cells by activating LXRα-ABCA1 signaling pathway.

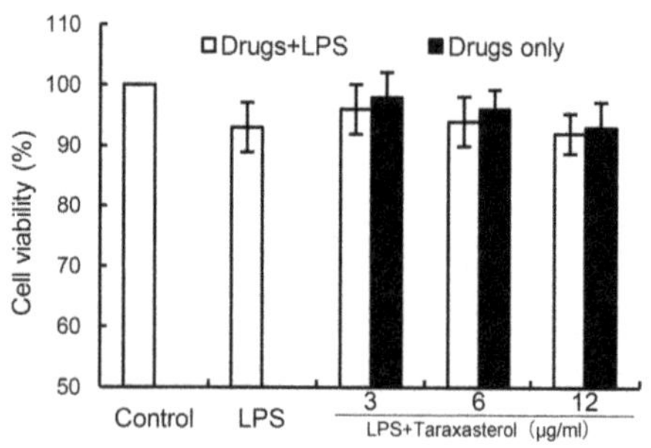

FIGURE 1 | Effects of taraxasterol on the cell viability of BV2 microglia cells. BV2 microglia cells (2 × 10^5 cells/ml) were seeded in 96 well plates and treated with different concentrations of taraxasterol and stimulated with LPS (0.5 μg/ml) for 24 h. The cell viability was determined by MTT assay. The values presented are the means ± SEM of three independent experiments.

MATERIALS AND METHODS

Materials

Taraxasterol (purity: > 98%) was purchased from Chengdu Preferred Biotechnology Co., Ltd. (Chengdu, China). LPS (*Escherichia coli* O55:B5) and MTT was purchased from Sigma (St. Louis, MO, United States). Enzyme-linked immunosorbent assay (ELISA) kits of TNF-α and IL-1β were purchased from Biolegend (CA, United States). Antibodies against LXRα and ABCA1 monoclonal antibodies were purchased from Santa Cruz Biotechnology Inc. (Santa Cruz, CA, United States). Antibodies against TLR4, NF-κB p65, IκBα, and β-actin monoclonal antibodies were purchased from Cell Signaling Technology (Danvers, MA, United States). FuGENE HD transfection reagent was purchased from Roche Applied Science (Indianapolis, IN, United States).

Cell Culture and Treatment

BV2 microglia cells were purchased from the Institute of Basic Medical Sciences of the China Science Academy. The cells were

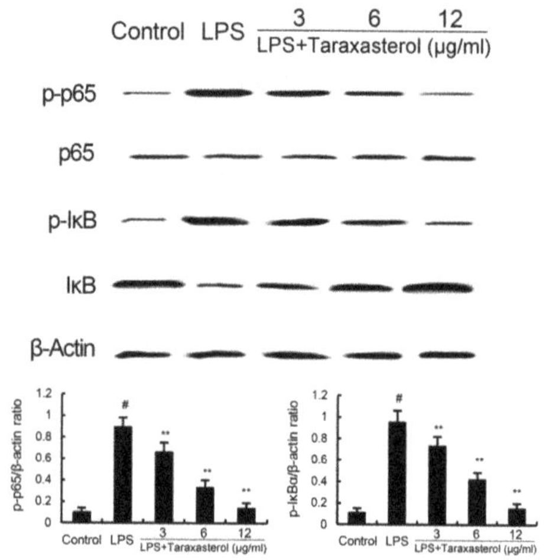

FIGURE 3 | Taraxasterol inhibits LPS-induced NF-κB activation. The values presented are the means ± SEM of three independent experiments. #$p < 0.05$ vs. control group; *$p < 0.05$, **$p < 0.01$ vs. LPS group.

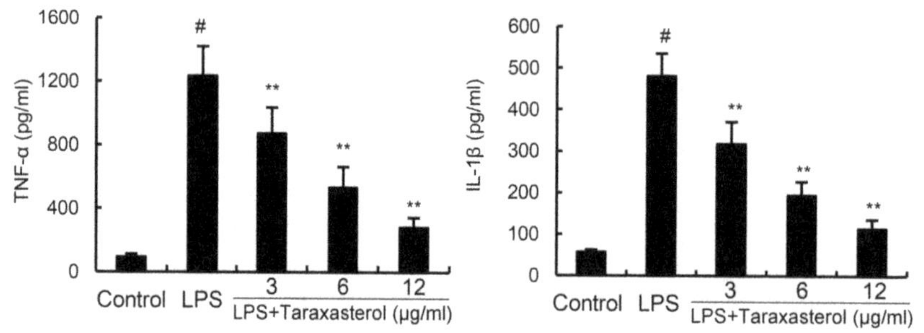

FIGURE 2 | Effects of taraxasterol on LPS-induced TNF-α and IL-1β production. The data presented are the means ± SEM of three independent experiments. #$p < 0.05$ vs. control group; *$p < 0.05$, **$p < 0.01$ vs. LPS group.

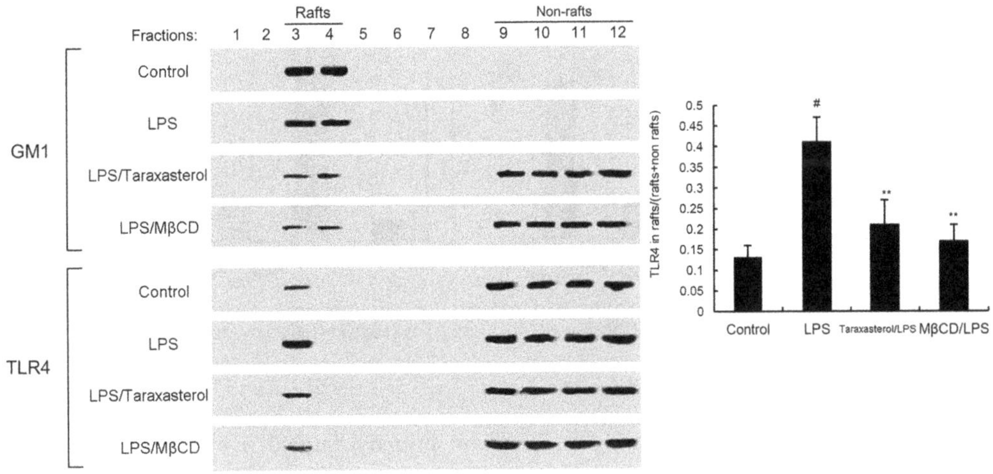

FIGURE 4 | The recruitment of TLR4 to lipid rafts was inhibited by taraxasterol. Fractions 3–4 correspond to lipid rafts. Representative blots of three separate experiments are shown. TLR4 content of macrophage lipid rafts was calculated as a percentage of total membrane TLR4 (lipid rafts + non-rafts). The values presented are the means ± SEM of three independent experiments. $^{\#}p < 0.05$ vs. control group; $^{*}p < 0.05$, $^{**}p < 0.01$ vs. LPS group.

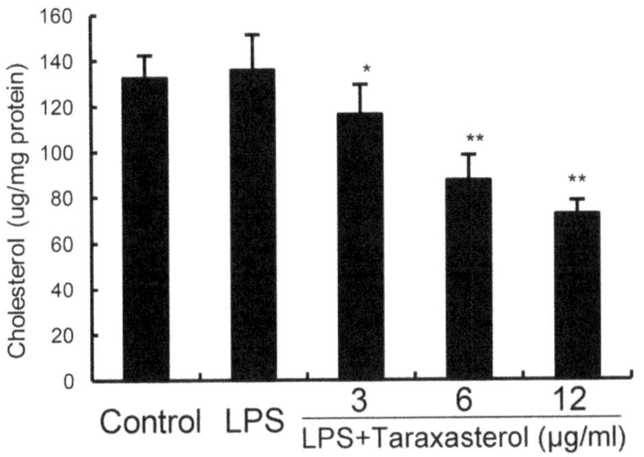

FIGURE 5 | Effects of taraxasterol on lipid rafts cholesterol levels. Cells were treated with taraxasterol (3, 6, 12 μg/ml) for 12 h. Membrane cholesterol levels were measured by gas–liquid chromatography and the results were plotted as μg cholesterol/mg protein. The values presented are the means ± SEM of three independent experiments. $^{\#}p < 0.05$ vs. control group; $^{*}p < 0.05$, $^{**}p < 0.01$ vs. LPS group.

cultured in DMEM supplemented with 10% heat-inactivated fetal bovine serum at 37°C in a humidified incubator under 5% CO_2. The cells were pretreated with taraxasterol (3, 6, 12 μg/ml) 12 h before LPS (0.5 μg/ml) treatment. The concentration of LPS used in this study was based on previous studies (Jeong et al., 2010; Wang et al., 2015).

Effects of Taraxasterol on Cell Viability

The potential cytotoxicity of taraxasterol on BV2 microglia was evaluated by MTT assay as described previously (Yu et al., 2015). Briefly, BV2 microglia cells (2×10^5 cells/ml) were seeded in 96 well plates and treated with different concentrations of taraxasterol and stimulated with LPS for 24 h. After the culture supernatants were removed, the resulting dark blue crystals were dissolved with DMSO. Absorbance was determined at 540 nm.

Effects of Taraxasterol on LPS-Induced TNF-α and IL-1β Production

The effects of taraxasterol on LPS-induced inflammatory cytokines production were measured by ELISA as described previously (Yu et al., 2015). BV2 microglia cells were pretreated with taraxasterol for 12 h and stimulated with LPS for 24 h. The levels of inflammatory cytokines TNF-α and IL-1β were detected by ELISA (Biolegend, CA, United States) according to the manufacturer's protocol.

Effects of Taraxasterol on Cholesterol Levels in Lipid Rafts

Lipid rafts were isolated as described previously (Fu et al., 2014a). The level of cholesterol in lipid raft was assayed by gas–liquid chromatography as previously described (Fu et al., 2014a).

Effects of Taraxasterol on Transcriptional Activity of LXRα

The effects of taraxasterol on transcriptional activity of LXRα were detected by LXR receptor gene assay as described previously (Fu et al., 2015). BV2 microglia were transfected with β-galactosidase control vector and LXRα luciferase reporter plasmid using FuGENE HD transfection reagent according to the manufacturer's instructions. Six hours after transfection, cells were treated with taraxasterol for 12 h. Luciferase activity was normalized by β-galactosidase activity.

Western Blot Analysis

Total proteins from cells were extracted by M-PER Mammalian Protein Extraction Reagent (Pierce, Rock ford, IL, United States).

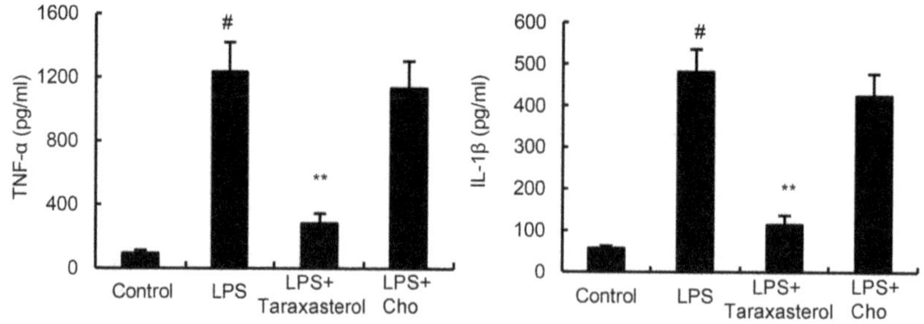

FIGURE 6 | Cholesterol replenishment prevents the anti-inflammatory effect of taraxasterol. The values presented are the means ± SEM of three independent experiments. $^{\#}p < 0.05$ vs. control group; $^{*}p < 0.05$, $^{**}p < 0.01$ vs. LPS group.

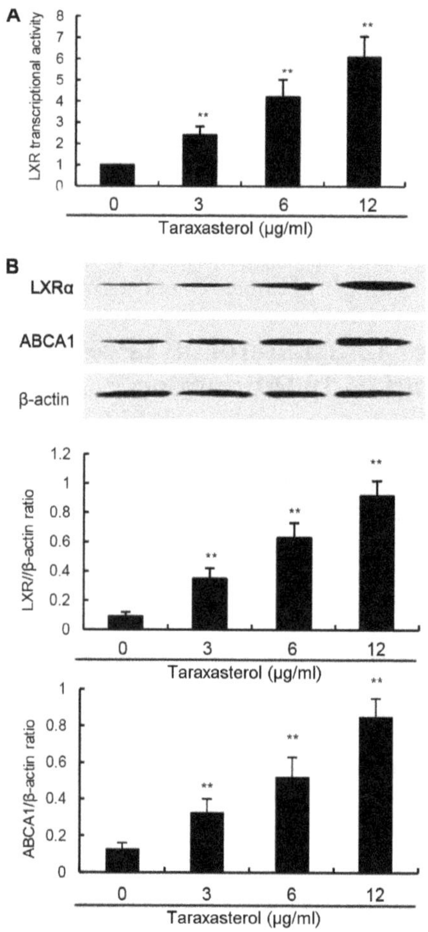

FIGURE 7 | (A) Effects of taraxasterol on LXR transcriptional activity. **(B)** Effects of taraxasterol on LXRα and ABCA1 expression. The values presented are the means ± SEM of three independent experiments. $^{\#}p < 0.05$ vs. control group; $^{*}p < 0.05$, $^{**}p < 0.01$ vs. LPS group.

Protein concentrations were determined by BCA method. Equal amount of protein (30 μg) were loaded and electrophoresed on a 12% SDS-PAGE and transferred onto PVDF membrane (Millipore, Cork, Ireland). The membrane was blocked with 5% fetal bovine serum. Then the membrane was probed with primary antibodies overnight at 4°C. Subsequently, the membranes were probed with HRP-conjugated secondary antibodies for 2 h at room temperature. The immunoreactive bands were visualized using an enhanced chemiluminescence system (Thermo Scientific, United States). Density value of the bands was quantified using Quantity One Software (Bio-Rad, United States) and the values obtained were used for statistical analysis.

LXRα siRNA Transfections

BV2 microglia cells were transfected with LXRα siRNA or control siRNA using FuGENE HD transfection reagent according to the manufacturer's instructions (Fu et al., 2014b). 36 h later, the cells were treated with taraxasterol and stimulated with LPS. 24 h later, the levels of TNF-α and IL-1β were detected by ELISA.

Statistical Analysis

All data were presented as means ± SEM of three independent experiments and analyzed using one-way ANOVA combined with Tukey's multiple comparison tests. $P < 0.05$ was taken as statistically significant.

RESULTS

Effects of Taraxasterol on Cell Viability

As shown in **Figure 1**, the results showed that LPS (0.5 μg/ml) did not affect the cell viability of BV2 microglia. Taraxasterol at the concentration up to 12 μg/ml had no cellular toxicity on BV2 microglia (**Figure 1**).

Effects of Taraxasterol on LPS-Induced TNF-α and IL-1β Production

As shown in **Figure 2**, treatment of BV2 microglia with LPS resulted in significant increases in cytokines TNF-α and IL-1β production. However, taraxasterol significantly inhibited LPS-induced TNF-α and IL-1β production.

Effects of Taraxasterol on LPS-Induced NF-κB Activation

The effects of taraxasterol on LPS-induced NF-κB activation were detected by Western blotting. As shown in **Figure 3**,

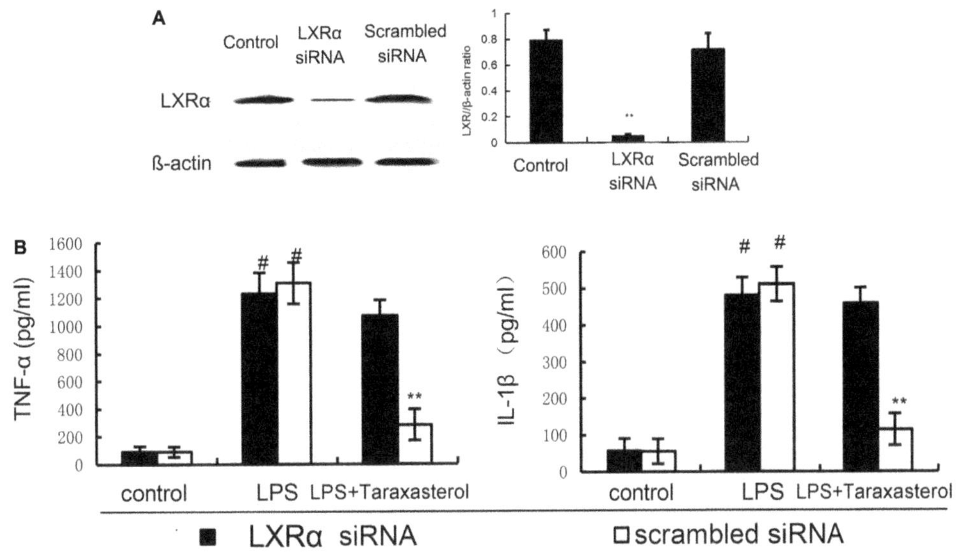

FIGURE 8 | (A) The effects of siRNA on LXRα expression. **(B)** Knockdown of LXRα abrogated the effects of taraxasterol on LPS induces inflammatory response in BV2 microglia cells. The data presented are the means ± SEM of three independent experiments. $^{\#}p < 0.05$ vs. control group; $^{*}p < 0.05$, $^{**}p < 0.01$ vs. LPS group.

LPS significantly up-regulated the expression of NF-κB. However, treatment of taraxasterol inhibited LPS-induced NF-κB activation in a dose-dependent manner.

Effects of Taraxasterol on LPS-Induced TLR4 Translocation Into Lipid Rafts

As shown in **Figure 4**, treatment of cells with LPS induced the translocation of TLR4 into lipid rafts. However, taraxasterol significantly suppressed LPS-induced TLR4 translocation into lipid rafts.

Taraxasterol Disrupts Lipid Rafts by Depleting Cholesterol

As shown in **Figure 5**, taraxasterol significantly decreased the level of cholesterol in lipid rafts which results in the disrupting of lipid rafts.

Cholesterol Replenishment Prevents the Anti-inflammatory Effects of Taraxasterol

Cholesterol replenishment experiments were carried out in this study to investigate the effects of cholesterol in the anti-inflammatory mechanism of taraxasterol. The results showed that when cholesterol were added, the anti-inflammatory effects of taraxasterol were reversed (**Figure 6**).

Effects of Taraxasterol on LXRα-ABCA1 Signaling Pathway

In this study, the effects of taraxasterol on LXRα-ABCA1 signaling pathway were detected in this study. As shown in **Figure 7A**, taraxasterol significantly up-regulated the transcriptional activity of LXRα. Furthermore, taraxasterol was found to up-regulate the expression of LXRα and ABCA1 in a dose-dependent manner (**Figure 7B**).

Taraxasterol Exerts Anti-inflammatory Activity Through Activating LXRα

To investigate whether activation of LXRα is responsible for the anti-inflammatory effect of taraxasterol, LXRα was knockdown by siRNA (**Figure 8A**). As shown in **Figure 8B**, the results showed that LXRα knockdown significantly reversed the inhibition of TNF-α and IL-1β production by taraxasterol.

DISCUSSION

Neurodegenerative diseases are accompanied by inflammation of the CNS (Amor et al., 2010). Studies showed that controlling of inflammation had the ability to treat neurodegenerative diseases (Gao et al., 2003; Carnevale et al., 2007). Taraxasterol, a pentacyclic-triterpene isolated from *T. officinale*, has been reported to have anti-inflammatory effects. In the present study, we investigated the effects of taraxasterol on LPS-induced inflammatory responses in BV2 microglia. The results showed that taraxasterol inhibited LPS-induced inflammatory cytokines production by activating LXRα-ABCA1 signaling pathway.

LPS, the main endotoxin produced by Gram-negative bacteria, has been identified as one of the most important factor that causes neurodegenerative diseases (Qin et al., 2007). Stimulating of microglia by LPS lead to the production of inflammatory cytokines such as TNF-α and IL-1ß (Brandenburg et al., 2010). These inflammatory cytokines initiate and amplify the inflammatory response and lead to development of neurodegenerative diseases (Lucas et al., 2006). Recent studies showed that inhibition of inflammatory cytokines production could attenuate the severity of neurodegenerative diseases (Arvin et al., 1996). In this study, our results showed that taraxasterol significantly inhibited LPS-induced inflammatory cytokines production. NF-κB is an important transcriptional factor that play a critical role in the regulation of TNF-α and IL-1ß production (Dong et al., 2010). Nowadays, NF-κB has been identified as the main target for the treatment of inflammatory diseases such as neurodegenerative diseases (Zipp and Aktas, 2006). In this study, our results showed that treatment of taraxasterol significantly inhibited LPS-induced NF-κB activation. These results suggested that taraxasterol inhibited LPS-induced inflammatory response by inhibiting NF-κB activation.

LPS stimulation induces TLR4 receptor dimerization and recruitment of TLR4 into lipid rafts, which subsequently induced the activation of NF-κB (Zhu et al., 2010). Lipid raft disruption leads to impairment in TLR4 signaling by preventing TLR4 translocation into lipid rafts (Fernandez-Lizarbe et al., 2008). To investigate the anti-inflammatory mechanism of taraxasterol, the effects of taraxasterol on LPS-induced recruitment of TLR4 into lipid rafts were detected by western blot analysis in this study. The results showed that taraxasterol significantly inhibited recruitment of TLR4 into lipid rafts. Furthermore, the effects of taraxasterol on cholesterol level in lipid rafts were detected in this study. Our results showed that taraxasterol disrupted the formation of lipid rafts by decreasing the level of cholesterol. These results suggested that taraxasterol disrupted the formation of lipid rafts by decreasing the level of cholesterol, thereby inhibited LPS-induced recruitment of TLR4 into lipid rafts and TLR4 signaling pathway.

The liver X receptors (LXRs) are members of the nuclear hormone receptor superfamily that are bound and activated by oxysterols (Lehmann et al., 1997). LXRα has previously been shown to regulate the metabolic conversion of cholesterol to bile acids (Peet et al., 1998). Activating of LXRα induces the expression of ABCA1, a lipid pump that effluxes cholesterol out of cells (Cavelier et al., 2006). Recent studies showed that many herbal compounds are the ligands of LXRα (Gong and Xie, 2004). In this study, our results showed that taraxasterol could activate LXRα and up-regulated the expression of LXRα and ABCA1, suggesting taraxasterol was a ligand of LXRα. To further confirm the anti-inflammatory mechanism of taraxasterol is through activating LXRα, LXRα was knockdown by siRNA. Our results showed that LXRα knockdown significantly reversed the inhibition of TNF-α and IL-1ß by taraxasterol. These results suggested that taraxasterol exerted anti-inflammatory effects via activating LXRα.

CONCLUSION

These results showed that taraxasterol inhibited LPS-induced inflammatory response By activating LXRα-ABCA1 signaling pathway, which subsequently disrupting lipid rafts and inhibiting TLR4 translocation into lipid rafts, thereby inhibiting LPS-induced inflammatory responses. Taraxasterol might be a valuable agent for the treatment of neurodegenerative diseases.

AUTHOR CONTRIBUTIONS

YF and FL designed the experiments. BL, JW, ZX, and YF did the experiments. BL and YF wrote the paper. YF and ZH revised the paper.

FUNDING

This study was supported by grants from the National Natural Science Foundation of China (No. 81320108025), China Postdoctoral Science Foundation funded project (2016M600233).

REFERENCES

Amor, S., Puentes, F., Baker, D., and van der Valk, P. (2010). Inflammation in neurodegenerative diseases. *Immunology* 129, 154–169. doi: 10.1111/j.1365-2567.2009.03225.x doi: 10.1111/j.1365-2567.2009.03225.x

Arvin, B., Neville, L. F., Barone, F. C., and Feuerstein, G. Z. (1996). The role of inflammation and cytokines in brain injury. *Neurosci. Biobehav. Rev.* 20, 445–452. doi: 10.1016/0149-7634(95)00026-7

Brandenburg, L. O., Kipp, M., Lucius, R., Pufe, T., and Wruck, C. J. (2010). Sulforaphane suppresses LPS-induced inflammation in primary rat microglia. *Inflamm. Res.* 59, 443–450. doi: 10.1007/s00011-009-0116-5

Cameron, B., and Landreth, G. E. (2010). Inflammation, microglia, and Alzheimer's disease. *Neurobiol. Dis.* 37, 503–509. doi: 10.1016/j.nbd.2009.10.006

Carnevale, D., De Simone, R., and Minghetti, L. (2007). Microglia-neuron interaction in inflammatory and degenerative diseases: role of cholinergic and noradrenergic systems. *CNS Neurol. Disord. Drug Targets* 6, 388–397. doi: 10.2174/187152707783399193

Cavelier, C., Lorenzi, I., Rohrer, L., and von Eckardstein, A. (2006). Lipid efflux by the ATP-binding cassette transporters ABCA1 and ABCG1. *Biochim. Biophys. Acta* 1761, 655–666. doi: 10.1016/j.bbalip.2006.04.012

Dong, X. R., Luo, M., Fan, L., Zhang, T., Liu, L., Dong, J. H., et al. (2010). Corilagin inhibits the double strand break-triggered NF-kappaB pathway in irradiated microglial cells. *Int. J. Mol. Med.* 25, 531–536.

Fernandez-Lizarbe, S., Pascual, M., Gascon, M. S., Blanco, A., and Guerri, C. (2008). Lipid rafts regulate ethanol-induced activation of TLR4 signaling in murine macrophages. *Mol. Immunol.* 45, 2007–2016. doi: 10.1016/j.molimm.2007.10.025

Fu, Y., Hu, X., Cao, Y., Zhang, Z., and Zhang, N. (2015). Saikosaponin a inhibits lipopolysaccharide-oxidative stress and inflammation in Human umbilical vein endothelial cells via preventing TLR4 translocation into lipid rafts. *Free Radic. Biol. Med.* 89, 777–785. doi: 10.1016/j.freeradbiomed.2015.10.407

Fu, Y., Wei, Z., Zhou, E., Zhang, N., and Yang, Z. (2014a). Cyanidin-3-O-β-glucoside inhibits lipopolysaccharide-induced inflammatory response in mouse mastitis model. *J. Lipid. Res.* 55, 1111–1119. doi: 10.1194/jlr.M047340

Fu, Y., Zhou, E., Wei, Z., Wang, W., Wang, T., Yang, Z., et al. (2014b). Cyanidin-3-O-beta-glucoside ameliorates lipopolysaccharide-induced acute lung injury by reducing TLR4 recruitment into lipid rafts. *Biochem. Pharmacol.* 90, 126–134. doi: 10.1016/j.bcp.2014.05.004

Gao, H. M., Liu, B., Zhang, W., and Hong, J. S. (2003). Novel anti-inflammatory therapy for Parkinson's disease. *Trends Pharmacol. Sci.* 24, 395–401. doi: 10.1016/S0165-6147(03)00176-7

Gong, H., and Xie, W. (2004). Orphan nuclear receptors, PXR and LXR: new ligands and therapeutic potential. *Expert Opin. Ther. Targets* 8, 49–54. doi: 10.1517/14728222.8.1.49

Jeong, J. W., Jin, C. Y., Kim, G. Y., Lee, J. D., Park, C., Kim, G. D., et al. (2010). Anti-inflammatory effects of cordycepin via suppression of inflammatory mediators in BV2 microglial cells. *Int. Immunopharmacol.* 10, 1580–1586. doi: 10.1016/j.intimp.2010.09.011

Kawai, T., and Akira, S. (2007). Signaling to NF-kappaB by Toll-like receptors. *Trends Mol. Med.* 13, 460–469. doi: 10.1016/j.molmed.2007.09.002

Lehmann, J. M., Kliewer, S. A., Moore, L. B., Smith-Oliver, T. A., Oliver, B. B., Su, J. L., et al. (1997). Activation of the nuclear receptor LXR by oxysterols defines a new hormone response pathway. *J. Biol. Chem.* 272, 3137–3140. doi: 10.1074/jbc.272.6.3137

Liu, J., Xiong, H., Cheng, Y., Cui, C., Zhang, X., Xu, L., et al. (2013). Effects of taraxasterol on ovalbumin-induced allergic asthma in mice. *J. Ethnopharmacol.* 148, 787–793. doi: 10.1016/j.jep.2013.05.006

Lucas, S. M., Rothwell, N. J., and Gibson, R. M. (2006). The role of inflammation in CNS injury and disease. *Br. J. Pharmacol.* 147(Suppl. 1), S232–S240. doi: 10.1038/sj.bjp.0706400

Peet, D. J., Turley, S. D., Ma, W., Janowski, B. A., Lobaccaro, J. M., Hammer, R. E., et al. (1998). Cholesterol and bile acid metabolism are impaired in mice lacking the nuclear oxysterol receptor LXR alpha. *Cell* 93, 693–704. doi: 10.1016/S0092-8674(00)81432-4

Piao, T., Ma, Z., Li, X., and Liu, J. (2015). Taraxasterol inhibits IL-1β-induced inflammatory response in human osteoarthritic chondrocytes. *Eur. J. Pharmacol.* 756, 38–42. doi: 10.1016/j.ejphar.2015.03.012

Qin, L., Li, G., Qian, X., Liu, Y., Wu, X., Liu, B., et al. (2005). Interactive role of the toll-like receptor 4 and reactive oxygen species in LPS-induced microglia activation. *Glia* 52, 78–84. doi: 10.1002/glia.20225

Qin, L., Wu, X., Block, M. L., Liu, Y., Breese, G. R., Hong, J. S., et al. (2007). Systemic LPS causes chronic neuroinflammation and progressive neurodegeneration. *Glia* 55, 453–462. doi: 10.1002/glia.20467

San, Z., Fu, Y., Li, W., Zhou, E., Li, Y., Song, X., et al. (2014). Protective effect of taraxasterol on acute lung injury induced by lipopolysaccharide in mice. *Int. Immunopharmacol.* 19, 342–350. doi: 10.1016/j.intimp.2014.01.031

Sun, G. Y., Shelat, P. B., Jensen, M. B., He, Y., Sun, A. Y., and Simonyi, A. (2010). Phospholipases A2 and inflammatory responses in the central nervous system. *Neuromolecular Med.* 12, 133–148. doi: 10.1007/s12017-009-8092-z

Wang, H. Y., Wang, H., Wang, J. H., Wang, Q., Ma, Q. F., and Chen, Y. Y. (2015). Protocatechuic acid inhibits inflammatory responses in LPS-stimulated BV2 microglia via NF-kappaB and MAPKs signaling pathways. *Neurochem. Res.* 40, 1655–1660. doi: 10.1007/s11064-015-1646-6

Xiong, H., Cheng, Y., Zhang, X., and Zhang, X. (2014). Effects of taraxasterol on iNOS and COX-2 expression in LPS-induced RAW 264.7 macrophages. *J. Ethnopharmacol.* 155, 753–757. doi: 10.1016/j.jep.2014.06.023

Yu, Z., Tang, L., Chen, L., Li, J., Wu, W., and Hu, C. (2015). Capillarisin suppresses lipopolysaccharide-induced inflammatory mediators in BV2 microglial cells by suppressing TLR4-mediated NF-kappaB and MAPKs signaling pathway. *Neurochem. Res.* 40, 1095–1101. doi: 10.1007/s11064-015-1567-4

Zhang, X., Xiong, H., Li, H., and Cheng, Y. (2014). Protective effect of taraxasterol against LPS-induced endotoxic shock by modulating inflammatory responses in mice. *Immunopharmacol. Immunotoxicol.* 36, 11–16. doi: 10.3109/08923973.2013.861482

Zhu, X., Owen, J. S., Wilson, M. D., Li, H., Griffiths, G. L., Thomas, M. J., et al. (2010). Macrophage ABCA1 reduces MyD88-dependent Toll-like receptor trafficking to lipid rafts by reduction of lipid raft cholesterol. *J. Lipid Res.* 51, 3196–3206. doi: 10.1194/jlr.M006486

Ziebell, J. M., and Morganti-Kossmann, M. C. (2010). Involvement of pro- and anti-inflammatory cytokines and chemokines in the pathophysiology of traumatic brain injury. *Neurotherapeutics* 7, 22–30. doi: 10.1016/j.nurt.2009.10.016

Zipp, F., and Aktas, O. (2006). The brain as a target of inflammation: common pathways link inflammatory and neurodegenerative diseases. *Trends Neurosci.* 29, 518–527. doi: 10.1016/j.tins.2006.07.006

12

Amelioration of Cognitive Deficit by Embelin in a Scopolamine-Induced Alzheimer's Disease-Like Condition in a Rat Model

Saatheeyavaane Bhuvanendran, Yatinesh Kumari*, Iekhsan Othman and Mohd Farooq Shaikh*

Neuropharmacology Research Laboratory, Jeffrey Cheah School of Medicine and Health Sciences, Monash University Malaysia, Bandar Sunway, Malaysia

***Correspondence:**
Yatinesh Kumari
yatinesh.kumari@monash.edu
Mohd Farooq Shaikh
farooq.shaikh@monash.edu;
shaikhmohdfarooq@gmail.com

Embelin (2,5-dihydroxy-3-undecyl-1,4-benzoquinone) is one of the active components (2.3%) found in *Embelia ribes* Burm fruits. As determined via *in vitro* AChE inhibition assay, embelin can inhibit the acetylcholinesterase enzyme. Therefore, embelin can be utilized as a therapeutic compound, after further screening has been conducted for its use in the treatment of Alzheimer's disease (AD). In this study, the nootropic and anti-amnesic effects of embelin on scopolamine-induced amnesia in rats were evaluated. Rats were treated once daily with embelin (0.3 mg/kg, 0.6 mg/kg, 1.2 mg/kg) and donepezil (1 mg/kg) intraperitoneally (i.p.) for 17 days. During the final 9 days of treatment, a daily injection of scopolamine (1 mg/kg) was administered to induce cognitive deficits. Besides that, behavioral analysis was carried out to assess the rats' learning and memory functions. Meanwhile, hippocampal tissues were extracted for gene expression, neurotransmitter, and immunocytochemistry studies. Embelin was found to significantly improve the recognition index and memory retention in the novel object recognition (NOR) and elevated plus maze (EPM) tests, respectively. Furthermore, embelin at certain doses (0.3 mg/kg, 0.6 mg/kg, and 1.2 mg/kg) significantly exhibited a memory-enhancing effect in the absence of scopolamine, besides improving the recognition index when challenged with chronic scopolamine treatment. Moreover, in the EPM test, embelin treated rats (0.6 mg/kg) showed an increase in inflection ratio in nootropic activity. However, the increase was not significant in chronic scopolamine model. In addition, embelin contributed toward the elevated expression of BDNF, CREB1, and scavengers enzymes (SOD1 and CAT) mRNA levels. Next, pretreatment of rats with embelin mitigated scopolamine-induced neurochemical and histological changes in a manner comparable to donepezil. These research findings suggest that embelin is a nootropic compound, which also possesses an anti-amnesic ability that is displayed against scopolamine-induced memory impairment in rats. Hence, embelin could be a promising compound to treat AD.

Keywords: embelin, Alzheimer's disease, cognition, neuroprotective, anti-amnesic effect

INTRODUCTION

Alzheimer's disease (AD) is known as the leading cause of dementia amongst people aged 65 and older (Ghumatkar et al., 2015). This age-related disease affects millions of individuals, and it is estimated that by 2050, 1 in 85 people worldwide will be suffering from AD (Brookmeyer et al., 2007). According to Tanzi and Bertram (2005), AD is a progressive and chronic neurodegenerative disorder which displays global cognitive decline involving memory, orientation, judgment, and reasoning. The key features of AD's pathogenesis are the gradual amassing of the protein fragment beta-amyloid (plaques) and twisted fibers of the protein tau (tangles), outside and inside neurons in the brain, respectively (Alzheimer's Association, 2017). Beta-amyloid plaques function as a neurotoxin by intervening in neuron-to-neuron communication at synapses. On the other hand, tau tangles prevent the passage of essential molecules and nutrients inside neurons, which causes axonal transport dysfunction and neuronal loss (Ali et al., 2015; Alzheimer's Association, 2017).

Apart from that, memory impairment is associated with cholinergic system dysfunction, which involves cholinergic neurons, neurotransmitters, and their receptors (Bartus et al., 1982; Lee et al., 2015). Cholinergic system dysfunction results from a loss of cholinergic neurons in the basal forebrain and hippocampus, which diminishes cognitive capability (Bartus et al., 1982; Lee et al., 2015). In healthy individuals, activation of the central cholinergic system enhances hippocampal neurogenesis through the cAMP response element-binding protein/brain-derived neurotrophic factor (CREB/BDNF) pathway (Lee et al., 2015). At present, one of the treatments for AD is a dispensation of acetylcholinesterase (AChE) inhibitors like tacrine or donepezil that increase the availability of acetylcholine at cholinergic synapses (Pandareesh et al., 2016). Moreover, oxidative stress plays an important role in AD, with some studies suggesting that beta-amyloid toxicity is linked to an increment in reactive oxygen species (ROS), including H_2O_2 (Butterfield and Lauderback, 2002), and lipid peroxidation in neuronal cultures (Yatin et al., 1999). High oxidative stress can cause memory deficits via impairment of hippocampal synaptic plasticity (Serrano and Klann, 2004) and oxidative damage in neurodegenerative diseases (Ding et al., 2007).

Current pharmacological options for AD, only have a partial effect and poor control over the disease-causing neurons linked with Alzheimer's symptoms and lethal complications (Alzheimer's Association, 2017). As such, the available drugs in the market mainly focus on the improving memory by inhibiting the AChE enzyme (Ghumatkar et al., 2015). However, AD is not a result of a single factor like AChE, but rather is a multifactorial condition and this needs to be considered when designing a drug. Other factors such as oxidative stress and synaptic dysfunction play a significant role in the cognitive deficits in AD. Natural products could be a source of neuroprotective drugs as they can maintain normal cellular interaction in the brain and reduce the loss of neuronal functions in pathological circumstances (Hritcu et al., 2014). Presently, many AD research groups have already explored the potential of using natural products as neuroprotective agents.

One such potential natural product is embelin (2,5-dihydroxy-3-undecyl-1,4-benzoquinone), which is the main active constituent in the fruits of *Embelia ribes* Burm (Family: Myrsinaceae), commonly known as "False Black Pepper" (Kundap et al., 2017a). The bright orange fruits of *E. ribes* have been utilized in traditional medicinal practice for treating central nervous system (CNS) disorders such as mental disorders and as a brain tonic (Poojari, 2014). Moreover, embelin has displayed anti-inflammatory, antioxidant, analgesic, antifertility, antitumor, wound healing, hepatoprotective, and antibacterial activities (Mahendran et al., 2011). Additionally, it has been reported that embelin is neuroprotective and possesses anticonvulsant ability when tested using animal models (Mahendran et al., 2011).

Embelin possesses all the features of a compound that can traverse the blood-brain barrier (BBB) and prompt a reaction in the CNS (Pathan et al., 2009; Kundap et al., 2017a). Even though embelin has various uses, there have been no studies of its neuropharmacological activities against AD-like conditions. Thus, in the present study, the anti-amnesic potential of embelin on memory deficits in a rat model of cognitive impairment caused by scopolamine was examined.

MATERIALS AND METHODS

Animal Care

In-house bred Sprague Dawley rats weighing between 180–200 g and between 6–8 weeks old were housed in the animal facility of the Jeffrey Cheah School of Medicine and Health Sciences, Monash University Malaysia. The rats were kept in cages and maintained under standard husbandry conditions (12:12 h light/dark cycle, controlled room temperature (23 ± 2°C), stress-free, *ad libitum* water, standard diets, and sanitary conditions). Before commencing the experiment, the rats were allowed to acclimatize for a period of 1 week to reduce stress. The Monash Animal Research Platform (MARP) Animal Ethics Committee in Australia approved all the animal experimentations conducted in this study.

Experimental Design

Drug Treatment

Embelin (98%) batch number (Yucca/EM/2015/01/01) was purchased from Yucca Enterprises, Mumbai, India. The range of doses for embelin was determined based on pre-screening results. Embelin was solubilized in DMSO and then dissolved in saline. Donepezil and scopolamine were prepared in saline. Normal control rats were administered saline throughout the experiment. The treatments were given intraperitoneally (i.p) at a volume corresponding to 0.1 ml/100 g of body weight.

All experiments were performed in a balanced design (9 animals/group) to avoid being influenced by order and time. The behavioral studies were divided into two categories namely the nootropic and scopolamine models.

Nootropic Model

(i) **Group 1**: Control (Saline) ($n = 9$);
(ii) **Group 2**: Positive control (donepezil (DPZ) 1 mg/kg);
(iii) **Group 3**: Low dose of embelin (EMB) 0.3 mg/kg;
(iv) **Group 4**: Medium dose of EMB 0.6 mg/kg;
(v) **Group 5**: High dose of EMB 1.2 mg/kg

For nootropic activity, all the groups received pretreatment via the intraperitoneal route, for 8 days. All these rats were subjected to a battery of behavioral tests from day six onward until day eight for NOR and EPM (**Figure 1**).

Scopolamine Model

(i) **Group 1**: Control (Saline) ($n = 9$);
(ii) **Group 2**: Negative control [scopolamine (SCP) 1 mg/kg] ($n = 9$);
(iii) **Group 3**: Positive control [donepezil (DPZ) 1 mg/kg] + (SCP 1 mg/kg) ($n = 9$);
(iv) **Group 4**: Low dose of embelin (EMB) 0.3 mg/kg + (SCP 1 mg/kg) ($n = 9$);
(v) **Group 5**: Medium dose of EMB 0.6 mg/kg + (SCP 1 mg/kg) ($n = 9$);
(vi) **Group 6**: High dose of EMB 1.2 mg/kg + (SCP 1 mg/kg) ($n = 9$)

For scopolamine, amnesia was induced in all the groups except the control group by daily intraperitoneal injections of scopolamine (1 mg/kg) for 9 days after embelin pre-treatment (day nine to day 17). Half an hour after scopolamine administration, NOR was conducted on day 15, and EPM was carried out on day 16 and 17 of the study. At the end of the experiment, the rats were sacrificed, and their brains were isolated for further biochemical and immunohistochemistry analysis.

Novel Object Recognition (NOR)

For the object recognition task, an open field box (40 × 40 × 20 cm) composed of black acrylic material was utilized as the experimental apparatus. This method is similar to that used by Ennaceur and Delacour (1988), with minor modifications. Besides that, behavioral testing was carried out between 9:00 am and 6:00 pm under red light illumination. The scrutinized objects were two similar transparent culture flasks containing water and a Lego toy of similar height as that of the flask (new object). Both objects types presented during the test session varied in texture, color, and size. This assessment has three phases: (i) habituation; (ii) training, and (iii) test. On the first day, each rat was allowed to become familiarized with the open field box without the presence of an object for about 10 min. On the second day, each rat was placed in the open field for 5 min and allowed to freely explore the two identical objects (transparent cultured flask with water). After an interval of 90 min post-training session, one of the old objects used was substituted with a new object and the rats were subjected to a 2 min test run. The time spent with each object was recorded and evaluated using SMART software version 3.0. The open field box was cleaned with 70% ethanol between runs to minimize scent trails. The recognition index was calculated using the formula [TB/(TA + TB)*100] where TA and TB are time spent exploring familiar object A and novel object B respectively (Batool et al., 2016). Exploration of an object was noted when a rat sniffed or touched the object with its nose and/or forepaws.

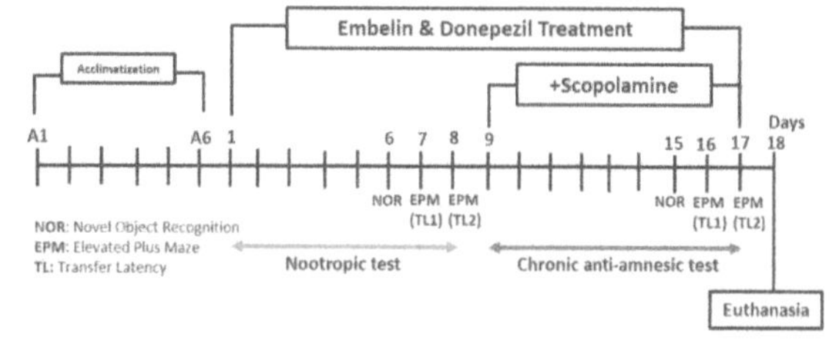

FIGURE 1 | Schematic representation of the experimental procedure.

Elevated Plus Maze (EPM)

The EPM device was comprised of four arms sharing the same dimensions, i.e., two open arms (50 × 10 cm) that crossed over two closed arms with 40 cm high walls. These arms were connected using a central square (10 × 10 cm), thus giving the apparatus plus sign look. Furthermore, the EPM was elevated 50 cm above floor level. This technique is almost similar to one reported by Halder et al. (2011). The behavioral testing was conducted between 9:00 am and 6:00 pm under dim red light illumination. Assessment of memory via EPM was done in two sessions. During the training phase, each rat was placed at the end of an open arm and by using a stopwatch, transfer latency time (s), which is the time each rat took to enter (with all four paws) into either closed arm, was noted. The maze was cleaned with 70% ethanol between runs to minimize scent trails. To evaluate memory retention, a test phase was conducted 24 h (retention) after a training session. The cut-off time for each rat to explore the maze in both the phases (training and test) was 90 s. A drop in transfer latency time during test sessions was taken as an index of memory improvement.

Tissue Processing

All the rats were sacrificed under ketamine and xylazine anesthesia 1 h after completing the behavioral test. In each group, five rat brains were fixed in 4% paraformaldehyde, and hippocampi of remaining four rats were used for real-time PCR and neurotransmitter analysis. One part of the hippocampus was used for isolation of RNA and another part of the hippocampus was homogenized on ice using methanol containing formic acid.

Total RNA Extraction and Real-Time PCR

Total RNA was extracted from the rat brain's hippocampal region and was similar to the method used by Kundap et al. (2017b), with some minor modifications. One part of the hippocampus tissue was momentarily homogenized in Trizole solution. The mixture was extracted using chloroform and centrifuged at 13,500 rpm at 4°C. Then, the aqueous phase was precipitated with isopropanol and followed by centrifugation at 13,500 rpm at 4°C. The volume of isopropanol added was same as the volume of the supernatant from the aqueous phase. After that, the alcohol was removed. The pellet on the other hand, was rinsed twice with 70% ethanol and resuspended in 20 µL of RNase free water. RNA concentration was ascertained via absorbance at 260 nm using a Nanodrop machine. The total RNA (500 ng) was then reverse transcribed to synthesize cDNA using a QuantiTect® Reverse Transcription Kit, according to the manufacturer's protocol. Next, the mRNA expression of genes encoding cAMP response element-binding protein (CREB1), brain-derived neurotrophic factor (BDNF), superoxide dismutase 1 (SOD1), catalase (CAT), and IMPDH2 in the hippocampus, was measured by real-time PCR using the StepOne Real-Time PCR system. Subsequently, cDNA from the reverse transcription reaction was subjected to real-time PCR using a QuantiNova™ SYBR® Green PCR kit according to manufacturer's protocol. A comparative threshold (C_T) cycle method was applied to normalize cDNA content of samples, which involves of normalization of a number of target gene copies against the endogenous reference gene, IMPDH2.

Neurotransmitter Analysis Using Liquid Chromatography-Tandem Mass Spectrometry (LC-MS/MS)

The brain levels of neurotransmitters like dopamine (DA), glutamate (Glu), norepinephrine (NE), and acetylcholine (ACh) were estimated using LC-MS/MS in a similar manner to that used by Kundap et al. (2017b), with some modifications. For all these standard neurotransmitters, stock solutions of 1 mg/ml were prepared in methanol (0.1% formic acid) and then stored at 4°C until use. Four calibration standards with the concentration ranges of 0.25–200.00, 250.00–20,000.00, 0.50–200.00, and 0.25–200.00 ng/mL were used for validation of DA, Glu, NE, and ACh respectively. In brief, hippocampal tissue was homogenized in ice-cold methanol containing formic acid. Then, the homogenate was vortex-mixed followed by centrifugation at 14,000 rpm for 10 min at 4°C. Finally, the supernatant was subjected to LC-MS/MS analysis, which was run on an Agilent 1290 Infinity UHPLC, coupled with an auto-sampler system comprising of Agilent 6410 Triple Quad LC/MS, ZORBAXEclipse plus C18 RRHD 2.1 × 150.0 mm and 1.8-micron (P/N959759-902) column (Agilent Technologies, Santa Clara, CA, United States). The mobile phase consisted of 0.1% formic acid in (i) water (Solvent A) and (ii) acetonitrile (Solvent B). It was used with a gradient elution: (i) 0–3 min, 50% B; (ii) 3–6 min, 95% B; (iii) 6–7 min, 95% B at a flow rate of 0.1 mL/min.

Immunohistochemical Stain Analysis

Immunohistochemical stain analysis was conducted via assessment of neurogenesis using Doublecortin (DCX) and lipid peroxidation with 4-hydroxy-2-nonenal (4HNE) staining in the hippocampus. Five brain samples from each group were immersed in 4% paraformaldehyde overnight. The samples were methodically cryoprotected in 10, 20, and 30% sucrose for 24 h. Next, the brains were embedded in 15% polyvinylpyrrolidone (PVP), frozen using dry ice, and cut into 40 µm frozen coronal sections using a Leica CM3050 cryostat. All sections were then stored in an anti-freeze buffer. Endogenous quenching using 1% H_2O_2 in methanol for 30 min was performed on the free-floating sections. After washing with phosphate buffered saline (PBS), the tissues were treated with blocking buffer (1.0% bovine serum albumin in PBS and 0.3% Triton X-100) for 1 h, followed by incubation with primary DCX (1:500, Abcam) and 4HNE (1:250, Abcam) antibodies overnight at 4°C. The tissues were then incubated with a biotinylated goat anti-rabbit secondary antibody (Abcam) for 2 h after being washed with PBS. Subsequently, the tissues were exposed for 2 h to an avidin-biotin-peroxidase complex (Vectastain ABC kit, Vector). Peroxidase activity was visualized using a stable diaminobenzidine solution (DAB, Sigma). All immunoreactions were monitored via a microscope (BX41, Olympus) and using the DigiAcquis 2.0 software, results were calculated.

Statistical Analysis

All findings were expressed as mean ± standard error of the mean (SEM). These data were analyzed using one-way analysis of variance (ANOVA) followed by Dunnett's tests. The *P*-values of $^{*}P < 0.05$, $^{**}P < 0.01$, and $^{***}P < 0.001$ were considered as statistically significant. All the experimental groups were compared with the SCP 1 mg/kg group.

RESULTS

Nootropic effect of Embelin

Findings obtained from the NOR test for embelin nootropic activity are illustrated in **Figure 2A**. The effect of different embelin doses on memory function were assessed following 7 days of pretreatment. The results were expressed as recognition index (%) for the novel object. Based on the outcomes, the pretreated groups of embelin showed an increase in recognition index for novel object compared with the control group and donepezil groups. Only 0.6 mg/kg of embelin showed statistically significant results with p value of <0.05. In EPM, the inflection ratio was significantly increased in 0.6 mg/kg embelin treated groups when compared with the control (**Figure 2B**). There was no significant difference in other treated groups.

Anti-amnesic Effect of Embelin in Rats With Scopolamine-Induced Amnesia

The NOR test showed a reduction in recognition index percentage for the negative group (SCP 1 mg/kg) in the chronic scopolamine model (**Figure 3A**). Moreover, the recognition index percentage for all the embelin treated groups were high and comparable with donepezil (1 mg/kg) group. A significant difference in the recognition index percentage was observed between all embelin treated and the negative group ($P < 0.05$). In EPM, inflection ratio analysis showed that there was an increase in retention memory in all embelin treated groups compared with the negative control group; however, it was statistically not significant (**Figure 3B**).

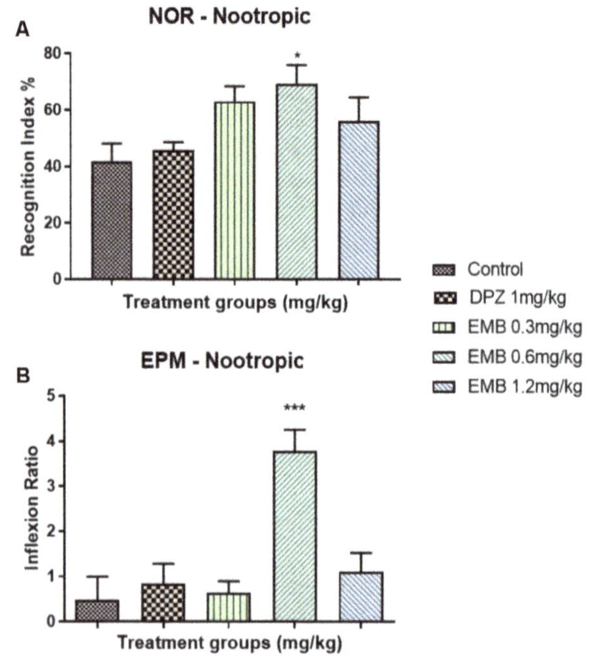

FIGURE 2 | Behavioral analysis for novel object recognition (NOR) and elevated plus maze (EPM). **(A)** represent the graph plot for the recognition indices in NOR for the nootropic model **(B)** represents the graph plot for the inflection ratios in EPM for the nootropic model. The behavioral analysis for **(A,B)** were compared to control group. Data are expressed as Mean ± SEM, $n = 9$ and statistical analysis by one-way ANOVA followed by Dunnett test *$P < 0.05$, **$P < 0.01$, and ***$P < 0.001$.

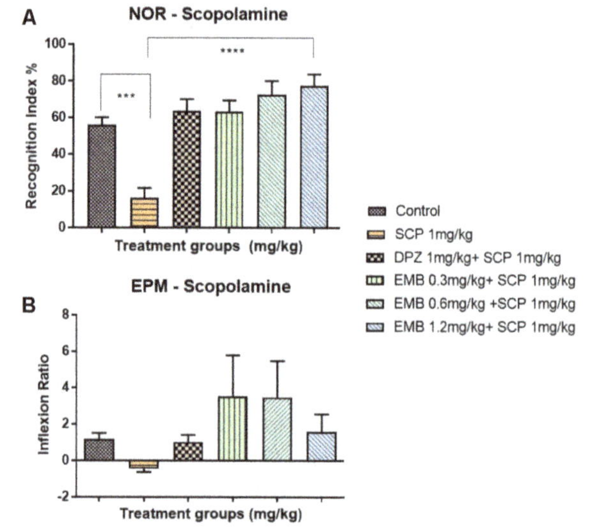

FIGURE 3 | Behavioral analysis for NOR and EPM. **(A)** represents the graph plot for the recognition indices in NOR for the scopolamine model **(B)** represents the graph plot for inflection ratios in EPM for the scopolamine model. The behavioral analysis for **(A,B)** were compared to negative control (SCP 1mg/kg). Data are expressed as Mean ± SEM, $n = 9$ and statistical analysis by one-way ANOVA followed by Dunnett test *$P < 0.05$, **$P < 0.01$, ***$P < 0.001$, and ****$P < 0.0001$.

Changes in mRNA Levels in the Hippocampus

BDNF mRNA levels were significantly down-regulated, approximately twofold in the hippocampus of the scopolamine group, compared with the positive control, $P < 0.01$. This down-regulation was ameliorated by embelin, in a dose-dependent manner, in comparison with the negative control, and a significant difference was revealed for the 1.2 mg/kg dose of embelin (**Figure 4A**). In addition, multiple exposures to scopolamine significantly down-regulated (twofold) the mRNA expression level of CREB1 in the negative control, compared with the positive control ($P < 0.001$). Embelin treatment increased CREB1 expression level in a dose-dependent manner, compared with the negative control, and it was significant for the 1.2 mg/kg embelin dose (**Figure 4B**). Furthermore, scopolamine depleted antioxidant mRNA in hippocampal tissues, including (CAT) (**Figure 4C**) and SOD1 gene expression (**Figure 4D**). The down-regulation of CAT mRNA was significantly ameliorated through embelin treatment compared to the negative control for the 1.2 mg/kg embelin group ($P < 0.05$). In SOD1, these changes were reversed by embelin pretreatment for all embelin treated groups, and the result was significant in the 0.6 mg/kg embelin group, with approximately a 1.5-fold change in comparison with the scopolamine treated group.

Estimation of Neurotransmitters by LC-MS/MS

Administration of scopolamine significantly altered the levels of ACh, DA, NE, and Glu in the rat brain's hippocampus. Specifically, the level of ACh ($P < 0.05$) decreased substantially whereas other neurotransmitters' levels increased significantly ($P < 0.05$ for DA and Glu; $P < 0.01$ for NE). Nevertheless, embelin treatment significantly normalized the level of all these neurotransmitters, and it was in a dose-dependent manner for ACh and DA (**Figures 5A–D**) (*$P < 0.05$, **$P < 0.01$, and ***$P < 0.001$).

Neurogenesis and Lipid Peroxidation in the Hippocampus

Scopolamine significantly inhibited adult neurogenesis via a reduction in the distribution of dendrites and neuron bodies in the dentate gyrus (DG) region, as shown by DCX staining in the subgranular zone (SGZ) (**Figure 6A**). Pretreatment with embelin totally ameliorated adult neurogenesis by enhancing immature neurons in the SGZ in a dose-dependent approach in comparison with the negative control ($P < 0.05$ for 0.3 mg/kg, $P < 0.01$ for 0.6 mg/kg and $P < 0.001$ for 1.2 mg/kg; **Figure 6B**). On the other hand, scopolamine injection significantly induced lipid peroxidation in the hippocampus, as represented by a deep brown color in the cornu ammonis 3 (CA3) regions through 4HNE staining. Pretreatment with embelin significantly lowered 4HNE-positive staining in the CA3 (threefold change) compared with the negative group ($P < 0.0001$ for all embelin groups; **Figures 7A,B**). Besides that, donepezil ameliorated these

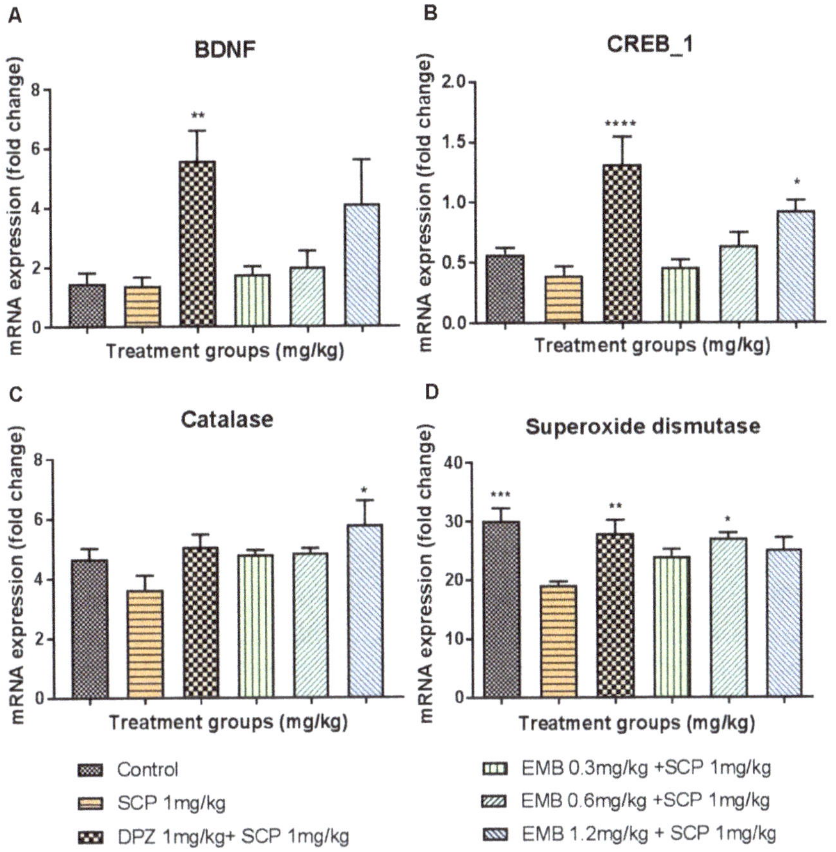

FIGURE 4 | Gene expression in the rat hippocampi determined by real time-PCR. The genes included are **(A)** BDNF, **(B)** CREB1, **(C)** Catalase, and **(D)** Superoxide Dismutase. All changes in the expressions levels were compared to the negative control group (SCP 1 mg/kg). Data are expressed as Mean ± SEM, $n = 4$ and statistical analysis by one-way ANOVA followed by Dunnett test $^{*}P < 0.05$, $^{**}P < 0.01$, $^{***}P < 0.001$, and $^{****}P < 0.0001$.

alterations triggered by scopolamine, as displayed through both DCX and 4-HNE staining.

DISCUSSION

This work aims to determine whether embelin has an anti-amnesic effect by modulating the cholinergic pathway. An animal model of hippocampal memory damage due to intraperitoneal injection of scopolamine was adopted to verify this hypothesis. The experiments comprised of two parts: Experiment 1 (pretreatment with embelin without scopolamine injection during training) to test embelin's nootropic effects on learning and memory process, and Experiment 2 (multiple exposures of scopolamine injection) to assess the effect of embelin on anti-amnesic activities and biochemical aspects during learning and memory process.

At the beginning of this experiment, we conducted a dose deciding study to find the therapeutic dose of embelin. A prior literature search determined that the range of embelin dose was between 2.5 mg/kg to 10 mg/kg for the intraperitoneal route in CNS related animal models (Mahendran et al., 2011; Afzal et al., 2012). However, our preliminary study using these range of embelin doses resulted in a neurobehavioral effect on coordination and motor activity whereby the treated rats were immobile and kept falling from the behavioral apparatus. Thus, we decided 1.2 mg/kg as the highest dose as the LD_{50} value for embelin was 44 mg/kg for intraperitoneal administration reported by Poojari (2014). Furthermore, we decided 0.3 mg/kg and 0.6 mg/kg would be the low dose and medium dose respectively, and all these 3 doses were effective therapeutic doses for our study as we noticed no side effects.

In this experiment, NOR and EPM were applied as behavioral models to evaluate learning and memory. The NOR test is particularly relevant in AD research as it allows the assessment of visual recognition memory, which is affected early in AD progression, involving brain regions similar to those affected by this devastating and debilitating neurodegenerative disease (Grayson et al., 2015). On the other hand, EPM is a behavioral test employed to study long-term spatial memory (Uddin et al., 2016b). Certain EPM parameters like retention transfer latency are utilized for the evaluation of memory. A decrease in transfer latency on the second day, which is after 24 h, indicates an improvement of memory and vice-versa (Dhingra and Kumar, 2012). The findings of this study showed that embelin at 0.6 mg/kg displayed nootropic activity in both the recognition

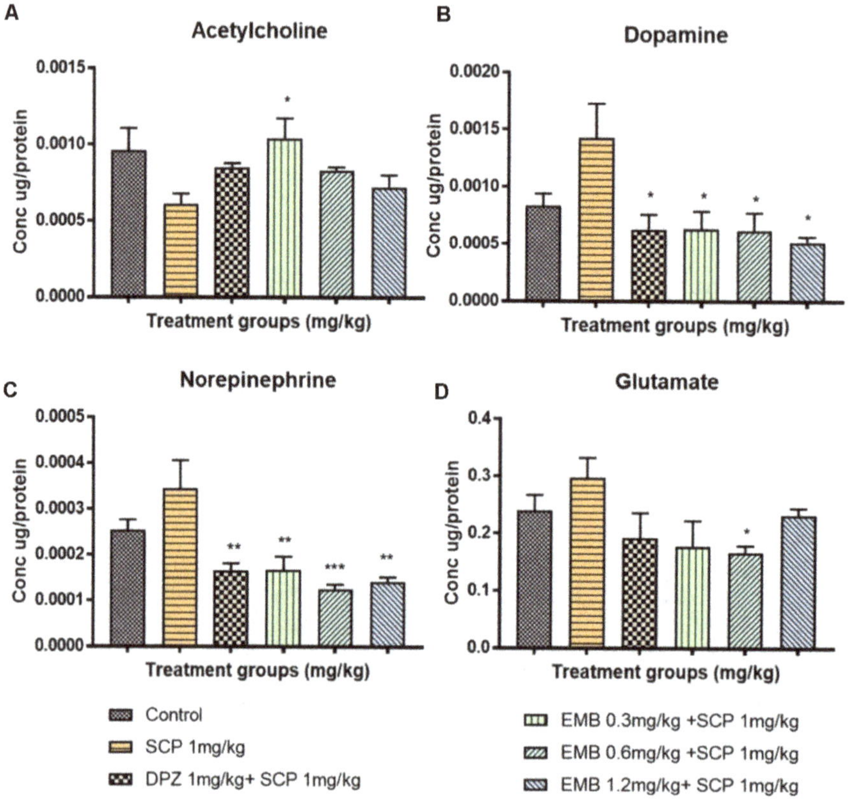

FIGURE 5 | The concentration of neurotransmitters in the rat hippocampi after chronic scopolamine. The figure represents the rat hippocampal neurotransmitter levels of **(A)** Acetylcholine, **(B)** Dopamine, **(C)** Norepinephrine, and **(D)** Glutamate. All changes in the neurotransmitter levels were compared to the negative control group (SCP 1 mg/kg). Data are expressed as Mean ± SEM, $n = 4$ and statistical analysis by one-way ANOVA followed by Dunnett test *$P < 0.05$, **$P < 0.01$, and ***$P < 0.001$.

index and inflection ratio in the NOR and EPM tests, respectively (**Figures 2A,B**). However, the nootropic activity of embelin in both behavioral paradigms was found to be dose independent. This could be explained that at a higher dose, the drug reaches its maximum effect so increasing the drug dosage does not increase its effectiveness, but on the contrary, effectiveness decreases. This theory is supported by the fact that CNS drugs such as antipsychotic drugs produce maximum dopaminergic blockage at high doses. However, further dose increments will not produce any dopamine blockage but eventually lead to other side effects such as anticholinergic activity (Bridges, 1981). It is possible that in this experiment, the 1.2 mg/kg embelin group has reached its maximum effect and therefore cognitive ability has declined. Based on the behavioral results obtained, it can be suggested that embelin is a nootropic drug that acts as a natural cognitive enhancer. These findings show that supplementation of embelin significantly amplified the rats' memory function and 0.6 mg/kg of embelin demonstrated significant nootropics effects. Nootropic drugs are used to treat cognition deficits in patients with AD, schizophrenia, stroke, attention deficit hyperactivity disorder (ADHD), and vascular dementia (VaD) (Birks and Grimley Evans, 2009; Froestl et al., 2012).

Scopolamine-induced dementia has been used extensively to assess potential therapeutic agents for treating AD (Kwon et al., 2009). Scopolamine is a nonselective muscarinic cholinergic receptor antagonist associated with cholinergic dysfunction, which causes performance deficits in learning and memory (Heo et al., 2014). Therefore, in this study, scopolamine was administered to rodents for 1 week to induce cholinergic neurodegeneration along with cognitive deficits. Following 6 days of scopolamine administration, the scopolamine treated group had less than 20% of the recognition index of other groups. Pretreatment with embelin ameliorated memory impairment caused by scopolamine (**Figure 3A**), with the recognition index being twofold more, in comparison with scopolamine treated group in a dose-dependent manner. These results exposed that embelin was as effective as the donepezil-treated group. Moreover, the findings showed that embelin treatment attenuated amnesic behavior in EPM, but it was insignificant (**Figure 3B**). Hence, these outcomes suggest that embelin had an anti-amnesic effect in the scopolamine model.

The brain is susceptible to oxidative stress because it consumes huge amounts of oxygen, has an abundant lipid content, and a low antioxidant level compared than other organs (Serrano and Klann, 2004). Furthermore, it is well known that the hippocampus region in the brain is crucial for learning and memory, and the formation of spatial memory (Huang et al., 2015; Lee et al., 2016). The scopolamine-induced memory

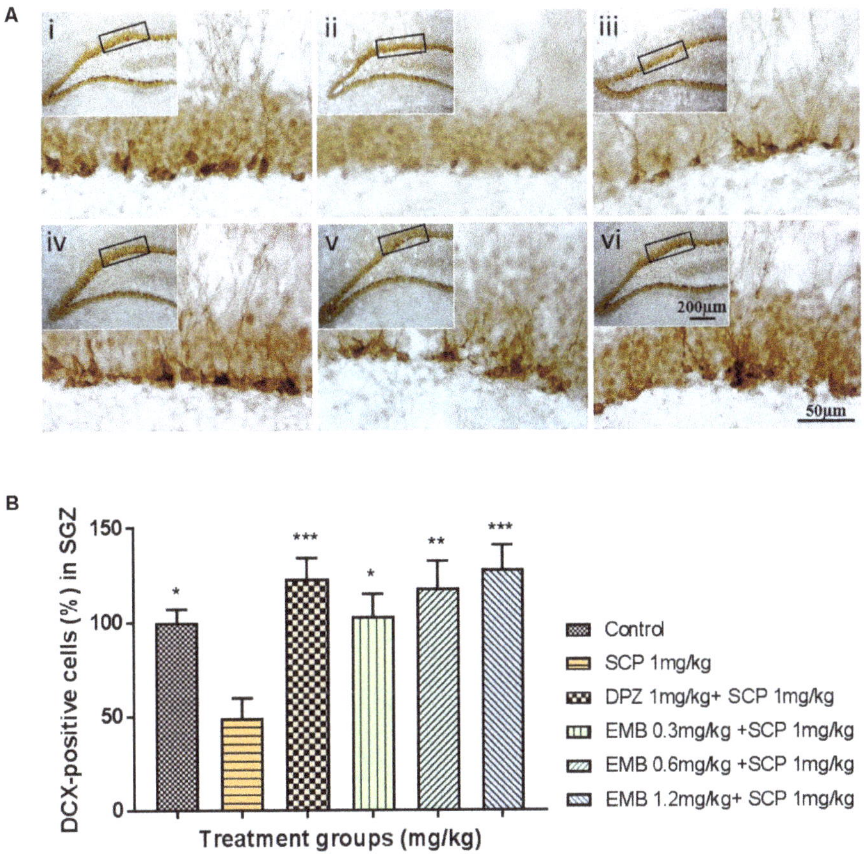

FIGURE 6 | DCX immunohistochemical analysis of the effects of embelin in improving scopolamine-induced suppression of neurogenesis in the dentate gyrus. **(A)** DCX-positive staining in immature neurons is shown in the subgranular zone of the dentate gyrus. Photomicrographs of the hippocampal section of treatment groups was (i) Control (ii) SCP 1 mg/kg alone (iii) DPZ 1 mg/kg + SCP 1 mg/kg (iv) EMB 0.3 mg/kg + SCP 1 mg/kg (v) EMB 0.6 mg/kg + SCP 1 mg/kg (vi) EMB 1.2 mg/kg + SCP 1 mg/kg. Representative photomicrographs were taken at magnifications of 40X and 200X. **(B)** Quantification of DCX population. Data are expressed as means Mean ± SEM, $n = 5$ and statistical analysis by one-way ANOVA followed by Dunnett test $^{*}P < 0.05$, $^{**}P < 0.01$, and $^{***}P < 0.001$.

deficit model demonstrated that prominent oxidative stress and memory deficits in a rodent model is similar to that in AD patients, even though the mechanism of action remains unclear (Lee et al., 2015). The change in the mRNA levels of antioxidants in the hippocampus after embelin pretreatment was examined using the scopolamine model in this present study. Scopolamine injection induced oxidative stress in the hippocampus, as evident by the decreased levels of CAT and SOD1 mRNA levels in the scopolamine alone treated negative group. To prevent or slow down the progression of free radical-mediated oxidative stress, brain antioxidant defense enzymes such as CAT and SOD play a vital role in protecting tissues against oxidative damage (Uddin et al., 2016a). Antioxidant mRNA alteration caused by scopolamine injection was significantly ameliorated for SOD1 via pretreatment with embelin. However, CAT mRNA level was decreased by scopolamine induction, but it was not significant (**Figures 4C,D**). Additionally, scopolamine-induced lipid peroxidation in the hippocampus's CA3 was shown as positively stained 4HNE cells. Nonetheless, pretreatment with embelin completely attenuated the over-production of 4HNE cells (**Figures 7A,B**). These results propose that the protective antioxidant gene response by embelin pretreatment reduced lipid peroxidation induced by scopolamine. An increase in 4HNE cells is a key histopathological feature of neurodegenerative diseases like AD (Serrano and Klann, 2004).

Expression of BDNF and CREB1 mRNA levels in scopolamine-induced hippocampal tissue were examined to investigate the role of embelin in neurogenesis and synaptic plasticity. In this study, hippocampal BDNF and CREB1 were markedly reduced due to scopolamine injection, and pretreatment with embelin increased the mRNA expression level of both BDNF and CREB1. A high dose of embelin at 1.2 mg/kg exhibited maximum protection by increasing the levels of BDNF and CREB1. Other than that, cAMP response element binding protein (CREB) plays a crucial role in neuronal growth, proliferation, differentiation, and survival (Lee et al., 2016). In our results, the explanation for the increased in dose dependency for both BDNF and CREB 1 could possibly be that embelin may be responsible for visual recognition memory in NOR through this BDNF/CREB pathway. We noticed that at the 1.2 mg/kg dose, embelin expressed high mRNA levels of BDNF and CREB1 and this could be the reason for a 60%

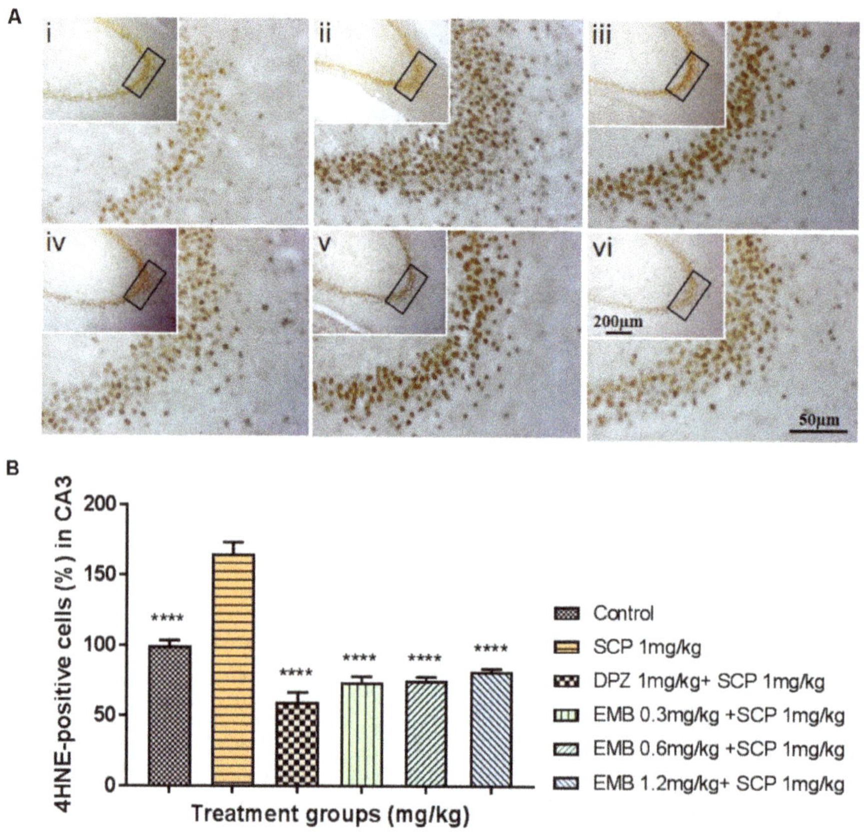

FIGURE 7 | 4HNE immunohistochemical analysis illustrating the inhibitory effects of embelin against scopolamine-induced lipid peroxidation in the hippocampus. **(A)** The 4HNE-positive stained cells in the CA3 region of the hippocampus are indicative of lipid peroxidation. Photomicrographs hippocampal section of treatment groups was (i) Control (ii) SCP 1 mg/kg alone (iii) DPZ 1 mg/kg + SCP 1 mg/kg (iv) EMB 0.3 mg/kg + SCP 1 mg/kg (v) EMB 0.6 mg/kg + SCP 1 mg/kg (vi) EMB 1.2 mg/kg + SCP 1 mg/kg. Representative photomicrographs were taken at magnifications of 40X, and 200X. **(B)** Quantification of 4HNE protein in CA3. Data are expressed as means Mean ± SEM, $n = 5$ and statistical analysis by one-way ANOVA followed by Dunnett test $*P < 0.05$, $**P < 0.01$, $***P < 0.001$, and $****P < 0.0001$.

increase in visual recognition index in NOR when compared with the scopolamine treated group. Thus, this validates the role of BDNF-CREB signaling in visual recognition memory, particularly for hippocampus-dependent learning.

Likewise, adult hippocampal neurogenesis plays a key role in hippocampal memory function (Mu and Gage, 2011). Altman and Das (1965) first reported on the continual production of new neurons in the adult hippocampus. These new neurons originated from adult neural stem cells (NSCs) residing in the SGZ of DG (Bonaguidi et al., 2011). In this present research, a significantly reduced level of immature neurons, revealed through DCX staining of scopolamine-induced rat hippocampus was determined, while pretreatment with embelin distinctly ameliorated repression of the SGZ region's neuronal precursor cells in a dose-dependent manner (**Figures 6A,B**).

Numerous studies have reported that most classical neurotransmitter systems such as ACh, NE, Glu, and DA, influence learning and memory (Myhrer, 2003). We adopted LC-MS/MS method as it is a simple, sensitive and simultaneously able to quantify the four major neurotransmitters from rat hippocampal tissue in a single run (Zheng et al., 2012). The extraction of the neurotransmitters from rat hippocampus was done with utmost care and prior to LC-MS/MS analysis to avoid any possibilities of sample degradation and oxidation as described by He et al. (2013). The neurotransmitters' concentrations were expressed as a ratio of total protein concentration in order to get correct value and to avoid possible variation in sample when subjected to LC-MS/MS. In AD patients, pathological changes affecting glutamatergic, cholinergic, noradrenergic, and serotonergic systems have been revealed (Francis et al., 1999). In this study, the effect of embelin on brain neurotransmitter levels in rats administered scopolamine was investigated. ACh plays an essential role in learning process and memory as a key transmitter in the cholinergic system (Chen et al., 2016). A decrease in ACh levels is reported in this study as a biomarker of scopolamine-induced cognitive impairment in the rat hippocampus. Embelin administered at a dose of 0.3 mg/kg significantly increased ACh levels, subsequently improving cholinergic function. Interestingly, Arora and Deshmukh (2017) reported that embelin treatment in a streptozotocin-induced rat model decreased AChE activity, which is the enzyme that metabolizes ACh

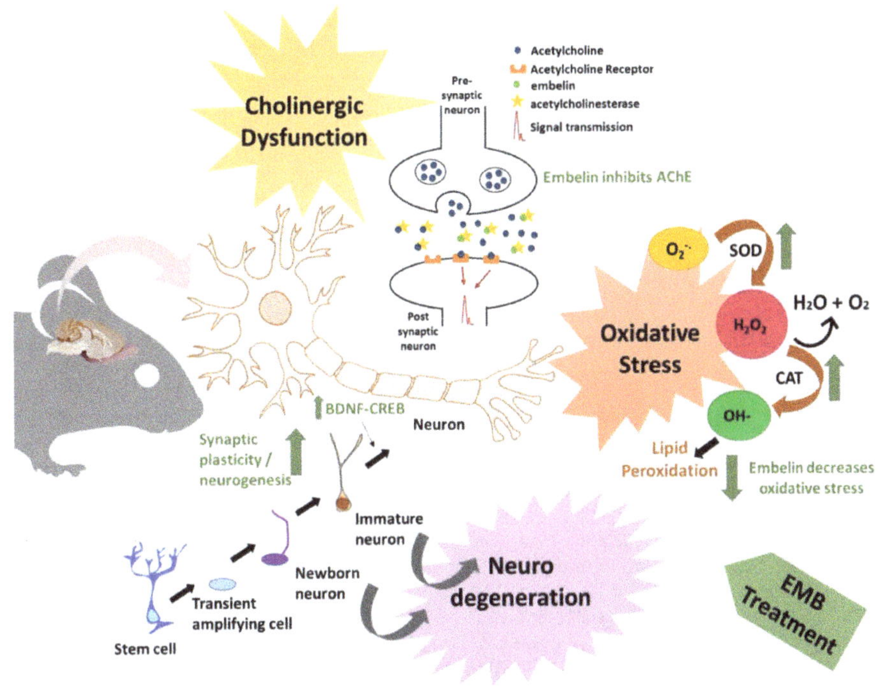

FIGURE 8 | Schematic diagram showing the effect of embelin in a diseased condition. The figure depicts cholinergic dysfunction, oxidative stress, and neurodegeneration which contributes to neuronal loss, synaptic dysfunction, and an AD-like condition. Embelin could act as memory enhancer by stimulating the cholinergic systems via acetylcholine release and inhibition of AChE. In the oxidative defense pathway, embelin reduces oxidative stress by increasing SOD and CAT mRNA levels and eventually reducing lipid peroxidation. In addition to these effects, a rise in DCX expression by embelin treatment contributes to neurogenesis and an increase in BDNF-CREB levels may contribute to synaptic plasticity.

into choline and acetate. Therefore, a reduction in AChE level indicates a high level of ACh as a result of embelin treatment, which is similar to our results. In the current research, Glu levels were raised after being treated with scopolamine. Similar outcomes were reported by Pandareesh et al. (2016) and Arora and Deshmukh (2017). Administration of 0.6 mg/kg embelin significantly lowered the level of Glu. A rise in Glu level has been reported to cause excitotoxic neuronal damage and loss of cognitive function (Arora and Deshmukh, 2017) and also associated with excitotoxicity in AD brains (Jackson, 2014). Scopolamine treatment also caused an increment in the levels of DA and NE in the hippocampus. Earlier reports suggests that an increase in DA and NE levels leads to amnesia and memory deficits. Wu et al.'s (2014) study, demonstrated that donepezil treatment can modulate the increase levels of DA and NE in disease control group. Interestingly, a similar protective effect was observed with embelin pre-treatment in amnesia condition.

In this scopolamine model, our results are unusual, with embelin causing different dose dependency in the behavioral model and neurotransmitters, particularly ACh when compared to other reported studies that utilized embelin. This could be explained by embelin being neuroprotective in a scopolamine-induced amnesia model via visual recognition memory but not in long-term spatial memory. This theory is supported by our results as there was a dose dependency in embelin treatment in NOR and the result of embelin is comparable with the donepezil group. However, we could not see this pattern in EPM. Whilst embelin improved visual recognition in dose dependency manner, it also reduced the level of ACh in a dose-dependent manner as well. This discrepancy could be because at a dose of 0.3 mg/kg, embelin might be effectively increasing the level of ACh but stops further production of ACh at 1.2 mg/kg. At this particular dose, embelin probably plays a different role in inhibiting the enzyme AChE. This could be the reason that at 1.2 mg/kg of embelin, we observed a high recognition index in NOR of scopolamine-induced amnesia rats.

CONCLUSION

In conclusion, the results from this study have demonstrated that embelin displays nootropic and neuroprotective abilities in scopolamine-induced amnesia in rats. Nootropic effects may be attributed to an increase in visual recognition and spatial memory in both NOR and EPM. Embelin possesses anti-amnesic effects, which could be mediated by an antioxidant gene response particularly though SOD1, the CREB-BDNF pathway, hippocampal neurogenesis, and cholinergic activity. The anti-amnesic effect of embelin is also comparable to that of donepezil at a specific concentration even though it is not in a dose-dependent manner in certain cases. Therefore, embelin could be a promising treatment for patients suffering from neurodegenerative diseases. **Figure 8** shows the potential mechanism of action of embelin in scopolamine-induced memory impairment in rodents.

AUTHOR CONTRIBUTIONS

SB performed all the experiments and was responsible for the writing of the manuscript in its entirety. YK helped in designing gene expression study, result analysis and figures in the manuscript. IO helped in LC-MS/MS method. MS helped in conceptualizing, designing the study, result analysis, and manuscript writing. All authors gave their final approval for the submission of the manuscript.

REFERENCES

Afzal, M., Gupta, G., Kazmi, I., Rahman, M., Upadhyay, G., Ahmad, K., et al. (2012). Evaluation of anxiolytic activity of embelin isolated from *Embelia ribes*. *Biomed. Aging Pathol.* 2, 45–47. doi: 10.1016/j.biomag.2012.03.003

Ali, T., Yoon, G. H., Shah, S. A., Lee, H. Y., and Kim, M. O. (2015). Osmotin attenuates amyloid beta-induced memory impairment, tau phosphorylation and neurodegeneration in the mouse hippocampus. *Sci. Rep.* 5:11708. doi: 10.1038/srep11708

Altman, J., and Das, G. D. (1965). Autoradiographic and histological evidence of postnatal hippocampal neurogenesis in rats. *J. Comp. Neurol.* 124, 319–335. doi: 10.1002/cne.901240303

Alzheimer's Association (2017). 2017 Alzheimer's disease facts and figures. *Alzheimers Dement.* 13, 325–373. doi: 10.1016/j.jalz.2017.02.001

Arora, R., and Deshmukh, R. (2017). Embelin attenuates intracerebroventricular streptozotocin-induced behavioral, biochemical, and neurochemical abnormalities in rats. *Mol. Neurobiol.* 54, 6670–6680. doi: 10.1007/s12035-016-0182-y

Bartus, R. T., Dean, R. L., Beer, B., and Lippa, A. S. (1982). The cholinergic hypothesis of geriatric memory dysfunction. *Science* 217, 408–414. doi: 10.1126/science.7046051

Batool, Z., Sadir, S., Liaquat, L., Tabassum, S., Madiha, S., Rafiq, S., et al. (2016). Repeated administration of almonds increases brain acetylcholine levels and enhances memory function in healthy rats while attenuates memory deficits in animal model of amnesia. *Brain Res. Bull.* 120, 63–74. doi: 10.1016/j.brainresbull.2015.11.001

Birks, J., and Grimley Evans, J. (2009). Ginkgo biloba for cognitive impairment and dementia. *Cochrane Database Syst. Rev.* CD003120. doi: 10.1002/14651858.CD003120.pub3

Bonaguidi, M. A., Wheeler, M. A., Shapiro, J. S., Stadel, R. P., Sun, G. J., Ming, G.-L., et al. (2011). In vivo clonal analysis reveals self-renewing and multipotent adult neural stem cell characteristics. *Cell* 145, 1142–1155. doi: 10.1016/j.cell.2011.05.024

Bridges, P. K. (1981). Disturbed behavior induced by high-dose antipsychotic drugs. *Br. Med. J. (Clin. Res. Ed.)* 282:313.

Brookmeyer, R., Johnson, E., Ziegler-Graham, K., and Arrighi, H. M. (2007). Forecasting the global burden of Alzheimer's disease. *Alzheimer's Dement.* 3, 186–191. doi: 10.1016/j.jalz.2007.04.381

Butterfield, D. A., and Lauderback, C. M. (2002). Lipid peroxidation and protein oxidation in Alzheimer's disease brain: potential causes and consequences involving amyloid β-peptide-associated free radical oxidative stress1, 2. *Free Radic. Biol. Med.* 32, 1050–1060. doi: 10.1016/S0891-5849(02)00794-3

Chen, L.-E., Wu, F., Zhao, A., Ge, H., and Zhan, H. (2016). Protection efficacy of the extract of *Ginkgo biloba* against the learning and memory damage of rats under repeated high sustained. *Evid. Based Complement. Alternat. Med.* 2016:6320586. doi: 10.1155/2016/6320586

Dhingra, D., and Kumar, V. (2012). Memory-enhancing activity of palmatine in mice using elevated plus maze and morris water maze. *Adv. Pharmacol. Sci.* 2012:357368. doi: 10.1155/2012/357368

Ding, Q., Dimayuga, E., and Keller, J. N. (2007). Oxidative damage, protein synthesis, and protein degradation in Alzheimer's disease. *Curr. Alzheimer Res.* 4, 73–79. doi: 10.2174/156720507779939788

Ennaceur, A., and Delacour, J. (1988). A new one-trial test for neurobiological studies of memory in rats. 1: behavioral data. *Behav. Brain Res.* 31, 47–59. doi: 10.1016/0166-4328(88)90157-X

Francis, P. T., Palmer, A. M., Snape, M., and Wilcock, G. K. (1999). The cholinergic hypothesis of Alzheimer's disease: a review of progress. *J. Neurol. Neurosurg. Psychiatry* 66, 137–147. doi: 10.1136/jnnp.66.2.137

Froestl, W., Muhs, A., and Pfeifer, A. (2012). Cognitive enhancers (nootropics). Part 1: drugs interacting with receptors. *J. Alzheimers Dis.* 32, 793–887. doi: 10.3233/JAD-2012-121186

Ghumatkar, P. J., Patil, S. P., Jain, P. D., Tambe, R. M., and Sathaye, S. (2015). Nootropic, neuroprotective and neurotrophic effects of phloretin in scopolamine induced amnesia in mice. *Pharmacol. Biochem. Behav.* 135, 182–191. doi: 10.1016/j.pbb.2015.06.005

Grayson, B., Leger, M., Piercy, C., Adamson, L., Harte, M., and Neill, J. C. (2015). Assessment of disease-related cognitive impairments using the novel object recognition (NOR) task in rodents. *Behav. Brain Res.* 285, 176–193. doi: 10.1016/j.bbr.2014.10.025

Halder, S., Mehta, A. K., Kar, R., Mustafa, M., Mediratta, P. K., and Sharma, K. K. (2011). Clove oil reverses learning and memory deficits in scopolamine-treated mice. *Planta Med.* 77, 830–834. doi: 10.1055/s-0030-1250605

He, B., Bi, K., Jia, Y., Wang, J., Lv, C., Liu, R., et al. (2013). Rapid analysis of neurotransmitters in rat brain using ultra-fast liquid chromatography and tandem mass spectrometry: application to a comparative study in normal and insomnic rats. *J. Mass Spectrom.* 48, 969–978. doi: 10.1002/jms.3243

Heo, Y.-M., Shin, M.-S., Lee, J.-M., Kim, C.-J., Baek, S.-B., Kim, K.-H., et al. (2014). Treadmill exercise ameliorates short-term memory disturbance in scopolamine-induced amnesia rats. *Int. Neurourol. J.* 18, 16–22. doi: 10.5213/inj.2014.18.1.16

Hritcu, L., Noumedem, J. A., Cioanca, O., Hancianu, M., Kuete, V., and Mihasan, M. (2014). Methanolic extract of Piper nigrum fruits improves memory impairment by decreasing brain oxidative stress in amyloid beta (1–42) rat model of Alzheimer's disease. *Cell Mol. Neurobiol.* 34, 437–449. doi: 10.1007/s10571-014-0028-y

Huang, T.-T., Leu, D., and Zou, Y. (2015). Oxidative stress and redox regulation on hippocampal-dependent cognitive functions. *Arch. Biochem. Biophys.* 576, 2–7. doi: 10.1016/j.abb.2015.03.014

Jackson, W. S. (2014). Selective vulnerability to neurodegenerative disease: the curious case of Prion protein. *Dis. Models Mech.* 7, 21–29. doi: 10.1242/dmm.012146

Kundap, U. P., Bhuvanendran, S., Kumari, Y., Othman, I., and Shaikh, M. F. (2017a). Plant derived phytocompound, embelin in CNS disorders: a systematic review. *Front. Pharmacol.* 8:76. doi: 10.3389/fphar.2017.00076

Kundap, U. P., Kumari, Y., Othman, I., and Shaikh, M. F. (2017b). Zebrafish as a model for epilepsy-induced cognitive dysfunction: a pharmacological, biochemical and behavioral approach. *Front. Pharmacol.* 8:515. doi: 10.3389/fphar.2017.00515

Kwon, S.-H., Kim, H.-C., Lee, S.-Y., and Jang, C.-G. (2009). Loganin improves learning and memory impairments induced by scopolamine in mice. *Eur. J. Pharmacol.* 619, 44–49. doi: 10.1016/j.ejphar.2009.06.062

Lee, J.-S., Hong, S.-S., Kim, H.-G., Lee, H.-W., Kim, W.-Y., Lee, S.-K., et al. (2016). Gongjin-Dan enhances hippocampal memory in a mouse model of scopolamine-induced amnesia. *PLoS One* 11:e0159823. doi: 10.1371/journal.pone.0159823

Lee, J.-S., Kim, H.-G., Lee, H.-W., Han, J.-M., Lee, S.-K., Kim, D.-W., et al. (2015). Hippocampal memory enhancing activity of pine needle extract against scopolamine-induced amnesia in a mouse model. *Sci. Rep.* 5:9651. doi: 10.1038/srep09651

Mahendran, S., Thippeswamy, B., Veerapur, V., and Badami, S. (2011). Anticonvulsant activity of embelin isolated from *Embelia ribes*. *Phytomedicine* 18, 186–188. doi: 10.1016/j.phymed.2010.04.002

Mu, Y., and Gage, F. H. (2011). Adult hippocampal neurogenesis and its role in Alzheimer's disease. *Mol. Neurodegener.* 6:85. doi: 10.1186/1750-1326-6-85

Myhrer, T. (2003). Neurotransmitter systems involved in learning and memory in the rat: a meta-analysis based on studies of four behavioral tasks. *Brain Res. Rev.* 41, 268–287. doi: 10.1016/S0165-0173(02)00268-0

Pandareesh, M., Anand, T., and Khanum, F. (2016). Cognition enhancing and neuromodulatory propensity of *Bacopa monniera* extract against scopolamine induced cognitive impairments in rat hippocampus. *Neurochem. Res.* 41, 985–999. doi: 10.1007/s11064-015-1780-1

Pathan, S. A., Iqbal, Z., Zaidi, S., Talegaonkar, S., Vohra, D., Jain, G. K., et al. (2009). CNS drug delivery systems: novel approaches. *Recent Pat. Drug Deliv. Formul.* 3, 71–89. doi: 10.2174/187221109787158355

Poojari, R. (2014). Embelin–a drug of antiquity: shifting the paradigm towards modern medicine. *Expert Opin. Investig. Drugs* 23, 427–444. doi: 10.1517/13543784.2014.867016

Serrano, F., and Klann, E. (2004). Reactive oxygen species and synaptic plasticity in the aging hippocampus. *Ageing Res. Rev.* 3, 431–443. doi: 10.1016/j.arr.2004.05.002

Tanzi, R. E., and Bertram, L. (2005). Twenty years of the Alzheimer's disease amyloid hypothesis: a genetic perspective. *Cell* 120, 545–555. doi: 10.1016/j.cell.2005.02.008

Uddin, M. S., Al Mamun, A., Hossain, M. S., Ashaduzzaman, M., Noor, M. A. A., Hossain, M. S., et al. (2016a). Neuroprotective effect of *Phyllanthus acidus* L. on learning and memory impairment in scopolamine-induced animal model of dementia and oxidative stress: natural wonder for regulating the development and progression of Alzheimer's disease. *Adv. Alzheimers Dis.* 5, 53–72. doi: 10.4236/aad.2016.52005

Uddin, M. S., Nasrullah, M., Hossain, M. S., Rahman, M. M., Sarwar, M. S., Amran, M. S., et al. (2016b). Evaluation of nootropic activity of *Persicaria flaccida* on cognitive performance, brain antioxidant markers and acetylcholinesterase activity in rats: implication for the management of Alzheimer's disease. *Am. J. Psychiatry Neurosci.* 4, 26–37. doi: 10.11648/j.ajpn.20160402.12

Wu, C.-R., Lin, H.-C., and Su, M.-H. (2014). Reversal by aqueous extracts of *Cistanche tubulosa* from behavioral deficits in Alzheimer's disease-like rat model: relevance for amyloid deposition and central neurotransmitter function. *BMC Complement. Altern. Med.* 14:202. doi: 10.1186/1472-6882-14-202

Yatin, S., Varadarajan, S., Link, C., and Butterfield, D. (1999). In vitro and in vivo oxidative stress associated with Alzheimer's amyloid ß-peptide (1–42). *Neurobiol. Aging* 20, 325–330.

Zheng, X., Kang, A., Dai, C., Liang, Y., Xie, T., Xie, L., et al. (2012). Quantitative analysis of neurochemical panel in rat brain and plasma by liquid chromatography-tandem mass spectrometry. *Anal. Chem.* 84, 10044–10051. doi: 10.1021/ac3025202

13

Isolation and Characterization of Two New Secondary Metabolites From *Quercus incana* and Their Antidepressant- and Anxiolytic-Like Potential

Rizwana Sarwar[1], Umar Farooq[1], Sadia Naz[1], Ajmal Khan[1,2*], Syed M. Bukhari[1], Haroon Khan[3], Nasiara Karim[4], Imran Khan[5], Ayaz Ahmed[6] and Ahmed Al-Harrasi[2]*

[1] Department of Chemistry, COMSATS Institute of Information Technology Abbottabad, Abbottabad, Pakistan, [2] UoN Chair of Oman's Medicinal Plants and Marine Natural Products, University of Nizwa, Nizwa, Oman, [3] Department of Pharmacy, Abdul Wali Khan University Mardan, Mardan, Pakistan, [4] Department of Pharmacy, University of Malakand, Chakdara, Pakistan, [5] Department of Pharmacy, University of Swabi, Swabi, Pakistan, [6] Dr. Panjwani Center for Molecular Medicine and Drug Research, International Center for Chemical and Biological Sciences, University of Karachi, Karachi, Pakistan

***Correspondence:**
Umar Farooq
umarf@ciit.net.pk
Ajmal Khan
ajmalkhan@ciit.net.pk;
ajmalchemist@yahoo.com

The ethyl acetate fraction of *Quercus incana* yielded two new compounds [**1** and **2**]. The characterization and structure elucidation of these compounds were carried out through various spectroscopic techniques such as mass spectrometry along with one- and two-dimensional NMR techniques. The structural formula was deduced to be 2-(4-hydroxybutan-2-yl)-5-methoxyphenol [**1**] and 4-hydroxy-3-(hydroxymethyl) pentanoic acid [**2**]. The elevated plus maze (EPM) and light–dark box (LDB) tests (classical mouse models) were performed in order to reveal the anxiolytic potential of both compounds [**1** and **2**]. Both compounds displayed dose-dependent increases in open-arm entries and time spent in open arms in EPM ($^{*}P < 0.05$, $^{**}P < 0.01$), and increased the time spent in the lit compartment and increased transitions between the two compartments in LDB test ($^{*}P < 0.05$, $^{**}P < 0.01$). Co-administration of selective benzodiazepine (BZP) receptor antagonist, flumazenil (2.5 mg/kg) with compounds [**1** and **2**] decreased the anxiolytic-like activity of both compounds in the EPM indicating BZP-binding site of GABA-A receptors are involved in the anxiolytic-like effect. Similarly, both compounds at the dose level of 10 and 30 mg/kg, i.p. exerted pronounced antidepressant-like effect in both forced swimming as well as tail suspension tests ($^{*}P < 0.05$, $^{**}P < 0.01$; ANOVA followed by Dunnett's *post hoc* test). The effect at 30 mg/kg was comparable to the reference drug imipramine (60 mg/kg).

Keywords: *Quercus incana*, aromatic acid, anxiolytic- and antidepressant-like effect, diazepam, flumazenil

INTRODUCTION

Stress is known to play a significant part in pathogenesis of mental dysfunctions (Kalueff and Tuohimaa, 2004). Anxiety, a common mental illness, from, which 20% of the adult population is suffering across the globe has become a significant research area in the field of psychopharmacology (Yadav et al., 2008; Sharmen et al., 2014). Anxiety is related to significant disability which may result in negative impacts on the patient's quality of life (Kudagi et al., 2012). Currently, benzodiazepines (BZPs) are used as the drug of choice for the treatment of several types of anxiety (Gupta et al., 2010). Despite the fact that BZPs are well known for their advantages, their side effects are high, which include sedation, myorelaxation, physical dependence, and anterograde amnesia (Barua et al., 2009).

Depression has been described as the mental disorder, which will become the second biggest global health problem after cardiovascular diseases by 2020 (Reddy, 2010). Depression can appear as comorbid symptom on several psychiatric conditions including response to stress, substance abuse, and chronic diseases including diabetes mellitus, cancer, and hypertension. Depression is also associated with disease causing pain, disability, deformity, and conditions, which may reduce patient's quality of life and life expectancy. A number of antidepressant drugs are now clinically available, which presumably act via different mechanisms, including the noradrenergic, serotonergic, and/or dopaminergic systems. These drugs include monoamine oxidase inhibitors, tricyclic antidepressant drugs, selective serotonin reuptake inhibitors (SSRIs), and serotonin–norepinephrine reuptake inhibitors (SNRIs) (Gonçalves et al., 2012; Khan et al., 2016). However, these agents have their limitations including inadequate effectiveness over a prolonged period and unwanted side effects (Berton and Nestler, 2006). Recently, there has been a renewed interest in natural compounds, particularly from plants that mitigate anxiety and depressive-like symptoms (González-Trujano et al., 2017).

Plant-derived constituents provide a large source of available pharmaceuticals in modern medicine, which are directly or indirectly derived from natural sources. In drug discovery process, the natural products are of great interest due to their natural diversity as well as leading development of desired therapeutic agents (Khan et al., 2016).

Quercus incana is a tree belonging to genus *Quercus* (oak), of family Fagaceae. There are approximately 900 species of genus *Quercus*, among them only six species are available in Pakistan (Nasir and Ali, 1976). The fruit (acorns) part of *Q. incana* has huge medicinal importance and has been used as astringent in digestive disorders, asthma, while the decoction of the bark is used for the treatment of diarrhea and dysentery (Manan et al., 2007). Fruit of *Q. incana* has analgesic effect and has been used for gastrointestinal activity (Sarwar et al., 2013). The leaves of *Q. incana* are known to possess antioxidant nature. These have also found to be effective against certain fungal as well as bacterial strains (Sarwar et al., 2015). Phytochemical study of *Q. incana* revealed the presence of phenolic compounds (Sadanandam and Christopher, 2010), condensed tannins (Jothimanivannan et al., 2010), proanthocyanidins (Kocyigit et al., 2010), and flavonoids (Thaina et al., 2009). Literature showed that the polar fractions from different parts of the genus *Quercus* possess antibacterial activities indicating their ethno-pharmacological use (Berahou et al., 2007).

In the current study, we are reporting the isolation and structure elucidation of new aromatic acid and aromatic alcohol and their anxiolytic- and antidepressant-like effects in mouse models of anxiety and depression.

MATERIALS AND METHODS

Chemicals and Drugs

The analytical grade solvents, flumazenil, imipramine, and the diazepam were purchased from Sigma (St. Louis, MO, United States).

Animals

Swiss albino male mice 25–30 g were obtained from the National Institute of Health (NIH), Islamabad, Pakistan and maintained in the animal house of the Department of Pharmacy, University of Malakand. The tested animals were acclimatized for a week prior the initiation of research work. Animals were housed in the Department of Pharmacy, University of Malakand's animal house with fresh water and standard food available *ad libitum*. The animals were maintained at 12 h light and dark cycle and with room temperature maintained at 22–25°C in the animal house. Experiments were conducted in accordance with the accepted guidelines of animal (Scientific Procedures) Act UK 1986. All drugs were dissolved in vehicle consisting of 95% saline, 4% DMSO, 1% Tween-20, and experiments were performed during day time (9 AM to 2 PM). The intraperitoneal administration of all treatments was carried out as 10 ml/kg body weight of mice.

Plant Extraction and Fractionation

Quercus incana leaves collection, extraction, and fractionation were done as reported in our previous study (Sarwar et al., 2015). Phytochemical analysis of ethyl acetate fraction through repeated column chromatography resulted in the isolation of two new compounds [**1** and **2**] as shown in **Figure 1**.

Experimental Procedures

Isolation and purification of compounds were performed by the help of column chromatography using silica gel (70–230 mesh and 230–400 E-Merck) as stationary phase. For TLC analysis, pre-coated (silica gel 60 F_{254}) plates were used. Also, IR and HR-EI-MS analysis of pure compounds were performed on UV-240 spectrophotometer JASCO-320-A and double-focusing Varian MAT-312 spectrometer, respectively. The NMR spectral

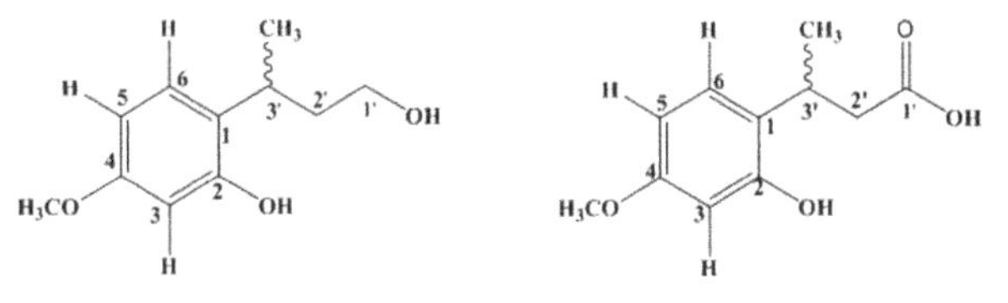

1 2

FIGURE 1 | Structure of compounds [**1** and **2**].

analysis (^{1}H and ^{13}C) was done by using Bruker AMX-300 spectrometer.

Pharmacological Experiments

Acute Toxicity Studies

The acute toxicity studies were performed according to the method described previously (Karim et al., 2015). Swiss albino male mice were divided into five groups with four mice in each group. Animals were deprived from food overnight but had access to water. After 12 h, animals in groups I and II were treated with compound **1** at the doses of 100 mg/kg, i.p. and 200 mg/kg, i.p. Similarly, groups III and IV received compound **2** at the dose level of 100 and 200 mg/kg, i.p. Animals in the control group received vehicle (10 ml/kg i.p.). Animals were keenly observed for any signs of toxicity for 6 h and then monitored for the next 24 h for changes in behaviors including sedation, convulsions, grooming, hyperactivity, respiratory arrest, increased or decreased motor activity, and mortality.

Assessment of Anxiolytic-Like Effect in Elevated Plus-Maze Test

Two open arms in EPM apparatus are connected with two closed arms by an open central platform. The assembly was lifted up from ground level at a height of 40 cm. An elevated edge, the height of which was 3 mm with a total thickness of 1 mm, encircled the open arms of the apparatus. The mice were distributed into 11 groups. Group I received vehicle (10 ml/kg) while diazepam (1 mg/kg, i.p.) was injected as reference to group II. The test compound **1** (1, 10, and 30 mg/kg, i.p.) was selected for treatment of groups III–V while test compound **2** (1, 10, and 30 mg/kg, i.p.) for groups VI–VIII.

After 20 min, animals were placed one by one in the central platform of the EPM facing an open arm and were allowed to explore the EPM for 5 min. An arm entry was defined when all four paws of the mouse were inside the arm. All sessions were recorded with a digital video camera positioned above the EPM. The behavioral parameters including the number of open-arm entries and time spent in open arms were noted at the end of the test from observing the recorded videos. The % open entries and the % time spent in the open arms were considered as a measure of state of anxiety. To evaluate the involvement of GABAergic system in the anxiolytic-like effects of these compounds, mice were pre-treated with either vehicle, flumazenil (2.5 mg/kg, i.p.), or PTZ (10 mg/kg, i.p.) before administration of compounds **1** and **2** or diazepam.

In order to avoid any cues associated with odor, the EPM was cleaned thoroughly with 70% ethanol after each session.

Assessment of Anxiolytic-Like Effect in Light/Dark Box Test

The light–dark box (LDB) test apparatus used in this study has been described previously (Karim et al., 2015). Briefly, it consists of a wooden box with 44 cm length, 21 cm width and height each. One-third of this box comprises small compartment whereas two-third of the box makes a large and illuminated compartment. The partition of the box has been done by a board made of wood possessing a 7 × 7 cm opening in the center linking both compartments. Inside walls of the small compartment was painted with black color whereas large compartment was painted white. The portion of the box comprising small compartment was covered with a lid made of wood whereas large compartment was covered with Plexiglas. The large compartment was getting light by a 60-watt bulb which was placed at a height of 30 cm above the test apparatus. A total eight groups of animals were created with six members in each group. Groups I and II were given vehicle (10 ml/kg) and diazepam (01 mg/kg, i.p.), respectively. Test compound **1** (01, 10, and 30 mg/kg, i.p.) was administered to Groups III–V and test compound **2** (01, 10, and 30 mg/kg, i.p.) to groups VI–VIII. Treated mice were given a total time of 20 min and were later placed one by one in illuminated compartment. It was assured that each animal faces the opening in the wooden board away from the dark section. For 5 min, the animal's behavior was recorded by video camera which was placed at a height of 1 m above the apparatus. The total time spent in illuminated section along with total number of times the animal passes between the two sections were the two parameters noted from the video records as a measure of anxiety. An increased exploration of the lit section and increased transitions between the two compartments of the box are associated with an anti-anxiety effect (Belzung et al., 1987; Bourin and Hascoët, 2003).

Antidepressant-Like Effect in the FST

The forced swim test (FST) was also conducted as described previously with minor modifications (Porsolt et al., 1978). The test is conducted in two phases. The pretest is conducted 24 h before the actual test. Imipramine (60 mg/kg) was used as reference drug. In pretest, mice were individually placed in transparent glass tanks (height × width = 45 cm × 18 cm) which were filled up to 25 cm with water and maintained at 25°C. Animals were allowed to swim for 15 min followed by their removal, drying by using a towel, and placement back in their respective cages. After 24 h, vehicle, imipramine, and compound **1** or compound **2** were administered intraperitoneally to the test animals. After 1 h of the compounds administration, the mice were subjected to similar experimental conditions as pretest session and the immobility duration was recorded for 5 min (Porsolt et al., 1978).

Antidepressant-Like Effect in the TST

This test was carried out as described earlier (Steru et al., 1985). Mice were administered with vehicle or imipramine (60 mg/kg) or compounds **1** or **2** at the dose level of 1, 10, and 30 mg/kg, i.p. Mice were suspended by their tails and the duration of immobility was recorded for a period of 6 min as described by Steru et al. (1985). The complete motionless suspension of test animals was referred to as a condition of immobility.

Approval from Research Ethics Committee

It is certified that the Departmental Research Ethics Committee (DREC) has reviewed the National Research Program for Universities (NRPU) research grants application of the project entitled "Anxiolytic and Antidepressant Activities of Selected

Natural product (Glycosides and Flavonoids)." The principal investigator of the project is Dr. Nasiara Karim, Assistant Professor, Department of Pharmacy, University of Malakand.

The committee approves (DAEC/Pharm/2017/01) the study to be conducted in the present form and expects to be informed about any revision in the protocol and subject/patient information/informed consent (where applicable).

Statistical Data Analysis

The data were expressed as mean ± standard error of the mean (SEM). Data were analyzed by one-way analysis of variance (ANOVA) followed by Dunnett's *post hoc* test using GraphPad Prism version 5.0. The analyzed values were statistically significant when $P < 0.05$.

RESULTS

Column Chromatography

Fraction obtained from ethyl acetate was taken up further to perform column chromatography. Stationary bed used for chromatography was silica gel and *n*-hexane was used as mobile phase, with a gradient of ethyl acetate up to 100% followed by methanol. It resulted in four fractions (fractions A–D). Further, fraction B was loaded on silica gel (flash silica 230-mesh) and eluted with EtOAc: *n*-hexane (70:30) to get compound **1** while compound **2** was purified at EtOAc: *n*-hexane (85:15), respectively.

Compound **1** was new rare class of aromatic alcohol isolated as colorless oil from ethyl acetate fraction of *Q. incana*. The structure was mainly elucidated by ^{1}H-NMR, ^{13}C-NMR, high resolution mass spectrometry, and supported by 2D-NMR techniques. The molecular ion peak of compound **1** appeared at *m/z* 196 $[M]^+$ both in HR-EI-MS and EI-MS spectra suggested molecular formula $C_{11}H_{16}O_3$, consistent with Δ^4 degree of unsaturation. In addition with its molecular ion peak, it showed characteristic fragments at *m/z* 181, 151, 137, and 91. The HR-EIMS gave exact mass of compound **1** at *m/z* 196.1006 (calcd. 196.1009 for $C_{11}H_{16}O_3$). The IR spectrum showed an absorption peak at 3383 cm^{-1} for the hydroxyl group. The ^{1}H-NMR spectrum revealed signals for three aromatic protons at δ_H 6.44 (1H, d, J = 2.4 Hz, H-3), δ_H 6.50 (1H, dd, J = 8.1, 2.4 Hz, H-5), and δ_H 7.06 (1H, d, J = 8.1 Hz, H-6), while the methoxy group at aromatic ring appeared at δ_H 3.77 (3H, s, OCH_3). The only methyl group appeared at δ_H 1.31 (3H, d, J = 7.1Hz, CH_3), while the methine signal centered at δ_H 3.20 (1H, m, H-3′) as shown in **Table 1**. Similarly, the methylene signal bearing hydroxyl group resonated at δ_H 3.39 (1H, m, H-1′), δ_H 3.68 (1H, m, H-1′) and the other methylene signal appeared at δ_H 1.53 (1H, m, H-2′), δ_H 2.01 (1H, m, H-2′). Methylene proton (H-5) showed *ortho* coupling with H-6 at δ_H 7.06 (1H, d, J = 8.1 Hz) and *meta* coupling with H-3 at δ_H 6.44 (1H, d, J = 2.4 Hz) characteristic of aromatic ring (Lal et al., 1987).

The ^{13}C-NMR spectra showed the presence of 11 carbon atom, including one methyl, one methoxy group, two methylene, four methine, and three quaternary carbons. The ^{13}C-NMR revealed the presence of aromatic carbon signal at δ_C 124 (C-1),

TABLE 1 | ^{1}H-NMR ($CDCl_3$, 300 MHz) data of compounds [**1** and **2**] in ppm, J in Hz.

Position	1	2
1	–	–
2	–	–
3	6.44 (d, J = 2.4 Hz)	6.45 (d, J = 2.5 Hz)
4	–	–
5	6.50 (dd, J = 8.1, 2.4 Hz)	6.52 (dd, J = 8.1, 2.5 Hz)
6	7.06 (d, J = 8.1 Hz)	7.06 (d, J = 8.1Hz)
7	–	–
8	–	–
9	–	–
10	–	–
1′	3.39, m 3.68, m	–
2′	1.53 m 2.01, m	2.90, m 3.08, m
3′	3.20, m	3.29, m
7-CH_3	1.31 (d, J = 7.1)	1.30 (d, J = 7.8)
8-OCH_3	3.77, s	3.74, s

155.1 (C-2), 102 (C-3), 158.6 (C-4), 106.9 (C-5), and 127.2 (C-6). Similarly, the signal for methoxy carbon appeared at δ_C 55.8, while methyl group resonated at δ_C 21.1. The downfield methylene appeared at δ_C 60.9 (C-1′) while other methylene signal was observed at δ_C 40.7 (C-2′). The HMBC spectrum confirmed the position of methoxy group at aromatic ring having HMBC correlation with C-4, C-5, and C-3. Similarly, the other data derived from ^{1}H-NMR and ^{13}C-NMR were supported by HMBC connectivity. The placement of the side chain at C-1 of the aromatic ring was supported by H-H-COSY and HMBC correlation (**Figure 2**). The HMBC correlation of the methine proton (δ_H 3.20) showed strong connectivity with aromatic carbon C-1, C-2, and C-6, and this proton was further correlated to CH_3, C-1′, and C-2′. Likewise the placement of CH_3 group at C-3′ was also suggested by HMBC which in turn showed correlation with C-2′, C-3′, and aromatic C-1. The structure proposed from spectral data for compound **1** was 2-(4-hydroxybutan-2-yl)-5-methoxyphenol.

The isolated compound **2** (colorless oil) was an aromatic acid. The EI–MS data which showed molecular ion peak at *m/z* 210 and HR-EI–MS gave the exact mass of compound **2** as *m/z* 210.0899 with molecular formula $C_{11}H_{14}O_4$, having Δ^5 degree of unsaturation. The compound **2** showed some characteristic mass fragments at *m/z* 192, 164, and 117. The IR absorption

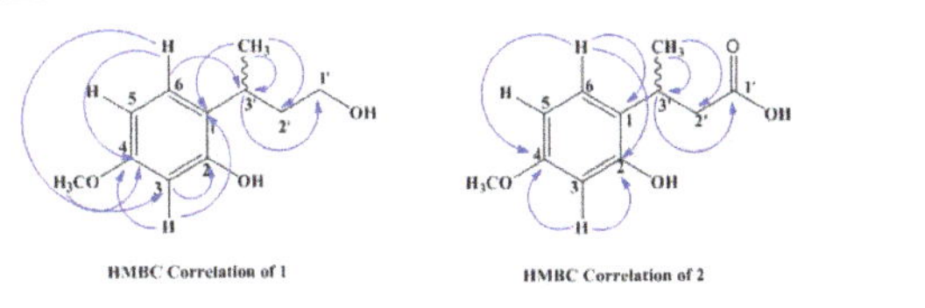

FIGURE 2 | Important HMBC correlation of compounds [**1** and **2**].

TABLE 2 | ^{13}C-NMR ($CDCl_3$, 75 MHz) data of compounds [**1** and **2**] in ppm.

Position	1	2
1	124.1	124.9
2	155.1	155.1
3	102.1	106.1
4	158.6	159.7
5	106.9	106.7
6	127.2	126.5
7	–	–
8	–	–
9	–	–
10	–	–
1′	60.9	178.4
2′	40.7	52.9
3′	26.3	26.1
7-CH_3	21.1	20.9
8-OCH_3	55.8	55.8

showed the presence of hydroxyl group signal at 3502 cm^{-1} and carboxyl group at 1721 cm^{-1}. The ^{1}H-NMR spectrum showed the presence of aromatic proton at position H-5 (δ_H 6.52, 1H, dd, J = 8.1, 2.5 Hz) having *ortho* and *meta* coupling with H-6 (δ_H 7.06, 1H, d, J = 8.1 Hz) and H-4 (δ_H 6.45, 1H, d, J = 2.5 Hz), respectively, quite identical to compound **2** (Lal et al., 1987). In addition, the methyl group resonated at δ_H 1.30 (3H, d, J = 7.8Hz, CH_3) and methine signal centered at δ_H 3.29 (1H, m, H-3′). The methylene signal appeared at δ_H 3.40 (1H, m, H-2′), δ_H 3.69 (1H, m, H-2′). The methoxy group in compound **2** at aromatic ring was resonated at δ_H 3.74 (3H, s, OCH_3) while the methylene signal appeared at δ_H 2.90 (1H, m, H-2′), δ_H 3.08 (1H, m, H-2′). The ^{13}C-NMR spectra showed the presence of 11 carbon atoms, including one methyl, one methoxy group, one methylene, three methine, and four quaternary carbons (as shown in **Table 2**).

The carbon spectrum showed aromatic signals at δ_C 124.9 (C-1), 155.1 (C-2), 106.1 (C-3), 159.7 (C-4), 106.7 (C-5), and 126.5 (C-6). Similarly, the signal for methoxy group appeared at δ_C 55.8, while methyl group resonated at 20.9 and downfield methylene appeared at δ_C 52.9 (C-2′). The HMBC correlations of compound **2** confirmed the position of methoxy group at aromatic ring having interactions with C-4, C-5, and C-3 (**Figure 2** and **Tables 1, 2**). All other data derived from ^{1}H-NMR and ^{13}C-NMR were supported by HMBC connectivity. The HMBC correlation of the methine proton δ_H 3.29 showed strong connectivity with C-1, C-2 and C-6, C-1′, C-2′, and CH_3. Likewise, position of CH_3 at C-3′ is also suggested through HMBC which in turn presents correlation with C-2′, C-3′, as well as aromatic C-1. Finally, the structure of compound **2** was found as 3-(2-hydroxy-4-methoxyphenyl) butanoic acid.

Characterization of Compound 1

Colorless oil: IR (KBr) υ_{max} 3383 cm^{-1}. EI–MS m/z: (rel. int.) 196 $[M]^+$ (35), 181 (20), 151 (100), 137 (25), 91 (37). HR-EI–MS: m/z 196.1006 (calcd. 196.1099 for $C_{11}H_{16}O_3$). ^{1}H-NMR ($CDCl_3$, 300 MHz): δ_H 6.44 (1H, d, J = 2.4 Hz, H-3), 6.50 (1H, dd, J = 8.1, 2.4 Hz, H-5), 7.06 (1H, d, J = 8.1 Hz, H-6), 3.20 (1H, m, H-1′), 1.53 (1H, m, H-2′), 2.01 (1H, m, H-2′), 3.68 (1H, m, H-3′), 3.39 (1H, m, H-3′), 1.31 (CH_3, d, J = 7.1 Hz, H-7), 3.77 (OCH_3, s). ^{13}C-NMR ($CDCl_3$, 75 MHz): δ_C 124.1 (C-1), 155.1 (C-2), 102.4 (C-3), 158.6 (C-4), 106.9 (C-5), 127.2 (C-6), 60.9 (C-1′), 40.7 (C-2′), 26.3 (C-3′), 21.1 (CH_3), 55.8 (OCH_3).

Characterization of Compound 2

Colorless oil: IR (KBr) υ_{max} 3502, 1761 cm^{-1}. EI–MS m/z: (rel. int.) 210 $[M]^+$ (11), 192 (40), 164 (33), 117 (65). HR-EI–MS: m/z 210.0899 (calcd. 210.0892 for $C_{11}H_{14}O_4$). ^{1}H-NMR ($CDCl_3$, 300 MHz): δ_H 6.45 (1H, d, J = 2.5 Hz, H-3), 6.52 (1H, dd, J = 8.1, 2.5 Hz, H-5), 7.06 (1H, d, J = 8.1 Hz, H-6), 1.30 (3H, d, J = 7.8 Hz, H-7), 3.74 (3H, s, H-8), 2.90, 3.08 (2H, m, H-2′), 3.29 (1H, m, H-3′), ^{13}C-NMR ($CDCl_3$, 75 MHz): δ_C 124.9 (C-1), 155.1 (C-2), 106.1 (C-3), 159.7 (C-4), 106.7 (C-5), 126.5 (C-6), 178.4 (C-1′), 52.9 (C-2′), 26.1 (C-3′), 20.9 (CH_3), 55.8 (OCH_3).

Acute Toxicity

No pronounced changes in the behavior of animals were evident by compounds [1 and 2] at dosage levels of 100 and 200 mg/kg. There had been observed no effect on sedation, respiration, convulsions and grooming, or muscle activity.

Anxiolytic-Like Effects in EPM Test

The effect of 3′-MeO6MF or diazepam in the behavior of mice in elevated plus maze (EPM) is given in **Figure 3**. Both diazepam and compounds **1** and **2** significantly reduced the anxiety in mice. Compound **1** at dose levels of 01, 10, and 30 mg/kg, i.p., effectively resulted in an increase of % open-arm entries as well as % time spent in open arms of the EPM ($^*P < 0.05$, $^*P < 0.01$, respectively, $n = 6$, one-way ANOVA followed by Dunnett's test). As shown in **Figure 3**, compound **2** at dose levels of 10 and 30 mg/kg also showed pronounced increase in open-arm entries and % increase in time spent within open arm ($^*P < 0.05$, $^*P < 0.01$, respectively, $n = 6$, one-way ANOVA followed by Dunnett's test). The standard reference drug diazepam at 1 mg/kg, i.p., also increased % open-arm entries and % time spent in open arms of the EPM ($^{**}P < 0.01$, $n = 6$, one-way ANOVA followed by Dunnett's test).

Effect of Flumazenil on the Anxiolytic-Like Activity of Compounds 1 and 2 in the EPM

In order to identify the involvement of BDZ-binding site, flumazenil was used to antagonize the effects of compounds **1** and **2**. As shown in **Figure 4**, flumazenil (2.5 mg/kg) completely abolished the increases in the number of open-arm entries and % increase in time spent in open arms by compounds **1** and **2**. This effect was similar to that of diazepam indicating that compounds **1** and **2** (10 mg/kg) were mediating its anxiolytic-like effect *via* the BDZ receptors (**Figure 4**).

Anxiolytic-Like Effects of Compounds 1 and 2 in Light Dark/Dark Box Test

The behavioral effects of diazepam, compounds **1** and **2**, or vehicle in the light–dark box (LDB) test are shown in **Figure 5**.

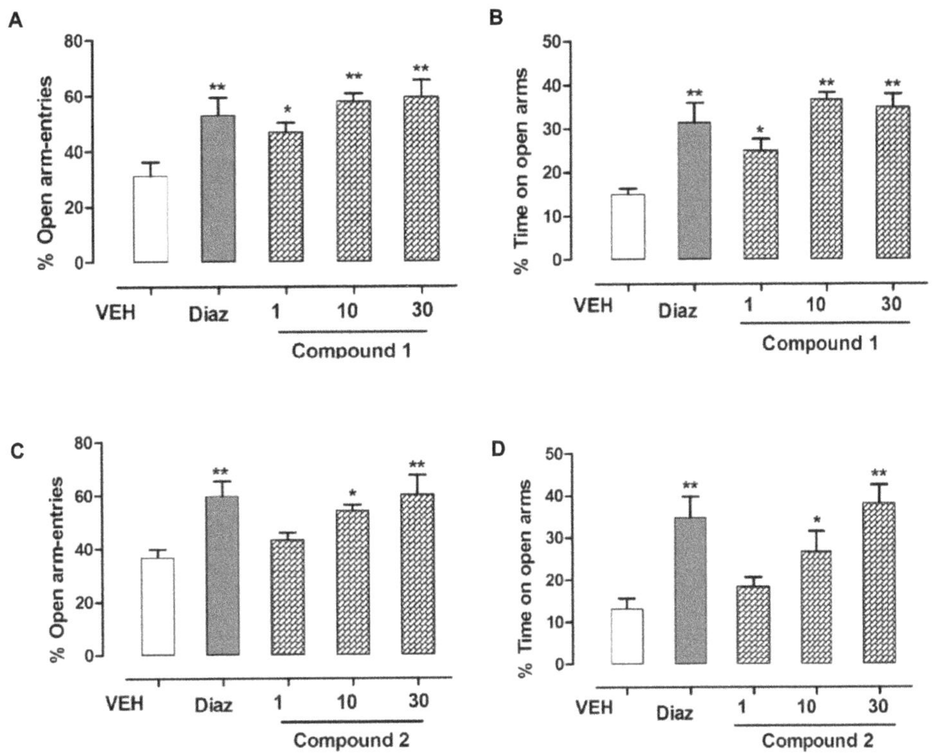

FIGURE 3 | Effect of compounds **1** and **2** and diazepam on the behavior of mice in the EPM. **(A)** % open-arm entries, **(B)** % time spent in open arms registered over a session of 5 min, after 20 min of an i.p. injection of compound **1** (1, 10, and 30 mg/kg), diazepam (1 mg/kg), or vehicle. **(C)** % open-arm entries **(D)** % time spent in open arms registered over a session of 5 min, after 20 min of an i.p. injection of compound **2** (1, 10, and 30 mg/kg), diazepam (1 mg/kg), or vehicle. Column represents mean ± SEM (n = 6/group). $^*P < 0.05$, $^{**}P < 0.01$, compared with vehicle group using one-way ANOVA followed by Dunnett's test.

Outcomes from ANOVA analysis revealed that compound **1**, at the dose levels (10 and 30 mg/kg, i.p), has not only effectively increased time spent in light compartment but also increased the transitions across two compartments ($^*P < 0.05$, $^{**}P < 0.01$, respectively, $n = 6$, one-way ANOVA followed by Dunnett's test). Similar results were obtained for compound **2** which also significantly enhanced time spent in light compartment as well as number of transitions across the two compartments ($^*P < 0.05$, $^{**}P < 0.01$, respectively, $n = 6$, one-way ANOVA followed by Dunnett's test) at dose levels of 10 and 30 mg/kg. The diazepam which was taken as reference drug (1 mg/kg, i.p.) also significantly ($^{**}P < 0.01$; n = 6, one-way ANOVA followed by Dunnett's test) enhanced time spent in light area of the light–dark box showing anti-anxiety potential, which confirmed the validity of paradigm.

Antidepressant-Like Effects in Forced Swimming Test

The effects of compounds **1** and **2** in mice FST were summarized in **Table 3**. Intraperitoneal administration of compounds **1** and **2** at doses of 10 and 30 mg/kg significantly decreased the immobility time in the FST compared to the control (vehicle) ($^*P < 0.05$; $^{**}P < 0.01$; one-way ANOVA, followed by Dunnett's test). Imipramine was used as a reference drug which also significantly decreased the immobility time in comparison with vehicle at a dose of 60 mg/kg ($^{***}P < 0.001$; one-way ANOVA followed by Dunnett's test).

Antidepressant-Like Effects in Tail Suspension Test

The effects of compounds **1** and **2** in the tail suspension test (TST) were shown in **Table 4**. Intraperitoneal administration of the reference drug, imipramine at the dose of 60 mg/kg, significantly decreased the immobility time compared to the vehicle ($^{***}P < 0.001$; one-way ANOVA, followed by Dunnett's test). Compounds **1** and **2** at the doses of 10 and 30 mg/kg also caused a significant decrease in the immobility time compared to the vehicle control group ($^*P < 0.05$; $^{**}P < 0.01$; one-way ANOVA, followed by Dunnett's test).

DISCUSSION

Anxiety and depression are the most prevalent health problems among other mood disorders worldwide. In this study, the anxiolytic- and antidepressant-like effects of compounds **1** and **2** had been studied in different animal models of anxiety and depression. In this study, compounds **1** and **2** exerted significant anxiolytic effects in both EPM and light dark tests (LDTs). In the EPM, compound **1** dose dependently increased the exploratory

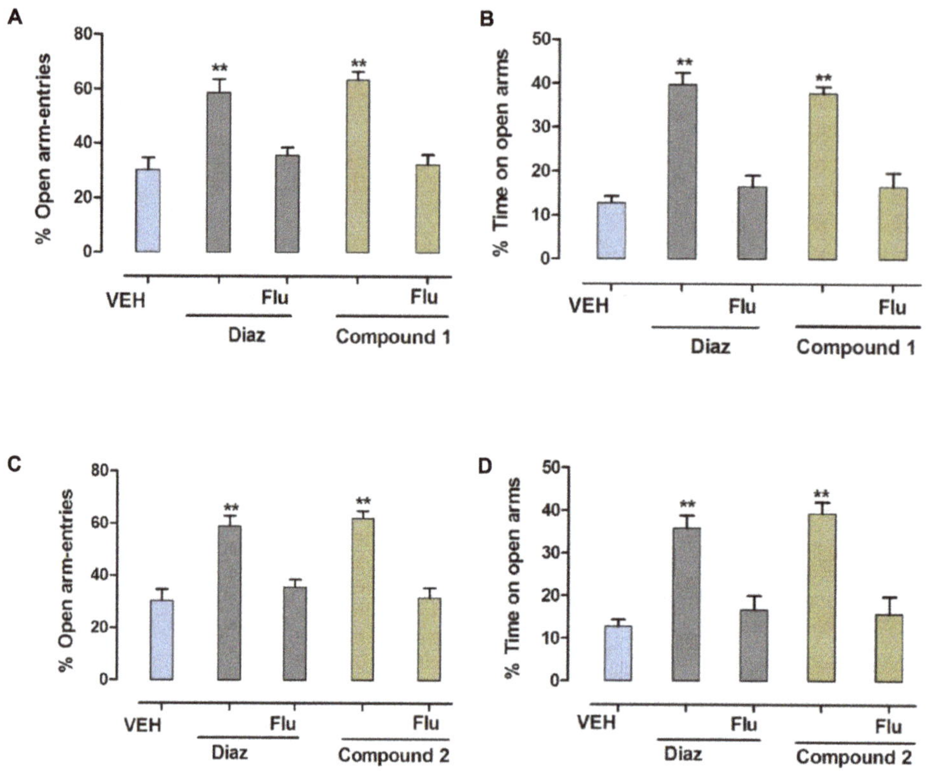

FIGURE 4 | Effect of flumazenil on the anxiolytic activity of compounds **1** and **2** in the EPM. **(A)** % entries in open arms, **(B)** % time spent in open arms registered over a session of 5 min, after 20 min of an i.p. injection of vehicle, diazepam (1 mg/kg), and compound **1** (10 mg/kg), **(C)** % entries in open arms, **(D)** % time spent in open arms registered over a session of 5 min, after 20 min of an i.p. injection of vehicle, diazepam (1 mg/kg), and compound **2** (10 mg/kg) in the presence of flumazenil (2.5 mg/kg). Columns express mean ± SEM (n = 6/group), n = 6 per group. $^{**}P < 0.01$, compared with vehicle control group using one-way ANOVA post-Dunnett's test. Co-administration of flumazenil (2.5 mg/kg) blocked the anti-anxiety action of compounds **1** and **2** (10 mg/kg showing the anxiolytic effect is mediated via the benzodiazepine site.

behavior of mice by increasing both the % open-arm entries and time spent on open arms ($^{*}P < 0.05$, $^{**}P < 0.01$, $^{***}P < 0.001$; $n = 6$). Similarly, compound **2** also significantly increased the % open-arm entries and time spent on open arms at the dose level of 10 and 30 mg/kg indicating anxiolytic-like effects ($^{*}P < 0.05$, $^{**}P < 0.01$; $n = 6$). Co-administration flumazenil (2.5 mg/kg) with compounds **1** and **2** (10 mg/kg) completely abolished the anxiolytic-like activity of compounds **1** and **2** indicating that the BZP site of GABAergic system was involved in the anxiolytic-like activity. In LDB test, the ANOVA analysis demonstrates that compound **1** at the dose level of 1–30 mg/kg exerted significant anxiolytic-like effect ($^{*}P < 0.05$, $^{**}P < 0.01$, $^{***}P < 0.001$; $n = 6$). Similarly, compound **2** showed significant anxiolytic activity at the dose level of 10 and 30 mg/kg ($^{*}P < 0.05$, $^{**}P < 0.01$; $n = 6$). The anxiolytic-like effect of both compounds at 30 mg/kg was comparable to the standard reference drug diazepam in both EPM and LDB tests.

The EPM and LDTs were the most important behavioral assays for the assessment of anxiolytic-like effect. Several studies have reported that GABAergic neurotransmission was involved in expression etiology and therapy of anxiety disorders (Chakraborty et al., 2010). The sensitivity of EPM to the effect of both anti-anxiety and anxiogenic drug acting at the $GABA_A$ BZP complex was very high (Nic Dhonnchadha et al., 2003). In EPM, normal animals were normally chosen to spend much of their allowed time in the closed arms. This orientation seems to reflect a distaste toward open arms that was produced by the anxiety of the open spaces. Drug like diazepam that enhances exploration on open arm are believed as anxiolytic and the opposite holds right for anxiogenics.

Administration of compounds **1** and **2** prior to test significantly decreased the total immobility time compared to the vehicle control. Similar results were obtained in TST, another primary screening test for detecting antidepressant substances. The TST also induces a state of despair in animals similar to that in FST (Steru et al., 1985). Both compounds [**1** and **2**] dose dependently decreased the immobility time in TST. The reduction in immobility time in both TST and FST was dose dependent with no effect at 1 mg/kg.

The tail suspension and forced swimming tests are the most validated animal models to evaluate substances with putative antidepressant-like effects (Porsolt et al., 1977; Steru et al., 1985). In FST, when rodents are forced to swim in a confined, they tend to become immobile after an initial period of struggling. This inescapable stressful situation is evaluated by assessing different behavioral parameters (Porsolt et al., 1978).

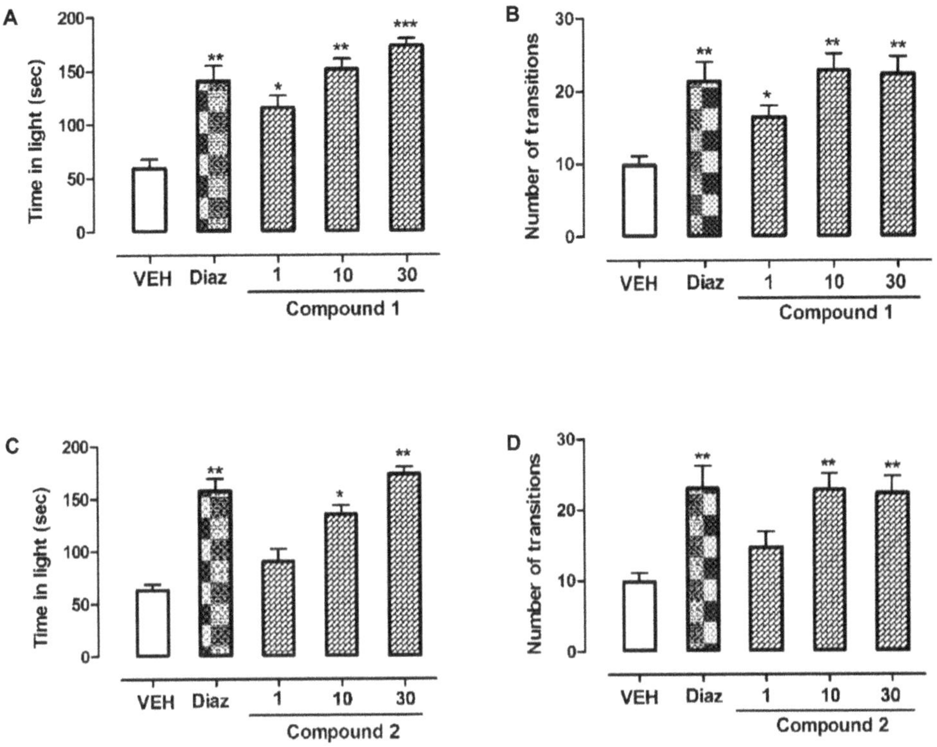

FIGURE 5 | Effect of compounds **1** and **2** and diazepam on the behavior of mice in the light–dark box test. **(A)** Time spent in lit area, **(B)** number of transitions recorded over a session of 5 min, after 20 min of an i.p. injection of compound **1** (1, 10, and 30 mg/kg), diazepam (1 mg/kg), or vehicle. **(C)** Time spent in lit area, **(D)** number of transitions recorded over a session of 5 min, after 20 min of an i.p. injection of compound **2** (1, 10, and 30 mg/kg), diazepam (1 mg/kg), or vehicle. Values express mean ± SEM (*n* = 6/group). **P* < 0.05, ***P* < 0.01, and ****P* < 0.001 compared with vehicle group using one-way ANOVA followed by Dunnett's test.

TABLE 3 | Effect of compounds **1** and **2** on immobility period (seconds) of mice using forced swimming test.

Treatment	Dose (mg/kg)	Immobility time (seconds)
Control	–	170.5 ± 8.5
Compound **1**	1	168.4 ± 6.5
	10	120.5 ± 5.5*
	30	85.3 ± 7.2**
Compound **2**	1	169.4 ± 4.4
	10	145.3 ± 4.5*
	30	105.5 ± 10.3**
Imipramine	60	75.5 ± 9.6***

*All values are expressed in mean ± SEM (n = 6). *P < 0.05, **P < 0.01, ***P < 0.001 compared to the vehicle group. Difference between groups was analyzed by ANOVA (one-way ANOVA followed by Dunnett's test).*

TABLE 4 | Effect of compounds 1 and 2 on immobility period (seconds) of mice using tail suspension test.

Treatment	Dose (mg/kg)	Immobility time (seconds)
Control	–	165.6 ± 12.5
Compound 1	1	159.4 ± 8.5
	10	130.5 ± 5.5*
	30	90.5 ± 4.2**
Compound 2	1	161.4 ± 8.4
	10	141.3 ± 6.5*
	30	96.5 ± 7.5**
Imipramine	60	80.5 ± 9.5***

*All values are expressed in mean ± SEM (n = 6). *P < 0.05, **P < 0.01, ***P < 0.001 compared to the vehicle group. Difference between groups was analyzed by ANOVA (one-way ANOVA followed by Dunnett's test).*

Several neurotransmitters have been implicated in the pathophysiology of depressive disorders including GABA, serotonin, noradrenalin, and dopamine (Dailly et al., 2004; Abdelhalim et al., 2015). Thus, depression has been believed to be due to deficiency of one or another of these neurotransmitters (Willner et al., 2005; Luscher et al., 2011). Furthermore, in the present study, flumazenil was able to antagonize the anxiolytic-like effect of compounds **1** and **2** in the EPM and LDB test suggests the involvement of these biogenic amines in the antidepressant-like effects of these compounds.

CONCLUSION

Compounds **1** and **2** exerted anxiolytic and antidepressant-like effects in classical mouse models of anxiety and depression. Additionally the results indicated that the anxiolytic-like effect may involve the BZP site of GABA-A receptors. Thus, this study provides valuable preliminary data on the anxiolytic and antidepressant-like effects of compounds **1** and **2** isolated from *Q. incana*. However, further studies are required to elucidate the antidepressant-like mechanisms and to conduct further preclinical and clinical studies of these compounds.

AUTHOR CONTRIBUTIONS

AK and UF conceived and designed the study. RS and SN performed the isolation and SB helped in the structure elucidation. NK and IK performed *in vivo* studies. HK and AA analyzed the data. UF, AK, and AA wrote the manuscript with inputs and comments from all co-authors. All authors read and approved the final version of the manuscript.

FUNDING

This research did not receive any specific grant from funding agencies in the public, commercial, or not-for-profit sectors.

REFERENCES

Abdelhalim, A., Karim, N., Chebib, M., Aburjai, T., Khan, I., Johnston, G. A., et al. (2015). Antidepressant, anxiolytic and antinociceptive activities of constituents from *Rosmarinus officinalis*. *J. Pharm. Pharm. Sci.* 18, 448–459.

Barua, C. C., Roy, J. D., Buragohain, B., Barua, A. G., Borah, P., and Lahkar, M. (2009). Anxiolytic effect of hydroethanolic extract of *Drymaria cordata* L Willd. *Indian J. Exp. Biol.* 47, 969–973.

Belzung, C., Misslin, R., Vogel, E., Dodd, R. H., and Chapouthier, G. (1987). Anxiogenic effects of methyl-β-carboline-3-carboxylate in a light/dark choice situation. *Pharmacol. Biochem. Behav.* 28, 29–33.

Berahou, A., Auhmani, A., Fdil, N., Benharref, A., Jana, M., and Gadhi, C. (2007). Antibacterial activity of *Quercus ilex* bark's extracts. *J. Ethnopharmacol.* 112, 426–429.

Berton, O., and Nestler, E. J. (2006). New approaches to antidepressant drug discovery: beyond monoamines. *Nat. Rev. Neurosci.* 7, 137–151.

Bourin, M., and Hascoët, M. (2003). The mouse light/dark box test. *Eur. J. Pharmacol.* 463, 55–65.

Chakraborty, A., Amudha, P., Geetha, M., and Singh, N. S. (2010). Evaluation of anxiolytic activity of methanolic extract of *Sapindus mukorossi* Gaertn. in mice. *Int. J. Pharmacol. Bio Sci.* 1, 1–8.

Dailly, E., Chenu, F., Renard, C. E., and Bourin, M. (2004). Dopamine, depression and antidepressants. *Fundam. Clin. Pharmacol.* 18, 601–607.

Gonçalves, A. E., Bürger, C., Amoah, S. K. S., Tolardo, R., Biavatti, M. W., and de Souza, M. M. (2012). The antidepressant-like effect of *Hedyosmum brasiliense* and its sesquiterpene lactone, podoandin in mice: evidence for the involvement of adrenergic, dopaminergic and serotonergic systems. *Eur. J. Pharmacol.* 674, 307–314. doi: 10.1016/j.ejphar.2011.11.009

González-Trujano, M. E., Hernández-Sánchez, L. Y., Muñoz Ocotero, V., Dorazco-González, A., Guevara Fefer, P., and Aguirre-Hernández, E. (2017). Pharmacological evaluation of the anxiolytic-like effects of *Lippia graveolens* and bioactive compounds. *Pharm. Biol.* 55, 1569–1576. doi: 10.1080/13880209.2017.1310908

Gupta, V., Bansal, P., Kumar, P., and Shri, R. (2010). Anxiolytic and antidepressant activities of different extracts from *Citrus paradisi* var. duncan. *Asian J. Pharm. Clin. Res.* 3, 98–100.

Jothimanivannan, C., Kumar, R., and Subramanian, N. (2010). Anti-inflammatory and analgesic activities of ethanol extract of aerial parts of *Justicia gendarussa* Burm. *Int. J. Pharmacol.* 6, 278–283.

Kalueff, A. V., and Tuohimaa, P. (2004). Experimental modeling of anxiety and depression. *Acta Neurobiol. Exp.* 64, 439–448.

Karim, N., Irshad, S., Khan, I., Mohammad, A., Anis, I., Shah, M. R., et al. (2015). GABA(A) receptor modulation and neuropharmacological activities of viscosine isolated from *Dodonaea viscosa* (Linn). *Pharmacol. Biochem. Behav.* 136, 64–72. doi: 10.1016/j.pbb.2015.07.006

Khan, I., Karim, N., Ahmad, W., Abdelhalim, A., and Chebib, M. (2016). GABA-A receptor modulation and anticonvulsant, anxiolytic, and antidepressant activities of constituents from *Artemisia indica* Linn. *Evid. Based Complement. Alternat. Med.* 2016:1215393. doi: 10.1155/2016/1215393

Kocyigit, I., Unal, A., Sipahioglu, M., Tokgoz, B., Oymak, O., and Utas, C. (2010). Peritoneal dialysis-related peritonitis due to *Neisseria weaveri*: the first case report. *Perit. Dial. Int.* 30, 116–117.

Kudagi, B., Kumar, R. P., and Basha, S. S. (2012). Evaluation of anti-anxiety, sedative and motor co-ordination properties of ganaxolone in comparison with diazepam in rodent models. *J. Dent. Med. Sci.* 1, 42–47.

Lal, K., Ghosh, S., and Salomon, R. G. (1987). Hydroxyl-directed regioselective monodemethylation of polymethoxyarenes. *J. Org. Chem.* 52, 1072–1078.

Luscher, B., Shen, Q., and Sahir, N. (2011). The GABAergic deficit hypothesis of major depressive disorder. *Mol. Psychiatry* 16, 383–406. doi: 10.1038/mp.2010.120

Manan, Z., Razzaq, A., and Islam, M. (2007). Diversity of medicinal plants in Wari subdivision district Upper Dir, Pakistan. *Pak. J. Plant Sci.* 45, 231–234.

Nasir, E., and Ali, S. I. (1976). *Flora of West Pakistan*. Rawalpindi: Botany Department.

Nic Dhonnchadha, B. A., Bourin, M., and Hascoët, M. (2003). Anxiolytic-like effects of 5-HT 2 ligands on three mouse models of anxiety. *Behav. Brain Res.* 140, 203–214.

Porsolt, R. D., Anton, G., Blavet, N., and Jalfre, M. (1978). Behavioural despair in rats: a new model sensitive to antidepressant treatments. *Eur. J. Pharmacol.* 47, 379–391.

Porsolt, R. D., Bertin, A., and Jalfre, M. (1977). Behavioral despair in mice: a primary screening test for antidepressants. *Arch. Int. Pharmacodyn. Ther.* 229, 327–336.

Reddy, M. S. (2010). Depression: the disorder and the burden. *Indian J. Psychol. Med.* 32, 1–2.

Sadanandam, A., and Christopher, T. (2010). Hypoglycemic activity of red kino tree in normal and streptozotocin induced diabetic rats. *Int. J. Pharmacol.* 6, 301–305.

Sarwar, G., Ibrar, M., Barkatullah, M. N., Muhammad, N., Sirajuddin, and Rauf, A. (2013). Evaluation of crude ethanolic extract of *Quercus incana* fruit for analgesic and gastrointestinal motility profile. *Middle East J. Sci. Res.* 13, 455–458.

Sarwar, R., Farooq, U., Khan, A., Naz, S., Khan, S., Khan, A., et al. (2015). Evaluation of antioxidant, free radical scavenging, and antimicrobial activity of *Quercus incana* Roxb. *Front. Pharmacol.* 6:277. doi: 10.3389/fphar.2015.00277

Sharmen, F., Mannan, A., Rahman, M. M., Chowdhury, M. A. U., Uddin, M. E., and Ahmed, A. A. (2014). Investigation of *in vivo* neuropharmacological effect of *Alpinia nigra* leaf extract. *Asian Pac. J. Trop. Biomed.* 4, 137–142. doi: 10.1016/S2221-1691(14)60222-7

Steru, L., Chermat, R., Thierry, B., and Simon, P. (1985). The tail suspension test: a new method for screening antidepressants in mice. *Psychopharmacology* 85, 367–370.

Thaina, P., Tungcharoen, P., Wongnawa, M., Reanmongkol, W., and Subhadhirasakul, S. (2009). Uterine relaxant effects of *Curcuma aeruginosa* Roxb. rhizome extracts. *J. Ethnopharmacol.* 121, 433–443. doi: 10.1016/j.jep.2008.10.022

Willner, P., Hale, A. S., and Argyropoulos, S. (2005). Dopaminergic mechanism of antidepressant action in depressed patients. *J. Affect. Disord.* 86, 37–45.

Yadav, A., Kawale, L., and Nade, V. (2008). Effect of *Morus alba* L. (mulberry) leaves on anxiety in mice. *Indian J. Pharmacol.* 40, 32–36. doi: 10.4103/0253-7613.40487

14

Plant Extracts and Phytochemicals Targeting α-Synuclein Aggregation in Parkinson's Disease Models

Hayate Javed[1], *Mohamed Fizur Nagoor Meeran*[2], *Sheikh Azimullah*[2], *Abdu Adem*[2*], *Bassem Sadek*[2] *and Shreesh Kumar Ojha*[2*]

[1] *Department of Anatomy, College of Medicine and Health Sciences, United Arab Emirates University, Al Ain, United Arab Emirates,* [2] *Department of Pharmacology and Therapeutics, College of Medicine and Health Sciences, United Arab Emirates University, Al Ain, United Arab Emirates*

***Correspondence:**
Abdu Adem
abdu.adem@uaeu.ac.ae
Shreesh Kumar Ojha
shreeshojha@uaeu.ac.ae

α-Synuclein (α-syn) is a presynaptic protein that regulates the release of neurotransmitters from synaptic vesicles in the brain. α-Syn aggregates, including Lewy bodies, are features of both sporadic and familial forms of Parkinson's disease (PD). These aggregates undergo several key stages of fibrillation, oligomerization, and aggregation. Therapeutic benefits of drugs decline with disease progression and offer only symptomatic treatment. Novel therapeutic strategies are required which can either prevent or delay the progression of the disease. The link between α-syn and the etiopathogenesis and progression of PD are well-established in the literature. Studies indicate that α-syn is an important therapeutic target and inhibition of α-syn aggregation, oligomerization, and fibrillation are an important disease modification strategy. However, recent studies have shown that plant extracts and phytochemicals have neuroprotective effects on α-syn oligomerization and fibrillation by targeting different key stages of its formation. Although many reviews on the antioxidant-mediated, neuroprotective effect of plant extracts and phytochemicals on PD symptoms have been well-highlighted, the antioxidant mechanisms show limited success for translation to clinical studies. The identification of specific plant extracts and phytochemicals that target α-syn aggregation will provide selective molecules to develop new drugs for PD. The present review provides an overview of plant extracts and phytochemicals that target α-syn in PD and summarizes the observed effects and the underlying mechanisms. Furthermore, we provide a synopsis of current experimental models and techniques used to evaluate plant extracts and phytochemicals. Plant extracts and phytochemicals were found to inhibit the aggregation or fibril formation of oligomers. These also appear to direct α-syn oligomer formation into its unstructured form or promote non-toxic pathways and suggested to be valuable drug candidates for PD and related synucleinopathy. Current evidences from *in vitro* studies require confirmation in the *in vivo* studies. Further studies are needed to ascertain their potential effects and safety in preclinical studies for pharmaceutical/nutritional development of these phytochemicals or dietary inclusion of the plant extracts in PD treatment.

Keywords: α-synuclein, plants, phytochemicals, Parkinson's disease, neuroprotective, natural products, neurotoxicity, bioactive agents

INTRODUCTION

Parkinson's disease (PD) is a progressive, debilitating neurodegenerative disease that often begins with the gradual loss of dopaminergic neurons in the substantia nigra pars compacta (SNc) (Herrera et al., 2017). It is a common age-related movement disorder that often appears sporadically (Collier et al., 2017). The pathogenesis of PD remains poorly understood, but emerging evidence implicates various genetic and environmental factors in the initiation and progression of PD (Cannon and Greenamyre, 2013). The multifactorial etiopathogensis of PD includes mitochondrial dysfunction, excitotoxicity, endoplasmic reticulum stress, oxidative/nitrosative stress, and inflammation, along with ubiquitin-proteasome system dysfunction (Moore et al., 2005; Lashuel et al., 2013; Ur Rasheed et al., 2016; Gelders et al., 2018). Altogether, these events lead to the accumulation of abnormal or misfolded α-synuclein (α-syn) protein (Moore et al., 2005; Lashuel et al., 2013; Ur Rasheed et al., 2016; Gelders et al., 2018). Numerous genetic, biochemical, cellular, pathological, and molecular studies indicate PD pathogenesis is associated with environments where α-syn is susceptible to polymerization, aggregation and fibril formation, and propagation (Moore et al., 2005; Hansen and Li, 2012; Lashuel et al., 2013; Gelders et al., 2018; Ghiglieri et al., 2018). The α-syn oligomers cause mitochondrial dysfunction and induce endoplasmic stress, oxidative stress, neuroinflammation, and inhibit proteasomal activity and autophagy (Ghiglieri et al., 2018).

Current PD treatment options, such as dopamine agonists, cholinesterase, and monoamine oxidase inhibitors provide only symptomatic relief (Ellis and Fell, 2017). Dopamine-based drugs have reduced effectiveness in relieving symptoms with disease progression (Ceravolo et al., 2016). The oligomerization and fibrillation of α-syn is linked with the onset and progression of PD (Hansen and Li, 2012), and is believed to be a unique and convincing disease-modification therapeutic strategy for PD, dementia with Lewy body (DLB), and related α-synucleinopathy (Kalia et al., 2015; Török et al., 2016; Brundin et al., 2017). Several molecules including antibodies (Bergström et al., 2016), polyamines (Büttner et al., 2014), heat shock proteins (Cox et al., 2016), chaperones (Friesen et al., 2017), and pharmaceuticals (Lauterbach et al., 2010) have been shown to affect different forms of α-syn (i.e., monomers, soluble oligomers, protofibrils, or fibrils) and oligomerization, fibrillation, and clearance. Therefore, targeting α-syn aggregation, oligomerization, fibrillation, and propagation to reduce α-syn toxicity emerged as an important therapeutic target for slowing or halting disease progression (Kalia et al., 2015; Török et al., 2016; Brundin et al., 2017).

Several recent reviews highlighted the neuroprotective potential of plant extracts and phytochemicals in PD through antioxidant and anti-inflammatory activities (Sarrafchi et al., 2016; da Costa et al., 2017; Mazo et al., 2017; Morgan and Grundmann, 2017; Wang et al., 2017; Zhang et al., 2017; Amro and Srijit, 2018). However, despite the enormous success of antioxidants (whether of synthetic or natural origin) in preclinical studies, coenzyme Q10 (Beal et al., 2014), creatine (Attia et al., 2017), and vitamin E (Ahlskog, 1994) either failed or showed marginal neuroprotection in patients. Recently, α-syn antibodies (PRX002) showed safety in phase 1 studies and were indicated for further phases of clinical studies (Schenk et al., 2017; Jankovic et al., 2018). Similarly, natural products (mainly plant extracts and phytochemicals) emerged to specifically target α-syn (Masuda et al., 2006; Meng et al., 2009, 2010; Caruana et al., 2011; Marchiani et al., 2013). Yet, no comprehensive review is available on these plant extracts and phytochemicals, or on how they target the different steps leading to α-syn oligomerization or fibrillation.

This review, therefore, focuses on the neuroprotective properties and mechanism of action of plant extracts, extract-based formulations, and plant-derived phytochemicals that target α-syn oligomerization, fibrillation, aggregation, and toxicity in various experimental PD models. Furthermore, we also elaborate on the suitability of biochemical, biophysical, and neurochemical techniques to evaluate plant extracts and phytochemicals that ameliorate α-syn neurotoxicity. The source of phytochemicals, the models used, and the effect/mechanisms observed are presented in **Tables 1–7**. The chemical structures of these phytochemicals are presented in **Figure 1**. A scheme on the action of the plant extracts and phytochemicals targeting α-syn is presented in **Figure 2**.

α-SYNUCLEIN AS A THERAPEUTIC TARGET FOR PD

α-syn, a 140-residue presynaptic protein in the brain, plays a key role in the trafficking and fusion of synaptic vesicles and it regulates dopamine release at presynaptic terminals (Burre et al., 2010; Bendor et al., 2013). The physiological concentration of α-syn is 1 μM in the normal human brain and 70 pM in cerebrospinal fluid (Borghi et al., 2000). It exists natively as an unfolded monomer and attains an α-helical secondary structure after binding lipid vesicles. Upon destabilization, this leads to the misfolding and aggregation of α-syn in neurons (Ruipérez et al., 2010; Bartels et al., 2011; Broersen et al., 2018). Monomeric α-syn is an intrinsically disordered protein found in different conformational states. It plays a significant role in many key biochemical processes (Tompa, 2005), as well as in a rising number of diseases involving misfolding, notably PD (Uversky and Dunker, 2010). In dopaminergic neurons, the intracytoplasmic inclusions of α-syn (Spillantini et al., 1998), synphilin-1 (Wakabayashi et al., 2000) and ubiquitin (Kuzuhara et al., 1988) form Lewy bodies, a pathological characteristic of PD. The cascade of α-syn aggregation begins with dimer formation, then tiny oligomers/protofibrils that lead to the development of β-sheet-rich α-syn fibrils. These eventually lead to end-stage fibrils and aggregated α-syn that are the major component of Lewy bodies (Ghiglieri et al., 2018). Thus, in the multistep process of α-syn-mediated neuronal toxicity, oligomerization of α-syn monomers is the primary phase that facilitates the development of intracytoplasmic inclusions and fibrils (Spillantini et al., 1997).

Numerous theories have been proposed on the role of α-syn in initiating dopaminergic neurodegeneration in PD (Herrera et al., 2017; Ghiglieri et al., 2018). These include the interaction of α-syn aggregates with biomolecules, impaired

TABLE 1 | The plant extracts and formulations providing neuroprotection in Parkinson's disease models by targeting α-synuclein.

Plant extract(s) (*Plant name,* family)	Experimental model system (s)	Effects and mechanisms observed	References
Acanthopanax senticosus harms (Siberian Ginseng, Araliaceae)	SH-SY5Y cells overexpressing wild-type or A53T mutant α-syn	▪ Inhibits α-syn, caspase-3, Akt, and p-GSK3β ▪ Reverses phospho-microtubule-associated tau in cells	Li et al., 2014
Alaria esculenta (Winged kelp, Araliaceae)	α-syn aggregation biochemical, biophysical assays	▪ Reduces the melting point of α-syn ▪ Inhibits aggregation and fibril formation by interacting with an unfolded form of α-syn	Giffin et al., 2017
Bacopa monnieri (Waterhyssop, Plantaginaceae)	*Caenorhabditis elegans* expressing human α-syn and 6-OHDA expressing GFP neurons	▪ Reduces α-syn aggregation ▪ Prevents dopaminergic cell death	Jadiya et al., 2011
Cinnamon zeylanicum (Cinnamon, Lauraceae)	α-syn aggregation assay and A53T α-syn expression in drosophila	▪ Inhibits α-syn aggregation, stabilizes soluble oligomers of α-syn and redirects to "off-pathway" oligomers ▪ Improves behavior and cognition	Shaltiel-Karyo et al., 2012
Centella asiatica (Asiatic pennywort, Apiaceae)	α-syn aggregation assay	▪ Inhibits α-syn aggregation and stabilizes oligomer ▪ Disintegrates preformed fibrils	Berrocal et al., 2014
Carthamus tinctorius (Safflower extract with flavonoids, Asteraceae)	6-OHDA-induced rat model of PD	▪ Improves behavioral performances ▪ Reduces α-syn aggregation and astrogliosis ▪ Decreases tortuosity and the rate constant of clearance	Ren et al., 2016
Crocus sativus L. (Saffron, Iridaceae)	α-syn aggregation, and α-syn fibril dissociation assays	▪ Prevents dissociation of fibrils and inhibit α-syn aggregation	Inoue et al., 2018
Chondrus crispus (Red seaweed or Irish Moss, Gigartinaceae)	6-OHDA-induced neurodegeneration in transgenic *Caenorhabditis elegans*	▪ Reduces α-syn accumulation ▪ Attenuates oxidatives stress and improved longevity	Liu et al., 2015
Corema album (Portuguese Crowberry, Ericaceae)	Cellular and *in vitro* models of α-syn toxicity and aggregation	▪ Promotes non-toxic α-syn and inhibits its aggregation ▪ Promotes autophagic flux and reduces oxidative stress	Macedo et al., 2015
Geum urbanum (Bennet, colewort, Rosaceae)	α-syn aggregation biochemical, biophysical assays	▪ Inhibits α-syn fibrillation dose dependent ▪ Disintegrates preformed α-syn fibrils	Lobbens et al., 2016
Opuntia ficus-indica (*Prickly pear*, Cactaceae) and *Padina pavonica* (Peacock's tail, brown algae, Dictyotaceae)	PD model of transgenic drosophila expressing human α-syn A53T	▪ Increases lifespan and correct behavioral deficit ▪ Inhibits fibrillogenesis, stabilize/remodeloligomers	Briffa et al., 2017
Panax ginseng (G115) (Asian ginseng, Araliaceae)	β-sitosterol β-d-glucoside-induced PD in rats	▪ Prevents dopaminergic loss and locomotor deficits ▪ Attenuates α-Syn aggregation, microgliosis, and apoptosis	Van Kampen et al., 2003
Polygala tenuifolia (Tenuigenin) (Chinese Senega, Polygalaceae)	SH-SY5Y cells transfected with wild-type or A53T mutant α-syn	▪ Improves cell viability ▪ Reduces α-syn phosphorylation and PLK3 levels	Zhou et al., 2013
S/B formulation (*Scutellaria baicalensis* Georgi; Baikal skullcap, Lamiaceae and *Bupleurum scorzonerifolfium* Willd)	α-syn aggregation in the infused substantia nigra of rats	▪ Attenuates inflammation, apoptosis, oxidative, mitochondrial and ER stress and preserves glutathione ▪ Attenuates astrocytosis/microgliosis, improve dopamine ▪ Inhibits α-syn aggregation in SNc	Lin et al., 2011
Rehmannia glutinosa Libosch (Chinese foxglove, Scrophulariaceae)	Monosodium L-glutamate induced-hippocampal changes in rats	▪ Polysaccharides show anxiolytic activity ▪ Inhibits down-regulation of β-Syn	Cui et al., 2013
Scutellaria pinnatifida (Skullcap, Lamiaceae)	PC12 and primary dopaminergic neurons	▪ Dichloromethane and n-butanol extract reduces α-SN aggregation and scavenges free radicals	Sashourpour et al., 2017
Tianma Gouteng Yin (Traditional Chinese medicine decoction)	Rotenone intoxicated and human α-syn transgenic drosophila and SH-SY5Y cells	▪ Enhances fly survival and locomotion ▪ Reduces the loss of dopaminergic neurons and cytotoxicity ▪ Inhibits α-syn and dopaminergic neurons degeneration	Liu et al., 2015

fusion, and trafficking of vesicles, excessive free radical generation, mitochondrial dysfunction, endoplasmic reticulum stress, and synaptic dysfunction (Herrera et al., 2017; Longhena et al., 2017; Ghiglieri et al., 2018). The α-syn protein consists of three distinct domains, where the central region is critical for α-syn fibril aggregation, a key component of Lewy bodies.

TABLE 2 | The phytochemicals targeting α-synuclein in the *in vitro* models of Parkinson's disease.

Phytochemicals (*Plant name*, family)	*In vitro* model system	Effects and mechanisms observed	References
3α-Acetoxyeudesma-1,4(15),11(13)-trien-12,6α-olide (*Laurus nobilis,* Lauraceae)	Dopamine-induction and α-syn formation in neuroblastoma cells (SH-SY5Y)	■ Inhibits apoptosis by decreasing ofcaspase-3 and p53 activation and increasing Bcl-2 ■ Suppresses tyrosinase activity and ROS generation ■ Suppresses quinoprotein and α-syn formation	Koo et al., 2011
Alpinin A and B (Diarylheptanoid from *Alpinia officinarum,* Zingiberaceae)	α-syn aggregation assay	■ Inhibits α-syn aggregation, respectively	Fu et al., 2017
Baicalein (*Scutellaria baicalensis,* Lamiaceae)	α-syn aggregation assay	■ Inhibits the formation of α-syn fibrils ■ Disaggregates α-syn fibrils involving Tyr	Zhu et al., 2004
Baicalein (Flavonoid from *Scutellaria baicalensis,* Lamiaceae)	Dopaminergic cell lines (SN4741) overexpressing wild-type α-syn or A53T mutant type α-syn	■ Inhibits α-syn fibrillation by binding covalently ■ Promotes degradation of α-syn fibrils and polymerization to reduce its propagation and transmission ■ Enhances cell viability and increased macroautophagy	Li et al., 2017
dl-3-n-Butylphthalide (*Apium graveolens,* Apiaceae)	MPP^+-induced cellular injury in PC12 cells	■ Reduces cytotoxicity and α-syn accumulation ■ Suppresses oxidative stress and mitochondrial permeability ■ Upregulates LC3-II and its colocalization with α-syn	Huang et al., 2010
Celastrol (*Tripterygium wilfordii* Celastraceae)	Rotenone-induced cell death in SH-SY5Y cells	■ Alleviates oxidative stress and protects from cell death ■ Activates autophagy and increases LC3-II/LC3 I ratio ■ Enhances α-syn clearance	Deng et al., 2013
Chlorogenic acid (*Coffee Arabica,* Rubiaceae)	α-syn-induced toxicity in PC12 cells	■ Inhibits oxidation of dopamine and its interaction with α-syn ■ Inhibits α-syn oligomerization, cytotoxicity, and apoptosis	Teraoka et al., 2012
Costunolide (*Laurus nobilis,* Lauraceae)	Human dopaminergic SH-SY5Y cells	■ Regulates dopamine metabolism-associated genes ■ Decreases α-syn levels and apoptosis	Ham et al., 2012a
Curcumin (*Curcuma longa,* Zingiberaceae)	α-syn aggregation assay and α-syn induced cytotoxicity in SH-SY5Y cells and induced A53T α-syn PC12 in cells	■ Increases α-syn solubility and prevents oligomerization ■ Attenuates apoptosis, ROS, and mitochondrial depolarization ■ Reduces formation, aggregation, and accumulation of α-syn ■ Downregulates mTOR/p70S6K signaling and recovers suppressed macroautophagy ■ Binds to preformed oligomers/fibrils, alter the hydrophobic surface ■ Binds specifically to oligomer intermediates and reduces numbers	Ono and Yamada, 2006; Pandey et al., 2008; Wang et al., 2010; Liu et al., 2011; Gadad et al., 2012; Jiang et al., 2013; Singh et al., 2013
Curcumin-glucoside	α-syn aggregation biochemical assay	■ Prevents oligomer and fibrilformation ■ Improves binding with oligomers and enhances α-syn solubility and prevents fibrillation of α-syn ■ Solubilizes oligomers by disintegrating preformed fibrils	Gadad et al., 2012
Curcumin derivatives: Dehydrozingerone, O-methyl, zingerone, biphenyl analogs	α-syn aggregation biochemical assay and PC12 cells model of PD	■ Biphenyl analogs of dehydrozingerone and O-methyl-dehydrozingerone inhibit α-syn aggregation process ■ Displays the best antioxidant properties	Marchiani et al., 2013
Curcumin pyrazole and curcumin isoxazole	α-syn aggregation biochemical, biophysical and cell based assays	■ Curcumin pyrazole and derivative exhibit better potency ■ Arrests fibrillization and disrupting preformed fibrils ■ Prevents A11 conformation in protein that imparts toxicity ■ Decreases fast aggregating A53T mutant form of α-syn	Ahsan et al., 2015
Curcumin	α-syn in genetic synucleinopathy mouse line overexpresses wild-type α-syn	■ Improves gait impairments ■ Increases phosphorylated α-syn in presynaptic terminals without affecting α-syn aggregation	Spinelli et al., 2015
Curcumin with β-cyclodextrin	α-syn aggregation assay	■ Inhibits aggregation and ■ Brakes up preformed aggregates, exhibit synergy in their action at low concentrations	Gautam et al., 2014
Curcumin, myricetin, rosmarinic acid, nordihydroguaiaretic acid, and ferulic acid	Biophysical assays for α-syn and electrophysiological assays for long-term potentiation in mouse hippocampal slices	■ Inhibits α-syn oligomerization and structure conversion ■ Directly bound to the N-terminal region of α-syn ■ Ameliorates α-syn aggregation and α-syn synaptic toxicity ■ Prevents process, reducing the neurotoxicity of αS oligomers ■ Ameliorates α-syn synaptic toxicity in long-term potentiation	Takahashi et al., 2015

(Continued)

TABLE 2 | Continued

Phytochemicals (*Plant name*, family)	***In vitro* model system**	**Effects and mechanisms observed**	**References**
Crocin-1,2, safranal and crocetin, and its analogs; hexadecanedioic acid, norbixin, and trans-muconic acid (*Crocus sativus* L., oIridaceae)	α-syn aggregation and fibril dissociation assays	▪ Prevent dissociation of fibrils and inhibit α-syn aggregation ▪ Crocetin appears most potent and thereafter norbixin ▪ Other analogs of crocetin fail to affect α-syn aggregation and dissociation	Inoue et al., 2018
(-)-Epigallocatechingallate (EGCG)	Oligomerization, fibrillization, and preformed fibrils of α-syn using biophysical techniques	▪ Inhibits α-syn aggregation concentration dependently ▪ Decreases fibrillar size and toxicity of oligomeric/fibrillar aggregates of α-syn	Jha et al., 2017
(-)-Epigallocatechingallate (EGCG)	Fe^{+3}-induced fibrillation of α-syn in transduced-PC12 cells	▪ Inhibits ROS and β-sheet-enriched α-syn fibrils by chelating Fe(III)	Zhao et al., 2017
(-)-Epigallocatechin-3-gallate (EGCG)	α-syn aggregation biochemical and biophysical assays	▪ Influences aggregate toxicity, morphology, seeding competence, stability, and conformational changes ▪ Affects aggregation kinetics, oligomeric aggregation, binds to cross-beta sheet aggregation intermediates	Andrich and Bieschke, 2015
(-)-Epi-gallocatechine gallate (EGCG)	Fibril formation in incubates; SNCA fluorophore α-syn-HiLyte488 binding to plated SNCA and α-syn-HiLyte488 binding to aggregated SNCA in post-mortem PD tissue	▪ Concentration-dependent inhibition of α-syn aggregation ▪ ED_{50} of EGCG inhibition of α-syn-HiLyte488 was 250 nM ▪ Blocks concentration dependently α-syn-HiLyte488 ▪ Binds to SNCA by instable hydrophobic interactions ▪ Appear remodeling agent of SNCA aggregates and a disease modifying agent for PD	Xu et al., 2016
3-*O*-demethyl swertipunicoside (*Swertia punicea*, Gentianaceae)	MPP^+-induced neurotoxicity in PC12 cells	▪ Alleviates oxidative stress by regulating SOD, MDA, and ROS ▪ Down-regulates Bax and involve a caspases-mediated pathway ▪ Inhibits AIF translocation and α-syn aggregation	Zhou et al., 2013
Fistein (*Polyphenolic compound*)	MPTP/MPP^+-induced neurotoxicity in PC12 cells	▪ Decreases cytotoxicity, apoptosis, and inflammation ▪ Decreases α-syn expression	Patel et al., 2012
Flavonoids (*48 polyphenolic compounds*)	α-syn aggregation assay	▪ Inhibits α-syn fibrillation and disaggregates preformed fibrils	Meng et al., 2009
Gallic acid (*Flavonoid of reference*)	Thioflavin T fluorescence assays and transmission electron microscopy imaging, ion mobility-mass spectrometry	▪ Inhibits the formation of α-syn mediated amyloid fibrils ▪ Interacts with α-syn transiently ▪ Stabilizes its native structure	Liu et al., 2014
Ginsenosides (Rb1) (*Panax ginseng*, Araliaceae)	α-syn aggregation and toxicity using biophysical, biochemical and cell-culture techniques	▪ Inhibits α-syn fibrillation and disaggregate preformed fibrils and inhibit the seeded polymerization of α-syn ▪ Stabilizes soluble non-toxic oligomers with no β-sheet content	Ardah et al., 2015
Isorhynchophylline (*Uncaria rhynchophylla Miq.*, Rubiaceae)	Neuronal cell lines, including N2a, SH-SY5Y, and PC12 cells, and primary cortical neurons	▪ Clears α-syn oligomers and α-syn/synphilin-1 aggresomes ▪ Activates autophagy-lysosome pathway independent of the mTOR pathway rather dependent on the function of Beclin 1 ▪ Decreases α-syn levels in dopaminergic neurons	Lu et al., 2012
Jatamanin11 (*Valeriana jatamansi*, Caprifoliaceae)	*In silico* analysis using Homo sapiens α-syn gi|49456267 from NCBI database	▪ Shows good interaction α-syn in homology modeling	Bagchi and Hopper, 2011
Kaempferol (*a polyphenolic compound*)	α-syn aggregation biochemical assay	▪ Inhibits the formation of α-syn ▪ Destabilizes preformed α-syn	Ono and Yamada, 2006
Luteolin (*Dietary flavonoid*)	Arsenite-induced apoptosis in the dopaminergic PC12 cells	▪ Scavenges ROS production, and promotes apoptosis ▪ Reduces α-syn aggregation	Wu et al., 2017
α-Mangostin (*Garcinia mangostana L.*, Guttiferae)	*In vitro* model of Parkinson's disease induced by rotenone in SH-SY5Y cells	▪ Reduces α-syn aggregation and TH loss ▪ Reduces reactive oxygen species and caspases 3 and 8 ▪ Restores mitochondrial membrane potential and cellular ATP	Hao et al., 2017
Moracenin D (*Morus alba*, Moraceae)	Dopamine-induction in neuroblastoma, SH-SY5Y cells	▪ Upregulates nurr1 levels and down-regulate α-syn levels	Ham et al., 2012b
Neferine (*Lotus seed embryo of Nelumbo nucifera*, Nelumbonaceae)	GFP-LC3 autophagy detection platform in PC-12 cells with mutant toxic proteins, including huntingtin or α-syn	▪ Induces autophagy through an AMPK-mTOR pathway ▪ Reduces expression and toxicity of mutant huntingtin by autophagy-related gene 7 (Atg7) dependent mechanism	Wong et al., 2015

(*Continued*)

TABLE 2 | Continued

Phytochemicals (*Plant name,* family)	***In vitro* model system**	**Effects and mechanisms observed**	**References**
Onjisaponin B (Triterpenoid saponin from *Radix Polygalae,* Polygalaceae)	Mutant α-syn in PC-12 cells	▪ Accelerates clearance of mutant A53T α-syn ▪ Induces autophagy via the AMPK-mTOR signaling pathway ▪ Reduces oligomerization of α-syn	Wu et al., 2013
Oxidized quercetin (Chalcantrione, benzyfuranone, quercetinchinone)	α-syn aggregation biochemical assay	▪ Inhibits fibrillation of α-syn ▪ Disaggregates α-syn fibrils ▪ Inhibits fibrillation and stabilizes oligomers	Zhu et al., 2013
Polyphenols with β-cyclodextrin (Baicalein, curcumin, EGCG, and resveratrol)	α-syn aggregation in mouse neuroblastoma cell lines (N2a cells)	▪ Inhibited α-syn aggregation and disaggregate fibrils ▪ CURCUMIN appears most efficient followed by baicalein, EGCG, and resveratrol	Gautam et al., 2017
Piceatannol, ampelopsin A and isohopeaphenol (Stilbene compounds)	α-syn aggregation biochemical and biophysical assays in PC12 cells	▪ Protects against α-syn-induced membrane damage ▪ Rescues against α-syn-induced toxicity ▪ Inhibits α-syn fibril formation and destabilizes preformed	Temsamani et al., 2016
Paeoniflorin (*Paeoniae alba,* Paeoniaceae)	MPP^+/acidosis-induced cytotoxicity in PC12 cells expressing α-syn	▪ Upregulates LC3-II expression showing autophagy ▪ Reduces MPP^+ cytotoxicity and α-syn accumulation ▪ Enhances autophagic degradation of α-syn	Suñ et al., 2011
Quercetin, (-)-Epigallocatechin gallate (EGCG) and cyanidin-3-glucoside (C3G)	Primary cortical neuron cultures exposed to oxidative insult	▪ EGCG crosses blood brain barrier faster, then C3G ▪ EGCG and C3G reduces necrosis and apoptosis by 30–40% ▪ Quercetin, EGCG, and C3G inhibited α-syn fibrillation ▪ EGCG appears most promising neuroprotective compound	Pogacnik et al., 2016
Rottlerin (Polyphenol from berry fruits or kamala tree, *Mallotus Philippinensis*, Euphorbiaceae)	α-syn aggregation biochemical assay	▪ Prevents aggregation of numerous amyloid precursors (α-syn, amyloid-β, prion proteins, and lysozyme)	Maioli et al., 2012
Resveratrol (*Red grapes,* Vitaceae)	Rotenone-treated human SH-SY5Y cells and wild-type α-syn, A30P, or A53T α-syn expressing PC12 cells	▪ Protects against apoptosis and enhanced degradation of α-syn ▪ Shows AMPK-SIRT1-mediated autophagy induction ▪ Activates SIRT1 and prevents α-syn aggregation	Albani et al., 2009; Wu et al., 2011
3,6-bis-O-di-O-galloyl-1,2,4-tri-O-galloyl-β-d-glucose (Tannin from *Rhus typhina,* Anacardiaceae)	α-syn aggregation biochemical and biophysical assays	▪ Interacts very strongly with human serum albumin through a "sphere of action" mechanism ▪ Time-dependent inhibition of α-synuclein aggregation	Sekowski et al., 2017
Strophanthidine (*Strophanthus Kombe & gratus,* Apocynaceae)	SNCA 5′UTR driven luciferase expression	▪ Blocks *SNCA* expression (~1 μM IC_{50}) in neural cells	Rogers et al., 2011
Theaflavins (TF1, TF2a, TF2b, and TF3) (*Camelia sinensis,* Theaceae)	α-syn aggregation biochemical assay	▪ Stimulates α-syn assembly into non-toxic, spherical aggregates	Grelle et al., 2011
Thymoquinone (*Nigella sativa,* Ranunculaceae)	α-syn-induced synaptic toxicity in rat hippocampal cells and human induced pluripotent stem cell (iPSC)-derived neurons	▪ Reduces the α-syn-induced loss of synaptophysin ▪ Enhances synaptic vesicles recycling in the presence of α-syn ▪ Protects iPSC-derived neurons and maintain firing activity ▪ Protects against mutated β-SynP123H-induced synaptic activity	Alhebshi et al., 2014

α-syn can adopt a wide range of conformational structures ranging from compact to fully extended (Winner et al., 2011). The interactions between the N- and C-termini of α-syn play a role in its stabilization into a compact, monomeric conformation that is non-toxic (Bertoncini et al., 2005). The agents that bind to α-syn and form a loop structure between the N- and C-terminus are believed to confer neuroprotection. In contrast, the agents which induce more compressed structures are considered neurotoxic in nature (Karpinar et al., 2009; Lashuel et al., 2013). Mutations in α-syn can contribute to multiple forms of PD including genetic and rare forms of PD with early onset (Singleton et al., 2003; Simon-Sanchez et al., 2009). Monomeric α-syn is a potential therapeutic target as it is an upstream form of the protein during the aggregation process and the etiopathogenesis of PD (Winner et al., 2011; Lashuel et al., 2013; Brundin et al., 2017; Ghiglieri et al., 2018). The agents stabilizing, promoting clearance, degrading misfolded proteins, solubilizing oligomers, or inhibiting the propagation of α-syn aggregates are pharmacologically appropriate and a clinically relevant therapeutic strategy for PD.

TABLE 3 | The phytochemicals showed neuroprotective effects in the *in vivo* models of Parkinson's disease by targeting α-synuclein.

Phytochemicals *(Plant name,* family)	***In vivo* animal model**	**Effects and mechanisms observed**	**References**
Apigenin *(Flavone found in fruits and vegetables)*	Unilateral stereotaxic intranigral infusion of ROT-induced PD in rats	▪ Improves behavioral, biochemical and mitochondrial enzymes ▪ Attenuates pro-inflammatory cytokines release and NF-κB expression ▪ Inhibits neurotrophic factors and α-syn aggregation ▪ Enhances TH and dopamine D2 receptor expression	Anusha et al., 2017
Acteoside (*Cistanche deserticola* or *Cistanche tubulosa*, Orobanchaceae)	Rotenone-induced PD in rats	▪ Inhibits α-syn, caspase-3 activity and microtubule-associated protein 2 (MAP2) downregulation ▪ Binds and inhibits caspase-3 *in silico* and showed neuroprotection	Yuan et al., 2016
Acacetin (O-methylated flavone from Asteraceae)	Caenorhabditis elegans model system	▪ Improves lifespan, survival, stress resistance ▪ Enhances antioxidant and stress resistance genes ▪ Inhibits α-syn aggregation and age pigment lipofuscin	Asthana et al., 2016
Acetylcorynoline *(Corydalis bungeana Turcz,* Papaveraceae)	Transgenic *C. elegans* (OW13) expressing human α-syn, GFP in dopaminergic neurons and 6-OHDA-induced PD	▪ Decreases 6-OHDA-induced DA neuron degeneration ▪ Prevents α-syn aggregation and recovers lipid content ▪ Restores food-sensing behavior in 6-OHDA-treated animals ▪ Suppresses apoptosis by decreasing egl-1 expression ▪ Increases rpn5 expression that enhances the activity of proteasomes	Fu et al., 2014a
Apocyanin (*Picrorhiza kurroa* Royle ex Benth, Plantains)	Lipolysaccharide-injection in substantia niagra-induced PD in rats	▪ Ameliorates proinflammatory cytokines, improves behavior ▪ Inhibits NADPH oxidase, caspase 3, 9 and TUNEL positivity ▪ Inhibits α-syn deposition and prevents dopaminergic neurons	Sharma et al., 2016
Acetylcorynoline (*Corydalis bungeana*, Papaveraceae)	*Caenorhabditis elegans* strain (BZ555) expresses the green fluorescent protein in dopaminergic neurons, and a transgenic strain (OW13) express h α-syn in muscle cells PD model	▪ Appears safe and devoid of adverse effect in animals ▪ Decreases dopaminergic degeneration in BZ555 strain ▪ Prevents α-syn aggregation and recovers lipid contents ▪ Restores food-sensing behavior, and dopamine levels ▪ Prolongs life-span in 6-OH-treated N2 strain ▪ Decreases egl-1 expression to suppress apoptosis pathways ▪ Increases rpn5 expression to enhance proteasomes activity	Fu et al., 2014a
Baicalein (Flavonoid from *Scutellaria baicalensis,* Lamiaceae)	Intranigral infusion of MPP^+ in rat brain	▪ Attenuates α-syn aggregation ▪ Inhibits inflammasome activation and cathepsin B production ▪ Inhibits apoptosis (caspases 9 and 12, and autophagy (LC3-II)	Hung et al., 2016
n-Butylidenephthalide (*Angelica sinensis,* Apiaceae)	*Caenorhabditis elegans* express green fluorescent protein in neurons, BZ555 and a transgenic expresses human α-syn (OW13)	▪ Attenuates dopaminergic degeneration and prolongs life-span ▪ Reduces α-syn accumulation ▪ Restores dopamine, lipid content and food-sensing behavior ▪ Blocks *egl-1* expression that inhibits apoptosis ▪ Enhances *rpn-6* expression to increase proteasomes activity	Fu et al., 2014b
Curcumin (*Curcuma longa*, Zingiberaceae)	Interaction of curcumin and α-syn in genetic synucleinopathy of α-syn-GFP mouse line overexpresses α-syn	▪ Chronic and acute curcumin treatment improves gait impairments and increases phosphorylated forms of α-syn at cortical presynaptic terminals in α-syn-GFP line ▪ Increases phosphorylated α-syn in terminals without affecting α-syn aggregation	Spinelli et al., 2015
Alginate-curcumin nanocomposite	Supplemented with diet to *Drosophila melangoster*	▪ Delays climbing disability in flies ▪ Reduces oxidative stress and apoptosis in the brain of PD flies	Siddique et al., 2013b
α-Linolenic acid	*Caenorhabditis elegans* wild type N2 and transgenic (UA44) exposed to 6-OHDA	▪ Improves locomotion, pharyngeal pumping, and lifespan ▪ Shows a visibly significant reduction in neuronal degeneration ▪ Increases GFP expression within in neurons	Shashikumar et al., 2015
Squamosamide (N-[2-(4-Hydroxy-phenyl)-ethyl]-2-(2,5-dimethoxy-phenyl)-3-(3-methoxy-4-hydroxy-phenyl) acrylamide) *(Annona glabra,* Annonaceae)	6-OHDA-induced PD in rats	▪ Improves motor dysfunction and behavior ▪ Enhances dopamine level and TH activity ▪ Decreases α-syn expression mediated by the Akt/mTOR pathway ▪ Reduces RTP801 expression, a protein in the pathogenesis of PD	Bao et al., 2012
Geraniol *(Monoterpene from rose oil, palmarosa oil, and citronella oil)*	MPTP-induced PD in C57BL/6 mice	▪ Reduces α-syn aggregation in dose dependent manner ▪ Improves nigral dopamine, TH and dopamineric terminals in striatum ▪ Improves neuromuscular disability and Lewy body aggregation	Rekha et al., 2013

(Continued)

TABLE 3 | Continued

Phytochemicals *(Plant name,* family)	*In vivo* animal model	Effects and mechanisms observed	References
Irisflorentin (*Belamcanda chinensis* L. DC., Iridaceae)	Transgenic or 6-hydroxydopamine-induced PD in *Caenorhabditis elegans*	▪ Prevents α-syn accumulation ▪ Improves dopaminergic neurons, food-sensing, and life-span ▪ Promotes rpn-3 expression to enhance the activity of proteasomes ▪ Down-regulates egl-1 expression to block apoptosis pathways	Chen et al., 2015a
Lycopene *(Red grapes, peanuts)*	Rotenone-induced PD in mouse	▪ Increases the TH content and decreases α-syn and LC3-B positive neurons	Liu et al., 2013
N-2-(4-hydroxy-phenyl)-ethyl]-2-(2, 5-dimethoxy-phenyl)-3-(3-methoxy-4-hydroxy-phenyl)-acrylamide) (FLZ, a novel synthetic derivative of squamosamide from a Chinese herb)	Chronic PD mouse model induced by MPTP combined with probenecid (MPTP/p) and subacute PD models	▪ Improves motor behavior and dopaminergic neuronal function ▪ Elevates dopaminergic neurons, dopamine level, and TH activity ▪ Decreases α-syn phosphorylation, nitration, and aggregation ▪ Decreases interaction between α-syn and TH, which eventually improved dopaminergic neuronal function ▪ Activates Akt/mTOR phosphorylation signaling pathway	Bao et al., 2015
Salidroside (Phenylpropanoid glycoside from *Rhodiola rosea* L., Crassulaceae)	MPTP/MPP(+) models of Parkinson's disease and 6-OHDA and overexpresssion of WT/A30P-α-syn in SH-SY5Y cells.	▪ Protects dopaminergic neurons and regulates apoptotic proteins caspase-3,6 and 9, cyt-c and Smac release and Bcl-2/Bax ▪ Reduces α-syn aggregation ▪ Protects cells and cell viability mainly through recovering the 20S proteasome activity ▪ Decreases pSer129-α-syn and promotes the clearance of α-syn	Wang et al., 2015b, Li et al., 2018
Shatavarin IV (Steroidal glucosides, syn: asparinin B in roots of *Asparagus racemosus,* Asparagaceae)	*Caenorhabditis elegans* model of PD	▪ Improves antioxidant and stress defense genes ▪ Raises dopamine levels, inhibits lipids ▪ Inhibits α-syn aggregation involving ubiquitin proteasomal system	Smita et al., 2017
2,3,5,4′-tetrahydroxy stilbene-2-O-β-D-glucoside *(Polygonum multiflori,* Polygonaceae)	APPV717I transgenic mice expressing α-syn in the hippocampus	▪ Prevents α-syn overexpression at an early and late stage in the hippocampus ▪ Inhibits production of dimer and tetramer of α-syn protein ▪ Reverses the increased expression of α-syn	Zhang et al., 2013
2,3,5,4′-tetrahydroxystilbene-2-O-β-D-glucoside *(Polygonum multiflori,* Polygonaceae)	Memory and movement functions and its mechanisms related to synapses and α-syn in aged mice	▪ Inhibits α-syn aggregation and α-syn levels in the hippocampus ▪ Improves memory, movement and protects synaptic ultrastructure ▪ Enhances synaptophysin, phosphorylated synapsin I and post-synaptic density protein 95 (PSD95) and calcium/calmodulin-dependent protein kinase II (p-CaMKII) expression	Shen et al., 2015
10-O-trans-p-Coumaroylcatalpol *(Premna integrifolia syn: Premna serratifolia,* Verbenaceae)	Transgenic *Caenorhabditis elegans* model of PD expressing α-syn	▪ Inhibits α-syn aggregation ▪ Extends life span, stress resistance and reduces oxidative stress ▪ Enhances longevity promoting transcription factors	Shukla et al., 2012
Withanolide A (Steroidal lactone from *Withania somnifera* L. Dunal, Solanaceae)	Transgenic *Drosophila melanogaster* model	▪ Improves lifespan and delays age-associated physiological changes ▪ Inhibits α-syn aggregation and modulation of acetylcholine.	Akhoon et al., 2016

MEDICINAL PLANTS TARGETING α-SYNUCLEIN CASCADE AND TOXICITY

Recently, many plant extracts appear to inhibit oligomerization and fibrillization of α-syn, an emerging therapeutic target in PD (Lobbens et al., 2016; Ren et al., 2016; Briffa et al., 2017; Cheon et al., 2017). The plant extracts, which were shown to be neuroprotective in PD, target various pathogenic stages of α-syn conformations ranging from fibrillation to oligomerization in experimental models and are listed in **Table 1.** Plants, such as *Acanthopanax senticosus [Eleutherococcus senticosus (Rupr. & Maxim.) Maxim.], Bacopa monnieri [Bacopa monnieri (L.) Wettst.], Cinnamon extract precipitate [Cinnamomum verum J. Presl], Centella asiatica [Centella asiatica (L.) Urb.], Panax ginseng [Panax ginseng C.A. Mey.], Polygala tenuifolia [Polygala tenuifolia Willd.], Rehmannia glutinosa [Rehmannia glutinosa (Gaertn.) DC.], Corema album [Trema micranthum (L.) Blume], Opuntia ficus-indica [Opuntia ficus-indica (L.) Mill.], Padina pavonica [Sagina japonica (Sw. ex Steud.) Ohwi], Carthamus tinctorius L.*, and *Crocus sativus L.* are neuroprotective in PD by targeting oligomerization, fibrillation, and disaggregation of preformed α-syn fibrils. A scheme is presented in **Figure 2** to

TABLE 4 | The phytochemicals showed neuroprotective effects in both, the *in vitro* and *in vivo* models of Parkinson's disease by targeting α-synuclein.

Phytochemicals (*Plant name*, family)	*In vitro* and *in vivo* models	Effects and observed mechanisms	References
Astaxanthin (3,3′-dihydroxy-β, β′-carotene-4, 4′-dione)	MPTP/MPP$^+$-induced PD in mouse and neuroblastoma cells (SH-SY5Y)	▪ Inhibits apoptosis regulating Bax, Bcl-2 and caspase-3 expression ▪ Reduces α-syn and argyrophilic neurons ▪ Increases TH+ve neurons and antioxidant activity	Lee et al., 2011
2-Cyano-3, 12-dioxooleana-1,9-dien-28-oic acid (*a derivative of oleanolic acid*)	MPTP-induced PD in mice and 3-NP-neurotoxicity in mice and SH-SY5Y cells	▪ Reduces oxidative/nitrosative stress and activate the Nrf2/ARE pathway ▪ Preserves dopaminergic neurons, reduced α-syn accumulation	Yang et al., 2009
Corynoxine B (*Uncaria rhynchophylla Miq.*, Rubiaceae)	Neuronal cell lines and N2a and SHSY-5Y cells and drosophila model of PD	▪ Promotes autophagosomes formation in fly fat bodies ▪ Enhances clearance of wild-type and A53T α-syn ▪ Induces autophagy by Akt/mTOR pathway	Chen et al., 2014
(-)-Epicatechin gallate (EGCG) (*Camelia sinensis*, Theaceae)	α-syn aggregation biochemical assays, A53T α-syn expressing SH-SY5Y cells, transgenic drosophila model expressing normal human α-syn	▪ Inhibits α-syn fibrillogenesis and disaggregates large, mature α-syn fibrils into smaller, amorphous protein aggregates and α-syn tandem repeat in the aggregation ▪ Blocks genomic responses and accumulation of α-syn in SNc ▪ Forms a new type of unstructured, non-toxic α-syn ▪ Shows a dose-dependent delay in the loss of climbing ability ▪ Reduces oxidative stress and apoptosis in the brain ▪ Remodels α-syn amyloid fibrils into disordered oligomers ▪ Inhibits preformed oligomers to permeabilize vesicles, induce cytotoxicity in cells and immobilizes C-terminal region and reduces binding of oligomers to membranes ▪ Does not affect oligomer size distribution or secondary structure ▪ Reduces membrane affinity of the oligomer to prevent cytotoxicity	Mandel et al., 2004; Ehrnhoefer et al., 2008; Bae et al., 2010; Bieschke et al., 2010; Ma et al., 2010; Yoshida et al., 2013; Lorenzen et al., 2014; Siddique et al., 2014
Eicosanoyl-5-hydroxytryptamide (*Coffee Arabica*, Lamiaceae)	MPTP-model of PD in mice and cultured primary microglia/astrocytes and MPP-induced PD model of SH-SY5Y cells	▪ Prevents oxidative stress, cytotoxicity, and neuroinflammation ▪ Preserves dopaminergic neurons and improves neuronal integrity ▪ Reduces JNK activation, striatal dopamine, and TH content ▪ Ameliorates MPP$^+$-demethylation of phosphoprotein phosphatase 2A, the key of the cellular phosphoregulatory network ▪ Ameliorates protein aggregation and phosphorylation	Lee et al., 2013
Ellagic acid	Cell-based and cell-independent *in vitro* showing nitrosative stress mediated S-nitrosylation (SNO), the SNO-PDI formation is linked to the aggregation of α-syn and α-syn:synphilin-1 deposits in the PD brain	▪ Scavenges NOx radicals and protect cells from SNO-PDI formation via rotenone insult both, cell-based and cell-independent *in vitro* ▪ Mitigates nitrosative-stress-induced aggregation of synphilin-1 but also α-syn and α-syn: synphilin-1 composites (Lewy-like neurites) in PC12 cells ▪ Lowers rotenone-instigated reactive oxygen species and reactive nitrogen species in PC12 cells ▪ Inhibits apoptosis and interferes with SNO-PDI formation	Kabiraj et al., 2014
Nordihydroguaiaretic acid (*Larrea tridentata*, Zygophyllaceae)	Drosophila expressing human α-syn and α-syn aggregation biochemical assay	▪ Delays loss of climbing ability of flies ▪ Inhibits the formation of α-syn ▪ Destabilizes preformed α-syn	Ono and Yamada, 2006; Caruana et al., 2012; Siddique et al., 2012
Reynosin (*Laurus nobilis*, Lauraceae)	DA-induced PD model in SH-SY5Y cells and 6-OHDA induced PD in rats	▪ Reverse E6-associated protein, α-syn levels ▪ Appears more potent than apomorphine	Ham et al., 2013
Tanshinone I & IIA (*Salvia miltiorrhiza*, Lamiaceae)	Transgenic *Caenorhabditis elegans* PD model (NL5901) and *in vitro*	▪ Disaggregates fibrils, the transformation of α-syn from unstructured coils to β-sheets and reduce oligomer/fibril formation ▪ Inhibits α-syn aggregation and alleviates aggregated α-syn induced membrane disruption and extends life span	Ji et al., 2016
Tea polyphenols (flavanol-related catechins in black/green tea)	MPTP-induced PD models in mouse and monkey and cultured dopaminergic cells	▪ Alleviates motor impairments and dopaminergic injury in monkeysinhibits α-syn oligomers in cultured cells, striatum, brain reduces intracellular α-syn oligomers in neurons treated with α-syn oligomers, MPTP and increases cell viability	Chen et al., 2015b
Trehalose (natural sugar in fungi and plants)	Autophagy-induction in NB69 cells and mice model of Lewy body disease	▪ Induces autophagy and increases autophagosomes ▪ Increases autophagic and chaperon molecules in mice brain ▪ Suppressesinsoluble α-syn and apoptosis	Tanji et al., 2015

TABLE 5 | The polyphenol compounds investigated for their action on α-synuclein fibrillation, aggregation, and cytotoxicity.

Polyphenolic compounds	References
Apigenin, baicalein, (-)-catechin, (-)-catechin gallate, chlorogenic acid, curcumin, cyaniding, daidzein, delphinidin, 2,2′-dihydroxybenzophenone, 4,4′-dihydroxybenzophenone, dopamine chloride, (-)-epicatechin, (-)-epicatechin 3-gallate, epigallocatechin, epigallocatechin gallate, exifone, (-)-gallocatechin, (-)-gallocatechin gallate, gingerol, gossypetin, hinokiflavone, hypericin, kaempferol, luteolin, myricetin, naringenin, 2,3,4,2′,4′-pentahydroxybenzophenone, procyanidin B1, procyanidin B2, Purpurogallin, quercetin, rosmarinic acid, rutin, (+)-taxifolin, 2,2′,4,4′-tetrahydroxybenzophenone, theaflavine, (+)-R-tocopherol, 2,3,4-trihydroxybenzophenone (39 polyphenols)	Masuda et al., 2006
Quercetin (3,5,7,3′,4′-Pentahydroxyflavone dehydrate), Fisetin (3,7,3′,4′-Tetrahydroxyflavone), T-601 (3′,4′-Dihydroxyflavonol), 22-344 (3,6,3′,4′-Tetrahydroxyflavone), 22-318 (3,6,2′,3′-Tetrahydroxyflavone), G-500/Gossypetin (3,5,7,8,3′,4′-Hexahydroxyflavone), C-101/Myricetin (3,5,7,3′,4′,5′-Hexahydroxyflavone), Rutin (Quercetin-3-rutinoside), K-102/Kaempferol (3,5,7,4′-Tetrahydroxyflavone), 020065/Isorhamnetin (3′-Methoxy-3,5,7,4′-Tetrahydroxyflavone), 020067/Galangin (3,5,7-Trihydroxyflavone), 021140S/Tamarixetin (4′-Methoxy-3,5,7,3′-Tetrahydroflavone), 22-324 (6,2′,3′-Trihydroxyflavone), D-406 (2′,3′-Dihydroxyflavone), D-258 (3′,4′-Dihydroxyflavone), D-116 (5,6-Dihydroxy-7-Methoxyflavone), 22-357 (5,6-Dihydroxyflavone), 22-336 (6,7,3′-Trihydroxyflavone), D-112 (6,7-Dihydroxyflavone), Luteolin (5,7,3′,4′-Tetrahydroxyflavone), 22-340/Tricetin (5,7,3′,4′,5′-Pentahydroxyflavone), 22-341 (7,3′,4′,5′-Tetrahydroxyflavone), 021165/6-HP (5,6,7,4′-Tetrahydroxyflavone), B-101/Baicalein (5,6,7-Trihydroxyflavone), 22-323 (6,2′,3′-Trimethoxyflavone), D-407 (2′,4′-Dihydroxyflavone), 021104S/Chrysoeriol (4′,5,7-Trihydroxy-3′-Methoxyflavone0, 021108S/Diosmetin (5,7,3′-Trihydroxy-4′-Methoxyflavone), Wogonin (5,7-Dihydroxy-8-Methoxyflavone), H-114 (3′-Hydroxy-5,6,7,4′-Tetramethoxyflavone), Epigallo Catechin Gallate (EGCG) [(2R,3R)-2-(3,4,5-Trihydroxyphenyl)-3,4-dihydro-1(2H)-benzopyran-3,5,7-triol 3-(3,4,5-trihydroxybenzoate)], Epicatechin gallate (ECG) [(2R,3R)-2-(3,4-Dihydroxyphenyl)-3,4-dihydro-1(2H)-benzopyran-3,5,7-triol 3-(3,4,5-trihydroxybenzoate)], 020976S/Catechin [(+)-3,3′4′,5,7-Flavanepentol (2H)-benzopyran-3,5,7-triol/(2R,3R)-2-(3,4-Dihydroxyphenyl)-3,4-dihydro-1], T-116 (6,7,4′-Trihydroxyisoflavone), T-415 (7,3′,4′-Trihydroxyisoflavone), 19-612 (3′,4′-Dimethoxy-7-hydroxyisoflavone), D-101/Daidzein (7,4″-Dihydroxyisoflavone), F-103/Formononetin (7-Hydroxy-4′-methoxyisoflavone), Biochanin A (5,7-Dihydroxy-4′-methoxyisoflavone), 020056/Eriodictyol (2-[3,4-Dihydroxyphenyl] 2,3-dihydro-5,7-dihydroxy-4H-1benzopyran-4-one), H-103/Hesperetin (5,7,3′-Trihydroxy-4′-methoxyflavanone), 020091/Homoeriodictyol (5,7,4′-Trihydroxy-5′-methoxyflavanone), Hesperidin/Hesperetin-7-O-rutinoside, 020411/Alizarin (1,2-Dihydroxyanthraquinone), Chrysophanol (1,8-Dihydroxy-3-methylanthraquinone), Emodin (1,3,8-Trihydroxy-6-methylanthraquinone), D-105/Fustin (3,7,3′,4′-Tetrahydroxyflavone), 021037 (3,3′,4′,5′,7-Pentahydroxyflavanone) (48 polyphenols)	Meng et al., 2010
Apigenin, baicalein, epigallocatechin gallate, genistein, ginkgolide B, morin, myricetin (Myr), nordihydroguaiaretic acid, purpurogallin trimethyl ether, quercetin, resveratrol, rosmarinic acid, scutellarein, tannic acid, theaflavins (14 polyphenols)	Caruana et al., 2011
Apigenin, baicalein, EGCG, genistein, ginkgolide B, morin, nordihydroguaiaretic acid, propyl gallate, purpurogallin trimethyl ether, resveratrol, scutellarein, and black tea extract (BTE; >80% theaflavins) (12 polyphenoilc compunds)	Caruana et al., 2012
Benzoic acid and derivatives, such as 2-Hydroxybenzoic acid (salicylic acid), 3-Hydroxybenzoic acid, 4-Hydroxybenzoic acid, 2,3-dihydroxybenzoic acid, 2,4-dihydroxybenzoic acid, 2,5-dihydroxybenzoic acid (gentisic acid), 2,6-dihydroxybenzoic acid, 3,4-dihydroxybenzoic acid, 3,5-dihydroxybenzoic acid, 2,4,6-trihydroxybenzoic acid, 3,4,5-trihydroxybenzoic acid (gallic acid), 3,4,5-trihfluorobenzoic acid, 3,4,5-trimethoxybenzoic acid, 4-methoxybenzoic acid (Benzoic acid derivatives)	Ardah et al., 2014
Myricetin, curcumin, rosmarinic acid, nordihydroguaiaretic acid, and ferulic acid	Takahashi et al., 2015
Curcumin, baicalein, (-)-epigallocatechin gallate, and resveratrol	Gautam et al., 2017

depict the potential mechanism of action of the plant extracts and phytochemicals on α-syn oligomerization, fibrillation, and aggregation.

Many plant extracts show (often *in vitro*) effects in experimental models of PD by targeting α-syn. However, the bioactive constituents attributing to this effect are not available. *Bacopa monnieri* prevents neurodegeneration in A53T α-syn-induced PD in *Caenorhabditis elegans* (Jadiya et al., 2011). However, the chemical constituents collectively known as bacosides have not been investigated in experimental PD models or their effect on α-syn. *Centella asiatica (L.) Urb.,* known as Asiatic pennywort, reportedly prevents α-syn aggregation *in vitro* (Berrocal et al., 2014). Yet, the principal constituent asiatic acid failed to prevent α-syn aggregation. Meanwhile, asiaticoside and madecassic acid have not been investigated for their effects on α-syn. Cinnamon extract precipitate reportedly inhibits α-syn aggregation and stabilizes oligomers *in vitro* and *in vivo* in A53T α-syn-induced PD in flies (Shaltiel-Karyo et al., 2012). However, cinnamaldehyde, a major ingredient of cinnamon extract has not yet been investigated. *Eucalyptus citriodora* improves climbing ability and attenuates oxidative stress in transgenic drosophila expressing human α-syn (Siddique et al., 2013a). The effects of the bioactive contents citronellol, linalool, and isopulegol of *Eucalyptus citriodora* on α-syn are not known. *Crocus sativus* L., popularly known as saffron, is widely used for its color, flavor, and aroma in food and beverages. Saffron and its constituents, such as crocin-1, crocin-2, crocetin, safranal, and the crocetin structural analogs hexadecanedioic acid, norbixin, and trans-muconic acid, were found to affect α-syn fibrillation and aggregation (Inoue et al., 2018). However, some crocetin analogs failed to affect α-syn aggregation and dissociation. *Sorbus alnifolia,* also known as Korean mountain ash, improved viability of rat pheochromocytoma (PC12) cells while also improving the longevity, food sensing, and reducing dopaminergic neurodegeneration in *Caenorhabditis elegans* model of PD (Cheon et al., 2017). However, the extract failed to alter α-syn aggregation in the NL5901 strain (Cheon et al., 2017).

From the perspective of traditional medicine, targeting α-syn with plant extracts containing phytochemicals could be

TABLE 6 | The bioanalytical techniques employed to determine α-synuclein oligomerization, fibrillation, and cytotoxicity.

Biochemical/biophysical techniques	Events monitored in the system	References
Fluorescence polarization technique	α-syn aggregation	Luk et al., 2007
Scanning for intensely fluorescent targets and atomic force microscopy	α-syn oligomers	Kostka et al., 2008
High performance liquid chromatography (HPLC), Circular dichroism (CD), Fourier transform infrared spectroscopy (FTIR), Size exclusion HPLC, small-angle X-ray scattering, and atomic force microscopy (AFM)	HPLC (stability), Fourier transform infrared spectroscopy and atomic force microscopy (oligomer stabilization and fibrillation), CD (structural assessment)	Hong et al., 2008
Extrinsic multiple-emission probe 4′-(diethylamino)-3-hydroxyflavone spectroscopy	Amyloid fibril formed by mutant α-syn	Celej et al., 2009
Peptide mapping, Mass spectrometric and Ultra-high-field Nuclear Magnetic Resonance analysis	α-syn dimerization and inhibitor binding	Yamaguchi et al., 2010
Fluorescence spectroscopy, Thioflavin T (Thio T) assay and Transmission electron microscopy (TEM)	α-syn fibrillation and preformed α-syn	Ono and Yamada, 2006
Thio T assay, Light scattering measurement, size-exclusion HPLC, AFM	α-syn aggregation	Zhu et al., 2013
Membrane potential-sensitive bis-oxonol fluorescent dye, DiBAC4(3) bio-sensing system	Cytotoxicity of C-terminal truncated α-syn 119 (α-syn119)	Kim et al., 2013
Thio T assay, AFM, Nuclear magnetic resonance, Vesicle leakage assay	Fibril disassembling (Thio-T assay)	da Silva et al., 2013
Lipid vesicle permeabilisation assay	Membrane damage by α-syn aggregates	Caruana et al., 2012
Confocal single-molecule fluorescence spectroscopy	α-syn oligomer formation	Caruana et al., 2011
Circular dichroism spectroscopy, Transmission electron microscopy, Atomic force microscopy, and Nuclear magnetic resonance analysis and Electrophysiological assays	α-syn oligomerization, NMR (binding to the N-terminal of α-syn)	Takahashi et al., 2015
Electrochemical and localized surface plasmon resonance (LSPR), Cyclic and differential pulse voltammetry using redox probe [Fe(CN)6], Thio T assay, Surface plasmon resonance imaging, Transmission electron microscopy	α-syn oligomers by electrochemical and LSPR and Voltametry to detect binding of inhibitors to α-syn	Cheng et al., 2015
Split firefly luciferase complementation assay with bioluminescence imaging	Visualizes oligomerization of α-syn in cell culture, striatum and SNc	Aelvoet et al., 2014
ThT assays, Circular dichroism, Turbidity, and Rayleigh scattering measurements, Atomic force microscopy and Transmission electron microscopy	α-syn fibril formation	Fazili and Naeem, 2015
CCK-8 staining on MPP(+)-induced SH-SYSY cells and Transmission electron microscopy, AO staining and western blotting in cells	Survival rate (CCK-8), autophagy (TEM), AO staining (lysosome), western (α-syn)	Wang et al., 2014

TABLE 7 | The experimental models used to evaluate plant extracts and phytochemicals against neurotoxicity mediating α-synuclein oligomerization, and fibrillation.

Experimental models	α-synuclein based pathogenesis	References
MPTP-intoxicated monkeys showing PD features	Accumulation α-syn oligomers in the striatum	Chen et al., 2015b
MPP(+)-induced toxicity in SH-SY5Y cells	Increased α-syn level and expression	Wang et al., 2014
Rotenone-induced neurotoxicity in cell lines	Increased α-syn aggregation and synphilin-1 deposits	Kabiraj et al., 2014
Rotenone-induced neurotoxicity in SH-SY5Y cells	Increased α-syn level and expression	Deng et al., 2013
Lipid vesicles and SH-SY5Y cells	Formation of Aβ42, α-syn and tau aggregate complexes	Camilleri et al., 2013
Cytotoxicity in catecholaminergic PC12 cells	Increased α-syn level and expression	Teraoka et al., 2012
MPTP/MPP+-induced neurotoxicity in PC12 cells	Increased α-syn level and expression	Patel et al., 2012
Dopamine-induction in SH-SY5Y cells	Increased α-syn expression	Ham et al., 2013
Rotenone-neurotoxicity in SH-SY5Y and PC12 cells	Enhanced degradation of α-syn	Wu et al., 2011
Transgenic Drosophila expressing human α-syn	Increased α-syn I expression	Long et al., 2009
Yeast-based model expressing α-syn	Increased α-syn fibrillation-induced neurotoxicity	Griffioen et al., 2006
MPTP and 6-OHDA-induced PD in rodents	Increased of α-syn expression in the SNpc	Mandel et al., 2004

considered beneficial using dietary intervention. This could be due to the synergy in action and superior therapeutic effects, along with polypharmacological properties (Wagner and Ulrich-Merzenich, 2009; Wu et al., 2013). The fraction that termed active from *Radix Polygalae* was found more potent than the constituent, where onjisaponin B increased mutant huntingtin removal and reduced α-syn aggregation. This plant could be a good source of phytochemicals and a template for novel small molecule inhibitors of α-syn (Wu et al., 2013). Plant-based formulations, such as S/B which contain extracts of

Scutellaria baicalensis Georgi and *Bupleurum scorzonerifolfium* and a traditional Chinese medicine decoction known as *Tianma Gouteng Yin,* were also found to diminish α-syn accumulation and aggregation in experimental PD models (Lin et al., 2011).

The majority of plant extracts used in traditional medicines are based on long-established knowledge of their health benefits, time tested safety due to ancient use, and potential therapeutic effects. However, some plants are not as beneficial as documented or are detrimental; the essential oil from *Myrtus communis,* which is popular in the Zoroastrian community for aroma (Morshedi and Nasouti, 2016), increases α-syn fibrillation and enhances α-syn toxicity in human neuroblastoma cells (Morshedi and Nasouti, 2016). This study suggests that essential oils used in aromatherapy should be investigated for their potential neurotoxicity or neurodegenerative ability.

The attenuation of α-syn toxicity by plant extracts validates traditional claims of medicinal plants. It may also provide the basis for dietary or nutritional inclusion of these plants in foods to achieve neuroprotective effects. This is not only based on antioxidant approaches but also inhibition of α-syn aggregation. However, in-depth studies are needed for a dietary or therapeutic recommendation on the use of plant extracts in humans.

PLANT EXTRACTS AND PHYTOCHEMICALS AS PHARMACOLOGICAL CHAPERONES FOR PD

Pharmacological chaperoning is emerging as a potential therapeutic approach for the treatment of numerous diseases associated with single gene mutations (Srinivasan et al., 2014). These chaperones are small molecules that bind proteins and stabilize them against proteolytic degradation or protect

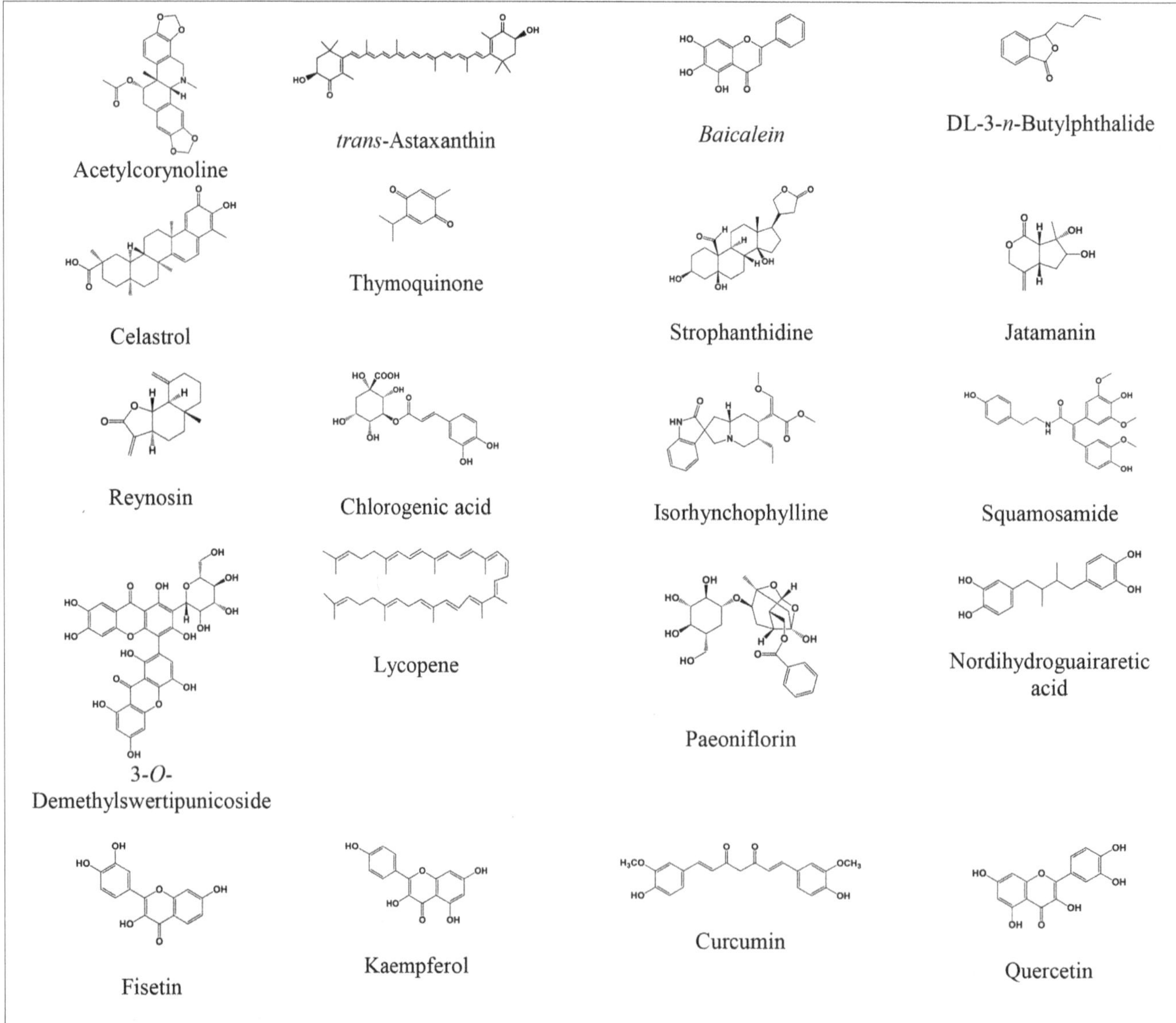

FIGURE 1 | (Continued)

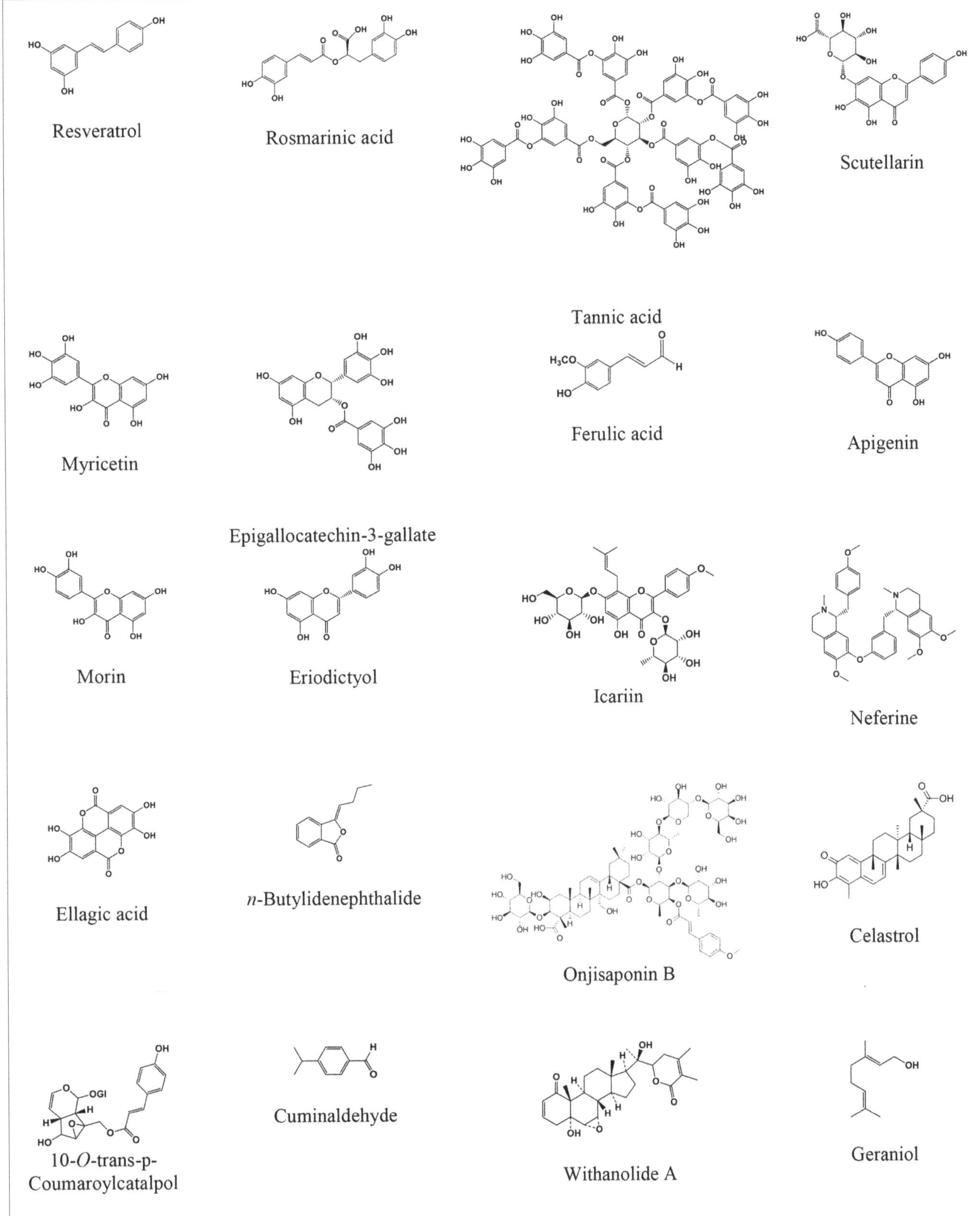

FIGURE 1 | (Continued)

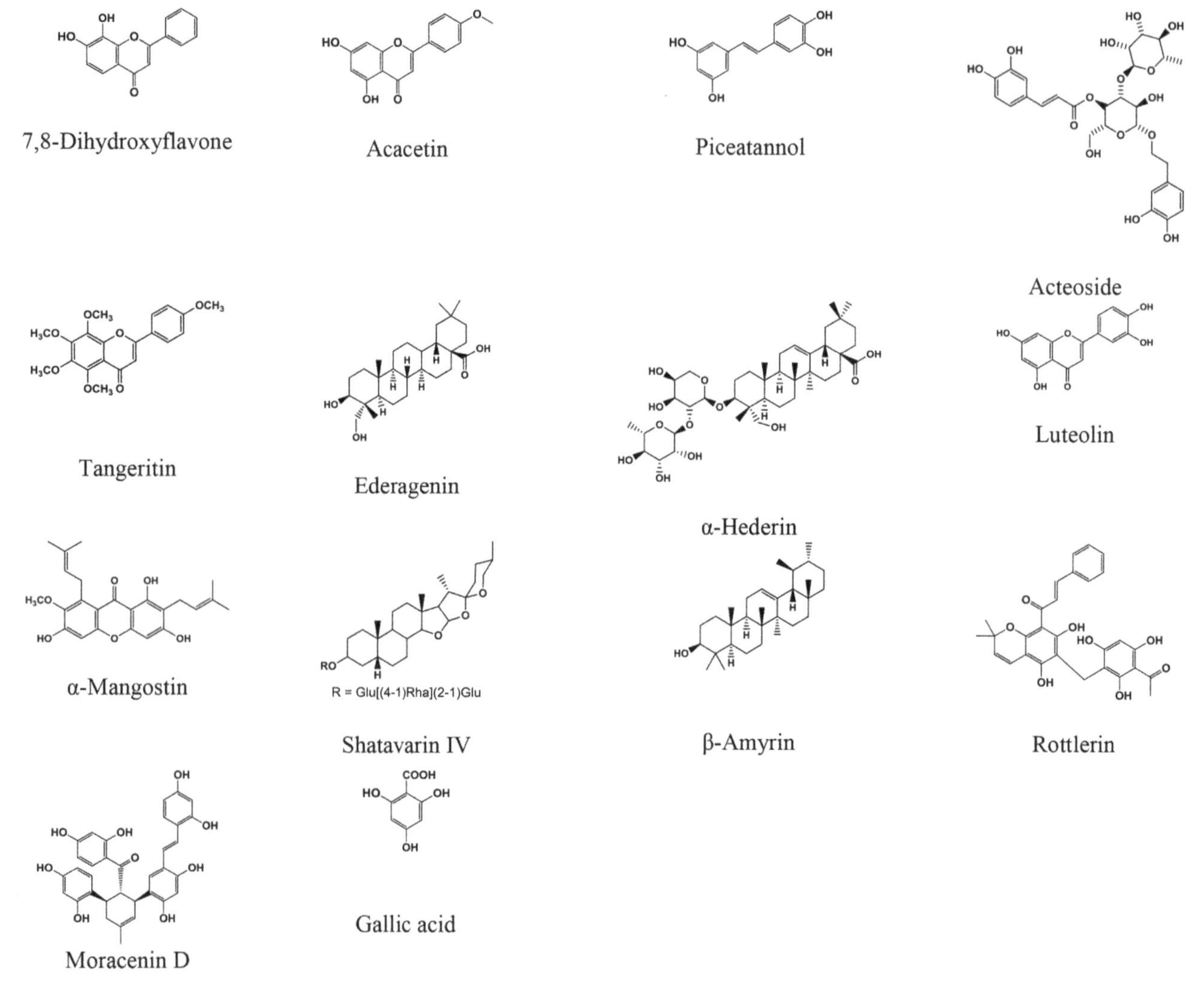

FIGURE 1 | Chemical structure of the phytochemicals attenuating α-synuclein activity in animal models of Parkinson's disease.

them from thermal denaturation. Furthermore, they assist in or prevent certain protein-protein assemblies similar to the molecular chaperones (Ringe and Petsko, 2009). Chaperoning is beneficial in cystic fibrosis (Chanoux and Rubenstein, 2012), Gaucher's disease (Sawkar et al., 2002), nephrogenic diabetes insipidus (Tamarappoo and Verkman, 1998), and retinitis pigmentosa (Noorwez et al., 2003). Mechanistically, ligand-mediated chaperoning is believed to correct receptor mislocalization and inhibit mutant proteins from forming toxic intracellular aggregates (Loo and Clarke, 2007). This has been shown to be successful with the pharmacological chaperone, tafamadis, in a clinical trial for the treatment of transthyretin familial amyloid polyneuropathy (Coelho et al., 2013). Several of the molecular chaperones, such as Hsp70, Hsp40, and torsin A either prevent the misfolding of proteins or promote the degradation and elimination of misfolded proteins; they provide a novel therapeutic approach in PD (Dimant et al., 2012).

Although molecular chaperoning is therapeutically significant in α-syn-associated neurodegeneration, the structural heterogeneity and deficiency of persistent structural components for α-syn creates a major issue in the discovery, design, and development of small molecules targeting α-syn (Lester et al., 2009). Plant-derived phytochaperones are a good source of molecules that target protein misfolding in neurotherapeutics (Bernd, 2008). In a chaperone-based approach, *Ginkgo biloba* is being utilized to search for lead molecules in drug discovery and in the development of protein-misfolding diseases leading to neurodegeneration (Kastenholz and Garfin, 2009). Thus, plant extracts and phytochemicals are a novel source of pharmacological chaperones for a disease-modifying approach that could be promising against neurodegenerative diseases. Following the reductionist approach of drug discovery from plant extracts, it is also important to characterize the bioactive constituents contributing to these pharmacological effects.

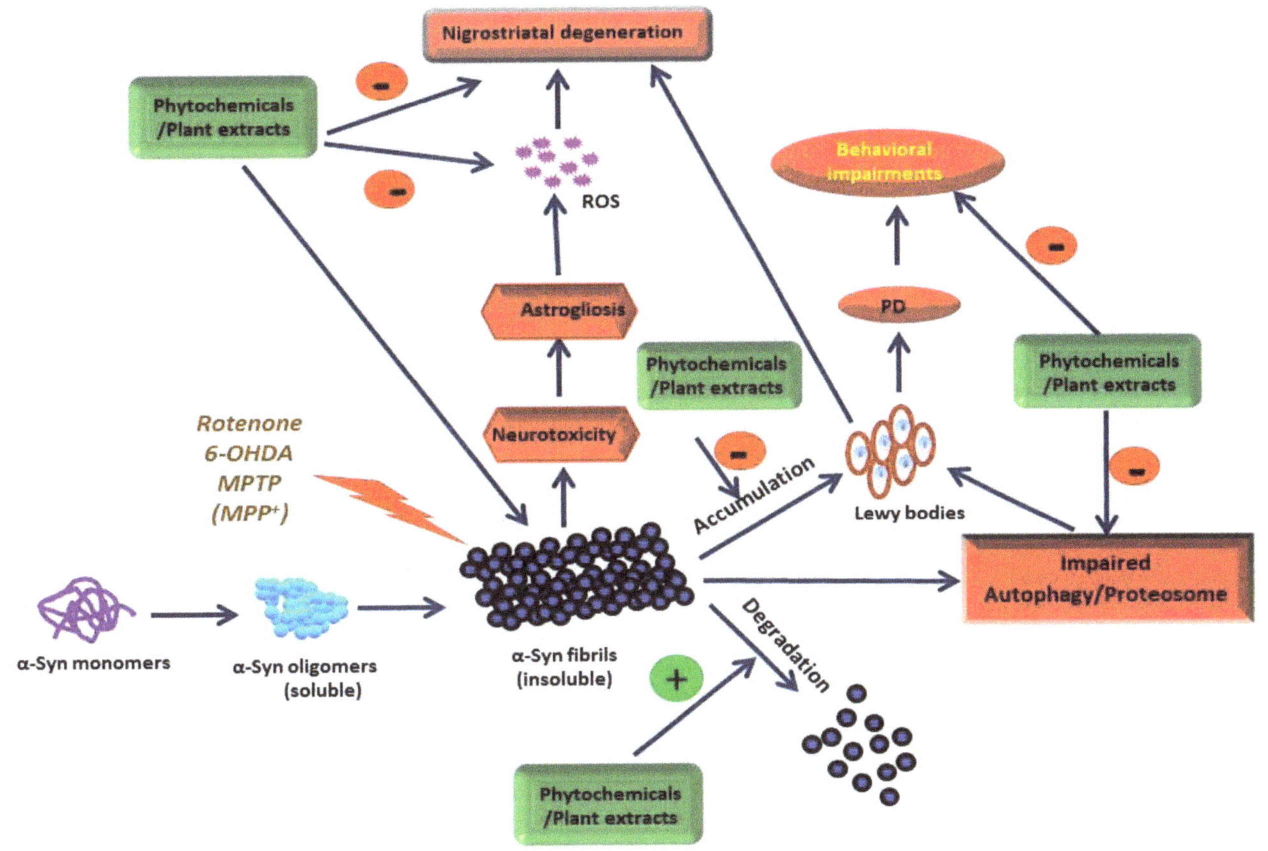

FIGURE 2 | The site of action of the phytochemicals and plant extracts on α-Syn.

PHYTOCHEMICALS TARGETING α-SYNUCLEIN ASSEMBLY AND TOXICITY

The phytochemicals are non-nutritive secondary metabolites that are heavily utilized for drug discovery and development; they remain an important source of drugs (Beutler, 2009; Henrich and Beutler, 2013). The phytochemicals that target α-syn at different stages of pathogenicity are represented in **Table 2** (*in vitro* studies), **Table 3** (*in vivo* studies), and **Table 4** (*in vitro* and *in vivo*, both studies), respectively. A benefit of the phytochemicals is their huge structural diversity that offers lead structures for drug discovery and development. They belong to many classes, such as alkaloids, saponins, carotenoids, lignans, glycosides, etc. Briefly, the alkaloids are a nitrogen-containing, structurally-diverse group of secondary metabolites that are protective against neurodegenerative diseases (Hussain et al., 2018). To name a few, galantamine is used in the pharmacotherapy of mild to moderate Alzheimer's disease. Many of the alkaloids, such as acetylcorynoline, 3α-acetoxyeudesma-1,4 (15),11 (13)-trien-12, 6α-olide, corynoxine B, dl-3-n-butylphthalide, isorhynchophylline, and squamosamide attenuate neurotoxicity in experimental models by directly inhibiting α-syn aggregation or fibril formation.

Saponins are an abundant group of secondary metabolites that can be classified as triterpenoids, steroids, and glycosides (Dinda et al., 2010). Their effects in neurodegenerative, neuropsychiatric, and affective disorders were recently reviewed (Sun et al., 2015). Saponins possess surface-active and amphipathic properties (Lorenzen et al., 2014) that may contribute to their membrane-permeabilizing actions and surfactant-based disruption of α-syn fibril formation. Many of the glucosides, such as 3-O-demethylswertipunicoside, jatamanin 11, paeoniflorin, 2,3,5,4′-tetrahydroxy stilbene-2-O-β-D-glucoside, 10-O-trans-p-coumaroylcatalpol and strophanthidine attenuate neurotoxicity in experimental models by directly inhibiting α-syn aggregation or fibril formation. Similarly, many terpenoids, such as celastrol, 2-cyano-3, 12-dioxo-oleana-1,9-dien-28-oic acid, geraniol, reynosin, thymoquinone, and ginkgolide A, B, and C attenuate neurotoxicity in experimental models by directly inhibiting α-syn aggregation or fibril formation. However, asiatic acid failed to prevent α-syn aggregation and protofibril formation (Masuda et al., 2006).

Dietary intake of polyphenolic compounds is protective against neurodegeneration as evidenced from many epidemiologic and experimental studies (Ho and Pasinetti, 2010; Caruana et al., 2016; da Costa et al., 2017). Popular polyphenols in food are curcumin (present in turmeric), oleuropein (present in olive oil), resveratrol (present in grapes), catechins (present in black and green tea), astaxanthin (a carotenoid present in vegetables and fruits) and lycopene (present in tomato) (da Costa et al., 2017). Polyphenols inhibit α-syn aggregation and fibrillation (Masuda et al., 2006; Caruana et al., 2011, 2012; Sivanesam and Andersen, 2016) and formation of amyloid protofilaments and fibrils (Kumar et al., 2012; Velander et al., 2017) and confer protective effects in neurodegenerative diseases. Masuda et al. (2006) tested 79 compounds from different chemical classes of compounds including polyphenols, benzothiazoles, terpenoids, steroids, porphyrins, lignans, phenothiazines, polyene macrolides, and Congo red and its derivatives for their potential to inhibit α-syn assembly. Out of 39 polyphenolic compounds tested, 26 were found to inhibit α-syn assembly. These findings establish that polyphenols constitute a major class of compounds that can inhibit the assembly of α-syn. Several of them inhibited α-syn filament assembly with IC50 values in the low micromolar range. Caruana et al. (2011) investigated 14 polyphenolic compounds and black tea extract containing theaflavins and found that baicalein, scutellarein, myricetin, (-)-epigallocatechin-3-gallate (EGCG), nordihydroguaiaretic acid and black tea extract are the ideal candidates to investigate in experimental models for their direct effect on the inhibition of α-syn oligomer formation. The polyphenolic compounds are believed to interact with receptors or plasma membrane transporters and activate intracellular signaling pathways. Among several polyphenols, EGCG associates with the laminin receptor on vascular cells (Tachibana et al., 2004). Currently, numerous polyphenolic compounds have been studied for their effect on α-syn aggregation, fibrillation, elongation, nitration, and oligomerization using biophysical and biochemical techniques (Meng et al., 2010; Caruana et al., 2011, 2012; Takahashi et al., 2015). The list of these compounds is presented in **Table 5**. A scheme is presented in **Figure 2** to depict the mechanism of action of the plant extracts and phytochemicals on α-syn oligomerization, fibrillation, and aggregation. An overview of some important phytochemicals which target α-syn aggregation and fibrillation and appear ideal candidates for further development is presented below.

Baicalein

Baicalein is a flavone isolated from the roots of *Scutellaria baicalensis* Georgi ("Huang Qin" in Chinese), a reputed plant in traditional Chinese medicine (Gasiorowski et al., 2011) and Scutellaria *pinnatifida* grown in Iran (Sashourpour et al., 2017). In many studies, baicalein was shown to prevent α-syn oligomerization and fibrillation (Bomhoff et al., 2006; Meng et al., 2009; Caruana et al., 2011; Gasiorowski et al., 2011; Sashourpour et al., 2017). Baicalein interacts with α-syn through a tyrosine residue. Following oxidation, it generates quinone metabolites that bind covalently with a lysine side chain in α-syn. It prevents fibril formation and degrades preformed fibrils at low micromolar concentrations (Zhu et al., 2004). In another study, its non-covalent binding with α-syn and covalent modification by the oxidized form restricts the conformational changes in the unfolded protein that results in α-syn monomer and oligomer stabilization (Meng et al., 2009). The oligomers cause impairment of neuronal membrane integrity that results in disruption or permeabilization of the membrane, impairment of calcium homeostasis, and cell death (Caruana et al., 2012).

Baicalein prevents α-syn fibrillation and protects against neurotoxicity by preventing α-syn oligomer formation in SH-SY5Y and HeLa cells (Lu et al., 2011). It also stabilizes the oligomers, prevents further fibrillation (Hong et al., 2008) and tandem repeats of α-syn in the aggregation process (Bae et al., 2010). Further, it prevents the formation of annular protofibrils of α-syn induced by copper and reduces the β-sheet contents (Zhang et al., 2015). In another study, using JC-1, a probe that binds the α-syn C-terminal region, baicalein differentiated the α-syn fibrillation states (monomeric, oligomeric intermediate, and fibrillar forms) and reconfirmed the defibrillation action of baicalein on α-syn (Lee et al., 2009). In PC12 cells, it ameliorates cytotoxicity, mitochondrial depolarization, and inhibits proteasome inhibition induced by E46K, an α-syn point mutation that mimics familial PD (Jiang et al., 2010). In a recent study, baicalein induces autophagy, increases cell viability and reduces α-syn in the media of dopaminergic cell lines (SN4741) overexpressing A53T-syn (Li et al., 2017). Baicalein diminished the transmission of α-syn and prompted the polymerization of α-syn to a big complex rather than promoting clearance (Li et al., 2017). A recent study in rotenone-induced PD in rats showed reduced α-syn oligomer formation along with behavioral improvement and neurotransmitters in the striatum. However, it failed to reduce α-syn mRNA expression but prevented the transition from α-syn monomers to oligomers (Hu et al., 2016). Furthermore, baicalein attenuated α-syn aggregate formation, induced autophagy, inhibited apoptosis, reduced inflammation, and restored dopamine in PD induced by MPP^+ infusion in the SNc of mice (Hung et al., 2016).

The baicalein derivative N′-benzylidene-benzohydrazide also attenuated oligomer formation (Kostka et al., 2008). Baicalein in combination with β-cyclodextrin (β-CD) synergistically inhibited α-syn aggregation and disaggregated preformed fibrils even at very low concentrations (Gautam et al., 2017). A combination of baicalein with specific proteolytic peptide sequences of α-syn was developed for targeted drug delivery and found to prevent α-syn fibrillation (Yoshida et al., 2013). Integrating evidence from *in vitro* and *in vivo* studies, baicalein appears to be a potential drug to inhibit α-syn aggregation, fibrillation, and propagation among the neurons.

Curcumin

Curcumin, chemically known as diferuloylmethane, is one of the most popular natural leads to drug discovery and development from turmeric (Molino et al., 2016). It is reputed for its dietary importance and health benefits and is the most studied phytochemical in experimental and clinical studies (Molino et al., 2016). It is a beneficial treatment in neurodegenerative diseases, including PD, and has antioxidant, anti-inflammatory, and antiapoptotic properties (Kim et al., 2012; Singh et al., 2013; Ji and Shen, 2014). Ono and Yamada (2006) found that curcumin possesses anti-fibrillogenic activity by inhibiting α-syn fibril formation and destabilizing preformed fibrils (Ono and Yamada, 2006). It was found to inhibit oligomerization of mutant α-syn into higher molecular weight aggregates (Pandey et al., 2008) and induce the dissociation of α-syn fibrils (Shoval et al., 2008). Curcumin treatment on mesencephalic cells did not affect α-syn fibril formation but enhanced LRRK2 mRNA and protein expression in rats (Ortiz-Ortiz et al., 2010). In neuroblastoma cells, curcumin attenuates cytotoxicity from aggregated α-syn, ROS generation, and diminished caspase-3 activation (Wang et al., 2010). In PC12 cells, curcumin ameliorates A53T mutant α-syn-induced PD (Liu et al., 2011). Further, curcumin reduces mutant α-syn accumulation by restoring macroautophagy, a process in the degradation pathway that clears proteins in cells by activating the mTOR/p70S6K signaling pathway (Jiang et al., 2013). Mechanistically, curcumin preferentially binds oligomeric intermediates rather than monomeric α-syn (Singh et al., 2013). Also, it binds strongly to the hydrophobic non-amyloid-β component of α-syn (Ahmad and Lapidus, 2012). The ordered structure is vital for effective binding and affects the extent of binding and potential in inhibiting oligomers or fibrils (Singh et al., 2013). The conformational and reconfiguration changes appear to govern the binding of curcumin to α-syn (Ahmad and Lapidus, 2012; Tavassoly et al., 2014). Curcumin, in combination with β-cyclodextrin, showed a synergistic inhibition of α-syn aggregation and degraded the preformed aggregates into monomers at very low concentrations (Gautam et al., 2014, 2017). Gautam et al. (2017) further demonstrated that a balanced arrangement of the phenolic groups, benzene rings, and flexibility attributes to the ability of curcumin. The phenolic groups enhance curcumin interactions with α-syn monomers as well as oligomers. In PC12 cells transfected with recombinant plasmids, α-syn-pEGFP-A53T downregulated α-syn expression or oligomer formation by regulating apoptosis-mediated mitochondrial membrane potential (Chen et al., 2015a). The effect of curcumin on α-syn observed *in vitro* was reconfirmed *in vivo* in genetic mouse models of synucleinopathy (Spinelli et al., 2015). Curcumin increased phosphorylated forms of α-syn at cortical presynaptic terminals but had no direct effect on α-syn aggregation. However, curcumin improved motor and behavioral performance (Spinelli et al., 2015).

Curcumin is less stable and soluble and has limited oral bioavailability. To improve its stability, solubility, and oral bioavailability, many nanoformulations or structural analogs have been developed (Gadad et al., 2012; Kundu et al., 2016; Taebnia et al., 2016). Curc-gluc, a modified curcumin preparation, inhibits α-syn oligomerization and fibrillation (Gadad et al., 2012). In another study, dehydrozingerone, zingerone; an O-methyl derivative of dehydrozingerone and their biphenyl analogs were investigated for their cytoprotective effects in PC12 cells challenged with H_2O_2, MPP^+, and $MnCl_2$ (Marchiani et al., 2013). The biphenyl analogs of dehydrozingerone and O-methyl-dehydrozingerone prevent α-syn aggregation; the biphenyl zingerone analog is the most potent inhibitor and has the most potent antioxidant activity. This activity was attributed to the hydroxylated biphenyl scaffold in the pharmacophore (Marchiani et al., 2013). In another study, stable curcumin analogs, such as curcumin pyrazole, curcumin isoxazole, and their derivatives, were evaluated against α-syn aggregation, fibrillation, and toxicity. Curcumin pyrazole and its derivative N-(3-Nitrophenyl pyrazole) curcumin reduces A53T-α-syn-induced neurotoxicity by preventing fibrillation and disrupting preformed fibrils (Ahsan et al., 2015). Taebnia et al. (2016) developed amine-functionalized mesoporous silica nanoparticles of curcumin to enhance its bioavailability and evaluated its effect against cytotoxicity and α-syn fibrillation (Taebnia et al., 2016). This nanoformulation showed interaction with α-syn species and prevented fibrillation with negligible effect on cytotoxicity (Taebnia et al., 2016). A nanoformulation containing curcumin and piperine with glyceryl monooleate nanoparticles coated with various surfactants was developed for targeted delivery to enhance its bioavailability in the brain (Kundu et al., 2016). The nanoformulation has been shown to attenuate oxidative stress, apoptosis, prevent α-syn oligomerization and fibrillation, and induce autophagy. Another nanoformulation prepared with lactoferrin by sol-oil chemistry ameliorates rotenone-induced neurotoxicity in dopaminergic SK-N-SH cells (Bollimpelli et al., 2016). This nanoformulation exhibited better availability, improved cell viability, attenuated oxidative stress, and reduced tyrosine hydroxylase and α-syn expression. Nine curcumin analogs were synthesized by substitution of groups on the aromatic ring which alters the hydrophobicity, promotes stability, and facilitates binding with the fibrils as well as oligomers (Jha et al., 2016). Some of the analogs showed improved stability and appeared to interact with oligomers and preformed fibrils. The analogs exhibited differential binding patterns and augmented α-syn aggregation, generating different kinds of amyloid fibrils. The liposomal nanohybrid of curcumin with polysorbate 80-modified cerasome was developed for targeted drug delivery in the striatum and showed better half-life and bioavailability (Zhang et al., 2018). This nanoformulation ameliorated motor deficits and improved dopamine and tyrosine hydroxylase expression by promoting α-syn clearance in a mouse model of MPTP-induced PD (Zhang et al., 2018). Curcumin inhibited α-syn aggregates in dopaminergic neurons and attenuated oxidative stress, inflammation, apoptosis, and motor deficits in a rat model of lipopolysaccharide-induced PD (Sharma and Nehru, 2018). These reports demonstrate the effect of curcumin on α-syn aggregation- and fibrillation-induced neurotoxicity but further studies are still needed to demonstrate therapeutic success.

Cuminaldehyde

Cuminaldehyde is isolated from many edible plants including *Artemisia salsoloides, Aegle marmelos*, and spices cumin *(Cuminum cyminum L.)* and is used as a food additive and flavoring agent in many cuisines in the Middle East, South Asia, and Mediterranean countries. Cuminaldehyde isolated from Iranian cumin showed to inhibit α-syn fibrillation (Morshedi et al., 2015). It prevented α-syn fibrillation even in the presence of seeds with negligible disaggregating effect on the preformed fibrils of α-syn. Interestingly, it was found to be superior to baicalein, a known inhibitor of α-syn fibrillation and blocked protein assembly into β-structural fibrils that were attributed to interaction with amine and aldehyde groups in the chemical structure (Morshedi and Nasouti, 2016).

Catechins, Theaflavins, and (-)-Epigallocatechin-3-Gallate (EGCG)

Catechins, the polyphenolic compounds present in black and green tea, are protective in neurodegenerative diseases (Caruana and Vassallo, 2015; Jha et al., 2017; Xu et al., 2017; Pervin et al., 2018). Theaflavins present in fermented black tea inhibits fibrillogenesis of α-syn and amyloid-β formation (Grelle et al., 2011). These compounds facilitate the assembly of amyloid-β and α-syn into non-toxic, spherical aggregates which are unable to undergo seeding to form amyloid plaques. They were also found to remodel the formed amyloid-β fibrils into non-toxic aggregates and these effects were comparable to EGCG. Theaflavins also appeared less vulnerable to oxidation in air and exhibited better activity in oxidizing environments in comparison with EGCG (Grelle et al., 2011).

One of the most popular catechins, (-)-Epigallocatechin 3-gallate (EGCG), is a flavonol compound predominantly present in green tea, a popular beverage across the world. EGCG inhibited α-syn aggregation and fibrillation in a concentration-dependent manner (Šneideris et al., 2015; Xu et al., 2017), and by disaggregating mature and large α-syn fibrils into smaller, non-toxic, amorphous aggregates (Ehrnhoefer et al., 2008). EGCG binds directly to the natively unfolded polypeptides and inhibits their conversion into toxic intermediates (Ehrnhoefer et al., 2008). It induces a conformational change without their disassembly into monomers or small diffusible oligomers (Bieschke et al., 2010). It appears to bind directly with β-sheet-rich aggregates and reduces its concentration required to induce conformational changes (Liu et al., 2018). Furthermore, it showed neuroprotection against free radicals and α-syn toxicity by chelating Fe (III) in PC12 cells transfected with α-syn and exposed to β-sheet-enriched α-syn fibrils (Zhao et al., 2017). EGCG appears to disaggregate α-syn fibrils by preventing the amyloid formation of α-syn tandem repeat and destabilizing α-syn fibrils into soluble amorphous aggregates (Bae et al., 2010). This study also revealed that the tandem repeat of α-syn may be used as a molecular model to study the mechanism of α-syn aggregation (Bae et al., 2010). Further, EGCG also prevents α-syn aggregation and accumulation by activating the hypoxia-inducible factor (HIF)-1 signaling mechanism that controls α-syn aggregation by regulating antioxidant and iron homeostasis (Weinreb et al., 2013).

Lorenzen et al. (2014) showed that EGCG has potential to prevent α-syn oligomer formation and attenuate the oligomer cytotoxicity by preventing vesicle permeabilization and blocking the membrane affinity of syn to bind and immobilize in the C-terminal region. Though, it failed to affect the oligomer size distribution or secondary structure. Recently, in primary cortical neuron cultures challenged with oxidative injury, quercetin, EGCG, and cyanidin-3-glucoside inhibited fibrillation of α-syn and apoptosis (Pogacnik et al., 2016). Further, it decreased amyloid fibril formation on the surface of liposomal membranes and generates compact oligomers following off-pathway, as well as facilitating the conversion of active oligomers into amyloid fibrils (Yang et al., 2017). A combination of EGCG with specific α-syn proteolytic peptide sequences was developed for targeted drug delivery and found to prevent the α-syn fibrillation (Yoshida et al., 2013). In combination, this evidence suggests EGCG could be a promising treatment in neurodegenerative diseases and a good candidate for pharmaceutical development and dietary inclusion.

Gallic Acid

Gallic acid, a type of phenolic acid chemically known as 3,4,5-trihydroxybenzoic acid, is found in free form or as part of the hydrolyzable tannins in many plants, such as gallnuts, sumac, witch hazel, tea leaves, and oak bark (Kosuru et al., 2018). Gallic acid and esters are well-known food additives, nutritional supplements, and a common reagent in the pharmaceutical analysis (Kosuru et al., 2018). Over the last few decades, many investigators showed the antioxidative, antiapoptotic, cardioprotective, neuroprotective and anticancer properties of gallic acid and gallates (Blainski et al., 2013; Choubey et al., 2018; Kosuru et al., 2018). It is used as a reference compound for the quantification of the phenolic contents in biochemical assays; Folin-Ciocalteau assay or Folin's phenol reagent or Folin-Denis reagent which determines the antioxidant power in gallic acid equivalents (Blainski et al., 2013). The polyphenolic compound gallic acid and its structurally similar benzoic acid derivatives elicit anti-aggregating effects (Ardah et al., 2014). Gallic acid impedes α-syn fibrillation and disaggregates the preformed fibrils of α-syn in a battery of biophysical, biochemical, and cell viability assays. In addition to inhibiting aggregation and disaggregation, it also binds to soluble and non-toxic oligomers devoid of β-sheet content and confers structural stability. Numerous benzoic acid derivatives have been developed using structure-activity relationship and all inhibit α-syn fibrillation (Ardah et al., 2014). The number of hydroxyl groups and their presence on the phenyl ring in these structural derivatives of gallic acid are believed to attribute to the potential mechanism in binding and inhibiting α-syn fibrillation. Furthermore, gallic acid prevents α-syn amyloid fibril formation, stabilizes the extended intrinsic structure of α-syn, and reacts rapidly in biochemical assays (Liu et al., 2014).

Ginsenosides

Ginseng, also known as red ginseng (*Panax ginseng*, Araliaceae), is a popular source of saponins and is reputed in the folk medicine of the Far East countries. It has shown neuroprotective effects in numerous neurodegenerative diseases including PD (Van Kampen et al., 2003; Chen et al., 2005; Luo et al., 2011). The ginseng extract, abbreviated as G115, confers neuroprotection against MPTP and its neurotoxic metabolite, MPP^+ in murine models of PD (Van Kampen et al., 2003). Van Kampen et al. (2014) reported that G115 treatment reduces dopaminergic cell loss, microgliosis, the buildup of α-syn aggregates, and improves locomotor activity and coordination in rats chronically exposed to the dietary phytosterol glucoside, β-sitosterol β-d-glucoside, which recapitulates features of PD.

Several studies identified the active constituents of ginseng known as ginsenosides, a group of 60 compounds that possess a wide range of pharmacological and physiological actions (Mohanan et al., 2018; Zheng et al., 2018). Several ginsenosides, Rg1, Rg3, and Rb1, were investigated for their effect on α-syn aggregation using biophysical and biochemical techniques (Ardah et al., 2015; Heng et al., 2016). Upon oral treatment, Rg1 attenuated neurodegeneration in a mouse model of

MPTP-induced PD by inhibiting pro-inflammatory cytokines; reducing mortality, behavioral defects, and dopamine neuron loss; and correcting ultrastructure changes in the SNc (Heng et al., 2016). Rg1 also reduced oligomeric, phosphorylated, and disease-related α-syn in the SNc. In contrast, a separate study identified only Rb1 as a strong inhibitor of α-syn fibrillation; it also disaggregated preformed fibrils and inhibited the seeded polymerization of α-syn (Ardah et al., 2015). Further, Rb1 binds to the oligomers and causes stabilization of soluble, non-toxic oligomers with negligible involvement of β-sheets that depicts a novel mechanism of action (Ardah et al., 2015). Although the authors did not find a significant effect of Rg1 and Rg3 on α-syn aggregation in cellular models (Ardah et al., 2015). In one of the study, Rg3, another ginsenoside present in *Panax ginseng*, reduced α-syn expression in stress models (Xu et al., 2013). The evidence of Rg3-mediated changes in α-syn in stress models needs to be investigated in PD (Xu et al., 2013). A detailed investigation is required to understand the observed differences in the *in vitro* and *in vivo* studies.

Resveratrol

Resveratrol, a natural phytoestrogen found in grapes and red wine, is reputed for its neuroprotective properties by attenuating oxidative stress, mitochondrial impairment, inducing apoptotic cell death and promoting autophagy (Caruana et al., 2016; Ur Rasheed et al., 2016). Wu et al. (2011) showed that resveratrol enhanced α-syn degradation in PC12 cells expressing α-syn by activating autophagy and mediating the induction of AMP-activated protein kinase (AMPK) mammalian silent information regulator 2 (SIRT1) signaling mechanism. This reduces protein levels of microtubule-associated protein 1 light chain 3 (LC3-II) and preserves neuronal cells. AMPK is a serine/threonine kinase which acts as a metabolic energy sensor to maintain energy balance; upon activation, it induces neuronal cell apoptosis and decreases SIRT1 leading to activation of the ubiquitin-proteasome pathway by enhancing ubiquitination and promoting SUMOylation that may be important in reducing the progression of neurodegeneration (Wu et al., 2011). The induction of autophagy and apoptotic pathways represents an important approach in the therapeutic targeting of α-syn (Ghavami et al., 2014). Further, in MPTP-induced PD in mice, resveratrol corrected the behavioral and motor deficits and attenuated neurodegeneration by inducing autophagy of α-syn via activation of SIRT1 and subsequent deacetylation of LC3 (Guo et al., 2016). Recently, in an effort to enhance the bioavailability to attain therapeutic benefits, resveratrol was prepared with β-CD; this combination was found synergistic in showing activity at very low concentrations to prevent α-syn aggregation as well as disaggregate preformed fibrils (Gautam et al., 2017). Resveratrol treatment reduced α-syn oligomers in S1/S2 transfected human H4 neuroglioma cells by activating peroxisome proliferator-activated receptor γ (PPARγ), which regulates energy metabolism and mitochondrial biogenesis, and plays a role in the pathogenesis of PD (Eschbach et al., 2015). At the molecular level, resveratrol downregulates α-syn expression mediating miR-214 in the MPTP-induced mouse model of PD and MPP^+ induced neurotoxicity in neuroblastoma cells (Wang et al., 2015a).

The phytochemicals that inhibit fibrils and oligomer formation along with the ability to stabilize the α-syn oligomers or disaggregate α-syn oligomers can be potential compounds for pharmaceutical development. The *in vitro* data reveals success with many phytochemicals in ameliorating the fibrils and oligomer formation of α-syn as well as inducing degradation of α-syn and promoting autophagy. However, many polyphenolic compounds showed difficulty in crossing the blood brain barrier due to their non-lipophilic nature. Therefore, they may not attain the required concentration to exert effects in the brain (Pandareesh et al., 2015; Pogacnik et al., 2016). Several factors, such as stability, solubility in an acidic environment at gastric pH, absorption pattern, gut microflora, enterohepatic circulation, first pass metabolism, and metabolic pattern either phase I or phase II play a key role in achieving the ideal bioavailability of the phytochemicals in the brain (Scholz and Williamson, 2007). Additionally, the inconsistency between the *in vitro* concentration and *in vivo* dose in certain models encourages systematic pharmacokinetic evaluations to understand the variation between the *in vitro* and *in vivo* data.

EXPERIMENTAL TECHNIQUES TO ASSESS THE α-SYN INHIBITORY ACTIVITY OF PHYTOCHEMICALS

Several biophysical and biochemical techniques used to assess the ability of phytochemicals and plant extracts in preventing α-syn oligomerization and fibrillation are represented in **Table 6**. These experimental techniques include surface plasmon resonance imaging (SPRi), Thioflavin-T (ThT) fluorescence, transmission electron microscopy (TEM), small angle X-ray scattering (SAXS), circular dichroism (CD) spectroscopy, fourier transform infrared spectroscopy (FTIR), nuclear magnetic resonance (NMR), and absorption spectroscopy of Congo red (CR) binding assay (Luk et al., 2007; Kostka et al., 2008; Celej et al., 2009; Yamaguchi et al., 2010; Giehm et al., 2011; da Silva et al., 2013; Aelvoet et al., 2014; Coelho-Cerqueira et al., 2014; Cheng et al., 2015; Fazili and Naeem, 2015; Takahashi et al., 2015; Pujols et al., 2017; Das et al., 2018). The biochemical and biophysical assays employed to measure the α-syn aggregation are efficient in providing a high-resolution structure of α-syn oligomers, but not free from the restrictions and misconceptions on their efficacy (Coelho-Cerqueira et al., 2014). The polyphenolic nature of phytochemicals may cause some variations in interferences in spectrophotometric and fluorescent assays used to measure α-syn formation (Coelho-Cerqueira et al., 2014). Coelho-Cerqueira et al. (2014) show the drawbacks related to the application of ThT assays to examine α-syn fibrillation as ThT reacts with disordered α-syn monomer and augments protein fibrillation *in vitro*. As a result, phytochemicals may also bias the ThT assay and ambiguous results may be interpreted from the application of ThT based real-time assays in the screening of anti-fibrillogenic compounds. Therefore, a battery of techniques is recommended to support or confirm the anti-aggregatory and anti-fibrillogenic activity in side-stepping the possible artifacts associated with the measure of ThT fluorescence (Coelho-Cerqueira et al., 2014).

The knowledge of the stage, form, nature, and propagation of α-syn that play a key role in enhanced toxicity in PD highlights the multitude of techniques needed to gauge α-syn disposition in experimental situations (Giehm et al., 2011; Pujols et al., 2017). Recently, Moree et al. (2015) developed a novel assay to recognize compounds that control the conformation of monomeric α-syn in a direct manner to reduce the encounters associated with conventional small molecule screening of α-syn. This novel assay may aid in understanding the role of α-syn oligomers in PD and opens new avenues to evaluate α-syn-based potential neuroprotective agents.

EXPERIMENTAL MODELS FOR SCREENING AGENTS TARGETING α-SYN TOXICITY

Apart from biophysical and biochemical assays, numerous models including cell lines *(in vitro)* and animal models (*in vivo*) have been developed to study the role of α-syn in the etiology and disease modification of PD and evaluate test compounds against α-syn (Skibinski and Finkbeiner, 2011; Javed et al., 2016; Visanji et al., 2016; Ko and Bezard, 2017; Lázaro et al., 2017). The experimental models showing α-syn fibrillation, oligomerization, and neurotoxicity are summarized in **Table 7**. The toxicant models and mutation-based *in vivo* models are popularly used to mimic sporadic and familial PD, respectively (Javed et al., 2016). The experimental models often present issues and challenges in separating the complexities of cellular and molecular mechanisms and are infeasible for high-throughput screening and other drug development stages, such as dose-response toxicology studies. Cell-based models including stem cells and primary neurons with features of dopaminergic neurons give important insights into the cellular mechanisms of PD for drug discovery (Lázaro et al., 2017). This enables the recognition of agents targeting α-syn and their molecular mechanisms. Some of the prominent human cell models for PD drug screening are SK-N-SH, SHSY5Y, and SK-N-MC (Skibinski and Finkbeiner, 2011; Lázaro et al., 2017). The development of α-syn-based experimental models of sporadic or familial PD that show progressive forms of the disease will elucidate the mechanisms of neurodegeneration and aid in the identification of phytochemicals modulating α-syn. The uptake of recombinant α-syn from the culture medium has been reported in many cellular models (Reyes et al., 2015). Recently, Reyes et al. (2015) established a culture system that is a physiologically appropriate assay for the characterization of genetic modifiers or small molecules which prevent cell-to-cell transfer or propagation of α-syn.

CONCLUDING REMARKS AND FUTURE PROSPECTS

This comprehensive review presents an overview of the plant extracts and phytochemicals specifically targeting α-syn oligomerization, fibrillation, and aggregation in different models of PD and their underlying mechanisms. It also discusses the experimental techniques and models used to evaluate the plant extracts and phytochemicals. The literature review suggests that many phytochemicals are promising in targeting α-syn in the *in vitro* studies; however, the actions observed *in vitro* need to be reconfirmed *in vivo*. Indeed, the screening of phytochemicals or plant extracts in cell lines often lacks clinical applicability due to physiological, biochemical, and pharmacological relevancy. The available literature from a convincing number of *in vitro* studies and few *in vivo* studies demonstrates that phytochemicals, such as baicalein, curcumin, resveratrol, and epigallocatechin gallate have promising therapeutic potential in inhibiting α-syn oligomerization, fibrillation, aggregation, and accumulation. All these promising compounds should be studied in the *in vivo* studies to proceed further for clinical studies and thereon.

The process of α-syn oligomerization and fibrillation were well-recognized but the triggers that induce α-syn aggregation are not yet well-established. Thus, for a fair translational disease modifying approach, evaluation of phytochemicals in animal models involving α-syn aggregation and mimicking the progressive nature of PD pathogenesis is desired as a proof of concept. Although the available preclinical studies are encouraging, they are markedly speculative for clinical success. The issues, such as bioavailability, stability, metabolism, as well as long-term safety and toxicity, should be resolved before pharmaceutical development and further testing in humans. Based on the available preclinical studies, it can be concluded that these phytochemicals could possibly be novel drug candidates for neurodegenerative diseases, such as PD.

AUTHOR CONTRIBUTIONS

All the authors provided important intellectual content, reviewed the content and approved the final version of this manuscript. AA and SO conceptualized the idea for this review. MFNM, SA, HJ, and SO performed the literature search. HJ and SO wrote the first draft of the manuscript. SO and AA thoroughly revised and edited the manuscript. BS drew the chemical structures.

ACKNOWLEDGMENTS

The authors sincerely acknowledge the research grant support from United Arab Emirates University awarded as University Program for Advanced Research and Center Based Interdisciplinary research grant #31R127.

REFERENCES

Aelvoet, S. A., Ibrahimi, A., Macchi, F., Gijsbers, R., Van den Haute, C., Debyser, Z., et al. (2014). Noninvasive bioluminescence imaging of α-synuclein oligomerization in mouse brain using split firefly luciferase reporters. *J. Neurosci.* 34, 16518–16532. doi: 10.1523/JNEUROSCI.4933-13.2014

Ahlskog, J. E. (1994). Treatment of Parkinson's disease. From theory to practice. *Postgrad. Med.* 95, 52–54, 57–58. doi: 10.1080/00325481.1994.11945830

Ahmad, B., and Lapidus, L. J. (2012). Curcumin prevents aggregation in α-synuclein by increasing reconfiguration rate. *J. Biol. Chem.* 287, 9193–9199. doi: 10.1074/jbc.M111.325548

Ahsan, N., Mishra, S., Jain, M. K., Surolia, A., and Gupta, S (2015). Curcumin pyrazole and its derivative (N-(3-Nitrophenylpyrazole) Curcumin inhibit aggregation, disrupt fibrils and modulate toxicity of wild type and mutant α-synuclein. *Sci. Rep.* 5:9862. doi: 10.1038/srep09862

Akhoon, B. A., Pandey, S., Tiwari, S., and Pandey, R. (2016). Withanolide A offers neuroprotection, ameliorates stress resistance and prolongs the life expectancy of Caenorhabditis elegans. *Exp. Gerontol.* 78, 47–56. doi: 10.1016/j.exger.2016.03.004

Albani, D., Polito, L., Batelli, S., De Mauro, S., Fracasso, C., Martelli, G., et al. (2009). The SIRT1 activator resveratrol protects SK-N-BE cells from oxidative stress and against toxicity caused by alpha-synuclein or amyloid-beta (1-42) peptide. *J. Neurochem.* 110, 1445–1456. doi: 10.1111/j.1471-4159.2009.06228.x

Alhebshi, A.H., Odawara, A., Gotoh, M., and Suzuki, I. (2014). Thymoquinone protects cultured hippocampal and human induced pluripotent stem cells-derived neurons against α-synuclein-induced synapse damage. *Neurosci. Lett.* 570, 126–131. doi: 10.1016/j.neulet.2013.09.049

Amro, M. S, Teoh, S. L, Norzana, A. G., and Srijit, D. (2018). The potential role of herbal products in the treatment of Parkinson's disease. *Clin. Ter.* 169, e23–e33. doi: 10.7417/T.2018.2050

Andrich, K., and Bieschke, J. (2015). The Effect of (-)-Epigallo-catechin-(3)-gallate on amyloidogenic proteins suggests a common mechanism. *Adv. Exp. Med. Biol.* 863, 139–161. doi: 10.1007/978-3-319-18365-7_7

Anusha, C., Sumathi, T., and Joseph, L.D. (2017). Protective role of apigenin on rotenone induced rat model of Parkinson's disease: suppression of neuroinflammation and oxidative stress mediated apoptosis. *Chem. Biol. Interact.* 269, 67–79. doi: 10.1016/j.cbi.2017.03.016

Ardah, M. T., Paleologou, K. E., Lv, G., Abul Khair, S. B., Kazim, A. S., Minhas, S. T., et al. (2014). Structure activity relationship of phenolic acid inhibitors of α-synuclein fibril formation and toxicity. *Front. Aging Neurosci.* 6:197. doi: 10.3389/fnagi.2014.00197

Ardah, M. T., Paleologou, K. E., Lv, G., Menon, S. A., Abul Khair, S. B., Lu, J.H., et al. (2015). Ginsenoside Rb1 inhibits fibrillation and toxicity of alpha-synuclein and disaggregates preformed fibrils. *Neurobiol. Dis.* 74, 89–101. doi: 10.1016/j.nbd.2014.11.007

Asthana, J., Mishra, B. N., and Pandey, R. (2016). Acacetin promotes healthy aging by altering stress response in Caenorhabditis elegans. *Free Radic. Res.* 50, 861–874. doi: 10.1080/10715762.2016.1187268

Attia, A. H., Gadelkarim, M., Morsi, M., Awad, K., Elnenny, M., Ghanem, E., et al. (2017). Meta-analysis of creatine for neuroprotection against Parkinson's disease. *CNS Neurol. Disord. Drug Targets* 16, 169–175. doi: 10.2174/1871527315666161104161855

Bae, S. Y., Kim, S., Hwang, H., Kim, H. K., Yoon, H. C., Kim, J. H., et al. (2010). Amyloid formation and disaggregation of α-synuclein and its tandem repeat (α-TR). *Biochem. Biophys. Res. Commun.* 400, 531–536. doi: 10.1016/j.bbrc.2010.08.088

Bagchi, P., and Hopper, W. (2011). "Virtual screening of compounds from Valeriana Jatamansi with α-Synuclein," in *2011 International Conference on Bioscience, Biochemistry, and Bioinformatics, IPCBEE*, Vol. 5. © (2011) (Singapore: IACSIT Press).

Bao, X. Q., Kong, X. C., Qian, C., and Zhang, D. (2012). FLZ protects dopaminergic neuron through activating protein kinase B/mammalian target of rapamycin pathway and inhibiting RTP801 expression in Parkinson's disease models. *Neuroscience* 202, 396–404. doi: 10.1016/j.neuroscience.2011.11.036

Bao, X. Q., Wu, L. Y., Wang, X. L., Sun, H., and Zhang, D. (2015). Squamosamide derivative FLZ protected tyrosine hydroxylase function in a chronic MPTP/probenecid mouse model of Parkinson's disease. *Naunyn Schmiedebergs. Arch. Pharmacol.* 388, 549–556. doi: 10.1007/s00210-015-1094-5

Bartels, T., Choi, J. G., and Selkoe, D. J. (2011). α-synuclein occurs physiologically as a helically folded tetramer that resists aggregation. *Nature* 477, 107–110. doi: 10.1038/nature10324

Beal, M. F., Oakes, D., Shoulson, I., Henchcliffe, C., Galpern, W. R., Haas, R., et al. (2014). Parkinson Study Group QE3 Investigators, a randomized clinical trial of high-dosage coenzyme Q10 in early Parkinson disease: no evidence of benefit. *JAMA Neurol.* 71, 543–552. doi: 10.1001/jamaneurol.2014.131

Bendor, J. T., Logan, T. P., and Edwards, R. H. (2013). The function of -synuclein. *Neuron* 79, 1044–1066. doi: 10.1016/j.neuron.2013.09.004

Bergström, A. L., Kallunki, P., and Fog, K. (2016). Development of passive immunotherapies for synucleinopathies. *Mov. Disord.* 31, 203–213. doi: 10.1002/mds.26481

Bernd, K. (2008). Phytochemical approach and bioanalytical strategy to develop chaperone-based medications. *Open Biochem. J.* 2, 44–48. doi: 10.2174/1874091X00802010044

Berrocal, R., Vasudevaraju, P., Indi, S. S., Sambasiva Rao, K. R., and Rao, K. S. (2014). *In vitro* evidence that an aqueous extract of *Centella asiatica* modulates α-synuclein aggregation dynamics. *J. Alzheimers Dis.* 39, 457–465. doi: 10.3233/JAD-131187

Bertoncini, C. W., Jung, Y.-S., Fernandez, C. O., Hoyer, W., Griesinger, C., Jovin, T. M., et al. (2005). Release of long-range tertiary interactions potentiates aggregation of natively unstructured α-synuclein. *Proc. Natl. Acad. Sci. U.S.A.* 102, 1430–1435. doi: 10.1073/pnas.0407146102

Beutler, J. A. (2009). Natural products as a foundation for drug discovery. *Curr. Protoc. Pharmacol.* 9, 9–11. doi: 10.1002/0471141755.ph0911s46

Bieschke, J., Russ, J., Friedrich, R. P., Ehrnhoefer, D. E., Wobst, H., Neugebauer, K., et al. (2010). EGCG remodels mature alpha-synuclein and amyloid-beta fibrils and reduces cellular toxicity. *Proc. Natl. Acad. Sci. USA.* 107, 7710–7715. doi: 10.1073/pnas.0910723107

Blainski, A., Lopes, G. C., and de Mello, J. C. (2013). Application and analysis of the Folin Ciocalteu method for the determination of the total phenolic content from *Limonium brasiliense* L. *Molecules* 18, 6852–6865. doi: 10.3390/molecules18066852

Bollimpelli, V. S., Kumar, P., Kumari, S., and Kondapi, A. K. (2016). Neuroprotective effect of curcumin-loaded lactoferrin nano particles against rotenone induced neurotoxicity. *Neurochem. Int.* 95, 37–45. doi: 10.1016/j.neuint.2016.01.006

Bomhoff, G., Sloan, K., McLain, C., Gogol, E. P., and Fisher, M. T. (2006). The effects of the flavonoid baicalein and osmolytes on the Mg^{2+} accelerated aggregation/fibrillation of carboxymethylated bovine 1SS-alpha-lactalbumin. *Arch. Biochem. Biophys.* 453, 75–86. doi: 10.1016/j.abb.2006.02.001

Borghi, R., Marchese, R., Negro, A., Marinelli, L., Forloni, G., Zaccheo, D., et al. (2000). Full length alpha-synuclein is present in cerebrospinal fluid from Parkinson's disease and normal subjects. *Neurosci. Lett.* 287, 65–67. doi: 10.1016/S0304-3940(00)01153-8

Briffa, M., Ghio, S., Neuner, J., Gauci, A. J., Cacciottolo, R., Marchal, C., et al. (2017). Extracts from two ubiquitous Mediterranean plants ameliorate cellular and animal models of neurodegenerative proteinopathies. *Neurosci. Lett.* 638, 12–20. doi: 10.1016/j.neulet.2016.11.058

Broersen, K., Ruiperez, V., and Davletov, B. (2018). Structural and aggregation properties of alpha-synuclein linked to phospholipase A2 action. *Protein Pept. Lett.* 25, 368–378. doi: 10.2174/0929866525666180326120052

Brundin, P., Dave, K. D., and Kordower, J. H. (2017). Therapeutic approaches to target alpha-synuclein pathology. *Exp. Neurol.* 298, 225–235. doi: 10.1016/j.expneurol.2017.10.003

Burre, J., Sharma, M., Tsetsenis, T., Buchman, V., Etherton, M. R., and Sudhof, T. C. (2010). α-synuclein promotes SNARE-complex assembly *in vivo* and *in vitro*. *Science* 329, 1663–1667. doi: 10.1126/science.1195227

Büttner, S., Broeskamp, F., Sommer, C., Markaki, M., Habernig, L., Alavian-Ghavanini, A., et al. (2014). Spermidine protects against α-synuclein neurotoxicity. *Cell Cycle* 13, 3903–3908. doi: 10.4161/15384101.2014.973309

Camilleri, A., Zarb, C., Caruana, M., Ostermeier, U., Ghio, S., Högen, T., et al. (2013). Mitochondrial membrane permeabilisation by amyloid aggregates and protection by polyphenols. *Biochim. Biophys. Acta* 1828, 2532–2543. doi: 10.1016/j.bbamem.2013.06.026

Cannon, J. R., and Greenamyre, J. T. (2013). Gene-environment interactions in Parkinson's disease: specific evidence in humans and mammalian models. *Neurobiol. Dis.* 57, 38–46. doi: 10.1016/j.nbd.2012.06.025

Caruana, M., Cauchi, R., and Vassallo, N. (2016). Putative role of red wine polyphenols against brain pathology in Alzheimer's and Parkinson's disease. *Front Nutr.* 3:31. doi: 10.3389/fnut.2016.00031

Caruana, M., Högen, T., Levin, J., Hillmer, A., Giese, A., and Vassallo, N. (2011). Inhibition and disaggregation of α-synuclein oligomers by natural polyphenolic compounds. *FEBS Lett.* 585, 1113–1120. doi: 10.1016/j.febslet.2011.03.046

Caruana, M., Neuner, J., Högen, T., Schmidt, F., Kamp, F., Scerri, C., et al. (2012). Polyphenolic compounds are novel protective agents against lipid membrane damage by α-synuclein aggregates *in vitro*. *Biochim. Biophys. Acta* 1818, 2502–2510. doi: 10.1016/j.bbamem.2012.05.019

Caruana, M., and Vassallo, N. (2015). Tea polyphenols in Parkinson's disease. *Adv. Exp. Med. Biol.* 863, 117–137. doi: 10.1007/978-3-319-18365-7_6

Celej, M. S., Caarls, W., Demchenko, A. P., and Jovin, T. M. (2009). A triple-emission fluorescent probe reveals distinctive amyloid fibrillar polymorphism of wild-type alpha-synuclein and its familial Parkinson's disease mutants. *Biochemistry* 48, 7465–7472. doi: 10.1021/bi9003843

Ceravolo, R., Rossi, C., Del Prete, E., and Bonuccelli, U. (2016). A review of adverse events linked to dopamine agonists in the treatment of Parkinson's disease. *Expert Opin. Drug Saf.* 15, 181–198. doi: 10.1517/14740338.2016.1130128

Chanoux, R. A., and Rubenstein, R. C. (2012). Molecular chaperones as targets to circumvent the cftr defect in cystic fibrosis. *Front. Pharmacol.* 3:137. doi: 10.3389/fphar.2012.00137

Chen, L. L., Song, J. X., Lu, J. H., Yuan, Z. W., Liu, L. F., Durairajan, S. S., et al. (2014). Corynoxine, a natural autophagy enhancer, promotes the clearance of alpha-synuclein via Akt/mTOR pathway. *J. Neuroimmune Pharmacol.* 9, 380–387. doi: 10.1007/s11481-014-9528-2

Chen, M., Wang, T., Yue, F., Li, X., Wang, P., Li, Y., et al. (2015b). Tea polyphenols alleviate motor impairments, dopaminergic neuronal injury, and cerebral α-synuclein aggregation in MPTP-intoxicated parkinsonian monkeys. *Neuroscience* 286, 383–392. doi: 10.1016/j.neuroscience.2014.12.003

Chen, X. C., Zhou, Y. C., Chen, Y., Zhu, Y. G., Fang, F., and Chen, L. M. (2005). Ginsenosdie Rgl reduces MPTP-induced substantia nigra neuron loss by suppressing oxidative stress. *Yao Xue Xue Bao* 26, 56–62. doi: 10.1111/j.1745-7254.2005.00019.x

Chen, Y. M., Liu, S. P., Lin, H. L., Chan, M. C., Chen, Y. C., Huang, Y. L., et al. (2015a). Irisflorentin improves α-synuclein accumulation and attenuates 6-OHDA-induced dopaminergic neuron degeneration, implication for Parkinson's disease therapy. *Biomedicine* 5:4. doi: 10.7603/s40681-015-0004-y

Cheng, X. R., Wallace, G. Q., Lagugné-Labarthet, F., and Kerman, K. (2015). Au nanostructured surfaces for electrochemical and localized surface plasmon resonance-based monitoring of α-synuclein-small molecule interactions. *ACS Appl. Mater. Interfaces* 7, 4081–4088. doi: 10.1021/am507972b

Cheon, S. M., Jang, I., Lee, M. H., Kim, D. K., Jeon, H., and Cha, D. S. (2017). *Sorbus alnifolia* protects dopaminergic neurodegeneration in *Caenorhabditis elegans*. *Pharm. Biol.* 55, 481–486. doi: 10.1080/13880209.2016.1251468

Choubey, S., Goyal, S., Varughese, L. R., Kumar, V., Sharma, A. K., and Beniwal, V (2018). Probing gallic acid for its broad spectrum applications. *Mini Rev. Med. Chem.* 18, 1283–1293. doi: 10.2174/1389557518666180330114010

Coelho, T., Maia, L. F., da Silva, A. M., Cruz, M. W., Plante-Bordeneuve, V., Suhr, O. B, et al. (2013). Long-term effects of tafamidis for the treatment of transthyretin familial amyloid polyneuropathy. *J. Neurol.* 260, 2802–2814. doi: 10.1007/s00415-013-7051-7

Coelho-Cerqueira, E., Pinheiro, A. S., and Follmer, C. (2014). Pitfalls associated with the use of Thioflavin-T to monitor anti-fibrillogenic activity. *Bioorg. Med. Chem. Lett.* 24, 3194–3198. doi: 10.1016/j.bmcl.2014.04.072

Collier, T. J., Kanaan, N. M., and Kordower, J. H. (2017). Aging and Parkinson's disease: different sides of the same coin? *Mov. Disord.* 32, 983–990. doi: 10.1002/mds.27037

Cox, D., Selig, E., Griffin, M. D., Carver, J. A., and Ecroyd, H. (2016). Small heat-shock proteins prevent α-synuclein aggregation via transient interactions and their efficacy is affected by the rate of aggregation. *J. Biol. Chem.* 291, 22618–22629. doi: 10.1074/jbc.M116.739250

Cui, Y., Rong, C., Wang, J., Cui, C., Wang, L., Feng, Z., et al. (2013). Mechanism-based anti-anxiety effects of polysaccharides extracted from shudihuang (radix rehmanniae preparata) by two-dimensional electrophoresis analysis in rat hippocampus proteins. *J. Tradit. Chin. Med.* 33, 524–530. doi: 10.1016/S0254-6272(13)60159-4

da Costa, I. M., Cavalcanti, J. R. L. P., de Queiroz, D. B., de Azevedo, E. P., do Rêgo, A. C. M., Araújo Filho, I., et al. (2017). Supplementation with herbal extracts to promote behavioral and neuroprotective effects in experimental models of Parkinson's disease: a systematic review. *Phytother. Res.* 31, 959–970. doi: 10.1002/ptr.5813

da Silva, F. L., Coelho Cerqueira, E., de Freitas, M. S., Gonçalves, D. L., Costa, L. T., and Follmer, C. (2013). Vitamins K interact with N-terminus, α-synuclein and modulate the protein fibrillization *in vitro*. Exploring the interaction between quinones, and α-synuclein. *Neurochem. Int.* 62, 103–112. doi: 10.1016/j.neuint.2012.10.001

Das, S., Pukala, T.L., and Smid, S.D. (2018). Exploring the structural diversity in inhibitors of α-synuclein amyloidogenic folding, aggregation, and neurotoxicity. *Front. Chem.* 6:181. doi: 10.3389/fchem.2018.00181

Deng, Y. N., Shi, J., Liu, J., and Qu, Q. M. (2013). Celastrol protects human neuroblastoma SH-SY5Y cells from rotenone-induced injury through induction of autophagy. *Neurochem. Int.* 63, 1–9. doi: 10.1016/j.neuint.2013.04.005

Dimant, H., Ebrahimi-Fakhari, D., and McLean, P. J. (2012). Molecular chaperones and co-chaperones in Parkinson disease. *Neuroscientist* 18, 589–601. doi: 10.1177/1073858412441372

Dinda, B., Debnath, S., Mohanta, B. C., and Harigaya, Y. (2010). Naturally occurring triterpenoid saponins. *Chem. Biodivers.* 7, 2327–2580. doi: 10.1002/cbdv.200800070

Ehrnhoefer, D. E., Bieschke, J., Boeddrich, A., Herbst, M., Masino, L., Lurz, R., et al. (2008). EGCG redirects amyloidogenic polypeptides into unstructured, off-pathway oligomers. *Nat. Struct. Mol. Biol.* 15, 558–566. doi: 10.1038/nsmb.1437

Ellis, J. M., and Fell, M. J. (2017). Current approaches to the treatment of Parkinson's disease. *Bioorg. Med. Chem. Lett.* 27, 4247–4255. doi: 10.1016/j.bmcl.2017.07.075

Eschbach, J., von Einem, B., Müller, K., Bayer, H., Scheffold, A., Morrison, B. E., et al. (2015). Mutual exacerbation of peroxisome proliferator-activated receptor γ coactivator 1α deregulation and α-synuclein oligomerization. *Ann. Neurol.* 77, 15–32. doi: 10.1002/ana.24294

Fazili, N. A., and Naeem, A. (2015). Anti-fibrillation potency of caffeic acid against an antidepressant induced fibrillogenesis of human α-synuclein: implications for Parkinson's disease. *Biochimie* 108, 178–185. doi: 10.1016/j.biochi.2014.11.011

Friesen, E. L., De Snoo, M. L., Rajendran, L., Kalia, L. V., and Kalia, S. K. (2017). Chaperone-based therapies for disease modification in Parkinson's disease. *Parkinsons Dis.* 2017:5015307. doi: 10.1155/2017/5015307

Fu, G., Zhang, W., Du, D., Ng, Y. P., Ip, F. C. F., Tong, R., et al. (2017). Diarylheptanoids from rhizomes of *Alpinia officinarum* inhibit aggregation of α-synuclein. *J. Agric. Food Chem.* 65, 6608–6614. doi: 10.1021/acs.jafc.7b02021

Fu, R. H., Harn, H. J, Liu, S. P., Chen, C. S., Chang, W. L., and Chen, Y. M., et al. (2014b). n-butylidenephthalide protects against dopaminergic neuron degeneration and α-synuclein accumulation in *Caenorhabditis elegans* models of Parkinson's disease. *PLoS ONE* 9:e85305. doi: 10.1371/journal.pone.0085305

Fu, R. H., Wang, Y. C., Chen, C. S., Tsai, R. T., Liu, S. P., Chang, W. L., et al. (2014a). Acetylcorynoline attenuates dopaminergic neuron degeneration and α-synuclein aggregation in animal models of Parkinson's disease. *Neuropharmacology* 82, 108–120. doi: 10.1016/j.neuropharm.2013.08.007

Gadad, B. S., Subramanya, P. K., Pullabhatla, S., Shantharam, I. S., and Rao, K. S. (2012). Curcumin-glucoside, a novel synthetic derivative of curcumin, inhibits α-synuclein oligomer formation: relevance to Parkinson's disease. *Curr. Pharm. Des.* 18, 76–84. doi: 10.2174/138161212798919093

Gasiorowski, K., Lamer-Zarawska, E., Leszek, J., Parvathaneni, K., Yendluri, B. B., Błach-Olszewska, Z., et al. (2011). Flavones from root of *Scutellaria baicalensis* Georgi: drugs of the future in neurodegeneration? *CNS Neurol. Disord. Drug Targets* 10, 184–191. doi: 10.2174/187152711794480384

Gautam, S., Karmakar, S., Batra, R., Sharma, P., Pradhan, P., Singh, J., et al. (2017). Polyphenols in combination with β-cyclodextrin can inhibit and disaggregate α-synuclein amyloids under cell mimicking conditions: a promising therapeutic alternative. *Biochim. Biophys. Acta* 1865, 589–603. doi: 10.1016/j.bbapap.2017.02.014

Gautam, S., Karmakar, S., Bose, A., and Chowdhury, P. K. (2014). β-cyclodextrin and curcumin, a potent cocktail for disaggregating and/or inhibiting amyloids: a case study with α-synuclein. *Biochemistry* 53, 4081–4083. doi: 10.1021/bi500642f

Gelders, G., Baekelandt, V., and Van der Perren, A. (2018). Linking neuroinflammation and neurodegeneration in Parkinson's disease. *J. Immunol. Res.* 2018:4784268. doi: 10.1155/2018/4784268

Ghavami, S., Shojaei, S., Yeganeh, B., Ande, S. R., Jangamreddy, J. R., Mehrpour, M., et al. (2014). Autophagy and apoptosis dysfunction in neurodegenerative disorders. *Prog. Neurobiol.* 112, 24–49. doi: 10.1016/j.pneurobio.2013.10.004

Ghiglieri, V., Calabrese, V., and Calabresi, P. (2018). Alpha-synuclein: from early synaptic dysfunction to neurodegeneration. *Front. Neurol.* 9:295. doi: 10.3389/fneur.2018.00295

Giehm, L., Lorenzen, N., and Otzen, D. E. (2011). Assays for α-synuclein aggregation. *Methods* 53, 295–305. doi: 10.1016/j.ymeth.2010.12.008

Giffin, J. C., Richards, R. C., Craft, C., Jahan, N., Leggiadro, C., Chopin, T., et al. (2017). An extract of the marine alga *Alaria esculenta* modulates α-synuclein folding and amyloid formation. *Neurosci. Lett.* 644, 87–93. doi: 10.1016/j.neulet.2017.02.055

Grelle, G., Otto, A., Lorenz, M., Frank, R. F., Wanker, E. E., and Bieschke, J. (2011). Black tea theaflavins inhibit formation of toxic amyloid-β and α-synuclein fibrils. *Biochemistry* 50, 10624–10636. doi: 10.1021/bi2012383

Griffioen, G., Duhamel, H., Van Damme, N., Pellens, K., Zabrocki, P., Pannecouque, C., et al. (2006). A yeast-based model of alpha-synucleinopathy identifies compounds with therapeutic potential. *Biochim. Biophys. Acta.* 1762, 312–318. doi: 10.1016/j.bbadis.2005.11.009

Guo, Y. J., Dong, S. Y., Cui, X. X., Feng, Y., Liu, T., Yin, M., et al. (2016). Resveratrol alleviates MPTP-induced motor impairments and pathological changes by autophagic degradation of α-synuclein via SIRT1-deacetylated LC3. *Mol. Nutr. Food Res.* 60, 2161–2175. doi: 10.1002/mnfr.201600111

Ham, A., Kim, D. W., Kim, K. H., Lee, S. J., Oh, K. B., Shin, J., et al. (2013). Reynosin protects against neuronal toxicity in dopamine-induced SH-SY5Y cells and 6-hydroxydopamine-lesioned rats as models of Parkinson's disease: reciprocal up-regulation of E6-AP and down-regulation of α-synuclein. *Brain Res.* 1524, 54–61. doi: 10.1016/j.brainres.2013.05.036

Ham, A., Lee, H. J., Hong, S. S., Lee, D., and Mar, W. (2012b). Moracenin D from Mori Cortex radicis protects SH-SY5Y cells against dopamine-induced cell death by regulating nurr1 and α-synuclein expression. *Phytother. Res.* 26, 620–624. doi: 10.1002/ptr.3592

Ham, A., Lee, S. J., Shin, J., Kim, K. H., and Mar, W. (2012a). Regulatory effects of costunolide on dopamine metabolism-associated genes inhibit dopamine-induced apoptosis in human dopaminergic SH-SY5Y cells. *Neurosci. Lett.* 507, 101–105. doi: 10.1016/j.neulet.2011.10.037

Hansen, C., and Li, J. Y. (2012). Beyond α-synuclein transfer: pathology propagation in Parkinson's disease. *Trends Mol. Med.* 18, 248–255. doi: 10.1016/j.molmed.2012.03.002

Hao, X. M., Li, L. D., Duan, C. L., and Li, Y. J. (2017). Neuroprotective effect of α-mangostin on mitochondrial dysfunction and α-synuclein aggregation in rotenone-induced model of Parkinson's disease in differentiated SH-SY5Y cells. *J. Asian Nat. Prod. Res.* 8, 833–845. doi: 10.1080/10286020.2017.1339349

Heng, Y., Zhang, Q. S., Mu, Z., Hu, J. F., Yuan, Y. H., and Chen, N. H. (2016). Ginsenoside Rg1 attenuates motor impairment and neuroinflammation in the MPTP-probenecid-induced parkinsonism mouse model by targeting α-synuclein abnormalities in the substantia nigra. *Toxicol. Lett.* 243, 7–21. doi: 10.1016/j.toxlet.2015.12.005

Henrich, C. J., and Beutler, J. A. (2013). Matching the power of high throughput screening to the chemical diversity of natural products. *Nat. Prod. Rep.* 30, 1284–1298. doi: 10.1039/c3np70052f

Herrera, A., Muñoz, P., Steinbusch, H. W. M., and Segura-Aguilar, J. (2017). Are dopamine oxidation metabolites involved in the loss of dopaminergic neurons in the nigrostriatal system in Parkinson's disease? *ACS Chem. Neurosci.* 8, 702–711. doi: 10.1021/acschemneuro.7b00034

Ho, L., and Pasinetti, G. M. (2010). Polyphenolic compounds for treating neurodegenerative disorders involving protein misfolding. *Expert Rev. Proteomics* 7, 579–589. doi: 10.1586/epr.10.69

Hong, D. P., Fink, A. L., and Uversky, V. N. (2008). Structural characteristics of alpha-synuclein oligomers stabilized by the flavonoid baicalein. *J. Mol. Biol.* 383, 214–223. doi: 10.1016/j.jmb.2008.08.039

Hu, Q., Uversky, V. N., Huang, M., Kang, H., Xu, F., Liu, X., et al. (2016). Baicalein inhibits α-synuclein oligomer formation and prevents progression of α-synuclein accumulation in a rotenone mouse model of Parkinson's disease. *Biochim. Biophys. Acta* 1862, 1883–1890. doi: 10.1016/j.bbadis.2016.07.008

Huang, J. Z., Chen, Y. Z., Su, M., Zheng, H. F., Yang, Y. P., Chen, J., et al. (2010). dl-3-n-Butylphthalide prevents oxidative damage and reduces mitochondrial dysfunction in an MPP(+)-induced cellular model of Parkinson's disease. *Neurosci. Lett.* 475, 89–94. doi: 10.1016/j.neulet.2010.03.053

Hung, K. C., Huang, H. J., Wang, Y. T., and Lin, A. M. (2016). Baicalein attenuates α-synuclein aggregation, inflammasome activation and autophagy in the MPP(+)-treated nigrostriatal dopaminergic system *in vivo*. *J. Ethnopharmacol.* 194, 522–529. doi: 10.1016/j.jep.2016.10.040

Hussain, G., Rasul, A., Anwar, H., Aziz, N., Razzaq, A., Wei, W., et al. (2018). Role of plant derived alkaloids and their mechanism in neurodegenerative disorders. *Int. J. Biol. Sci.* 14, 341–357. doi: 10.7150/ijbs.23247

Inoue, E., Shimizu, Y., Masui, R., Hayakawa, T., Tsubonoya, T., Hori, S., et al. (2018). Effects of saffron and its constituents, crocin-1, crocin-2, and crocetin on α-synuclein fibrils. *J. Nat. Med.* 72, 274–279. doi: 10.1007/s11418-017-1150-1

Jadiya, P., Khan, A., Sammi, S. R., Kaur, S., Mir, S. S., Nazira, A., et al. (2011). Anti-Parkinsonian effects of *Bacopa monnieri*: insights from transgenic and pharmacological *Caenorhabditis elegans* models of Parkinson's disease. *Biochem. Biophys. Res. Commun.* 413, 605–610. doi: 10.1016/j.bbrc.2011.09.010

Jankovic, J., Goodman, I., Safirstein, B., Marmon, T. K., Schenk, D. B., Koller, M., et al. (2018). Safety and tolerability of multiple ascending doses of PRX002/RG7935, an anti-α-synuclein monoclonal antibody, in patients with parkinson disease: a randomized clinical trial. *JAMA Neurol.* 75, 1206–1214. doi: 10.1001/jamaneurol.2018.1487

Javed, H., Kamal, M. A., and Ojha, S. (2016). An overview on the role of α-synuclein in experimental models of Parkinson's disease from pathogenesis to therapeutics. *CNS Neurol. Disord. Drug Targets* 15, 1240–1252. doi: 10.2174/1871527315666160920160512

Jha, N. N., Ghosh, D., Das, S., Anoop, A., Jacob, R. S., Singh, P. K., et al. (2016). Effect of curcumin analogs on α-synuclein aggregation and cytotoxicity. *Sci. Rep.* 6:28511. doi: 10.1038/srep28511

Jha, N. N., Kumar, R., Panigrahi, R., Navalkar, A., Ghosh, D., Sahay, S., et al. (2017). Comparison of α-synuclein fibril inhibition by four different amyloid inhibitors. *ACS Chem. Neurosci.* 20, 2722–2733. doi: 10.1021/acschemneuro.7b00261

Ji, H. F., and Shen, L. (2014). The multiple pharmaceutical potential of curcumin in Parkinson's disease. *CNS Neurol. Disord. Drug Targets* 13, 369–373. doi: 10.2174/18715273113129990077

Ji, K., Zhao, Y., Yu, T., Wang, Z., Gong, H., Yang, X., et al. (2016). Inhibition effects of tanshinone on the aggregation of α-synuclein. *Food Funct.* 7, 409–416. doi: 10.1039/C5FO00664C

Jiang, M., Porat-Shliom, Y., Pei, Z., Cheng, Y., Xiang, L., and Sommers, K. (2010). Baicalein reduces E46K alpha-synuclein aggregation *in vitro* and protects cells against E46K alpha-synuclein toxicity in cell models of familiar Parkinsonism. *J. Neurochem.* 114, 419–429. doi: 10.1111/j.1471-4159.2010.06752.x

Jiang, T. F., Zhang, Y. J., Zhou, H. Y., Wang, H. M., Tian, L. P, and Liu, J. (2013). Curcumin ameliorates the neurodegenerative pathology in A53T α-synuclein cell model of Parkinson's disease through the downregulation of mTOR/p70S6K signaling and the recovery of macroautophagy. *J. Neuroimmune Pharmacol.* 8, 356–369. doi: 10.1007/s11481-012-9431-7

Kabiraj, P., Marin, J. E., Varela-Ramirez, A., Zubia, E., and Narayan, M. (2014). Ellagic acid mitigates SNO-PDI induced aggregation of Parkinsonian biomarkers. *ACS Chem. Neurosci.* 5, 1209–1220. doi: 10.1021/cn500214k

Kalia, L. V., Kalia, S. K., and Lang, A. E. (2015). Disease-modifying strategies for Parkinson's disease. *Mov. Disord.* 30, 1442–1450. doi: 10.1002/mds.26354

Karpinar, D. P., Balija, M. B., Kügler, S., Opazo, F., Rezaei-Ghaleh, N., Wender, N., et al. (2009). Pre-fibrillar α-synuclein variants with impaired β-structure increase neurotoxicity in Parkinson's disease models. *EMBO J.* 28, 3256–3268. doi: 10.1038/emboj.2009.257

Kastenholz, B., and Garfin, D. E. (2009). Medicinal plants: a natural chaperones source for treating neurological disorders. *Protein Pept. Lett.* 16, 116–120. doi: 10.2174/092986609787316234

Kim, D. S., Kim, J. Y., and Han, Y. (2012). Curcuminoids in neurodegenerative diseases. *Recent Pat. CNS Drug Discov.* 7, 184–204. doi: 10.2174/157488912803252032

Kim, J., Sasaki, Y., Yoshida, W., Kobayashi, N., Veloso, A. J., Kerman, K., et al. (2013). Rapid cytotoxicity screening platform for amyloid inhibitors using a membrane-potential sensitive fluorescent probe. *Anal. Chem.* 85, 185–192. doi: 10.1021/ac302442q

Ko, W. K. D., and Bezard, E. (2017). Experimental animal models of Parkinson's disease: a transition from assessing symptomatology to α-synuclein targeted disease modification. *Exp. Neurol.* 298, 172–179. doi: 10.1016/j.expneurol.2017.07.020

Koo, U., Nam, K. W., Ham, A., Lyu, D., Kim, B., Lee, S. J., et al. (2011). Neuroprotective effects of 3α-acetoxyeudesma-1,4(15),11(13)-trien-12,6α-olide against dopamine-induced apoptosis in the human neuroblastoma SH-SY5Y cell line. *Neurochem. Res.* 36, 1991–2001. doi: 10.1007/s11064-011-0523-1

Kostka, M., Högen, T., Danzer, K. M., Levin, J., Habeck, M., Wirth, A., et al. (2008). Single particle characterization of iron-induced pore-forming alpha-synuclein oligomers. *J. Biol. Chem.* 83, 10992–11003. doi: 10.1074/jbc.M709634200

Kosuru, R. Y., Roy, A., Das, S. K., and Bera, S. (2018). Gallic acid and gallates in human health and disease: do mitochondria hold the key to success? *Mol. Nutr. Food Res.* 62. doi: 10.1002/mnfr.201700699

Kumar, S., Okello, E. J., and Harris, J. R. (2012). Experimental inhibition of fibrillogenesis and neurotoxicity by amyloid-beta (Aβ) and other disease-related peptides/proteins by plant extracts and herbal compounds. *Subcell. Biochem.* 65, 295–326. doi: 10.1007/978-94-007-5416-4_13

Kundu, P., Das, M., Tripathy, K., and Sahoo, S. K. (2016). Delivery of dual drug loaded lipid based nanoparticles across the blood-brain barrier imparts enhanced neuroprotection in a rotenone induced mouse model of Parkinson's disease. *ACS Chem. Neurosci.* 7, 1658–1670. doi: 10.1021/acschemneuro.6b00207

Kuzuhara, S., Mori, H., Izumiyama, N., Yoshimura, M., and Ihara, Y. (1988). Lewy bodies are ubiquitinated. A light and electron microscopic immunocytochemical study. *Acta Neuropathol.* 75, 345–353. doi: 10.1007/BF00687787

Lashuel, H. A., Overk, C. R., Oueslati, A., and Masliah, E. (2013). The many faces of α-synuclein: from structure and toxicity to therapeutic target. *Nat. Rev. Neurosci.* 14, 38–48. doi: 10.1038/nrn3406

Lauterbach, E. C., Victoroff, J., Coburn, K. L., Shillcutt, S. D., Doonan, S. M., and Mendez, M. F. (2010). Psychopharmacological neuroprotection in neurodegenerative disease: assessing the preclinical data. *J. Neuropsychiatry Clin. Neurosci.* 22, 8–18. doi: 10.1176/jnp.2010.22.1.8

Lázaro, D. F., Pavlou, M. A. S., and Outeiro, T. F. (2017). Cellular models as tools for the study of the role of alpha-synuclein in Parkinson's disease. *Exp. Neurol.* 298, 162–171. doi: 10.1016/j.expneurol.2017.05.007

Lee, D. H., Kim, C. S., and Lee, Y. J. (2011). Astaxanthin protects against MPTP/MPP+-induced mitochondrial dysfunction and ROS production *in vivo* and *in vitro*. *Food Chem. Toxicol.* 49, 271–280. doi: 10.1016/j.fct.2010.10.029

Lee, J. H., Lee, I. H., Choe, Y. J., Kang, S., Kim, H. Y., Gai, W. P., et al. (2009). Real-time analysis of amyloid fibril formation of alpha-synuclein using a fibrillation-state-specific fluorescent probe of JC-1. *Biochem. J.* 418, 311–323. doi: 10.1042/BJ20081572

Lee, K. W., Im, J. Y., Woo, J. M., Grosso, H., Kim, Y. S., Cristovao, A. C., et al. (2013). Neuroprotective and anti-inflammatory properties of a coffee component in the MPTP model of Parkinson's disease. *Neurotherapeutics* 10, 143–153. doi: 10.1007/s13311-012-0165-2

Lester, H. A., Xiao, C., Srinivasan, R., Son, C. D., Miwa, J., Pantoja, R., et al. (2009). Nicotine is a selective pharmacological chaperone of acetylcholine receptor number and stoichiometry. Implications for drug discovery. *AAPS J.* 11, 167–177. doi: 10.1208/s12248-009-9090-7

Li, T., Feng, Y., Yang, R., Wu, L., Li, R., Huang, L., et al. (2018). Salidroside promotes the pathological α-synuclein clearance through ubiquitin-proteasome system in SH-SY5Y cells. *Front. Pharmacol.* 9:377. doi: 10.3389/fphar.2018.00377

Li, X., Zhang, G., Nie, Q., Wu, T., Jiao, L., Zheng, M., et al. (2017). Baicalein blocks α-synuclein secretion from SN4741 cells and facilitates α-synuclein polymerization to big complex. *Neurosci. Lett.* 655, 109–114. doi: 10.1016/j.neulet.2017.06.031

Li, X. Z., Zhang, S. N., Wang, K. X., Liu, H. Y., Yang, Z. M., Liu, S. M., et al. (2014). Neuroprotective effects of extract of *Acanthopanax senticosus* harms on SH-SY5Y cells overexpressing wild-type or A53T mutant α-synuclein. *Phytomedicine* 21, 704–711. doi: 10.1016/j.phymed.2013.10.012

Lin, A. M., Ping, Y. H., Chang, G. F., Wang, J. Y., Chiu, J. H., Kuo, C. D., et al. (2011). Neuroprotective effect of oral S/B remedy (*Scutellaria baicalensis* Georgi and *Bupleurum scorzonerifolfium* Willd) on iron-induced neurodegeneration in the nigrostriatal dopaminergic system of rat brain. *J. Ethnopharmacol.* 134, 884–891. doi: 10.1016/j.jep.2011.01.056

Liu, C. B., Wang, R., Pan, H. B., Ding, Q. F., and Lu, F. B. (2013). Effect of lycopene on oxidative stress and behavioral deficits in rotenone induced model of Parkinson's disease. *Zhongguo Ying Yong Sheng Li Xue Za Zhi.* 29, 380–384.

Liu, L. F., Song, J. X., Lu, J. H., Huang, Y. Y., Zeng, Y., Chen, L. L., et al. (2015). Tianma Gouteng Yin, a Traditional Chinese Medicine decoction, exerts neuroprotective effects in animal and cellular models of Parkinson's disease. *Sci. Rep.* 5:16862. doi: 10.1038/srep16862

Liu, X., Zhou, S., Shi, D., Bai, Q., Liu, H., and Yao, X. (2018). Influence of EGCG on α-synuclein (αS) aggregation and identification of their possible binding mode: a computational study using molecular dynamics simulation. *Chem. Biol. Drug Des.* 91, 162–171. doi: 10.1111/cbdd.13067

Liu, Y., Carver, J. A., Calabrese, A. N., and Pukala, T. L. (2014). Gallic acid interacts with α-synuclein to prevent the structural collapse necessary for its aggregation. *Biochim. Biophys. Acta* 1844, 1481–1485. doi: 10.1016/j.bbapap.2014.04.013

Liu, Z., Yu, Y., Li, X., Ross, C. A., and Smith, W. W. (2011). Curcumin protects against A53T alpha-synuclein-induced toxicity in a PC12 inducible cell model for Parkinsonism. *Pharmacol. Res.* 63, 439–444. doi: 10.1016/j.phrs.2011.01.004

Lobbens, E. S., Breydo, L., Skamris, T., Vestergaard, B., Jäger, A. K., Jorgensen, L., et al. (2016). Mechanistic study of the inhibitory activity of *Geum urbanum* extract against α-synuclein fibrillation. *Biochim. Biophys. Acta* 1864, 1160–1169. doi: 10.1016/j.bbapap.2016.06.009

Long, J., Gao, H., Sun, L., Liu, J., and Zhao-Wilson, X. (2009). Grape extract protects mitochondria from oxidative damage and improves locomotor dysfunction and extends lifespan in a Drosophila Parkinson's disease model. *Rejuvenation Res.* 12, 321–331. doi: 10.1089/rej.2009.0877

Longhena, F., Faustini, G., Missale, C., Pizzi, M., Spano, P., and Bellucci, A. (2017). The contribution of α-synuclein spreading to Parkinson's disease synaptopathy. *Neural Plast.* 2017:5012129. doi: 10.1155/2017/5012129

Loo, T. W., and Clarke, D. M. (2007). Chemical and pharmacological chaperones as new therapeutic agents. *Expert Rev. Mol. Med.* 9, 1–18. doi: 10.1017/S1462399407000361

Lorenzen, N., Nielsen, S. B., Yoshimura, Y., Vad, B. S., Andersen, C. B., Betzer, C., et al. (2014). How epigallocatechin gallate can inhibit α-synuclein oligomer toxicity *in vitro*. *J. Biol. Chem.* 289, 21299–212310. doi: 10.1074/jbc.M114.554667

Lu, J. H., Ardah, M. T., Durairajan, S. S., Liu, L. F., Xie, L. X., Fong, W. F., et al. (2011). Baicalein inhibits formation of α-synuclein oligomers within living cells and prevents Aβ peptide fibrillation and oligomerisation. *Chembiochem* 12, 615–624. doi: 10.1002/cbic.201000604

Lu, J. H., Tan, J. Q., Durairajan, S. S., Liu, L. F., Zhang, Z. H., Ma, L., et al. (2012). Isorhynchophylline, a natural alkaloid, promotes the degradation of alpha-synuclein in neuronal cells via inducing autophagy. *Autophagy* 8, 98–108. doi: 10.4161/auto.8.1.18313

Luk, K. C., Hyde, E. G., Trojanowski, J. Q., and Lee, V. M. (2007). Sensitive fluorescence polarization technique for rapid screening of alpha-synuclein oligomerization/fibrillization inhibitors. *Biochemistry* 46, 12522–12529. doi: 10.1021/bi701128c

Luo, F. C., Wang, S. D., Qi, L., Song, J. Y., Lv, T., and Bai, J. (2011). Protective effect of panaxatriol saponins extracted from Panax notoginseng against MPTP-induced neurotoxicity *in vivo*. *J. Ethnopharmacol.* 133, 448–453. doi: 10.1016/j.jep.2010.10.017

Ma, L., Cao, T. T., Kandpal, G., Warren, L., Fred Hess, J., Seabrook, G. R., et al. (2010). Genome-wide microarray analysis of the differential neuroprotective effects of antioxidants in neuroblastoma cells overexpressing the familial Parkinson's disease alpha-synuclein A53T mutation. *Neurochem. Res.* 35, 130–142. doi: 10.1007/s11064-009-0038-1

Macedo, D., Tavares, L., McDougall, G. J., Vicente Miranda, H., Stewart, D., Ferreira, R. B., et al. (2015). (Poly)phenols protect from α-synuclein toxicity by reducing oxidative stress and promoting autophagy. *Hum. Mol. Genet.* 24, 1717–1732. doi: 10.1093/hmg/ddu585

Maioli, E., Torricelli, C., and Valacchi, G. (2012). Rottlerin and curcumin: a comparative analysis. *Ann. N. Y. Acad. Sci.* 1259, 65–76. doi: 10.1111/j.1749-6632.2012.06514.x

Mandel, S., Weinreb, O., Amit, T., and Youdim, M. B. (2004). Cell signaling pathways in the neuroprotective actions of the green tea polyphenol (-)-epigallocatechin-3-gallate: implications for neurodegenerative diseases. *J. Neurochem.* 88, 1555–1569. doi: 10.1046/j.1471-4159.2003.02291.x

Marchiani, A., Mammi, S., Siligardi, G., Hussain, R., Tessari, I., Bubacco, L., et al. (2013). Small molecules interacting with α-synuclein: antiaggregating and cytoprotective properties. *Amino Acids* 45, 327–338. doi: 10.1007/s00726-013-1503-3

Masuda, M., Suzuki, N., Taniguchi, S., Oikawa, T., Nonaka, T., Iwatsubo, T., et al. (2006). Small molecule inhibitors of α-synuclein filament assembly. *Biochemistry* 45, 6085–6094. doi: 10.1021/bi0600749

Mazo, N. A., Echeverria, V., Cabezas, R., Avila-Rodriguez, M., Tarasov, V. V., Yarla, N. S., et al. (2017). Medicinal plants as protective strategies against Parkinson's disease. *Curr. Pharm. Des.* 23, 4180–4188. doi: 10.2174/1381612823666170316142803

Meng, F., Abedini, A., Plesner, A., Verchere, C. B., and Raleigh, D. P. (2010). The flavanol (-)-epigallocatechin 3-gallate inhibits amyloid formation by islet amyloid polypeptide, disaggregates amyloid fibrils, and protects cultured cells against IAPP-induced toxicity. *Biochemistry* 49, 8127–8133. doi: 10.1021/bi100939a

Meng, X., Munishkina, L. A., Fink, A. L., and Uversky, V. N. (2009). Molecular mechanisms underlying the flavonoid-induced inhibition of alpha-synuclein fibrillation. *Biochemistry* 48, 8206–8224. doi: 10.1021/bi900506b

Mohanan, P., Subramaniyam, S., Mathiyalagan, R., and Yang, D. C. (2018). Molecular signaling of ginsenosides Rb1, Rg1, and Rg3 and their mode of actions. *J. Ginseng Res.* 42, 123–132. doi: 10.1016/j.jgr.2017.01.008

Molino, S., Dossena, M., Buonocore, D., Ferrari, F., Venturini, L., Ricevuti, G., et al. (2016). Polyphenols in dementia: From molecular basis to clinical trials. *Life Sci.* 61, 69–77. doi: 10.1016/j.lfs.2016.07.021

Moore, D. J., West, A. B., Dawson, V. L., and Dawson, T. M. (2005). Molecular pathophysiology of Parkinson's disease. *Annu. Rev. Neurosci.* 28, 57–87. doi: 10.1146/annurev.neuro.28.061604.135718

Moree, B., Yin, G., Lázaro, D. F., Munari, F., Strohäker, T., Giller, K., et al. (2015). Small molecules detected by second-harmonic generation modulate the conformation of monomeric α-synuclein and reduce its aggregation in cells. *J. Biol. Chem.* 290, 27582–27593. doi: 10.1074/jbc.M114.636027

Morgan, L. A., and Grundmann, O. (2017). Preclinical and potential applications of common western herbal supplements as complementary treatment in Parkinson's disease. *J. Diet. Suppl.* 14, 453–466. doi: 10.1080/19390211.2016.1263710

Morshedi, D., Aliakbari, F., Tayaranian-Marvian, A., Fassihi, A., Pan-Montojo, F., and Pérez-Sánchez, H. (2015). Cuminaldehyde as the major component of *Cuminum cyminum*, a natural aldehyde with inhibitory effect on alpha-synuclein fibrillation and cytotoxicity. *J. Food Sci.* 80, H2336–2345. doi: 10.1111/1750-3841.13016

Morshedi, D., and Nasouti, M. (2016). Essential oils may lead α-synuclein towards toxic fibrils formation. *Parkinsons. Dis.* 2016:6219249. doi: 10.1155/2016/6219249

Noorwez, S. M., Kuksa, V., Imanishi, Y., Zhu, L., Filipek, S., Palczewski, K., et al. (2003). Pharmacological chaperone-mediated *in vivo* folding and stabilization of the p23h-opsin mutant associated with autosomal dominant retinitis pigmentosa. *J. Biol. Chem.* 278, 14442–14450. doi: 10.1074/jbc.M300 087200

Ono, K., and Yamada, M. (2006). Antioxidant compounds have potent anti-fibrillogenic and fibril-destabilizing effects for alpha-synuclein fibrils *in vitro*. *J. Neurochem.* 97, 105–115. doi: 10.1111/j.1471-4159.2006.03707.x

Ortiz-Ortiz, M. A., Morán, J. M., Ruiz-Mesa, L. M., Niso-Santano, M., Bravo-SanPedro, J. M., Gómez-Sánchez, R., et al. (2010). Curcumin exposure induces expression of the Parkinson's disease-associated leucine-rich repeat kinase 2 (LRRK2) in rat mesencephalic cells. *Neurosci. Lett.* 468, 120–124. doi: 10.1016/j.neulet.2009.10.081

Pandareesh, M. D., Mythri, R. B., and Srinivas Bharath, M. M. (2015). Bioavailability of dietary polyphenols: Factors contributing to their clinical application in CNS diseases. *Neurochem. Int.* 89, 198–208. doi: 10.1016/j.neuint.2015.07.003

Pandey, N., Strider, J., Nolan, W. C., Yan, S. X., and Galvin, J. E. (2008). Curcumin inhibits aggregation of alpha-synuclein. *Acta Neuropathol.* 115, 479–489. doi: 10.1007/s00401-007-0332-4

Patel, M. Y., Panchal, H. V., Ghribi, O., and Benzeroual, K. E. (2012). The neuroprotective effect of fisetin in the MPTP model of Parkinson's disease. *J. Parkinsons Dis.* 2, 287–302. doi: 10.3233/JPD-012110

Pervin, M., Unno, K., Ohishi, T., Tanabe, H., Miyoshi, N., and Nakamura, Y. (2018). Beneficial effects of green tea catechins on neurodegenerative diseases. *Molecules.* 23:E1297. doi: 10.3390/molecules23061297

Pogacnik, L., Pirc, K., Palmela, I., Skrt, M., Kim, K. S., Brites, D., et al. (2016). Potential for brain accessibility and analysis of stability of selected flavonoids in relation to neuroprotection *in vitro*. *Brain Res.* 1651, 17–26. doi: 10.1016/j.brainres.2016.09.020

Pujols, J., Peña-Díaz, S., Conde-Giménez, M., Pinheiro, F., Navarro, S., Sancho, J., et al. (2017). High-throughput screening methodology to identify alpha-synuclein aggregation inhibitors. *Int. J. Mol. Sci.* 18:E478. doi: 10.3390/ijms18030478

Rekha, K. R., Selvakumar, G. P., Santha, K., and Inmozhi Sivakamasundari, R. (2013). Geraniol attenuates α-synuclein expression and neuromuscular impairment through increase dopamine content in MPTP intoxicated mice by dose dependent manner. *Biochem. Biophys. Res. Commun.* 440, 664–670. doi: 10.1016/j.bbrc.2013.09.122

Ren, R., Shi, C., Cao, J., Sun, Y., Zhao, X., Guo, Y., et al. (2016). Neuroprotective effects of a standardized flavonoid extract of safflower against neurotoxin-induced cellular and animal models of Parkinson's disease. *Sci. Rep.* 6:22135. doi: 10.1038/srep22135

Reyes, J. F., Olsson, T. T., Lamberts, J. T., Devine, M. J., Kunath, T., and Brundin, P. (2015). A cell culture model for monitoring α-synuclein cell-to-cell transfer. *Neurobiol. Dis.* 77, 266–275. doi: 10.1016/j.nbd.2014.07.003

Ringe, D., and Petsko, G. A. (2009). What are pharmacological chaperones and why are they interesting? *J. Biol.* 8:80. doi: 10.1186/jbiol186

Rogers, J. T., Mikkilineni, S., Cantuti-Castelvetri, I., Smith, D. H., Huang, X., Bandyopadhyay, S., et al. (2011). The alpha-synuclein 5′untranslated region targeted translation blockers: anti-alpha synucleinefficacy of cardiac glycosides and Posiphen. *J. Neural Transm. (Vienna)* 118, 493–507. doi: 10.1007/s00702-010-0513-5

Ruipérez, V., Darios, F., and Davletov, B. (2010). Alpha-synuclein, lipids and Parkinson's disease. *Prog. Lipid Res.* 49, 420–428. doi: 10.1016/j.plipres.2010.05.004

Sarrafchi, A., Bahmani, M., Shirzad, H., and Rafieian-Kopaei, M. (2016). Oxidative stress and Parkinson's disease: new hopes in treatment with herbal antioxidants. *Curr. Pharm. Des.* 22, 238–246. doi: 10.2174/1381612822666151112151653

Sashourpour, M., Zahri, S., Radjabian, T., Ruf, V., Pan-Montojo, F., and Morshedi, D. (2017). A study on the modulation of alpha-synuclein fibrillation by *Scutellaria pinnatifida* extracts and its neuroprotective properties. *PLoS ONE* 12:e0184483. doi: 10.1371/journal.pone.0184483

Sawkar, A. R., Cheng, W. C., Beutler, E., Wong, C. H., Balch, W. E., and Kelly, J. W. (2002). Chemical chaperones increase the cellular activity of n370s beta-glucosidase: a therapeutic strategy for gaucher disease. *Proc. Natl. Acad. Sci. U.S.A.* 99, 15428–15433. doi: 10.1073/pnas.192582899

Schenk, D. B., Koller, M., Ness, D. K., Griffith, S. G., Grundman, M., Zago, W., et al. (2017). First-in-human assessment of PRX002, an anti-α-synuclein monoclonal antibody, in healthy volunteers. *Mov. Disord.* 32, 211–218. doi: 10.1002/mds.26878

Scholz, S., and Williamson, G. (2007). Interactions affecting the bioavailability of dietary polyphenols *in vivo*. *Int. J. Vitam. Nutr. Res.* 77, 224–235. doi: 10.1024/0300-9831.77.3.224

Sekowski, S., Ionov, M., Abdulladjanova, N., Makhmudov, R., Mavlyanov, S., Milowska, K., et al. (2017). Interaction of α-synuclein with *Rhus typhina* tannin–implication for Parkinson's disease. *Colloids Surf. B Biointerfaces* 155, 159–165. doi: 10.1016/j.colsurfb.2017.04.007

Shaltiel-Karyo, R., Davidi, D., Frenkel-Pinter, M., Ovadia, M., Segal, D., and Gazit, E. (2012). Differential inhibition of α-synuclein oligomeric and fibrillar assembly in parkinson's disease model by cinnamon extract. *Biochim. Biophys. Acta* 1820, 1628–1635. doi: 10.1016/j.bbagen.2012.04.021

Sharma, N., Kapoor, M., and Nehru, B. (2016). Apocyanin, NADPH oxidase inhibitor prevents lipopolysaccharide induced α-synucleinaggregation and ameliorates motor function deficits in rats: possible role of biochemical and inflammatory alterations. *Behav. Brain Res.* 296, 177–190. doi: 10.1016/j.bbr.2015.09.012

Sharma, N., and Nehru, B. (2018). Curcumin affords neuroprotection and inhibits α-synuclein aggregation in lipopolysaccharide-induced Parkinson's disease model. *Inflammopharmacology* 26, 349–360. doi: 10.1007/s10787-017-0402-8

Shashikumar, S., Pradeep, H., Chinnu, S., Rajini, P. S., and Rajanikant, G. K. (2015). Alpha-linolenic acid suppresses dopaminergic neurodegeneration induced by 6-OHDA in *Caenorhabditis elegans*. *Physiol. Behav.* 151, 563–569. doi: 10.1016/j.physbeh.2015.08.025

Shen, C., Sun, F. L., Zhang, R. Y., Zhang, L., Li, Y. L., Zhang, L., et al. (2015). Tetrahydroxystilbene glucoside ameliorates memory and movement functions, protects synapses and inhibits α-synuclein aggregation in hippocampus and striatum in aged mice. *Restor. Neurol. Neurosci.* 33, 531–541. doi: 10.3233/RNN-150514

Shoval, H., Weiner, L., Gazit, E., Levy, M., Pinchuk, I., and Lichtenberg, D. (2008). Polyphenol-induced dissociation of various amyloid fibrils results in a methionine-independent formation of ROS. *Biochim. Biophys. Acta* 1784, 1570–1577. doi: 10.1016/j.bbapap.2008.08.007

Shukla, V., Phulara, S. C., Yadav, D., Tiwari, S., Kaur, S., Gupta, M. M., et al. (2012). Iridoid compound 10-O-trans-p-coumaroylcatalpol extends longevity and reduces α synucleinaggregation in *Caenorhabditis elegans*. *CNS Neurol. Disord. Drug Targets* 11, 984–992. doi: 10.2174/1871527311211080007

Siddique, Y. H., Ara, G., Jyoti, S., and Afzal, M. (2012). The dietary supplementation of nordihydroguaiaretic acid (NDGA) delayed the loss of climbing ability in Drosophila model of Parkinson's disease. *J. Diet. Suppl.* 9, 1–8. doi: 10.3109/19390211.2011.630716

Siddique, Y. H., Jyoti, S., and Naz, F (2014). Effect of epicatechin gallate dietary supplementation on transgenic Drosophila model of Parkinson's disease. *J. Diet. Suppl.* 11, 121–130. doi: 10.3109/19390211.2013.859207

Siddique, Y. H., Khan, W., Singh, B. R., and Naqvi, A. H. (2013b). Synthesis of alginate-curcumin nanocomposite and its protective role in transgenic Drosophila model of Parkinson's disease. *ISRN Pharmacol.* 2013:794582. doi: 10.1155/2013/794582

Siddique, Y. H., Mujtaba, S. F., Jyoti, S., and Naz, F (2013a). GC-MS analysis of *Eucalyptus citriodora* leaf extract and its role on the dietary supplementation in transgenic Drosophila model of Parkinson's disease. *Food Chem Toxicol.* 55, 29–35. doi: 10.1016/j.fct.2012.12.028

Simon-Sanchez, J., Schulte, C., Bras, J. M., Sharma, M., Gibbs, J. R., Berg, D., et al. (2009). Genome-wide association study reveals genetic risk underlying Parkinson's disease. *Nat. Genet.* 41, 1308–1312. doi: 10.1038/ng.487

Singh, P. K., Kotia, V., Ghosh, D., Mohite, G. M., Kumar, A., and Maji, S. K. (2013). Curcumin modulates α-synuclein aggregation and toxicity. *ACS Chem. Neurosci.* 4, 393–407. doi: 10.1021/cn3001203

Singleton, A. B., Farrer, M., Johnson, J., Singleton, A., Hague, S., Kachergus, J., et al. (2003). α-Synuclein locus triplication causes Parkinson's disease. *Science* 302:841. doi: 10.1126/science.1090278

Sivanesam, K., and Andersen, N. H. (2016). Modulating the amyloidogenesis of α-synuclein. *Curr. Neuropharmacol.* 14, 226–237. doi: 10.2174/1570159X13666151030103153

Skibinski, G., and Finkbeiner, S. (2011). Drug discovery in Parkinson's disease–update and developments in the use of cellular models. *Int. J. High Throughput Screen.* 2011, 15–25. doi: 10.2147/IJHTS.S8681

Smita, S. S., Raj Sammi, S., Laxman, T. S., Bhatta, R. S., and Pandey, R. (2017). Shatavarin IV elicits lifespan extension and alleviates Parkinsonism in *Caenorhabditis elegans*. *Free Radic. Res.* 51, 954–969. doi: 10.1080/10715762.2017.1395419

Šneideris, T., Baranauskiene, L., Cannon, J.G., Rutkiene, R., Meškys, R., and Smirnovas, V. (2015). Looking for a generic inhibitor of amyloid-like fibril formation among flavone derivatives. *Peer J.* 3:e1271. doi: 10.7717/peerj.1271

Spillantini, M. G., Crowther, R. A., Jakes, R., Hasegawa, M., and Goedert, M. (1998). Alpha-synuclein in filamentous inclusions of Lewy bodies from Parkinson's disease and dementia with lewy bodies. *Proc. Natl. Acad. Sci. U.S.A.* 95, 6469–6473. doi: 10.1073/pnas.95.11.6469

Spillantini, M. G., Schmidt, M. L., Lee, V. M., Trojanowski, J. Q., Jakes, R., Goedert, M., et al. (1997). Alpha-synuclein in Lewy bodies. *Nature* 388, 839–840. doi: 10.1038/42166

Spinelli, K. J., Osterberg, V. R., Meshul, C. K., Soumyanath, A., and Unni, V. K. (2015). Curcumin treatment improves motor behavior in α-synuclein transgenic mice. *PLoS ONE* 10:e0128510. doi: 10.1371/journal.pone.0128510

Srinivasan, R., Henderson, B. J., Lester, H. A., and Richards, C. I. (2014). Pharmacological chaperoning of nAChRs: a therapeutic target for Parkinson's disease. *Pharmacol. Res.* 83, 20–29. doi: 10.1016/j.phrs.2014.02.005

Sun, A., Xu, X., Lin, J., Cui, X., and Xu, R. (2015). Neuroprotection by saponins. *Phytother. Res.* 29,187–200. doi: 10.1002/ptr.5246

Sun, X., Cao, Y. B., Hu, L. F., Yang, Y. P., Li, J., Wang, F., et al. (2011). ASICs mediate the modulatory effect by paeoniflorin on α-synuclein autophagic degradation. *Brain Res.* 1396,77–87. doi: 10.1016/j.brainres.2011.04.011

Tachibana, H., Koga, K., Fujimura, Y., and Yamada, K. (2004). A receptor for green tea polyphenol EGCG. *Nat. Struct. Mol. Biol.* 11, 380–381. doi: 10.1038/nsmb743

Taebnia, N., Morshedi, D., Yaghmaei, S., Aliakbari, F., Rahimi, F., and Arpanaei, A. (2016). Curcumin-loaded amine-functionalized mesoporous silica nanoparticles inhibit α-synuclein fibrillation and reduce its cytotoxicity-associated effects. *Langmuir* 32, 13394–13402. doi: 10.1021/acs.langmuir.6b02935

Takahashi, R., Ono, K., Takamura, Y., Mizuguchi, M., Ikeda, T., Nishijo, H., et al (2015). Phenolic compounds prevent the oligomerization of α-synuclein and reduce synaptic toxicity. *J. Neurochem.* 134, 943–955. doi: 10.1111/jnc.13180

Tamarappoo, B. K., and Verkman, A. S. (1998). Defective aquaporin-2 trafficking in nephrogenic diabetes insipidus and correction by chemical chaperones. *J. Clin. Invest.* 101, 2257–2567. doi: 10.1172/JCI2303

Tanji, K., Miki, Y., Maruyama, A., Mimura, J., Matsumiya, T., Mori, F., et al. (2015). Trehalose intake induces chaperone molecules along with autophagy in a mouse model of Lewy body disease. *Biochem. Biophys. Res. Commun.* 465, 746–752. doi: 10.1016/j.bbrc.2015.08.076

Tavassoly, O., Kakish, J., Nokhrin, S., Dmitriev, O., and Lee, J. S. (2014). The use of nanopore analysis for discovering drugs which bind to α-synuclein for treatment of Parkinson's disease. *Eur. J. Med. Chem.* 88, 42–54. doi: 10.1016/j.ejmech.2014.07.090

Temsamani, H., Krisa, S., Decossas-Mendoza, M., Lambert, O., Mérillon, J.M., and Richard, T. (2016). Piceatannol and other wine stilbenes: a pool of inhibitors against α-synuclein aggregation and cytotoxicity. *Nutrients* 8:E367. doi: 10.3390/nu8060367

Teraoka, M., Nakaso, K., Kusumoto, C., Katano, S., Tajima, N., Yamashita, A., et al. (2012). Cytoprotective effect of chlorogenic acid against α-synuclein-related toxicity in catecholaminergic PC12 cells. *J. Clin. Biochem. Nutr.* 51, 122–127. doi: 10.3164/jcbn.D-11-00030

Tompa, P. (2005). The interplay between structure and function in intrinsically unstructured proteins. *FEBS Lett.* 579, 3346–3354. doi: 10.1016/j.febslet.2005.03.072

Török, N., Majláth, Z., Szalárdy, L., and Vécsei, L. (2016). Investigational α-synuclein aggregation inhibitors: hope for Parkinson's disease. *Expert Opin. Investig. Drugs* 25, 1281–1294. doi: 10.1080/13543784.2016.1237501

Ur Rasheed, M. S., Tripathi, M. K., Mishra, A. K., Shukla, S., and Singh, M. P. (2016). Resveratrol protects from toxin-induced Parkinsonism: a plethora of proofs hitherto petty translational value. *Mol. Neurobiol.* 53, 2751–2760. doi: 10.1007/s12035-015-9124-3

Uversky, V. N., and Dunker, A. K. (2010). Understanding protein non-folding. *Biochim. Biophys. Acta* 1804, 1231–1264. doi: 10.1016/j.bbapap.2010.01.017

Van Kampen, J., Robertson, H. A., Hagg, T., and Drobitch, R. (2003). Neuroprotective actions of the ginseng extract G115 in two rodent models of Parkinson's disease. *Exp. Neurol.* 184, 521–529. doi: 10.1016/j.expneurol.2003.08.002

Van Kampen, J. M., Baranowski, D. B., Shaw, C. A., and Kay, D. G. (2014). Panax ginseng is neuroprotective in a novel progressive model of Parkinson's disease. *Exp. Gerontol.* 50, 95–105. doi: 10.1016/j.exger.2013.11.012

Velander, P., Wu, L., Henderson, F., Zhang, S., Bevan, D. R., and Xu, B. (2017). Natural product-based amyloid inhibitors. *Biochem. Pharmacol.* 139, 40–55. doi: 10.1016/j.bcp.2017.04.004

Visanji, N. P., Brotchie, J. M., Kalia, L. V., Koprich, J. B., Tandon, A., and Watts, J. C. (2016). α-synuclein based animal models of parkinson's disease: challenges and opportunities in a new era. *Trends Neurosci.* 39, 750–762. doi: 10.1016/j.tins.2016.09.003

Wagner, H., and Ulrich-Merzenich, G. (2009). Synergy research: approaching a new generation of phytopharmaceuticals. *Phytomedicine* 16, 97–110. doi: 10.1016/j.phymed.2008.12.018

Wakabayashi, K., Engelender, S., Yoshimoto, M., Tsuji, S., Ross, C. A., and Takahashi, H. (2000). Synphilin-1 is present in Lewy bodies in Parkinson's disease. *Ann. Neurol.* 47, 521–523. doi: 10.1002/1531-8249(200004)47:4<521::AID-ANA18>3.0.CO;2-B

Wang, M. S., Boddapati, S., Emadi, S., and Sierks, M. R. (2010). Curcumin reduces alpha-synuclein induced cytotoxicity in Parkinson's disease cell model. *BMC Neurosci.* 11:57. doi: 10.1186/1471-2202-11-57

Wang, S., He, H., Chen, L., Zhang, W., Zhang, X., and Chen, J (2015b). Protective effects of salidroside in the MPTP/MPP(+)-induced model of Parkinson's disease through ROS-NO-related mitochondrion pathway. *Mol Neurobiol.* 51, 718–728. doi: 10.1007/s12035-014-8755-0

Wang, X. C., Wang, X., and Li, Q. L. (2014). Effect of chaperone-mediated autophagy in MPP^+ -induced SH-SY5Y cells and interventional effect of puerarin. *Zhongguo Zhong Yao Za Zhi.* 39, 106–112.

Wang, Z. H., Zhang, J. L., Duan, Y. L., Zhang, Q. S., Li, G. F., and Zheng, D. L. (2015a). MicroRNA-214 participates in the neuroprotective effect of resveratrol via inhibiting α-synuclein expression in MPTP-induced Parkinson's disease mouse. *Biomed. Pharmacother.* 74, 252–256. doi: 10.1016/j.biopha.2015.08.025

Wang, Z. Y., Liu, J. Y., Yang, C. B., Malampati, S., Huang, Y. Y., Li, M. X., et al. (2017). Neuroprotective natural products for the treatment of Parkinson's disease by targeting the autophagy-lysosome pathway: a systematic review. *Phytother. Res.* 31, 1119–1127. doi: 10.1002/ptr.5834

Weinreb, O., Mandel, S., Youdim, M. B. H., and Amit, T. (2013). Targeting dysregulation of brain iron homeostasis in Parkinson's disease by iron chelators. *Free Radic. Biol. Med.* 62, 52–64. doi: 10.1016/j.freeradbiomed.2013.01.017

Winner, B., Jappelli, R., Maji, S. K., Desplats, P. A., Boyer, L., Aigner, S., et al. (2011). *In vivo* demonstration that α-synuclein oligomers are toxic. *Proc. Natl. Acad. Sci. U.S.A.* 108, 4194–4199. doi: 10.1073/pnas.1100976108

Wong, V. K., Wu, A. G., Wang, J. R., Liu, L., and Law, B. Y. (2015). Neferine attenuates the protein level and toxicity of mutant huntingtin in PC-12 cells via induction of autophagy. *Molecules* 20, 3496–3514. doi: 10.3390/molecules20033496

Wu, A. G., Wong, V. K., Xu, S. W., Chan, W. K., Ng, C. I., Liu, L., et al. (2013). Onjisaponin B derived from *Radix polygalae* enhances autophagy and accelerates the degradation of mutant α-synuclein and huntingtin in PC-12 Cells. *Int. J. Mol. Sci.* 14, 22618–22641. doi: 10.3390/ijms141122618

Wu, Y., Jiang, X., Yang, K., Xia, Y., Cheng, S., Tang, Q., et al. (2017). Inhibition of α-Synuclein contributes to the ameliorative effects of dietary flavonoids luteolin on arsenite-induced apoptotic cell death in the dopaminergic PC12 cells. *Toxicol. Mech. Methods* 27, 598–608. doi: 10.1080/15376516.2017.1339155

Wu, Y., Li, X., Zhu, J. X., Xie, W., Le, W., and Fan, Z. (2011). Resveratrol-activated AMPK/SIRT1/autophagy in cellular models of Parkinson's disease. *Neurosignals* 19, 163–174. doi: 10.1159/000328516

Xu, Q., Langley, M., Kanthasamy, A. G., and Reddy, M. B. (2017). Epigallocatechin gallate has a neurorescue effect in a mouse model of Parkinson disease. *J. Nutr.* 147, 1926–1931. doi: 10.3945/jn.117.255034

Xu, Y., Zhang, P., Wang, C., Shan, Y., Wang, D., Qian, F., et al. (2013). Effect of ginsenoside Rg3 on tyrosine hydroxylase and related mechanisms in the forced swimming-induced fatigue rats. *J. Ethnopharmacol.* 150, 138–147. doi: 10.1016/j.jep.2013.08.016

Xu, Y., Zhang, Y., Quan, Z., Wong, W., Guo, J., Zhang, R., et al. (2016). Epigallocatechin gallate (EGCG) inhibits alpha-synuclein aggregation: a potential agent for Parkinson's disease. *Neurochem. Res.* 41, 2788–2796. doi: 10.1007/s11064-016-1995-9

Yamaguchi, Y., Masuda, M., Sasakawa, H., Nonaka, T., Hanashima, S., Hisanaga, S., et al. (2010). Characterization of inhibitor-bound alpha-synuclein dimer: role of alpha-synuclein N-terminal region in dimerization and inhibitor binding. *J. Mol. Biol.* 395, 445–456. doi: 10.1016/j.jmb.2009.10.068

Yang, F., Yang, Y. P., Mao, C. J., Cao, B. Y., Cai, Z. L., Shi, J. J., et al. (2009). Role of autophagy and proteasome degradation pathways in apoptosis of PC12 cells overexpressing human alpha-synuclein. *Neurosci. Lett.* 454, 203–218. doi: 10.1016/j.neulet.2009.03.027

Yang, J. E., Rhoo, K. Y., Lee, S., Lee, J. T., Park, J. H., Bhak, G., et al. (2017). EGCG-mediated protection of the membrane disruption and cytotoxicity caused by the 'active oligomer' of α-synuclein. *Sci. Rep.* 7:17945. doi: 10.1038/s41598-017-18349-z

Yoshida, W., Kobayashi, N., Sasaki, Y., Ikebukuro, K., and Sode, K. (2013). Partial peptide of α-synuclein modified with small-molecule inhibitors specifically inhibits amyloid fibrillation of α-synuclein. *Int. J. Mol. Sci.* 14, 2590–2600. doi: 10.3390/ijms14022590

Yuan, J., Ren, J., Wang, Y., He, X., and Zhao, Y. (2016). Acteoside binds to caspase-3 and exerts neuroprotection in the rotenone rat model of Parkinson's disease. *PLoS ONE* 11:e0162696. doi: 10.1371/journal.pone.0162696

Zhang, H., Bai, L., He, J., Zhong, L., Duan, X., Ouyang, L., et al. (2017). Recent advances in discovery and development of natural products as source for anti-Parkinson's disease lead compounds. *Eur. J. Med. Chem.* 141, 257–272. doi: 10.1016/j.ejmech.2017.09.068

Zhang, H., Rochet, J. C., and Stanciu, L. A. (2015). Cu(II) promotes amyloid pore formation. *Biochem. Biophys. Res. Commun.* 464, 342–347. doi: 10.1016/j.bbrc.2015.06.156

Zhang, L., Yu, S., Zhang, R., Xing, Y., Li, Y., and Li, L. (2013). Tetrahydroxystilbene glucoside antagonizes age-related α-synuclein overexpression in the hippocampus of APP transgenic mouse model of Alzheimer's disease. *Restor. Neurol. Neurosci.* 31, 41–52. doi: 10.3233/RNN-120260

Zhang, N., Yan, F., Liang, X., Wu, M., Shen, Y., Chen, M., et al. (2018). Localized delivery of curcumin into brain with polysorbate 80-modified cerasomes by ultrasound-targeted microbubble destruction for improved Parkinson's disease therapy. *Theranostics* 8, 2264–2277. doi: 10.7150/thno.23734

Zhao, J., Xu, L., Liang, Q., Sun, Q., Chen, C., Zhang, Y., et al. (2017). Metal chelator EGCG attenuates Fe(III)-induced conformational transition of α-synuclein and protects AS-PC12 cells against Fe(III)-induced death. *J. Neurochem.* 143, 136–146. doi: 10.1111/jnc.14142

Zheng, M., Xin, Y., Li, Y., Xu, F., Xi, X., Guo, H., et al. (2018). Ginsenosides: a potential neuroprotective agent. *Biomed. Res. Int.* 2018:8174345. doi: 10.1155/2018/8174345

Zhou, J. X., Zhang, H. B., Huang, Y., He, Y., Zheng, Y., Anderson, J. P., et al. (2013). Tenuigenin attenuates α-synuclein-induced cytotoxicity by down-regulating polo-like kinase 3. *CNS Neurosci. Ther.* 19, 688–694. doi: 10.1111/cns.12124

Zhu, M., Han, S., and Fink, A. L. (2013). Oxidized quercetin inhibits α-synuclein fibrillization. *Biochim. Biophys. Acta* 1830, 2872–2881. doi: 10.1016/j.bbagen.2012.12.027

Zhu, M., Rajamani, S., Kaylor, J., Han, S., Zhou, F., and Fink, A. L. (2004). The flavonoid baicalein inhibits fibrillation of alpha-synuclein and disaggregates existing fibrils. *J. Biol. Chem.* 279, 26846–26857. doi: 10.1074/jbc.M403129200

15

Naturally Occurring Acetylcholinesterase Inhibitors and Their Potential Use for Alzheimer's Disease Therapy

Thaiane Coelho dos Santos[1,2], *Thaís Mota Gomes*[1], *Bruno Araújo Serra Pinto*[1,2], *Adriana Leandro Camara*[1] *and Antonio Marcus de Andrade Paes*[1,2*]

[1] *Laboratory of Experimental Physiology, Department of Physiological Sciences, Biological and Health Sciences Centre, Federal University of Maranhão, São Luís, Brazil,* [2] *Health Sciences Graduate Program, Biological and Health Sciences Centre, Federal University of Maranhão, São Luís, Brazil*

***Correspondence:**
Antonio Marcus de Andrade Paes
marcuspaes@ufma.br

Alzheimer's disease (AD) is a main cause of dementia, accounting for up to 75% of all dementia cases. Pathophysiological processes described for AD progression involve neurons and synapses degeneration, mainly characterized by cholinergic impairment. This feature makes acetylcholinesterase inhibitors (AChEi) the main class of drugs currently used for the treatment of AD dementia phase, among which galantamine is the only naturally occurring substance. However, several plant species producing diverse classes of alkaloids, coumarins, terpenes, and polyphenols have been assessed for their anti-AChE activity, becoming potential candidates for new anti-AD drugs. Therefore, this mini-review aimed to recapitulate last decade studies on the anti-AChE activity of plant species, their respective extracts, as well as isolated compounds. The anti-AChE activity of extracts prepared from 54 plant species pertaining 29 families, as well as 36 isolated compounds were classified and discussed according to their anti-AChE pharmacological potency to highlight the most prominent ones. Besides, relevant limitations, such as proper antioxidant assessment, and scarcity of toxicological and clinical studies were also discussed in order to help researchers out with the bioprospection of potentially new AChEi.

Keywords: Alzheimer's disease, acetylcholinesterase inhibitors, anti-cholinesterase, plant species, secondary metabolites

INTRODUCTION

Alzheimer's disease (AD) is a main cause of dementia, accounting for up to 75% of all dementia cases and has become a population aging-related concern for policymakers and public health systems around the world by its both direct and indirect costs (Takizawa et al., 2015; Fiest et al., 2016; Scheltens et al., 2016). Nowadays, AD prevalence among people over 60 years old is estimated in 40.2 per 1000, while its incidence proportion is 34.1 per 1,000 (Prince, 2015; Fiest et al., 2016). Those values mean that over 45 million people is suffering from AD symptoms worldwide, whereas this scenario is expected to double every 20 years until at least 2050 (Scheltens et al., 2016). AD is mainly characterized by progressive neurodegenerative disorder, clinically demonstrated by cognitive and memory decline, progressive impairment of daily activities, and a variety of neuropsychiatric symptoms and behavioral disturbances (Tarawneh and Holtzman, 2012).

Pathophysiological processes described for AD progression involve neurons and synapses degeneration resulting from beta-amyloid (Aβ) protein aggregation and neurofibrillary tangles, as well as, neuroinflammation, mitochondrial damage, oxidative stress and excitotoxicity, which interfere with several neurotransmitters signaling pathways (Madeo and Elsayad, 2013; Godyn et al., 2016; Henstridge et al., 2016). Among the latter, cholinergic dysfunction is the most studied and has been closely associated with the early cognitive decline found in AD patients (Craig et al., 2011). In fact, early in the 70's, it was observed that cholinergic neurons were prematurely lost in AD process, arising the Alzheimer's Cholinergic Hypothesis (Bartus et al., 1982). This hypothesis was further corroborated by observations that cholinergic neurons in basal forebrain are severely damaged during AD progression (Bartus, 2000).

Despite the huge research on AD, supportive care from family and other caregivers is still the mainstay treatment, though pharmacotherapy has importantly evolved during the last decade. Four drugs are currently used for the treatment of the dementia phase: the acetylcholinesterase (AChE) inhibitors (AChEi)–donepezil, rivastigmine, and galantamine–and the glutamate antagonist memantine. AChEi increase synaptic acetylcholine (ACh) levels and improve cholinergic function in the brain (Anand and Singh, 2013; Andrieu et al., 2015). Amongst those clinically relevant AChEi, galantamine is the only naturally occurring substance, consisting of an alkaloid extracted from Amaryllidaceae family (Heinrich, 2010; Murray et al., 2013). Galantamine reversibly and competitively inhibits AChE (Thomsen and Kewitz, 1990) and allosterically modulates nicotinic ACh receptors (Schrattenholz et al., 1996). Notwithstanding, besides its anti-AChE activity, most of natural AChEi molecules generally present additional pharmacological properties, particularly antioxidant, which enable them to be applied as multi-target strategies against AD onset and progression (Orhan et al., 2011; Ayaz et al., 2017; Sahoo et al., 2018).

Several studies have been carried out toward identification and isolation of natural molecules applicable for design and development of new anti-AD drugs, particularly those pertaining to the classes of alkaloids, terpenes, coumarins and polyphenols (Huang et al., 2013). Therefore, this mini-review recapitulates last decade studies on the anti-AchE activity of plant species, their respective extracts, as well as isolated compounds, in order to settle down the state-of-the-art in the field and to help researchers out with the bioprospection of potentially new AChEi candidates applicable for anti-AD drug design and pharmacotherapy.

METHODOLOGY

This mini-review revises published studies available in Pubmed between 2007 and 2018 (1st semester), which were retrieved by using the following descriptors combination: "anti-acetylcholinesterase and plant extract" and "acetylcholinesterase inhibitors and plant extract and Alzheimer." The only criterion for inclusion was that anti-AChE activity of the plant extract and/or isolated compounds had been assessed by Ellman's methodology (Ellman et al., 1961), which is considered a gold standard for AChEi screening (Holas et al., 2012). On the other hand, two criteria for exclusion were applied: the lack of reliable positive controls, which might include but are not limited to galantamine, huperzine A and B, or physostigmine (Mehta et al., 2012); and the absence of half maximal inhibitory concentration (IC_{50}) assessment, which allow us to compare the anti-AChE potencies among different plant extracts and/or isolated compounds (Colovic et al., 2013).

A total of 207 original studies were retrieved, from which 71 were considered appropriate. All the species Latin names were validated at The Plant List (2013); version 1.1.; http://www.theplantlist.org/ (accessed 15th August, 2018). When the Latin name provided by the study diverged from that accepted at The Plant List, the species was identified by the accepted one followed by the former, which was reported as synonym, between parenthesis. To improve the readability of the text, the identity of the plant taxonomist(s) for each species is informed only in **Table 1**, excepting those mentioned as the source of isolated compounds, but whose extracts were not assayed.

PLANT SPECIES WITH ANTI-ACETYLCHOLINESTERASE ACTIVITY

Amaryllidaceae is the leading family of genera holding anti-AChE activity, particularly *Galanthus* spp., which are the primordial source of galantamine (Heinrich, 2010). However, subsequently to galantamine's approval for the treatment of mild-to-moderate AD in 2001, a plethora of species have been assessed in a pursuit of new AChEi. In our survey timeframe, a total of 39 studies reporting the anti-AChE activity for 51 species, from 29 different families, were considered. The most prevalent families were Amaryllidaceae, Lycopodiaceae, and Polygonaceae, contributing with 5, 5, and 4 species, respectively. Noteworthy, *Huperzia* spp. keep drawing ethnopharmacology researchers' attention, despite the consistent basic and clinical evidence already available for Huperzine A on AD treatment (Ha et al., 2011; Sahoo et al., 2018).

Table 1 summarizes the contemplated species, which were classified in three categories, in accordance to the IC_{50} values determined for their respective extracts/fractions: high potency, $IC_{50} < 20\,\mu g/mL$; moderate potency, $20 < IC_{50} < 200\,\mu g/mL$; and low potency, $200 < IC_{50} < 1{,}000\,\mu g/mL$. Those cutoffs were set according to the average IC_{50} value described for galantamine in the literature ($\sim 2\,\mu M$ or $0.575\,\mu g/mL$) multiplied by a factor of 10 (Lopez et al., 2002; Ingkaninan et al., 2003; Berkov et al., 2008). Similar criteria have been previously applied by Murray et al. (2013), excepting that they included studies reporting only the maximal anti-AChE inhibitory activity and set the cutoff for low potency at $IC_{50} > 500\,\mu g/mL$.

Twenty-four plant species fell into high potency category, with IC_{50} values varying from $0.3\,\mu g/mL$ for ethyl acetate bulb extract of *Scadoxus puniceus* (Amaryllidaceae), ethyl acetate root extract of *Lannea schweinfurthii* (Anacardiaceae; Adewusi and Steenkamp, 2011), and ethyl acetate root fraction of

TABLE 1 | Plant extracts with *in vitro* anticholinesterase activity assessed by Ellman's Method reported in Pubmed from 2007 to 2018 (1st semester).

Plant species (Families)	Type of extract or fraction (plant's part)	IC_{50} (μg/mL)	Toxicological assessment[#]	References
Scadoxus puniceus (L.) Friis & Nordal (Amaryllidaceae)	Ethyl acetate extract (bulb)	0.3	Not assessed	Adewusi and Steenkamp, 2011
Lannea schweinfurthii Engl. (Anacardiaceae)	Ethyl acetate extract (root)	0.3	Not assessed	Adewusi and Steenkamp, 2011
Carpolobia lutea G. Don (Polygalaceae)	Ethyl acetate fraction (root)	0.3	≤100 μg/mL	Nwidu et al., 2017
Xysmalobium undulatum (L.) W. T. Aiton (Apocynaceae)	Ethyl acetate extract (root)	0.5	Not assessed	Adewusi and Steenkamp, 2011
Phlegmariurus tetragonus (Hook. & Grev.) B. Øllg. (Lycopodiaceae)*	Alkaloidal fraction (aerial parts)	0.9	Not assessed	Armijos et al., 2016
Esenbeckia leiocarpa Engl. (Rutaceae)	Alkaloidal fraction (stems)	1.6	Not assessed	Cardoso-Lopes et al., 2010
Melissa officinalis L. (Lamiaceae)	Ethanolic extract (leaves)	1.7	Not assessed	Dastmalchi et al., 2009
Carpolobia lutea G. Don (Polygalaceae)	Aqueous fraction (root)	2	≤100 μg/mL	Nwidu et al., 2017
Crinum bulbispermum (Burm. f.) Milne-Redh. & Schweick. (Amaryllidaceae)	Ethyl acetate extract (bulb)	2.1	Not assessed	Adewusi and Steenkamp, 2011
Morus alba L. (Moraceae)	Ethyl acetate fraction (root-bark)	2.5	Not assessed	Kuk et al., 2017
Angelica decursiva (Miq.) Franch. & Sav. (Apiaceae)	Aqueous fraction (whole plant)	2.6	Not assessed	Ali et al., 2015
Carpolobia lutea G. Don (Polygalaceae)	Methanolic extract (root)	3	≤100 μg/mL	Nwidu et al., 2017
Buchanania axillaris (Desr.) Ramamoorthy (Anacardiaceae)	Methanolic extract (aerial parts)	4.9	Not assessed	Penumala et al., 2018
Salvia miltiorrhiza Bunge (Lamiaceae)	Ethanolic extract (whole plant)	5.0	Not assessed	Lin et al., 2008
Huperzia serrata (Thunb.) Trevis. (Lycopodiaceae)	Alkaloids fraction (whole plant)	6.0	Not assessed	Ohba et al., 2015
Esenbeckia leiocarpa Engl. (Rutaceae)	Hexanic fraction (stems)	6.0	Not assessed	Cardoso-Lopes et al., 2010
Angelica decursiva (Miq.) Franch. & Sav. (Apiaceae)	Buthanolic fraction (whole plant)	6.0	Not assessed	Ali et al., 2015
Berberis aetnensis C. Presl (Berberidaceae)	Methanolic fraction (root)	7.6	Not assessed	Bonesi et al., 2013
Senna obtusifolia (L.) H. S. Irwin & Barneby. (Leguminosae)	Ethyl acetate fraction (leaves)	9.4	Not assessed	Jung et al., 2016
Angelica decursiva (Miq.) Franch. & Sav. (Apiaceae)	Ethyl acetate fraction (whole plant)	9.7	Not assessed	Ali et al., 2015
Senna obtusifolia (L.) H.S. Irwin & Barneby. (Leguminosae)	Buthanolic fraction (leaves)	9.9	Not assessed	Jung et al., 2016
Zanthoxylum davyi Waterm. (Rutaceae)	Methanolic extract (roots)	10	Not assessed	Adewusi and Steenkamp, 2011
Ziziphus mucronata Willd. (Rhamnaceae)	Ethyl acetate extract (root)	11.2	Not assessed	Adewusi and Steenkamp, 2011
Morus alba L. (Moraceae)	Methanolic extract (root-bark)	11.4	Not assessed	Kuk et al., 2017
Zanthoxylum davyi Waterm. (Rutaceae)	Ethyl acetate extract (roots)	11.6	Not assessed	Adewusi and Steenkamp, 2011
Buchanania axillaris (Desr.) Ramamoorthy (Anacardiaceae)	Chloroform fraction (aerial parts)	12.3	Not assessed	Penumala et al., 2018
Senna obtusifolia (L.) H.S. Irwin & Barneby. (Leguminosae)	Chloroform fraction (leaves)	12.7	Not assessed	Jung et al., 2016
Morus alba L. (Moraceae)	Chloroform fraction (root-bark)	13.4	Not assessed	Kuk et al., 2017
Angelica decursiva (Miq.) Franch. & Sav. (Apiaceae)	Chloroform fraction (whole plant)	13.7	Not assessed	Ali et al., 2015
Senna obtusifolia (L.) H. S. Irwin & Barneby. (Leguminosae)	Aqueous fraction (leaves)	14.5	Not assessed	Jung et al., 2016

(Continued)

TABLE 1 | Continued

Plant species (Families)	Type of extract or fraction (plant's part)	IC_{50} (μg/mL)	Toxicological assessment#	References
Crinum bulbispermum (Burm. f.) Milne-Redh. & Schweick. (Amaryllidaceae)	Methanolic extract (bulb)	14.8	Not assessed	Adewusi and Steenkamp, 2011
Scabiosa arenaria Forssk. (Caprifoliaceae)	Ethyl acetate fraction (stem and leaves)	16	Not assessed	Besbes Hlila et al., 2013
Angelica decursiva (Miq.) Franch. & Sav. (Apiaceae)	Methanolic extract (whole plant)	16.6	Not assessed	Ali et al., 2015
Berberis libanotica Ehrenb. ex C.K. Schneid. (Berberidaceae)	Methanolic fraction (root)	16.9	Not assessed	Bonesi et al., 2013
Pavetta indica L. (Rubiaceae)	Methanolic extract (aerial parts)	17.8	Not assessed	Penumala et al., 2017
Zephyranthes carinata Herb. (Amaryllidaceae)	Alkaloidal fraction (bulb)	18.0	Not assessed	Cortes et al., 2015
Crinum jagus (J. Thomps.) Dandy (Amaryllidaceae)	Alkaloidal fraction (bulb)	18.3	≤28.7 μg/mL	Cortes et al., 2015
Adenia gummifera (Harv.) Harms (Passifloraceae)	Ethyl acetate extract (root)	18.9	Not assessed	Adewusi and Steenkamp, 2011
Berberis libanotica Ehrenb. ex C.K. Schneid. (Berberidaceae)	Methanolic extract (root)	21.7	Not assessed	Bonesi et al., 2013
Huperzia squarrosa (G. Forst.) Trevis. (Lycopodiaceae)	Ethyl acetate fraction (aerial parts)	23.4	Not assessed	Tung et al., 2017
Berberis aetnensis C. Presl (Berberidaceae)	Alkaloidal fraction (root)	24.5	Not assessed	Bonesi et al., 2013
Ochna obtusata DC. (Ochnaceae)	Chloroform fraction (aerial parts)	25.7	Not assessed	Penumala et al., 2017
Gossypium herbaceum L. (Malvaceae)	Hydroalcoholic extracts (flowers)	28.1	Not assessed	Zhao et al., 2013
Hippeastrum puniceum (Lam.) Voss. (Amaryllidaceae)	Alkaloid fraction (bulb)	28.1	≤28.7 μg/mL	Cortes et al., 2015
Hemidesmus indicus (L.) R. Br. ex Schult. (Apocynaceae)	Chloroform fraction (aerial part)	28.1	Not assessed	Penumala et al., 2018
Scabiosa arenaria Forssk. (Caprifoliaceae)	Buthanolic fraction (stems and leaves)	29.0	Not assessed	Besbes Hlila et al., 2013
Senna obtusifolia (L.) H.S. Irwin & Barneby. (Leguminosae)	Methanolic fraction (leaves)	29.2	Not assessed	Jung et al., 2016
Morus alba L. (Moraceae)	Buthanolic fraction (root-bark)	36.6	Not assessed	Kuk et al., 2017
Ficus sur Forssk. (Moraceae)	Ethyl acetate extract (fruit)	31.9	Not assessed	Adewusi and Steenkamp, 2011
Rumex hastatus D. Don (Polygonaceae)	Essential Oils (aerial parts)	32.5	Not assessed	Ahmad et al., 2016
Acalypha alnifolia Klein ex Willd. (Euphorbiaceae)	Chloroform fraction (aerial parts)	32.9	Not assessed	Penumala et al., 2017
Olax nana Wall. ex Benth. (Olacaceae)	Methanolic extract (leaves)	33.2	Not assessed	Ovais et al., 2018
Nelumbo nucifera Gaertn. (Nelumbonaceae)	Buthanolic fraction (leaves)	33.2	Not assessed	Jung et al., 2015
Persicaria hydropiper (L.) Delarbre. (Polygonaceae)**	Hexanic fraction (whole plant)	35.0	Not assessed	Ayaz et al., 2014
Berberis aetnensis C. Presl (Berberidaceae)	Hexanic fraction (root)	36.5	Not assessed	Bonesi et al., 2013
Crinum bulbispermum (Burm. f.) Milne-Redh. & Schweick. (Amaryllidaceae)	Ethyl acetate extract (root)	39.3	Not assessed	Adewusi and Steenkamp, 2011
Huperzia brevifolia (Grev. & Hook.) Holub (Lycopodiaceae)	Alkaloidal fraction (aerial parts)	39.6	Not assessed	Armijos et al., 2016
Piper capense L. f. (Piperaceae)	Ethyl acetate extract (root)	40.7	Not assessed	Adewusi and Steenkamp, 2011

(Continued)

TABLE 1 | Continued

Plant species (Families)	Type of extract or fraction (plant's part)	IC_{50} (µg/mL)	Toxicological assessment[#]	References
Searsia mysorensis (G. Don) Moffett. (Anacardiaceae)	Chloroform fraction (aerial part)	41.3	Not assessed	Penumala et al., 2018
Morus alba L. (Moraceae)	Aqueous fraction (root-bark)	43.0	Not assessed	Kuk et al., 2017
Hemidesmus indicus (L.) R. Br. ex Schult. (Apocynaceae)	Methanolic extract (aerial part)	48.6	Not assessed	Penumala et al., 2018
Huperzia squarrosa (G. Forst.) Trevis. (Lycopodiaceae)	Buthanolic fraction (aerial parts)	50.1	Not assessed	Tung et al., 2017
Esenbeckia leiocarpa Engl. (Rutaceae)	Ethanolic extract (stems)	50.7	Not assessed	Cardoso-Lopes et al., 2010
Scabiosa arenaria Forssk. (Caprifoliaceae)	Ethyl Acetate fraction (flowers)	51.0	Not assessed	Besbes Hlila et al., 2013
Pavetta indica L. (Rubiaceae)	Chloroform fraction (aerial parts)	52.1	Not assessed	Penumala et al., 2017
Polygonum hydropiper L. (Polygonaceae)	Chloroform fraction (whole plant)	55.0	Not assessed	Ayaz et al., 2014
Acalypha alnifolia Klein ex Willd. (Euphorbiaceae)	Methanolic extrac (aerial parts)	59.2	Not assessed	Penumala et al., 2017
Carpolobia lutea G. Don (Polygalaceae)	Chloroform fraction (leaves)	60.0	≤100 µg/mL	Nwidu et al., 2017
Pavetta indica L. (Rubiaceae)	Buthanolic fraction (aerial parts)	60.1	Not assessed	Penumala et al., 2017
Nelumbo nucifera Gaertn. (Nelumbonaceae)	Ethylacetate fraction (leaves)	61.1	Not assessed	Jung et al., 2015
Huperzia compacta (Hook.) Trevis. (Lycopodiaceae)	Alkaloid fraction (aerial parts)	62.4	Not assessed	Armijos et al., 2016
Acalypha alnifolia Klein ex Willd. (Euphorbiaceae)	Aqueous fraction (aerial parts)	64.8	Not assessed	Penumala et al., 2017
Nelumbo nucifera Gaertn. (Nelumbonaceae)	Chloroform fraction (leaves)	67.3	Not assessed	Jung et al., 2015
Buchanania axillaris (Desr.) Ramamoorthy (Anacardiaceae)	Buthanolic fraction (aerial parts)	67.5	Not assessed	Penumala et al., 2018
Scabiosa arenaria Forssk. (Caprifoliaceae)	Buthanolic fraction (flowers)	74.0	Not assessed	Besbes Hlila et al., 2013
Rumex hastatus D. Don (Polygonaceae)	Chloroform fraction (whole plant)	75.0	Not assessed	Ahmad et al., 2015
Scabiosa arenaria Forssk. (Caprifoliaceae)	Methanolic extract (flowers)	80.0	Not assessed	Besbes Hlila et al., 2013
Carpolobia lutea G. Don (Polygalaceae)	Ethanolic fraction (leaves)	81.0	≤100 µg/mL	Nwidu et al., 2017
Ochna obtusata DC. (Ochnaceae)	Methanolic extrac (aerial parts)	82.2	Not assessed	Penumala et al., 2017
Berberis libanotica Ehrenb. ex C.K. Schneid. (Berberidaceae)	Alkaloidal extract (root)	82.4	Not assessed	Bonesi et al., 2013
Searsia mysorensis (G. Don) Moffett. (Anacardiaceae)	Buthanolic fraction (aerial part)	83.5	Not assessed	Penumala et al., 2018
Searsia mysorensis (G. Don) Moffett. (Anacardiaceae)	Aqueous fraction (aerial part)	93.7	Not assessed	Penumala et al., 2018
Berberis libanotica Ehrenb. ex C.K. Schneid. (Berberidaceae)	Hexanic extract (root)	95.5	Not assessed	Bonesi et al., 2013
Jatropha gossypifolia L. (Euphorbiaceae)	Ethyl acetate fraction (leaves)	95.7	Not assessed	Saleem et al., 2016
Polygonum hydropiper L. (Polygonaceae)	Aqueous fraction (whole plant)	100.0	Not assessed	Ayaz et al., 2014
Pavetta indica L. (Rubiaceae)	Aqueous fraction (aerial parts)	100.4	Not assessed	Penumala et al., 2017
Stemona sessilifolia (Miq.) Miq. (Stemonaceae)	Alkaloidal extracts (root)	102.6	Not assessed	Lai et al., 2013
Huperzia squarrosa (G. Forst.) Trevis. (Lycopodiaceae)	Ethanolic extract (aerial parts)	112.2	Not assessed	Tung et al., 2017

(Continued)

TABLE 1 | Continued

Plant species (Families)	Type of extract or fraction (plant's part)	IC_{50} (µg/mL)	Toxicological assessment[#]	References
Hemidesmus indicus(L.) R. Br. ex Schult. (Apocynaceae)	Buthaolic fraction (aerial part)	113.5	Not assessed	Penumala et al., 2018
Rumex hastatus D. Don (Polygonaceae)	Ethyl acetate fraction (whole plant)	115.0	Not assessed	Ahmad et al., 2015
Nelumbo nucifera Gaertn. (Nelumbonaceae)	Aqueous fraction (leaves)	119.6	Not assessed	Jung et al., 2015
Persicaria hydropiper (L.) Delarbre. (Polygonaceae)***	Essential Oils (leaves)	130.0	Not assessed	Ayaz et al., 2015
Hemidesmus indicus(L.) R. Br. ex Schult. (Apocynaceae)	Aqueous fraction (aerial part)	129.4	Not assessed	Penumala et al., 2018
Buchanania axillaris (Desr.) Ramamoorthy (Anacardiaceae)	Aqueous fraction (aerial parts)	136.2	Not assessed	Penumala et al., 2018
Carpolobia lutea G. Don (Polygalaceae)	Ethanolic extract (stem-bark)	140.0	≤100 µg/mL	Nwidu et al., 2017
Carpolobia lutea G. Don (Polygalaceae)	Hexanic fraction oil (stem)	140.0	≤100 µg/mL	Nwidu et al., 2017
Carpolobia lutea G. Don (Polygalaceae)	Methanolic fraction (stem)	142.0	≤100 µg/mL	Nwidu et al., 2017
Elatostema papillosum Wedd. (Urticaceae)	Methanolic extract (leaves)	165.4	Not assessed	Reza et al., 2018
Scabiosa arenaria Forssk. (Caprifoliaceae)	Aqueous fraction (flowers)	170	Not assessed	Besbes Hlila et al., 2013
Ochna obtusata DC. (Ochnaceae)	Buthanolic fraction (aerial parts)	174.4	Not assessed	Penumala et al., 2017
Jatropha gossypifolia L. (Euphorbiaceae)	Dichloromethane extract (root)	176.0	Not assessed	Saleem et al., 2016
Nelumbo nucifera Gaertn. (Nelumbonaceae)	Methanolic fraction (leaves)	184.5	Not assessed	Jung et al., 2015
Rumex hastatus D. Don (Polygonaceae)	Methanolic extract (whole plant)	218.0	Not assessed	Ahmad et al., 2015
Jatropha gossypifolia L. (Euphorbiaceae)	Methanolic extract (root)	222.0	Not assessed	Saleem et al., 2016
Polygonum hydropiper L. (Polygonaceae)	Essential Oils (flowers)	225.0	Not assessed	Ayaz et al., 2015
Scabiosa arenaria Forssk. (Caprifoliaceae)	Methanolic extract (stems and leaves)	230.0	Not assessed	Besbes Hlila et al., 2013
Diplotaxis simplex Asch. ex Rohlfs (Brassicaceae)	Aqueous extract (seeds)	233.0	Not assessed	Bahloul et al., 2016
Persicaria minor (Huds.) Opiz. (Polygonaceae)****	Aqueous extract (leaves)	234.0	Not assessed	Ahmad et al., 2014
Scabiosa arenaria Forssk. (Caprifoliaceae)	Buthanolic fraction (fruits)	240.0	Not assessed	Besbes Hlila et al., 2013
Polygonum hydropiper L. (Polygonaceae)	Buthanolic fraction (whole plant)	240.0	Not assessed	Ayaz et al., 2014
Huperzia squarrosa (G. Forst.) Trevis. (Lycopodiaceae)	Hexanic fraction (aerial parts)	257.0	Not assessed	Tung et al., 2017
Acalypha alnifolia Klein ex Willd. (Euphorbiaceae)	Buthanolic fraction (aerial parts)	257.5	Not assessed	Penumala et al., 2017
Atriplex laciniata L. (Amaranthaceae)	Aqueous fraction (whole plant)	267.0	Not assessed	Kamal et al., 2015
Scabiosa arenaria Forssk. (Caprifoliaceae)	Methanolic extract (fruits)	270.0	Not assessed	Besbes Hlila et al., 2013
Atriplex laciniata L. (Amaranthaceae)	Ethyl acetate fraction (whole plant)	270.0	Not assessed	Kamal et al., 2015
Atriplex laciniata L. (Amaranthaceae)	Methanolic extract (whole plant)	280.0	Not assessed	Kamal et al., 2015
Jatropha gossypifolia L. (Euphorbiaceae)	Dichloromethane extract (leaves)	289.0	Not assessed	Saleem et al., 2016
Justicia adhatoda L. (Acanthaceae)	Methanolic extract (leaves)	294.0	Not assessed	Ali et al., 2013

(Continued)

TABLE 1 | Continued

Plant species (Families)	Type of extract or fraction (plant's part)	IC_{50} (µg/mL)	Toxicological assessment#	References
Polygonum hydropiper L. (Polygonaceae)	Ethyl acetate fraction (whole plant)	310.0	Not assessed	Ayaz et al., 2014
Atriplex laciniata L. (Amaranthaceae)	Hexanic fraction (whole plant)	310.0	Not assessed	Kamal et al., 2015
Diplotaxis harra (Forssk.) Boiss. (Brassicaceae)	Aqueous extract (seeds)	313.0	Not assessed	Bahloul et al., 2016
Polygonum hydropiper L. (Polygonaceae)	Methanolic extract (whole plant)	330.0	Not assessed	Ayaz et al., 2014
Polygonum minus Huds. (Polygonaceae)	Methanolic extract (leaves)	342.8	Not assessed	Ahmad et al., 2014
Ochna obtusata DC. (Ochnaceae)	Aqueous fraction (aerial parts)	369.1	Not assessed	Penumala et al., 2017
Atriplex laciniata L. (Amaranthaceae)	Chloroform fraction (whole plant)	390.0	Not assessed	Kamal et al., 2015
Scabiosa arenaria Forssk. (Caprifoliaceae)	Aqueous fraction (stems and leaves)	410.0	Not assessed	Besbes Hlila et al., 2013
Diplotaxis simplex Asch. ex Rohlfs (Brassicaceae)	Aqueous extract (flowers)	420.0	Not assessed	Bahloul et al., 2016
Salsola vermiculata L. (Amaranthaceae)	Methanol extract (roots)	450.0	Not assessed	Rasheed et al., 2013
Polygonum minus Huds. *(Polygonaceae)*	Dichloromethane extract (leaves)	478.0	Not assessed	Ahmad et al., 2014
Scabiosa arenaria Forssk. (Caprifoliaceae)	Ethyl acetate fraction (fruits)	500.0	Not assessed	Besbes Hlila et al., 2013
Polygonum minus Huds. (Polygonaceae)	Aqueous extract (stem)	581.0	Not assessed	Ahmad et al., 2014
Salvia leriifolia Benth. (Lamiaceae)	Hexane fraction (leaves)	590.0	Not assessed	Loizzo et al., 2010
Jacaranda caroba (Vell.) DC. (Bignoniaceae)	Aqueous extract (leaves)	670.2	Not assessed	Ferreres et al., 2013
Polygonum minus Huds. *(Polygonaceae)*	Dichloromethane extract (leaves)	770.0	Not assessed	Ahmad et al., 2014
Diplotaxis harra (Forssk.) Boiss. (Brassicaceae)	Aqueous extract (flowers)	760.0	Not assessed	Bahloul et al., 2016
Polygonum minus Huds. (Polygonaceae)	Methanolic extract (stem)	809.0	Not assessed	Ahmad et al., 2014
Salvia leriifolia Benth. (Lamiaceae)	Dichloromethane fraction (leaves)	840.0	Not assessed	Loizzo et al., 2010
Salvia leriifolia Benth. (Lamiaceae)	Ehtyl acetate fraction (leaves)	870.0	Not assessed	Loizzo et al., 2010
Rhizophora lamarckii Montrouz. (Rhizophoraceae)	Methanol extract (leaves)	910.0	Not assessed	Suganthy et al., 2009
Polygonum minus Huds. *(Polygonaceae)*	Ethanolic extract (leaves)	910.0	Not assessed	Ahmad et al., 2014
Polygonum minus Huds. *(Polygonaceae)*	Ethanolic extract (stem)	930.0	Not assessed	Ahmad et al., 2014
Jacaranda caroba (Vell.) DC. (Bignoniaceae)	Hydromethanolic extracts (leaves)	1000.4	Not assessed	Ferreres et al., 2013

AChE, acetylcholinesterase; IC_{50}, half maximal inhibition concentration.

**Syn, Huperzia tetragona (Hook. & Grev.) Trevis. **Syn, Polygonum hydropiper L. ***Syn, Polygonum hydropiper L. ****Syn, Polygonum minus Huds. #Maximal concentration assessed for the absence of cytotoxicity.*

Plant species and their respective extracts were classified in accordance with the criteria described at Section Plant Species With Anti-Acetylcholinesterase Activity in: high potency (green background), moderate potency (orange background), and low potency (red background).

Carpolobia lutea G. Don (Polygalaceae; Nwidu et al., 2017); to 18.9 µg/mL for the ethyl acetate root extract of *Adenia gummifera (Harv.) Harms (Passifloraceae;* Adewusi and Steenkamp, 2011; **Table 1**). Both *S. puniceus* and *L. schweinfurthii* ethyl acetate extracts showed very-limited antioxidant activity, leading the authors to attribute the strong anti-AChE activity to the extract alkaloid-content (Adewusi and Steenkamp, 2011). However, primary extraction with ethyl acetate hardly renders alkaloid-rich extracts, which demands an extraction scheme outlined to adjustable acid and basic pH values during partitioning (Sarker et al., 2005), therefore further validation for those species is advisable. Notwithstanding, analyzing the solvents employed for preparation of the potent extracts within this category (**Table 1**), there is no direct correlation between solvent polarity and anti-AChE activity, supporting the assumption that non-alkaloidal secondary metabolites, such as terpenoids, flavonoids and other phenolic compounds, would be as active as the classic alkaloidal AChEi (Murray et al., 2013).

For instance, the ethyl acetate root fraction of *Carpolobia lutea* (Polygalaceae)–whose total phenolic content was 296.5 mg EAG/g–presented $IC_{50} = 0.3\,\mu g/mL$ (Nwidu et al., 2017); virtually the same value determined to the essential oil from *Salvia leriifolia* (Lamiaceae) aerial parts, which presented $IC_{50} = 0.32\,\mu L/mL$ and had camphor (10.5%), 1,8-cineole (8.6%), camphene (6.2%) and α-pinene (4.7%) as main components (Loizzo et al., 2009). Contrarily, the n-Hexane whole plant fraction of *Polygonum hydropiper* (Polygonaceae) crude extract presented moderate anti-AChE activity with $IC_{50} = 35\,\mu g/mL$ (Ayaz et al., 2014), meanwhile the essential oil from its leaves showed a potency nearly four times lower ($IC_{50} = 120\,\mu g/mL$; Ayaz et al., 2015). The alkaloid fraction of *Esenbeckia leiocarpa* (Rutaceae), obtained by acid-base partition of the ethanol stem extract, presented $IC_{50} = 1.6\,\mu g/mL$, which corresponded to an inhibitory potency 30-fold higher than the original crude extract ($IC_{50} = 50.7\,\mu g/mL$; Cardoso-Lopes et al., 2010). Still, the assessment of anti-AChE activity of *Berberis aetnensis* and *Berberis libanotica* root extracts, whose major constituent was the alkaloid berberine, showed 3-fold higher activity for the methanol fraction ($IC_{50} = 7.6$ and $16.9\,\mu g/mL$, respectively) than for alkaloid-rich fraction ($IC_{50} = 24.5$ and $82.4\,\mu g/mL$, respectively), supporting the synergy between alkaloid and non-alkaloid components within methanol fraction from both species (Bonesi et al., 2013).

Huperzia spp. (Lycopodiaceae) have been used for over 1,000 years in China for diverse neuronal- and cognitive-based illnesses (Ma et al., 2007), becoming of major interest for the pharmaceutical industry upon the isolation of the alkaloid Huperzine A from *H. serrata* (Liu et al., 1986). Thenceforth, huge research has focused on the isolation of Huperzine A and other Lycopodium alkaloids from *Huperzia* spp. and other Lycopodiaceae species (Ha et al., 2011; Damar et al., 2016; Sahoo et al., 2018). In spite of that, our survey retrieved recent relevant studies on anti-AChE activity of five *Huperzia* spp.: *H. serrata* (Ohba et al., 2015), *H. squarrosa* (Tung et al., 2017), *H. brevifolia*, *H. compacta*, and *H. tetragona* (Armijos et al., 2016; **Table 1**). In the study by Ohba et al. (2015), alkaloid enriched fraction of *H. serrata* aerial parts, whose major alkaloidal constituent was Huperzine A (~0.5%), presented $IC_{50} = 5.96\,\mu g/mL$. On the other hand, in the study by Armijos et al. (2016), alkaloid fraction of *H. tetragona* aerial parts strongly inhibited AChE ($IC_{50} = 0.9\,\mu g/mL$), meanwhile *H. brevifolia* and *H. compacta* presented moderate potency ($IC_{50} = 39.6$ and $62.4\,\mu g/mL$, respectively). The authors ascribed the high potency of *H. tetragona* to other Lycopodium alkaloids, mainly lycopodine, 6-OH-lycopodine and des-*N*-methyl-α-obscurine, since Huperzine A was not detected in any of the assessed species. Tung et al. (2017) assessed anti-AChE activity in three different fractions obtained from the ethanol extract of *H. squarrosa* aerial parts. EtOAc and BuOH fractions presented moderated activity, whose IC_{50} values were 23.44 and $50.11\,\mu g/mL$, respectively. The n-hexane fraction otherwise presented the lowest AChE inhibitory activity ($IC_{50} = 257.03\,\mu g/mL$).

As showed in the abovementioned studies, anti-AChE activity of plant extracts is significantly variable regardless of the predominant secondary metabolite class or the polarity of the extracting solvent. To cope with these limitations and still screen potentially applicable species, most researchers have also assessed the extracts antioxidant capacity, in order to demonstrate their dual efficacy. Although the present mini-review does not aim to discuss antioxidant aspects, it is noticeable that most studies cited in **Table 1** have either quantified total phenolic content or measured antioxidant capacity in their extracts. Such assessments require appropriate methods that address the mechanism of antioxidant activity and focus on the kinetics of the reactions involving the antioxidants (Amorati and Valgimigli, 2018). Contrariwise, phenolic content was predominantly measured by Folin-Ciocalteu method, which also quantifies nonphenolic compounds, such as aromatic amino acids, sugars, ascorbic acid, and organic acids (Pueyo and Calvo, 2009), reason why it is not advisable for total phenol quantification. Similarly, antioxidant capacity was mostly assessed by trapping of the radicals $DPPH^{\bullet}$ and $ABTS^{\bullet +}$, which are non-biologically relevant oxidants (Amorati and Valgimigli, 2018). Thus, most plant extracts propelled as dually efficient (Anti-AChE and antioxidant) much probably deserve a biological approach to characterize their preventive instead of scavengering antioxidant capacity.

NATURAL AChEi COMPOUNDS

The active site of AChE contains two main subsites, the "esteratic" and "anionic" subsites, corresponding to the catalytic machinery and the choline-binding pocket, respectively. As illustrated in **Figure 1A**, the "esteratic" subsite consists in a histidine residue (His_{447}), whereas the "anionic" subsite is an tryptophan residue (Trp_{84}) able to bind quaternary ligands, which may act as competitive inhibitors (Dvir et al., 2010). Most of natural AChEi reported during our delimited survey period belong to the alkaloid group. Anti-AChE activity of alkaloids is ascribed to their complex nitrogen structures, which once positively charged bind to the "anionic" subsite on AChE active site (Hostettmann et al., 2006; Houghton et al., 2006). For instance, galantamine inhibits AChE by stably binding to Trp_{84}, as well as phenylalanine residues on the acyl-binding pocket (Greenblatt et al., 1999). On the other hand, non-alkaloidal AChEi, which include terpenes, flavonoids and other phenolic compounds, seem to act as non-competitive inhibitors that bind to peripheral anionic sites (PAS) mainly represented by the residues Tyr_{70}, Asp_{74}, Try_{121}, Trp_{279}, and Tyr_{334} (Johnson and Moore, 2006).

Figure 1B shows the isolated compounds identified as potential natural AChEi, which were classified in three categories, in accordance to their IC_{50} values: high potency, $IC_{50} < 15\,\mu M$; moderate potency, $15 < IC_{50} < 50\,\mu M$; and low potency, $50 < IC_{50} < 1{,}000\,\mu M$. As a comparative reasoning, IC_{50} values described for galantamine in the surveyed studies where it was used as positive control were averaged, resulting in

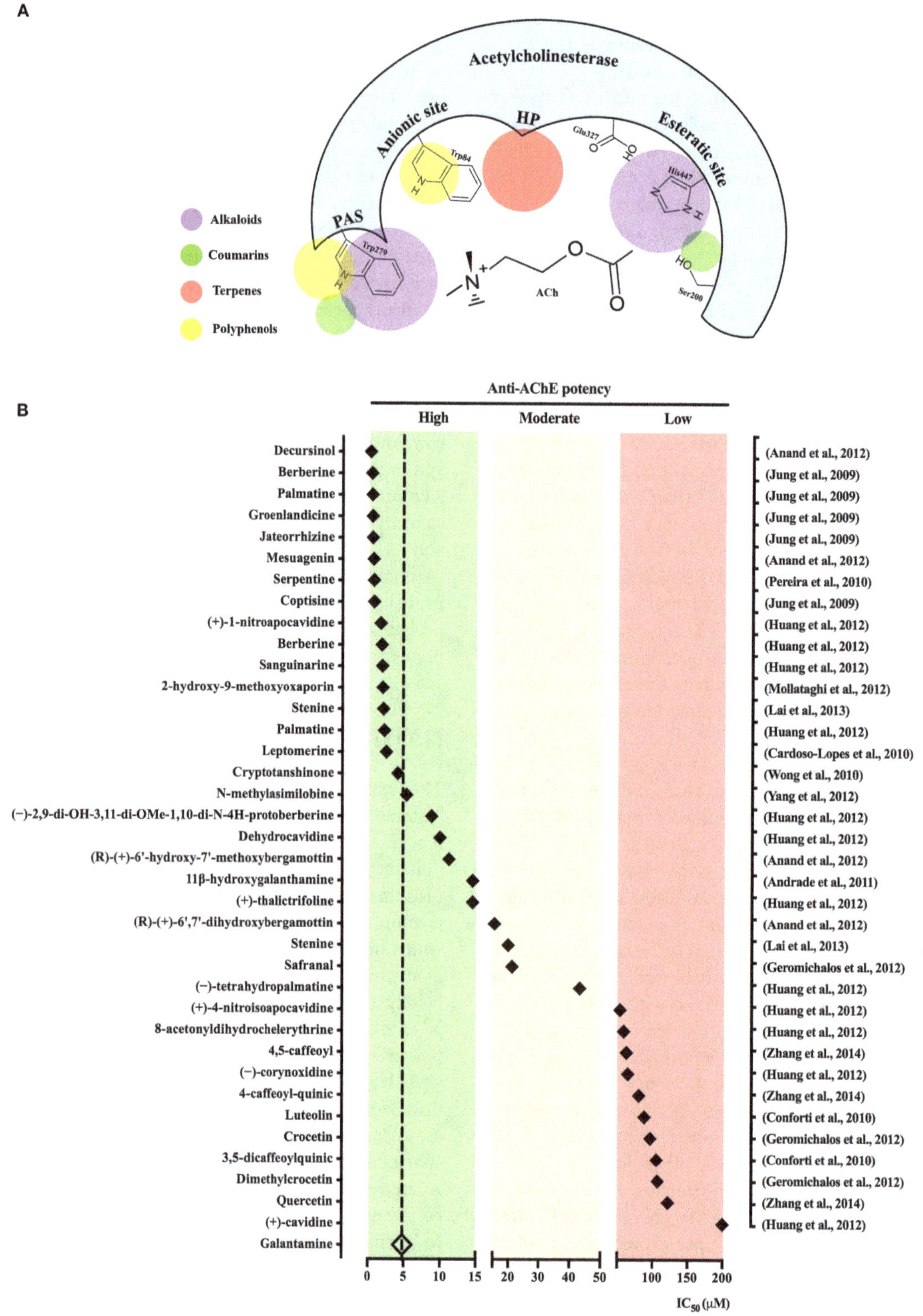

FIGURE 1 | Schematic view of acetylcholinesterase active binding sites for the main natural acetylcholinesterase inhibitors (AChEi) classes. **(A)** Acetylcholinesterase gorge pocket composed by the following binding sites: esteratic site, anionic site, peripheral anionic site (PAS), as well as hydrophobic pocket (HP) is shown. Colored circles represent the main binding sites for compounds pertaining to the indicated classes. **(B)** Natural AChEi reported in Pubmed from 2007 to 2018 (1st semester) were classified in accordance with the criteria described at Section Natural AChEi Compounds in: high potency (green background), moderate potency (orange background), and low potency (red background). The diamond symbol represents the IC_{50} value for each compound (in the left) as described in the respective study (in the right).

IC_{50} = 4.82 ± 1.29 μM. Studies describing discrepant IC_{50} values for galantamine were not considered. Sixteen compounds presented anti-AChE potency higher than galantamine, which include 01 terpene, 2 coumarins, and 13 alkaloids. Other 20 compounds, additionally pertaining to flavonoids and phenolic acids, were also selected with IC_{50} ranging from 5.33 to >200 μM (**Figure 1B**). The dihydropyranocoumarin decursinol isolated from *Angelica gigas* Nakai (Apiaceae) was the most potent AChEi (IC_{50} = 0.28 μM; Anand et al., 2012), such high potency had been previously attributed to characteristics of cyclization of the isoprenyl unit at C-6 and the functional groups attached to the coumarin nucleus, which differ from other coumarins (Kang et al., 2001).

The major alkaloids with recognized anti-AChE activity are the classical galantamine and huperzine A, which have been elegantly reviewed by Gulcan et al. (2015) and Qian and Ke (2014), respectively. However, other recently described alkaloids of various subclasses deserve special emphasis because of their important inhibitory action on AChE. Jung et al. (2009) assessed the anti-AChE activity of five protoberberine alkaloids isolated from the rhizome of *Coptis* spp. (berberine, palmatine, groenlandicine, jateorrhizine, and coptisine), with IC_{50} ranging from 0.44 to 0.80 μM. Interestingly, groenlandicine also strongly inhibited the enzyme responsible for cleaving the β-site of the amyloid precursor protein, adding an important property against AD pathogenesis (Jung et al., 2009). The potentialities of protoberberines alkaloids as natural AChEi were further supported by isolation of 12 isoquinoline alkaloids, including two new nitrotetrahydroprotoberberines (2,9-dihydroxy-3,11-dimethoxy-1,10-dinitrotetrahydroprotoberberine and 4-nitroisoapocavidine), from *Corydalis saxicola* Bunting (Papaveraceae). All the alkaloids were selectively active against AChE with IC_{50} < 10 μM. Structure-activity relationship study indicated that potency differences were related to the presence of phenolic hydroxy groups, which could reduce the anti-AChE activity, whereas nitro substitutions at ring A, especially at C-1, in the tetrahedroprotoberberines could increase it (Huang et al., 2012).

Studies on the molecular mechanisms by which natural AChEi interact with AChE binding subsites are still scant. Nevertheless, some studies have offered important insights on this matter. Serpentine, the main alkaloid found in the roots of *Catharanthus roseus* (L.) G. Don (Apocynaceae) presented high anti-AChE potency (IC_{50} = 0.77 μM), which was attributed to the binding of its quaternary nitrogen to an Asp residue at AChE peripheral anionic site (Pereira et al., 2010). Lai et al. (2013) when evaluating alkaloids from *Stemona sessilifolia* (Miq.) Miq. roots (Stemonaceae) identified the AChEi stenine B (IC_{50} = 2.10 μM) and stenine (IC_{50} = 19.8 μM). Authors attributed the stronger activity of stenine B to its ability to build hydrogen bonds with Tyr_{130}, similarly to huperzine A. Lastly, bioactivity-guided chromatographic fractionation of *Nelumbo nucifera* Gaertn. (Nelumbonaceae) leaf extract led to isolation of three aporphine-type alkaloids, an important subclass of natural inhibitors of AChE. Amongst them, N-methylasimilobine displayed a significant anti-AChE activity with IC_{50} = 5.33 μM. According to their *in silico* studies, such potency was due to a hydroxyl group at the alkaloid C-2 position, which makes hydrogen bond with a carbonyl group on Ser_{293} in association with another hydrogen bond between its alkaloidal quaternary nitrogen and the hydroxyl group of Tyr_{124} (Yang et al., 2012).

Salvia spp. (Lamiaceae) have been used for centuries for its beneficial effects on memory disorders (Hamidpour et al., 2014). Wong et al. (2010) demonstrated that the diterpene cryptotanshinone extracted from the root of *Salvia miltiorrhiza* Bunge is a reversible inhibitor of human AChE (IC_{50} = 4.09 μM) and that chronic oral administration can reverse cognitive deficits induced by scopolamine in rats. Flavonoids, a heterogeneous group of polyphenols, are currently considered a prominent source of anti-AD compounds (Khan et al., 2018) because of their potential AChE inhibitory activity allied to the well-known antioxidant activity and low toxicity (Uriarte-Pueyo and Calvo, 2011). However, our survey did not identify any highly potent, and consequently prominent AChEi pertaining to the flavonoid class (**Figure 1**). For instance, luteolin and 3,5-dicaffeoylquinic acid, phenolic compounds extracted from *Phagnalon saxatile* Cass. (Compositae) exhibited low activity against AChE with an IC_{50} of 88.00 and 105 μM, respectively (Conforti et al., 2010).

CLINICAL STUDIES

Besides galantamine, huperzine A is the most clinically studied alkaloidal AChEi (Qian and Ke, 2014). The efficacy of huperzine A was demonstrated in the treatment of 447 patients with age-related memory impairment or dementia (Shu, 1998; Ma et al., 2007). However, in another phase II study, the results were not conclusive on its beneficial cognitive effects for patients with moderate AD, requiring further investigation (Rafii et al., 2011). A clinical trial with *Salvia officinalis* L. administered to patients with mild to moderate AD for a 16-weeks period led to improved cognitive performance (Perry et al., 2003). Of importance, *S. officinalis* also attenuated cognitive impairment in patients suffering from moderate to severe AD when used for up to 1 year. However, authors recognized that long-term efficacy, safety and administration strategy still require further investigation (Tune, 2001). *Salvia* spp. are particularly rich in terpenes, whose anti-AChE capacity has been assessed through enough pre-clinical tests, but are awaiting clinical trials (Rollinger et al., 2004; Kennedy and Scholey, 2006). On the other hand, a 22-weeks randomized, double-blind, multicenter trial, including 54 individuals suffering from mild-to-moderate AD, showed that daily intake of *Crocus sativus* L. (Iridaceae) dried extract (30 mg/day) significantly improved cognitive capacity comparable to that observed in donepezil-treated patients (Akhondzadeh et al., 2010).

TOXICOLOGICAL STUDIES

A recent systematic review and meta-analysis of 43 randomized placebo-controlled clinical trials showed that AChEi improved cognitive function, global symptomatology, and functional capacity, as well as decreased patients' mortality (Blanco-Silvente et al., 2017). However, patients taking AChEi presented higher discontinuation due to adverse events, denoting an important issue on anti-AChE therapy. As showed in **Table 1**, the majority of the plant extract-based studies mentioned in this mini-review has not assessed their toxicity in animals or humans, although species like *S. officinalis* (Kennedy and Scholey, 2006) and *P. hydropiper* (Huq et al., 2014) have been considered as non-toxic. Amongst the main natural AChEi compounds herein mentioned, berberine and safranal seem to ally more advantages than disadvantages. Nevertheless, berberine has been shown to cause mild gastrointestinal reactions, including diarrhea and constipation, besides other less frequent side effects (Imenshahidi and Hosseinzadeh, 2016); and safranal has toxic effects on hematological and biochemical indices, as well as induced embryonic malformation in animal's models at high doses (Bostan et al., 2017).

CLOSING REMARKS AND PERSPECTIVES

The present mini-review demonstrated that during last decade several plant species and their potentially active compounds have been screened for anti-AChE activity. Amongst the most active extracts (**Table 1**), it is noticeable the use of extracting solvents of distinct polarities, which suggests that their active compounds might pertain to a wide range of secondary metabolites classes. However, having a look at the isolated substances summarized in **Figure 1B**, most high potent compounds assessed during this period pertain to alkaloid class, exception made to the highest potent decursinol, a dihydropyranocoumarin. Alkaloids indisputably are the most studied class of natural AChEi, what seemly has trapped the researcher's attention in this class when in pursuit of new potential AChEi candidates, a vision that urges to be changed. Notwithstanding, the search for secondary AD-relevant pharmacological properties, such as antioxidant, deserves experimental approaches addressing their capacity to prevent oxidants generation and oxidative damage, instead of their mere scavengering capacity.

Finally, despite the undoubted relevance of new AChEi discovery for AD palliative pharmacotherapy, there is scanty knowledge on their structure-activity relationships, as well as toxicological assessments that would enable them to phase II studies. For instance, berberine and related protoberberine alkaloids have been consistently assessed for their anti-AChE activity, but no phase II study has been conducted so far. Such knowledge is capital both to promote higher safety and to guide the design of new (semi-) synthetic AChEi. Thus, given the plethora of plant species and compounds already described, their assessment through clinical trials certainly represent the main barrier to be transposed in order to expand and improve the pharmacological care of AD patients.

AUTHOR CONTRIBUTIONS

TS conceived the proposal, discussed mini-review's structure, surveyed and selected relevant articles, tabulated the data and drafted the manuscript. TG surveyed and selected relevant articles, tabulated the data. BP supervised articles selection, analysis and data tabulation. AC discussed mini-review's structure, supervised articles selection, analysis and data tabulation. AP conceived the proposal, discussed mini-review's structure, oriented the selection of relevant articles, analyzed tabulated data, and drafted the manuscript. All authors read and approved the final format of the manuscript.

ACKNOWLEDGMENTS

Authors are thankful to Foundation for the Support of Research, Scientific, and Technological Development of the State of Maranhão–FAPEMA, which has importantly funded their research on ethnopharmacology of regional plant species for AD therapy through the grant Universal-00651/15.

REFERENCES

Adewusi, E. A., and Steenkamp, V. (2011). *In vitro* screening for acetylcholinesterase inhibition and antioxidant activity of medicinal plants from southern Africa. *Asian Pacif. J. Trop. Med.* 4, 829–835. doi: 10.1016/S1995-7645(11)60203-4

Ahmad, R., Baharum, S. N., Bunawan, H., Lee, M., Mohd Noor, N., Rohani, E. R., et al. (2014). Volatile profiling of aromatic traditional medicinal plant, Polygonum minus in different tissues and its biological activities. *Molecules* 19, 19220–19242. doi: 10.3390/molecules191119220

Ahmad, S., Ullah, F., Ayaz, M., Sadiq, A., and Imran, M. (2015). Antioxidant and anticholinesterase investigations of Rumex hastatus D. Don: potential effectiveness in oxidative stress and neurological disorders. *Biol. Res.* 48:20. doi: 10.1186/s40659-015-0010-2

Ahmad, S., Ullah, F., Sadiq, A., Ayaz, M., Imran, M., Ali, I., et al. (2016). Chemical composition, antioxidant and anticholinesterase potentials of essential oil of Rumex hastatus D. Don collected from the North West of Pakistan. *BMC Complement. Altern. Med.* 16:29. doi: 10.1186/s12906-016-0998-z

Akhondzadeh, S., Shafiee Sabet, M., Harirchian, M. H., Togha, M., Cheraghmakani, H., Razeghi, S., et al. (2010). A 22-week, multicenter, randomized, double-blind controlled trial of Crocus sativus in the treatment of mild-to-moderate Alzheimer's disease. *Psychopharmacology* 207, 637–643. doi: 10.1007/s00213-009-1706-1

Ali, M. Y., Jung, H. A., and Choi, J. S. (2015). Anti-diabetic and anti-Alzheimer's disease activities of Angelica decursiva. *Arch. Pharmacal. Res.* 38, 2216–2227. doi: 10.1007/s12272-015-0629-0

Ali, S. K., Hamed, A. R., Soltan, M. M., Hegazy, U. M., Elgorashi, E. E., El-Garf, I. A., et al. (2013). *In-vitro* evaluation of selected Egyptian traditional herbal medicines for treatment of Alzheimer disease. *BMC Complement. Alter. Med.* 13:121. doi: 10.1186/1472-6882-13-121

Amorati, R., and Valgimigli, L. (2018). Methods to measure the antioxidant activity of phytochemicals and plant extracts. *J. Agric. Food Chem.* 66, 3324–3329. doi: 10.1021/acs.jafc.8b01079

Anand, P., and Singh, B. (2013). A review on cholinesterase inhibitors for Alzheimer's disease. *Arch. Pharmacal Res.* 36, 375–399. doi: 10.1007/s12272-013-0036-3

Anand, P., Singh, B., and Singh, N. (2012). A review on coumarins as acetylcholinesterase inhibitors for Alzheimer's disease. *Bioorg. Med. Chem.* 20, 1175–1180. doi: 10.1016/j.bmc.2011.12.042

Andrieu, S., Coley, N., Lovestone, S., Aisen, P. S., and Vellas, B. (2015). Prevention of sporadic Alzheimer's disease: lessons learned from clinical trials and future directions. *Lancet Neurol.* 14, 926–944. doi: 10.1016/S1474-4422(15)00153-2

Armijos, C., Gilardoni, G., Amay, L., Lozano, A., Bracco, F., Ramirez, J., et al. (2016). Phytochemical and ethnomedicinal study of Huperzia species used in the traditional medicine of Saraguros in Southern Ecuador; AChE and MAO inhibitory activity. *J. Ethnopharmacol.* 193, 546–554. doi: 10.1016/j.jep.2016.09.049

Ayaz, M., Junaid, M., Ahmed, J., Ullah, F., Sadiq, A., Ahmad, S., et al. (2014). Phenolic contents, antioxidant and anticholinesterase potentials of crude extract, subsequent fractions and crude saponins from *Polygonum hydropiper* L. *BMC Complement. Altern. Med.* 14:145. doi: 10.1186/1472-6882-14-145

Ayaz, M., Junaid, M., Ullah, F., Sadiq, A., Khan, M. A., Ahmad, W., et al. (2015). Comparative chemical profiling, cholinesterase inhibitions and anti-radicals properties of essential oils from Polygonum hydropiper L: a preliminary anti-Alzheimer's study. *Lipids Health Dis.* 14:141. doi: 10.1186/s12944-015-0145-8

Ayaz, M., Sadiq, A., Junaid, M., Ullah, F., Subhan, F., and Ahmed, J. (2017). Neuroprotective and anti-aging potentials of essential oils from aromatic and medicinal plants. *Front. Aging Neurosci.* 9:168. doi: 10.3389/fnagi.2017.00168

Bahloul, N., Bellili, S., Aazza, S., Chérif, A., Faleiro, M. L., Antunes, M. D., et al. (2016). Aqueous extracts from tunisian diplotaxis: phenol content, antioxidant and anti-acetylcholinesterase activities, and impact of exposure to simulated gastrointestinal fluids. *Antioxidants* 5:12. doi: 10.3390/antiox5020012

Bartus, R. T. (2000). On neurodegenerative diseases, models, and treatment strategies: lessons learned and lessons forgotten a generation following the cholinergic hypothesis. *Exp. Neurol.* 163, 495–529. doi: 10.1006/exnr.2000.7397

Bartus, R. T., Dean, R. L., Beer, B., and Lippa, A. S. (1982). The cholinergic hypothesis of geriatric memory dysfunction. *Science* 217, 408–414. doi: 10.1126/science.7046051

Berkov, S., Codina, C., Viladomat, F., and Bastida, J. (2008). N-Alkylated galanthamine derivatives: potent acetylcholinesterase inhibitors from Leucojum aestivum. *Bioorg. Med. Chem. Lett.* 18, 2263–2266. doi: 10.1016/j.bmcl.2008.03.008

Besbes Hlila, M., Omri, A., Ben Jannet, H., Lamari, A., Aouni, M., and Selmi, B. (2013). Phenolic composition, antioxidant and anti-acetylcholinesterase activities of the Tunisian Scabiosa arenaria. *Pharmaceutical. Biol.* 51, 525–532. doi: 10.3109/13880209.2012.746713

Blanco-Silvente, L., Castells, X., Saez, M., Barcelo, M. A., Garre-Olmo, J., Vilalta-Franch, J., et al. (2017). Discontinuation, efficacy, and safety of cholinesterase inhibitors for Alzheimer's disease: a meta-analysis and meta-regression of 43 randomized clinical trials enrolling 16 106 patients. *Int. J. Neuropsychopharmacol.* 20, 519–528. doi: 10.1093/ijnp/pyx012

Bonesi, M., Loizzo, M. R., Conforti, F., Passalacqua, N. G., Saab, A., Menichini, F., et al. (2013). Berberis aetnensis and B. *libanotica:* a comparative study on the chemical composition, inhibitory effect on key enzymes linked to Alzheimer's disease and antioxidant activity. *J. Pharmacy Pharmacol.* 65, 1726–1735. doi: 10.1111/jphp.12172

Bostan, H. B., Mehri, S., and Hosseinzadeh, H. (2017). Toxicology effects of saffron and its constituents: a review. *Iran J. Basic Med. Sci.* 20, 110–121. doi: 10.22038/ijbms.2017.8230

Cardoso-Lopes, E. M., Maier, J. A., Silva, M. R. D., Regasini, L. O., Simote, S. Y., Lopes, N. P., et al. (2010). Alkaloids from stems of *Esenbeckia leiocarpa* Engl. (Rutaceae) as potential treatment for Alzheimer disease. *Molecules* 15, 9205–9213. doi: 10.3390/molecules15129205

Colovic, M. B., Krstic, D. Z., Lazarevic-Pasti, T. D., Bondzic, A. M., and Vasic, V. M. (2013). Acetylcholinesterase inhibitors: pharmacology and toxicology. *Curr. Neuropharmacol.* 11, 315–335. doi: 10.2174/1570159X11311030006

Conforti, F., Rigano, D., Formisano, C., Bruno, M., Loizzo, M. R., Menichini, F., et al. (2010). Metabolite profile and *in vitro* activities of *Phagnalon saxatile* (L.) Cass. relevant to treatment of Alzheimer's disease. *J. Enz. Inhibit. Med. Chem.* 25, 97–104. doi: 10.3109/14756360903018260

Cortes, N., Posada-Duque, R. A., Alvarez, R., Alzate, F., Berkov, S., Cardona-Gómez, G. P., et al. (2015). Neuroprotective activity and acetylcholinesterase inhibition of five Amaryllidaceae species: a comparative study. *Life Sci.* 122, 42–50. doi: 10.1016/j.lfs.2014.12.011

Craig, L. A., Hong, N. S., and Mcdonald, R. J. (2011). Revisiting the cholinergic hypothesis in the development of Alzheimer's disease. *Neurosci. Biobehav. Rev.* 35, 1397–1409. doi: 10.1016/j.neubiorev.2011.03.001

Damar, U., Gersner, R., Johnstone, J. T., Schachter, S., and Rotenberg, A. (2016). Huperzine A as a neuroprotective and antiepileptic drug: a review of preclinical research. *Expert Rev. Neurother.* 16, 671–680. doi: 10.1080/14737175.2016.1175303

Dastmalchi, K., Ollilainen, V., Lackman, P., Af Gennäs, G. B., Dorman, H. D., Järvinen, P. P., et al. (2009). Acetylcholinesterase inhibitory guided fractionation of *Melissa officinalis* L. *Bioorg. Med. Chem.* 17, 867–871. doi: 10.1016/j.bmc.2008.11.034

Dvir, H., Silman, I., Harel, M., Rosenberry, T. L., and Sussman, J. L. (2010). Acetylcholinesterase: from 3D structure to function. *Chem. Biol. Interact.* 187, 10–22. doi: 10.1016/j.cbi.2010.01.042

Ellman, G. L., Courtney, K. D., Andres V. Jr., and Featherstone, R. M. (1961). A new and rapid colorimetric determination of acetylcholinesterase activity. *Biochem. Pharmacol.* 7, 88–95. doi: 10.1016/0006-2952(61)90145-9

Ferreres, F., Grosso, C., Gil-Izquierdo, A., Valentão, P., and Andrade, P. B. (2013). Phenolic compounds from Jacaranda caroba (Vell.) A. *DC.*: approaches to neurodegenerative disorders. *Food Chem. Toxicol.* 57, 91–98. doi: 10.1016/j.fct.2013.03.012

Fiest, K. M., Roberts, J. I., Maxwell, C. J., Hogan, D. B., Smith, E. E., Frolkis, A., et al. (2016). The prevalence and incidence of dementia due to Alzheimer's disease: a systematic review and meta-analysis. *Can. J. Neurol. Sci.* 43, S51–S82. doi: 10.1017/cjn.2016.36

Godyn, J., Jonczyk, J., Panek, D., and Malawska, B. (2016). Therapeutic strategies for Alzheimer's disease in clinical trials. *Pharmacol. Rep.* 68, 127–138. doi: 10.1016/j.pharep.2015.07.006

Greenblatt, H. M., Kryger, G., Lewis, T., Silman, I., and Sussman, J. L. (1999). Structure of acetylcholinesterase complexed with (-)-galanthamine at 2.3 A resolution. *FEBS Lett.* 463, 321–326. doi: 10.1016/S0014-5793(99)01637-3

Gulcan, H. O., Orhan, I. E., and Sener, B. (2015). Chemical and molecular aspects on interactions of galanthamine and its derivatives with cholinesterases. *Curr. Pharm. Biotechnol.* 16, 252–258. doi: 10.2174/1389201015666141202105105

Ha, G. T., Wong, R. K., and Zhang, Y. (2011). Huperzine a as potential treatment of Alzheimer's disease: an assessment on chemistry, pharmacology, and clinical studies. *Chem. Biodivers.* 8, 1189–1204. doi: 10.1002/cbdv.201000269

Hamidpour, M., Hamidpour, R., Hamidpour, S., and Shahlari, M. (2014). Chemistry, pharmacology, and medicinal property of sage (Salvia) to prevent and cure illnesses such as obesity, diabetes, depression, dementia, lupus, autism, heart disease, and cancer. *J. Tradit. Complement. Med.* 4, 82–88. doi: 10.4103/2225-4110.130373

Heinrich, M. (2010). Galanthamine from galanthus and other amaryllidaceae–chemistry and biology based on traditional use. *Alkaloids Chem. Biol.* 68, 157–165. doi: 10.1016/S1099-4831(10)06804-5

Henstridge, C. M., Pickett, E., and Spires-Jones, T. L. (2016). Synaptic pathology: a shared mechanism in neurological disease. *Ageing Res. Rev.* 28, 72–84. doi: 10.1016/j.arr.2016.04.005

Holas, O., Musilek, K., Pohanka, M., and Kuca, K. (2012). The progress in the cholinesterase quantification methods. *Expert Opin. Drug Discov.* 7, 1207–1223. doi: 10.1517/17460441.2012.729037

Hostettmann, K., Borloz, A., Urbain, A., and Marston, A. (2006). Natural product inhibitors of acetylcholinesterase. *Curr. Org. Chem.* 10, 825–847. doi: 10.2174/138527206776894410

Houghton, P. J., Ren, Y., and Howes, M.-J. (2006). Acetylcholinesterase inhibitors from plants and fungi. *Nat. Product Rep.* 23, 181–199. doi: 10.1039/b508966m

Huang, L., Su, T., and Li, X. (2013). Natural products as sources of new lead compounds for the treatment of Alzheimer's disease. *Curr. Top. Med. Chem.* 13, 1864–1878. doi: 10.2174/15680266113139990142

Huang, Q.-Q., Bi, J.-L., Sun, Q.-Y., Yang, F.-M., Wang, Y.-H., Tang, G.-H., et al. (2012). Bioactive isoquinoline alkaloids from Corydalis saxicola. *Planta Med.* 78, 65–70. doi: 10.1055/s-0031-1280126

Huq, A. K., Jamal, J. A., and Stanslas, J. (2014). Ethnobotanical, phytochemical, pharmacological, and toxicological aspects of persicaria hydropiper (l.) delarbre. *Evid. Based Complement. Alternat. Med.* 2014:782830. doi: 10.1155/2014/782830

Imenshahidi, M., and Hosseinzadeh, H. (2016). Berberis vulgaris and berberine: an update review. *Phytother. Res.* 30, 1745–1764. doi: 10.1002/ptr.5693

Ingkaninan, K., Temkitthawon, P., Chuenchom, K., Yuyaem, T., and Thongnoi, W. (2003). Screening for acetylcholinesterase inhibitory activity in plants used in Thai traditional rejuvenating and neurotonic remedies. *J. Ethnopharmacol.* 89, 261–264. doi: 10.1016/j.jep.2003.08.008

Johnson, G., and Moore, S. W. (2006). The peripheral anionic site of acetylcholinesterase: structure, functions and potential role in rational drug design. *Curr. Pharm. Des.* 12, 217–225. doi: 10.2174/138161206775193127

Jung, H. A., Ali, M. Y., Jung, H. J., Jeong, H. O., Chung, H. Y., and Choi, J. S. (2016). Inhibitory activities of major anthraquinones and other constituents from *Cassia obtusifolia* against β-secretase and cholinesterases. *J. Ethnopharmacol.* 191, 152–160. doi: 10.1016/j.jep.2016.06.037

Jung, H. A., Karki, S., Kim, J. H., and Choi, J. S. (2015). BACE1 and cholinesterase inhibitory activities of Nelumbo nucifera embryos. *Arch. Pharm. Res.* 38, 1178–1187. doi: 10.1007/s12272-014-0492-4

Jung, H. A., Min, B.-S., Yokozawa, T., Lee, J.-H., Kim, Y. S., and Choi, J. S. (2009). Anti-Alzheimer and antioxidant activities of Coptidis Rhizoma alkaloids. *Biol. Pharm. Bull.* 32, 1433–1438. doi: 10.1248/bpb.32.1433

Kamal, Z., Ullah, F., Ayaz, M., Sadiq, A., Ahmad, S., Zeb, A., et al. (2015). Anticholinesterse and antioxidant investigations of crude extracts, subsequent fractions, saponins and flavonoids of *Atriplex laciniata* L.: potential effectiveness in Alzheimer's and other neurological disorders. *Biol. Res.* 48:21. doi: 10.1186/s40659-015-0011-1

Kang, S. Y., Lee, K. Y., Sung, S. H., Park, M. J., and Kim, Y. C. (2001). Coumarins isolated from Angelica gigas inhibit acetylcholinesterase: structure-activity relationships. *J. Nat. Prod.* 64, 683–685. doi: 10.1021/np000441w

Kennedy, D. O., and Scholey, A. B. (2006). The psychopharmacology of European herbs with cognition-enhancing properties. *Curr. Pharm. Design* 12, 4613–4623. doi: 10.2174/138161206779010387

Khan, H., Amin, S., Kamal, M. A., and Patel, S. (2018). Flavonoids as acetylcholinesterase inhibitors: current therapeutic standing and future prospects. *Biomed. Pharmacother.* 101, 860–870. doi: 10.1016/j.biopha.2018.03.007

Kuk, E. B., Jo, A. R., Oh, S. I., Sohn, H. S., Seong, S. H., Roy, A., et al. (2017). Anti-Alzheimer's disease activity of compounds from the root bark of *Morus alba* L. *Arch. Pharm. Res.* 40, 338–349. doi: 10.1007/s12272-017-0891-4

Lai, D.-H., Yang, Z.-D., Xue, W.-W., Sheng, J., Shi, Y., and Yao, X.-J. (2013). Isolation, characterization and acetylcholinesterase inhibitory activity of alkaloids from roots of Stemona sessilifolia. *Fitoterapia* 89, 257–264. doi: 10.1016/j.fitote.2013.06.010

Lin, H. Q., Ho, M. T., Lau, L. S., Wong, K. K., Shaw, P. C., and Wan, D. C. (2008). Anti-acetylcholinesterase activities of traditional chinese medicine for treating Alzheimer's disease. *Chem. Biol. Interact.* 175, 352–354. doi: 10.1016/j.cbi.2008.05.030

Liu, J.-S., Zhu, Y.-L., Yu, C.-M., Zhou, Y.-Z., Han, Y.-Y., Wu, F.-W., et al. (1986). The structures of huperzine A and B, two new alkaloids exhibiting marked anticholinesterase activity. *Can. J. Chem.* 64, 837–839. doi: 10.1139/v86-137

Loizzo, M. R., Menichini, F., Tundis, R., Bonesi, M., Conforti, F., Nadjafi, F., et al. (2009). *In vitro* biological activity of Salvia leriifolia Benth essential oil relevant to the treatment of Alzheimer's disease. *J. Oleo Sci.* 58, 443–446. doi: 10.5650/jos.58.443

Loizzo, M. R., Tundis, R., Conforti, F., Menichini, F., Bonesi, M., Nadjafi, F., et al. (2010). *Salvia leriifolia* Benth (Lamiaceae) extract demonstrates *in vitro* antioxidant properties and cholinesterase inhibitory activity. *Nutri. Res.* 30, 823–830. doi: 10.1016/j.nutres.2010.09.016

Lopez, S., Bastida, J., Viladomat, F., and Codina, C. (2002). Acetylcholinesterase inhibitory activity of some Amaryllidaceae alkaloids and Narcissus extracts. *Life Sci.* 71, 2521–2529. doi: 10.1016/S0024-3205(02)02034-9

Ma, X., Tan, C., Zhu, D., Gang, D. R., and Xiao, P. (2007). Huperzine A from Huperzia species—an ethnopharmacolgical review. *J. Ethnopharmacol.* 113, 15–34. doi: 10.1016/j.jep.2007.05.030

Madeo, J., and Elsayad, C. (2013). The role of oxidative stress in Alzheimer's disease. *J. Alzheimers Dis. Parkinsonism* 3, 116–121. doi: 10.4172/2161-0460.1000116

Mehta, M., Adem, A., and Sabbagh, M. (2012). New acetylcholinesterase inhibitors for Alzheimer's disease. *Int. J. Alzheimers Dis.* 2012:728983. doi: 10.1155/2012/728983

Murray, A. P., Faraoni, M. B., Castro, M. J., Alza, N. P., and Cavallaro, V. (2013). Natural AChE inhibitors from plants and their contribution to Alzheimer's disease therapy. *Curr. Neuropharmacol.* 11, 388–413.doi: 10.2174/1570159X11311040004

Nwidu, L. L., Elmorsy, E., Thornton, J., Wijamunige, B., Wijesekara, A., Tarbox, R., et al. (2017). Anti-acetylcholinesterase activity and antioxidant properties of extracts and fractions of Carpolobia lutea. *Pharm. Biol.* 55, 1875–1883. doi: 10.1080/13880209.2017.1339283

Ohba, T., Yoshino, Y., Ishisaka, M., Abe, N., Tsuruma, K., Shimazawa, M., et al. (2015). Japanese Huperzia serrata extract and the constituent, huperzine A, ameliorate the scopolamine-induced cognitive impairment in mice. *Biosci. Biotechnol. Biochem.* 79, 1838–1844. doi: 10.1080/09168451.2015.1052773

Orhan, I. E., Orhan, G., and Gurkas, E. (2011). An overview on natural cholinesterase inhibitors–a multi-targeted drug class–and their mass production. *Mini. Rev. Med. Chem.* 11, 836–842. doi: 10.2174/138955711796575434

Ovais, M., Ayaz, M., Khalil, A. T., Shah, S. A., Jan, M. S., Raza, A., et al. (2018). HPLC-DAD finger printing, antioxidant, cholinesterase, and α-glucosidase inhibitory potentials of a novel plant Olax nana. *BMC Complement. Alter. Med.* 18:1. doi: 10.1186/s12906-017-2057-9

Penumala, M., Zinka, R. B., Shaik, J. B., and Amooru Gangaiah, D. (2017). *In vitro* Screening of three indian medicinal plants for their phytochemicals, anticholinesterase, antiglucosidase, antioxidant, and neuroprotective effects. *Biomed. Res. Int.* 2017:5140506. doi: 10.1155/2017/5140506

Penumala, M., Zinka, R. B., Shaik, J. B., Mallepalli, S. K. R., Vadde, R., and Amooru, D. G. (2018). Phytochemical profiling and *in vitro* screening for anticholinesterase, antioxidant, antiglucosidase and neuroprotective effect of three traditional medicinal plants for Alzheimer's disease and diabetes mellitus dual therapy. *BMC Complement. Alter. Med.* 18:77. doi: 10.1186/s12906-018-2140-x

Pereira, D. M., Ferreres, F., Oliveira, J. M., Gaspar, L., Faria, J., Valentão, P., et al. (2010). Pharmacological effects of Catharanthus roseus root alkaloids in acetylcholinesterase inhibition and cholinergic neurotransmission. *Phytomedicine* 17, 646–652. doi: 10.1016/j.phymed.2009.10.008

Perry, N. S., Bollen, C., Perry, E. K., and Ballard, C. (2003). Salvia for dementia therapy: review of pharmacological activity and pilot tolerability clinical trial. *Pharmacol. Biochem. Behav.* 75, 651–659. doi: 10.1016/S0091-3057(03)00108-4

Prince, M. J. (2015). *World Alzheimer Report 2015: The Global Impact of Dementia: An Analysis of Prevalence, Incidence, Cost and Trends.* London: Alzheimer's Disease International.

Pueyo, I. U., and Calvo, M. I. (2009). Assay conditions and validation of a new UV spectrophotometric method using microplates for the determination of polyphenol content. *Fitoterapia* 80, 465–467. doi: 10.1016/j.fitote.2009.06.008

Qian, Z. M., and Ke, Y. (2014). Huperzine A: is it an effective disease-modifying drug for Alzheimer's disease? *Front. Aging Neurosci.* 6:216. doi: 10.3389/fnagi.2014.00216

Rafii, M., Walsh, S., Little, J., Behan, K., Reynolds, B., Ward, C., et al. (2011). A phase II trial of huperzine A in mild to moderate Alzheimer disease. *Neurology* 76, 1389–1394. doi: 10.1212/WNL.0b013e318216eb7b

Rasheed, D. M., El Zalabani, S. M., Koheil, M. A., El-Hefnawy, H. M., and Farag, M. A. (2013). Metabolite profiling driven analysis of Salsola species and their anti-acetylcholinesterase potential. *Nat. Prod. Res.* 27, 2320–2327. doi: 10.1080/14786419.2013.832676

Reza, A. A., Hossain, M. S., Akhter, S., Rahman, M. R., Nasrin, M. S., Uddin, M. J., et al. (2018). *In vitro* antioxidant and cholinesterase inhibitory activities of Elatostema papillosum leaves and correlation with their phytochemical profiles: a study relevant to the treatment of Alzheimer's disease. *BMC Complement. Alter. Med.* 18:123. doi: 10.1186/s12906-018-2182-0

Rollinger, J. M., Hornick, A., Langer, T., Stuppner, H., and Prast, H. (2004). Acetylcholinesterase inhibitory activity of scopolin and scopoletin discovered by virtual screening of natural products. *J. Med. Chem.* 47, 6248–6254. doi: 10.1021/jm049655r

Sahoo, A. K., Dandapat, J., Dash, U. C., and Kanhar, S. (2018). Features and outcomes of drugs for combination therapy as multi-targets strategy to combat Alzheimer's disease. *J. Ethnopharmacol.* 215, 42–73. doi: 10.1016/j.jep.2017.12.015

Saleem, H., Ahmad, I., Shahid, M. N., Gill, M., Nadeem, M. F., Mahmood, W., et al. (2016). *In vitro* acetylcholinesterase and butyrylcholinesterase inhibitory potentials of Jatropha gossypifolia plant extracts. *Acta Poloniae Pharmaceut. Drug Res.* 73, 419–423.

Sarker, S. D., Latif, Z., and Gray, A. I. (2005). *Natural Products Isolation.* Totowa, NJ: Humana Press.

Scheltens, P., Blennow, K., Breteler, M. M., De Strooper, B., Frisoni, G. B., Salloway, S., et al. (2016). Alzheimer's disease. *Lancet* 388, 505–517. doi: 10.1016/S0140-6736(15)01124-1

Schrattenholz, A., Pereira, E. F., Roth, U., Weber, K. H., Albuquerque, E. X., and Maelicke, A. (1996). Agonist responses of neuronal nicotinic acetylcholine receptors are potentiated by a novel class of allosterically acting ligands. *Mol. Pharm.* 49, 1–6.

Shu, Y.-Z. (1998). Recent natural products based drug development: a pharmaceutical industry perspective. *J. Nat. Prod.* 61, 1053–1071. doi: 10.1021/np9800102

Suganthy, N., Pandian, S. K., and Devi, K. P. (2009). Cholinesterase inhibitory effects of rhizophora lamarckii, avicennia officinalis, sesuvium portulacastrum and suaeda monica: mangroves inhabiting an Indian coastal area (Vellar Estuary). *J. Enz. Inhibit. Med. Chem.* 24, 702–707. doi: 10.1080/14756360802334719

Takizawa, C., Thompson, P. L., Van Walsem, A., Faure, C., and Maier, W. C. (2015). Epidemiological and economic burden of Alzheimer's disease: a systematic literature review of data across Europe and the United States of America. *J. Alzheimers Dis.* 43, 1271–1284. doi: 10.3233/JAD-141134

Tarawneh, R., and Holtzman, D. M. (2012). The clinical problem of symptomatic Alzheimer disease and mild cognitive impairment. *Cold Spring Harbor Perspect. Med.* 2:a006148. doi: 10.1101/cshperspect.a006148

Thomsen, T., and Kewitz, H. (1990). Selective inhibition of human acetylcholinesterase by galanthamine *in vitro* and *in vivo*. *Life Sci.* 46, 1553–1558. doi: 10.1016/0024-3205(90)90429-U

Tune, L. E. (2001). Anticholinergic effects of medication in elderly patients. *J. Clin. Psychiatry* 62, 11–14.

Tung, B. T., Hai, N. T., and Thu, D. K. (2017). Antioxidant and acetylcholinesterase inhibitory activities *in vitro* of different fraction of *Huperzia* squarrosa (Forst.) Trevis extract and attenuation of scopolamine-induced cognitive impairment in mice. *J. Ethnopharmacol.* 198, 24–32. doi: 10.1016/j.jep.2016.12.037

Uriarte-Pueyo, I., and Calvo, M. (2011). Flavonoids as acetylcholinesterase inhibitors. *Curr. Med. Chem.* 18, 5289–5302. doi: 10.2174/092986711798 184325

Wong, K. K.-K., Ho, M. T.-W., Lin, H. Q., Lau, K.-F., Rudd, J. A., Chung, R. C.-K., et al. (2010). Cryptotanshinone, an acetylcholinesterase inhibitor from *Salvia miltiorrhiza*, ameliorates scopolamine-induced amnesia in Morris water maze task. *Planta Med.* 76, 228–234. doi: 10.1055/s-0029-11 86084

Yang, Z.-D., Zhang, X., Du, J., Ma, Z.-J., Guo, F., Li, S., et al. (2012). An aporphine alkaloid from *Nelumbo nucifera* as an acetylcholinesterase inhibitor and the primary investigation for structure–activity correlations. *Nat. Prod Res.* 26, 387–392. doi: 10.1080/14786419.2010.487188

Zhao, Y., Dou, J., Wu, T., and Aisa, H. A. (2013). Investigating the antioxidant and acetylcholinesterase inhibition activities of *Gossypium herbaceam*. *Molecules* 18, 951–962. doi: 10.3390/molecules18010951

16

Neuroprotective Effect of Quercetin Against the Detrimental Effects of LPS in the Adult Mouse Brain

*Amjad Khan, Tahir Ali, Shafiq Ur Rehman, Muhammad Sohail Khan, Sayed Ibrar Alam, Muhammad Ikram, Tahir Muhammad, Kamran Saeed, Haroon Badshah and Myeong Ok Kim**

Division of Applied Life Science (BK 21), College of Natural Science, Gyeongsang National University, Jinju, South Korea

***Correspondence:**
Myeong Ok Kim
mokim@gnu.ac.kr

Chronic neuroinflammation is responsible for multiple neurodegenerative diseases, such as Alzheimer's disease, Parkinson's disease, and Huntington's disease. Lipopolysaccharide (LPS) is an essential component of the gram-negative bacterial cell wall and acts as a potent stimulator of neuroinflammation that mediates neurodegeneration. Quercetin is a natural flavonoid that is abundantly found in fruits and vegetables and has been shown to possess multiple forms of desirable biological activity including anti-inflammatory and antioxidant properties. This study aimed to evaluate the neuroprotective effect of quercetin against the detrimental effects of LPS, such as neuroinflammation-mediated neurodegeneration and synaptic/memory dysfunction, in adult mice. LPS [0.25 mg/kg/day, intraperitoneally (I.P.) injections for 1 week]-induced glial activation causes the secretion of cytokines/chemokines and other inflammatory mediators, which further activate the mitochondrial apoptotic pathway and neuronal degeneration. Compared to LPS alone, quercetin (30 mg/kg/day, I.P.) for 2 weeks (1 week prior to the LPS and 1 week cotreated with LPS) significantly reduced activated gliosis and various inflammatory markers and prevented neuroinflammation in the cortex and hippocampus of adult mice. Furthermore, quercetin rescued the mitochondrial apoptotic pathway and neuronal degeneration by regulating Bax/Bcl2, and decreasing activated cytochrome c, caspase-3 activity and cleaving PARP-1 in the cortical and hippocampal regions of the mouse brain. The quercetin treatment significantly reversed the LPS-induced synaptic loss in the cortex and hippocampus of the adult mouse brain and improved the memory performance of the LPS-treated mice. In summary, our results demonstrate that natural flavonoids such as quercetin can be beneficial against LPS-induced neurotoxicity in adult mice.

Keywords: lipopolysaccharide, natural flavonoids, quercetin, activated gliosis, neuroinflammation, neurotoxicity, memory performance

INTRODUCTION

Inflammation is a biological response initiated by various types of tissue upon sensing any foreign particle; the purposes of the response are to prevent further tissue harm and injury, to clear and repair damaged tissue, and to eliminate pathogenic elements. However, if inflammation is prolonged, then it becomes chronic inflammation and leads to progressive degeneration.

The central nervous system (CNS) contains glial cells, including astrocytes and microglia, that serve as an immune system for the CNS, defending it against pathogens and maintaining the normal structure of neurons (Witte et al., 2010; Badshah et al., 2015b). Tissue damage and systemic inflammation lead to glial cell activation, which releases inflammatory mediators and induces inflammatory diseases in the brain, such as meningitis and multiple sclerosis, as well as non-inflammatory diseases, such as Alzheimer's disease (AD), Parkinson's disease (PD) and Huntington's disease (HD) (Qin et al., 2007; Di Filipopo et al., 2010; Tajuddin et al., 2014). Numerous studies have reported that the activation of glial cells releases harmful mediators such as reactive oxygen species (ROS), nitric oxide, cytokines and inflammatory mediators, which ultimately lead to neuroinflammation-mediated neuronal degeneration (Di Filippo et al., 2008; Chen W.W. et al., 2016; Kempuraj et al., 2016, 2017). Lipopolysaccharide (LPS) is an essential component of the cell wall of gram-negative bacteria and acts as a potent stimulator of immune cells, including glial cells, inducing the expression of proinflammatory cytokines (Sheng et al., 2003; Biesmans et al., 2013). Various *in vitro* and *in vivo* studies have reported that LPS activates glial cells, leading to neuroinflammation followed by neurodegeneration (Johansson et al., 2014; Qin et al., 2015; Khan et al., 2017).

Flavonoids are a large group of natural polyphenolic plant pigments that are ubiquitous in many commonly consumed vegetables, fruits, grains, herbs, and beverages. Flavonoids have shown many forms of bioactivity, such as anticancer, cardiovascular, antioxidant, neuroprotective, and anti-inflammatory properties (Mennen et al., 2004; Yao et al., 2004; Hooper et al., 2008; Hwang et al., 2012). Most importantly, polyphenolic flavonoids play a key neuroprotective role against various neurotoxic conditions and paradigms (Dajas et al., 2003; Gopinath et al., 2011; Scapagnini et al., 2011; Prakash et al., 2013; Prakash and Sudhandiran, 2015; Ahmad et al., 2016; Khan et al., 2016; Ali et al., 2018). Quercetin (3,5,7,3′,4′-pentahydroxyflavone) is a well-known natural flavonoid abundantly found in fruits and vegetables such as apples, berries, onions and capers; a normal human diet includes a daily intake of up to 25 mg of this compound. Quercetin possesses multiple forms of biological activity, including antitumoral, antithrombotic, anti-inflammatory and antiapoptotic activities (Dajas et al., 2003; Zhang et al., 2011; Costa et al., 2016). Quercetin exerts anti-inflammatory activity by inhibiting the proinflammatory cytokines that are released by glial cells. It has been reported that quercetin protects against neuroinflammation by inhibiting nitric oxide (NO) production in microglial cells, which further leads to the inhibition of NF-κB signals and prevents inflammatory-related neuronal injury (Chen W.W. et al., 2016; Rao et al., 2005; Kao et al., 2010; Liao and Lin, 2015). Similarly, quercetin ameliorated activated astrocytes and prevented zidovudine-induced neuroinflammation in the CNS (Yang et al., 2018). Activated astrocytes and microglia mediate the activation of cytokines and reactive oxygen species, which further affect neuronal cells and trigger the degeneration of neurons (Hong, 2017; Shal et al., 2018). It has been reported that quercetin attenuates manganese-induced neurotoxicity by preventing neuroinflammation-mediated neurodegeneration, which it accomplishes via regulating the heme oxygenase-1 (HO-1)/nuclear factor erythroid 2-related factor 2 (Nrf2) and nuclear factor kappa B (NF-kB) pathway (Bahar et al., 2017). Furthermore, it has been found that quercetin has a neuroprotective effect against neurodegeneration in various *in vitro* and *in vivo* mouse models (Bureau et al., 2008; Yang et al., 2014; Lei et al., 2015; Pogacnik et al., 2016; Shveta et al., 2016). The present study was conducted to explore the neuroprotective effect of quercetin against LPS-induced neuroinflammation-mediated neurodegeneration in the adult mouse cortex and hippocampus.

MATERIALS AND METHODS

Mouse Strain, Housing and Ethical Considerations

Wild-type male C57BL/6N mice (age 8 weeks, body mass 25–30 g) were purchased from Samtako Bio (South Korea). The mice were acclimatized for 1 week in the university animal house under a 12-h/12-h light/dark cycle at 23°C with 60 ± 10% humidity and provided with food and water *ad libitum*. The maintenance and treatment of the mice were carried out in accordance with the Institutional Animal Care and Use Committee (IACUC) guidelines issued by the Division of Applied Life Science, Gyeongsang National University, South Korea. All efforts were made to minimize the suffering of animals. The experimental methods with mice were carried out in accordance with the approved guidelines (Approval ID: 125), and all experimental protocols were approved by the IACUC of the Division of Applied Life Science, Gyeongsang National University, South Korea.

Animal Grouping and Treatments

The schematic presentation of animal grouping and treatment is indicated in **Figure 1**. After acclimatization, the mice were placed in the following groups: (1) Control mice injected with saline [intraperitoneally (I.P.)] as vehicle for 2 weeks; (2) Mice injected with LPS (0.25 mg/kg/day, I.P.) for 1 week; and (3) Mice injected with LPS (0.25 mg/kg/day, I.P.) for 1 week and quercetin (30 mg/kg/day, I.P.) for 2 weeks (1 week prior to the LPS and 1 week cotreated with LPS).

The dosage of quercetin was selected in accordance with previously reported studies that quercetin at a 30 mg/kg body weight dose induced more significant and beneficial effects than 10 or 20 mg/kg (Haleagrahara et al., 2009; Yang et al., 2014; Park et al., 2018). Quercetin was dissolved in dimethyl sulfoxide (DMSO) to prepare the stock solution. Each day, fresh quercetin solution was prepared in normal saline according to the required volume of injection (250 μl/mouse/day). LPS dissolved in normal saline, and the same volume was administered I.P. to the mice. Every day at the same time, the mice were brought to the injection room for the injections.

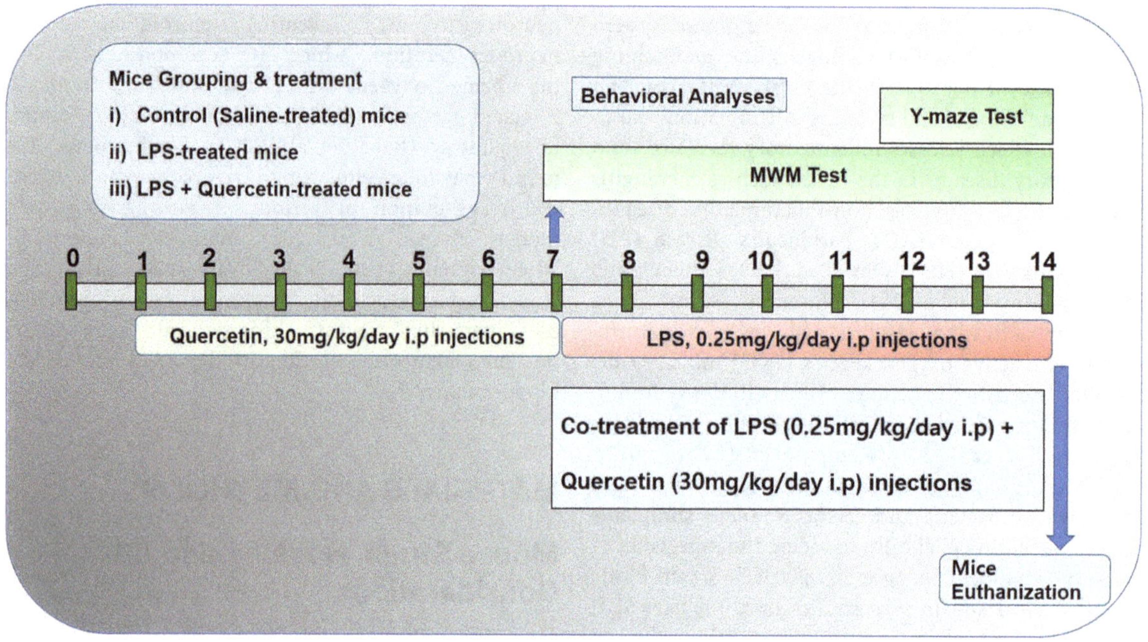

FIGURE 1 | Schematic of the experimental schedule. (1) Control paradigm mice (Cont) treated with saline as vehicle for 2 weeks. (2) Mice treated with vehicle for 1 week and LPS 0.25 mg/kg/day for 1 week. (3) Mice treated with LPS 0.25 mg/kg/day for 1 week and quercetin 30 mg/kg/day for 2 weeks (1 week before the LPS and 1 week cotreated with LPS). After behavioral analyses on the 14th day, the adult mice were euthanized and further subjected to western blotting and morphological analyses.

Behavioral Study

To investigate the effect of quercetin on memory functions, we performed a behavioral study ($n = 15$/group) using a Morris water maze (MWM) task and a Y-maze task.

The MWM test is a parameter task to evaluate memory functions. The experimental apparatus consisted of a circular water tank (100 cm in diameter, 40 cm in height) containing water (23 ± 1°C) to a depth of 15.5 cm, which was rendered opaque by adding white paint. A transparent escape platform (10 cm in diameter, 20 cm in height) was hidden 1 cm below the water surface and placed at the midpoint of one quadrant. The MWM test was started on day 7 and completed on the 13th day of the experimental schedule (**Figure 1**). Each mouse received training each day for 6 consecutive days using a single hidden platform in one quadrant with three rotating starting quadrants. Latency to escape from the water maze (finding the submerged escape platform) was calculated for each trial. On day seven, final escape latency and probe tests were performed to evaluate memory consolidation. The probe test was performed by removing the platform and allowing each mouse to swim freely for 60 s. The time the mice spent in the target quadrant (where the platform was located during hidden platform training) was measured. The time spent in the target quadrant is considered to represent the degree of memory consolidation that has taken place after learning. All data were recorded using video-tracking software (SMART, Panlab Harvard Apparatus Bioscience Company, United States).

The Y-maze was built from wood that had been painted black. Each arm of the maze was 50 cm long, 20 cm high, and 10 cm wide at the bottom and top. The Y-maze was started on day 12 and completed on day 14 of the experimental schedule (**Figure 1**). Each mouse was placed at the center of the apparatus and allowed to move freely through the maze for three 8-min sessions. The series of arm entries was visually observed. Spontaneous alteration was defined as the successive entry of the mice into the three arms in overlapping triplet sets. Alteration behavior (%) was calculated as follows: [successive triplet sets (entries into three different arms consecutively)/total number of arm entries-2] × 100.

Protein Extraction From Mouse Brain

After behavioral studies, all mice were brought to the surgical room and anesthetized with 0.05 ml/100 g body weight Rompun (Xylazine) and 0.1 ml/100 g body weight Zoletil (ketamine). After anesthesia, the mice were euthanized via decapitation, and brain tissue was immediately removed, and the cortex and hippocampus were separated and stored at −80°C. The cortical and hippocampal tissues were homogenized in PRO-PREP^{TM} protein extraction solution according to the manufacturer's instructions (iNtRON Biotechnology, Inc.). The samples were then centrifuged at 13000 rpm at 4°C for 25 min. The supernatants were collected and stored at −80°C.

Western Blot Analysis

Western blotting was performed as described previously (Ali et al., 2018). Briefly, the protein concentrations in the samples were measured (BioRad protein assay kit, BioRad Laboratories, CA, United States). Equal amounts of protein

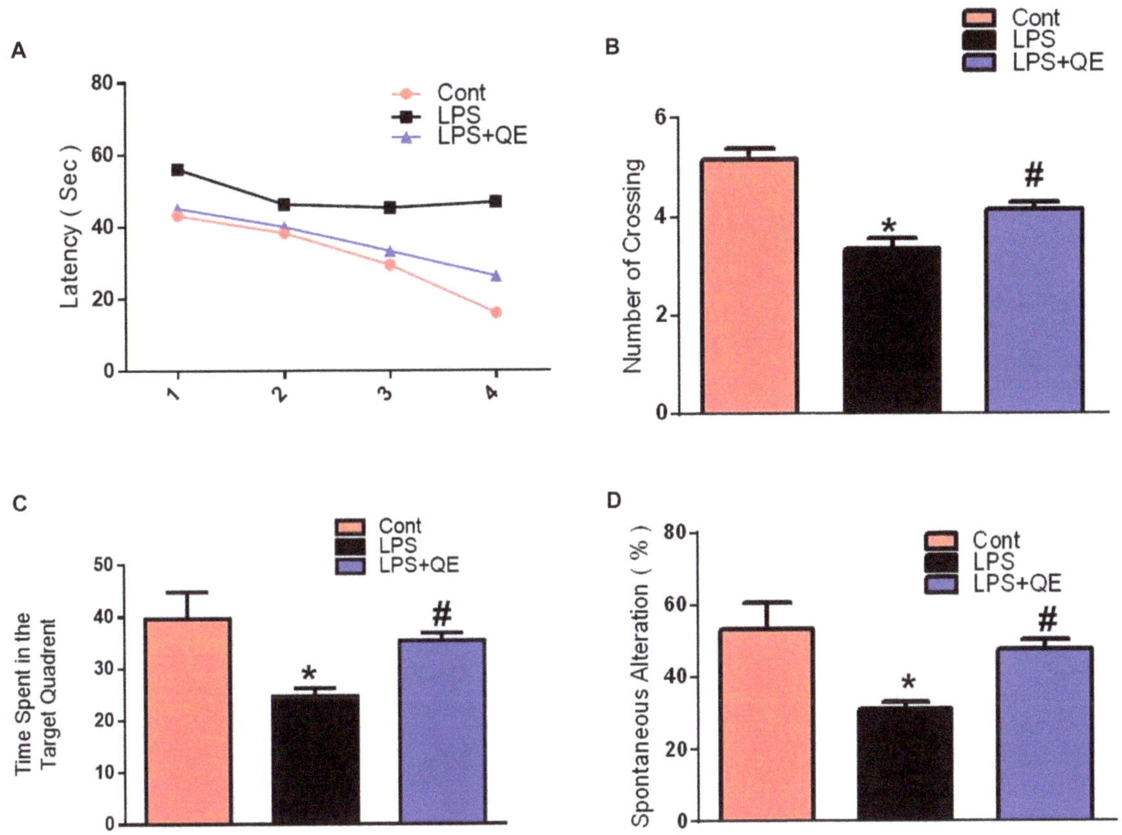

FIGURE 2 | Quercetin improved the memory function of the LPS-treated mice. For the behavioral analyses, the MWM and Y-maze tests were used to investigate and evaluate the memory functions of the control, LPS and LPS+quercetin group mice. **(A)** Average escape latency time for experimental mice to reach the hidden platform from 1 to 4 days. **(B)** The average number of crossings at the hidden platform during the probe test of the MWM test. **(C)** Time spent in the platform quadrant, where the hidden platform was placed during the trial session. **(D)** Spontaneous alteration behavior % of the mice during the Y-maze test. Histograms indicate the means ± SEM for the mice (n = 15/group). * Significantly different from the control; # significantly different from LPS-treated group. Significance: $P < 0.05$.

(15–30 μg) were electrophoresed on a 12–15% SDS-PAGE gel and transferred to a polyvinylidene difluoride (PVDF) membrane. A protein marker (GangNam-STAIN, iNtRON Biotechnology) was run in parallel for detection of the molecular weights of the proteins. To reduce the non-specific binding membrane, the membranes were blocked using 5% skim milk and incubated with primary antibodies anti-ionized calcium binding adapter molecule 1 (Iba-1), anti-glial fibrillary acidic protein (GFAP), anti-phosphorylated-nuclear factor kappa B (p-NF-kB) 65, anti-toll-like receptor-4 (TLR-4), anti-postsynaptic density protein (PSD)-95, anti-synaptophysin (Synap), anti-tumor necrosis factor-α (TNF-α), anti-nitric oxide synthase-2 (NOS-2), anti-cyclooxygenase-2 (COX-2), anti-caspase-3, anti-poly (ADP-ribose) polymerase-1 (PARP-1), anti- cytochrome c (Cyto. c), anti-Bax, anti-Bcl2, and anti-β-actin from Santa Cruz Biotechnology, Dallas, TX, United States, overnight at 4°C at 1:1000 dilution (**Table 1**). Immunoreaction was detected using chemiluminescence (Amersham ECL Advance Western Blotting Detection Reagent). The X-ray films were scanned, and the optical densities of the bands were measured using Computer-based Sigma Gel software (SPSS, Chicago, IL, United States).

Brain Tissue Collection and Sample Preparation for the Immunohistofluorescence Staining

After behavioral studies, all mice were brought to the surgical room and anesthetized with 0.05 ml/100 g body weight Rompun (Xylazine) and 0.1 ml/100 g body weight Zoletil (ketamine). The mice were perfused transcardially with 0.9% normal saline solution and 4% paraformaldehyde. The mice were euthanized via decapitation, and brain tissue was immediately removed from all mice and fixed with ice-cold paraformaldehyde at 4°C for 72 h, then submerged in 20% sucrose phosphate buffer for 72 h. All brains were frozen in O.C.T. compound (A.O., United States) and then cut into 14-μm coronal sections using a CM 3050C cryostat (Leica, Germany). The sections were thaw mounted on ProbeOn Plus charged slides (Fisher, United States).

Immunofluorescence Staining

The immunofluorescence staining proceeded as described previously with some modifications (Badshah et al., 2016). Briefly, slides containing brain sections were washed twice for 10 min each in 0.01 M PBS, 1X proteinase K was added to the tissue, and the slides were incubated at room temperature for 5 min. The slides were washed twice for 5 min each, followed by incubation for 1 h in blocking solution containing 2% normal serum and 0.3% Triton X-100 in 0.01 M PBS according to the antibody treatment. After the slides were blocked, they were incubated overnight at 4°C with primary antibodies GFAP, p-NF-kB, IL-1β, caspase-3 and SNAP23 from Santa Cruz Biotechnology, Dallas, TX, United States, diluted 1:100 in blocking solution. Following incubation with primary antibodies, the sections were incubated for 2 h in the secondary tetramethyl rhodamine isothiocyanate (TRITC)/fluorescein isothiocyanate (FITC)-labeled antibodies (1:50) (Santa Cruz Biotechnology, Dallas, TX, United States). After incubation with the TRITC/FITC-labeled antibodies, the slides were mounted with DAPI and Prolong Antifade Reagent. The images were captured using a FluoView FV 1000 laser confocal microscope equipped with FV10-ASW 3.1 Viewer (Olympus, Tokyo, Japan). The number of original confocal images per tissue was five per group, and the images were converted into TIF images. The fluorescence intensity of the same region of the cortex/total area and hippocampus/total area of the TIF images for all groups were measured using ImageJ software via the following method. The TIF image background was optimized according to the threshold intensity, and the immunofluorescence intensity, analyzed at the same threshold intensity for all groups, was expressed as the relative integrated density of the samples relative to the control.

Nissl Staining

To analyze neuronal loss and survival, Nissl staining was used as previously described with minor changes (Ali et al., 2015b; Badshah et al., 2015a). In brief, all slide sections were washed twice for 10–15 min in PBS (0.01 M) and incubated in 0.5% cresyl violet solution containing a few drops of glacial acetic acids for 10–15 min. The tissues were washed with distilled water and dehydrated in graded ethanol (70, 95, and 100%). After graded dehydration, the tissues were placed in xylene twice for 3 min each. The tissues were covered with a coverslip using mounting medium. Immunohistochemical TIF images were captured with a fluorescence light microscope. The number of images per slide was five for each group. The immunohistochemical intensity for the number of surviving neurons in the cortex/total area and hippocampus/total area (CA1) of the brain was counted using ImageJ software via the following method. The TIF image background was optimized according to the threshold intensity and analyzed the survival neuronal cells at the same threshold intensity for all groups and was expressed as the relative integrated density for the number of surviving neurons of the samples relative to the control.

Chemicals

LPS, quercetin [2-(3, 4-Dihydroxyphenyl)-3, 5, 7-trihydroxy-4H-1-benzopyran-4-one] and DMSO were purchased from Sigma-Aldrich Chemical Co. (St. louis, MO, United States).

Data and Statistical Analyses

Western blot bands were scanned and analyzed by densitometric analyses using the Sigma Gel System (SPSS, Chicago, IL, United States). ImageJ software (National Institutes of Health, Bethesda, MD, United States) was used for the densitometric analyses of the immunofluorescence and immunohistofluorescence images. All histograms were made using GraphPad Prism 5/6 (GraphPad Software, San Diego, CA, United States). For comparisons among the treatment groups and the control groups, statistical analyses were performed using one-way analysis of variance (ANOVA) followed by a two-tailed independent Student's *t-test* and Tukey's multiple comparison test where appropriate. The expressed data are presented as the means ± SEM of the three independent experiments. Statistical significance = $P < 0.05$*. Significantly different compared with

TABLE 1 | Primary antibodies information.

	Host	Application	Manufacturer	Catalog number	Concentration
Iba-1	Rabbit	WB	Santa Cruz Biotechnology, United States	SC 98468	1:1000
GFAP	Mouse	WB/IF	=	SC: 33673	1:1000/1:100
TLR-4	Goat	WB	=	SC: 16240	1:1000
p-NF-kB	Mouse	WB/IF	=	SC 8008	1:1000/1:100
TNF-α	Mouse	WB	=	SC: 8436	1:1000
COX-2	Rabbit	WB	=	SC:7951	1:1000
NOS-2	Rabbit	WB	=	SC:651	1:1000
IL-Iβ	Mouse	IF	=	SC: 32294	1:100
Bax	Mouse	WB	=	SC: 7480	1:1000
Bcl-2	Mouse	WB	=	SC: 7382	1:1000
Cyto. c	Mouse	WB	=	SC: 13156	1:1000
PARP-1	Mouse	WB	=	SC: 8007	1:1000
Caspase-3	Mouse	WB/IF	=	SC: 7272	1:1000/1:100
PSD-95	Mouse	WB	=	SC:71933	1:1000
Synap	Rabbit	WB	=	SC: 17750	1:1000
SNAP-23	Mouse	IF	=	SC: 374215	1:100

the control group; # significantly different compared with the LPS-injected mice.

RESULTS

Quercetin Improved the Memory Function of the LPS-Injected Mice

Mounting studies have supported the evidence that natural-derived substances, particularly flavonoids, have a promising role in the enhancement of learning, and memory functions (Scapagnini et al., 2011; Prakash et al., 2013; Liu et al., 2014; Ahmad et al., 2016; Ali et al., 2018). Quercetin also has a beneficial effect on memory and cognitive functions (Sriraksa et al., 2012; Ashrafpour et al., 2015). However, numerous studies have investigated that systemic LPS administration induces memory and cognitive dysfunction (Qin et al., 2007; Badshah et al., 2016; Khan et al., 2016, 2017). Therefore, to assess the memory-enhancing effect of quercetin against systemic LPS, we designed a dosage regimen of quercetin at a 30 mg/kg body weight dose for 2 weeks (1 week prior and 1 week cotreated with LPS) via the I.P route. Other studies also recommended a quercetin dose of 30 mg/kg/day I.P. for a short period of time induce beneficial effects (Haleagrahara et al., 2009; Yang et al., 2014; Park et al., 2018). We evaluated the memory functions of the mice using MWM and Y-maze tests. Initially, we trained all animals in an MWM task where they were required to find a submerged hidden platform and then analyzed the time required to reach the hidden platform. The LPS-injected animals took more time to find the hidden platform compared to the control mice (**Figure 2A**). However, quercetin treatment reversed the LPS effect and significantly improved memory function, as indicated by the animals taking less time to reach the hidden platform compared to the LPS-injected mice. Furthermore, a probe test showed that quercetin reversed the LPS effect and led to a significant increase in the number of platform crossings and an increase in the time spent in the target quadrant in which the hidden platform was previously located (**Figures 2B,C**). These results demonstrated that quercetin reversed the detrimental effect of LPS and significantly improved memory performance.

The Y-maze results also indicated that LPS triggered short-term spatial memory dysfunction compared to the control group. Quercetin treatment significantly enhanced the spontaneous alteration behavior percentage (a parameter for the enhancement of spatial working memory functions), indicating that quercetin improved the spatial working memory function of the LPS-injected mice (**Figure 2D**).

Quercetin Protects Against LPS-Induced Synaptic Dysfunction

Mounting studies have reported that flavonoids are beneficial for synaptic and memory functions (Ahmad et al., 2016; Matias et al., 2017; Ali et al., 2018; Khan et al., 2018). Because synaptic (pre- and postsynaptic) proteins have been associated with the decline of memory and cognitive functions. Therefore, we also examined the effects of quercetin on synaptic expression levels by western blot and confocal microscopy. The western blot (**Figures 3A,B**) results show that the group of mice that received LPS had decreased expression levels of PSD-95 and Synap in the cortex and hippocampus compared to the control group of adult mice. Treatment with quercetin along with LPS significantly reversed the LPS-induced synaptic deficit by increasing the expression of PSD95 and Synap in the cortex and hippocampus of adult mice (**Figures 3A,B**). To further verify the effect of quercetin on synaptic function, we examined SNAP-23 expression levels using confocal microscopy. The immunofluorescence images showed reduced reactivity in the LPS-treated mice compared to the control group. Quercetin treatment significantly increased the immunofluorescence reactivity of SNAP-23 in the cortex and DG region of the hippocampus compared to the LPS-treated group of adult mice (**Figure 3C**).

Quercetin Attenuates the LPS-Induced Activation of Microglia and Astrocytes

Microglia and astrocytes in the CNS respond rapidly to complaints such as infections, stress, and injury, which makes them important modulators of neuroinflammation responses (Witte et al., 2010; Chen et al., 2012; Badshah et al., 2015b). Studies have reported that in systemic LPS administration, activated microglia and astrocytes are responsible for neuroinflammation-mediated neurodegeneration (Qin et al., 2007; Badshah et al., 2015b, 2016; Khan et al., 2016; Rehman et al., 2018). GFAP protein and Iba-1 are specific markers for activated astrocytes and microglia, respectively. Flavonoids, on the other hand, have been reported to have multiple neuroprotective properties, including potent anti-inflammatory effects. Quercetin, a natural flavonoid, also shows a strong anti-inflammatory action by suppressing activated astrocytosis and microgliosis (Chen et al., 2005; Bureau et al., 2008; Kao et al., 2010; Rinwa and Kumar, 2013; Yang et al., 2018). To analyze the expression of GFAP and Iba-1, we found through western blotting that LPS treatment significantly increased the expression of these two proteins in the adult mouse cortex and hippocampus compared to the control group of mice. Treatment with quercetin along with LPS significantly decreased the expression of these proteins in the adult mouse cortex and hippocampus (**Figures 4A,B**). In addition, the GFAP expression level was also analyzed using immunofluorescence staining. The immunofluorescence results showed the increased intensity of GFAP-positive cells and immunofluorescence reactivity in the LPS-treated group compared to the control groups. Quercetin treatment along with LPS significantly reduced the GFAP-positive cells and immunofluorescence reactivity compared to LPS-treated mice (**Figure 4C**).

Quercetin Halts the LPS-Induced Activated TLR4/NFKB Pathway

Mounting studies have demonstrated that LPS is known to activate microglia in several animal models, which leads

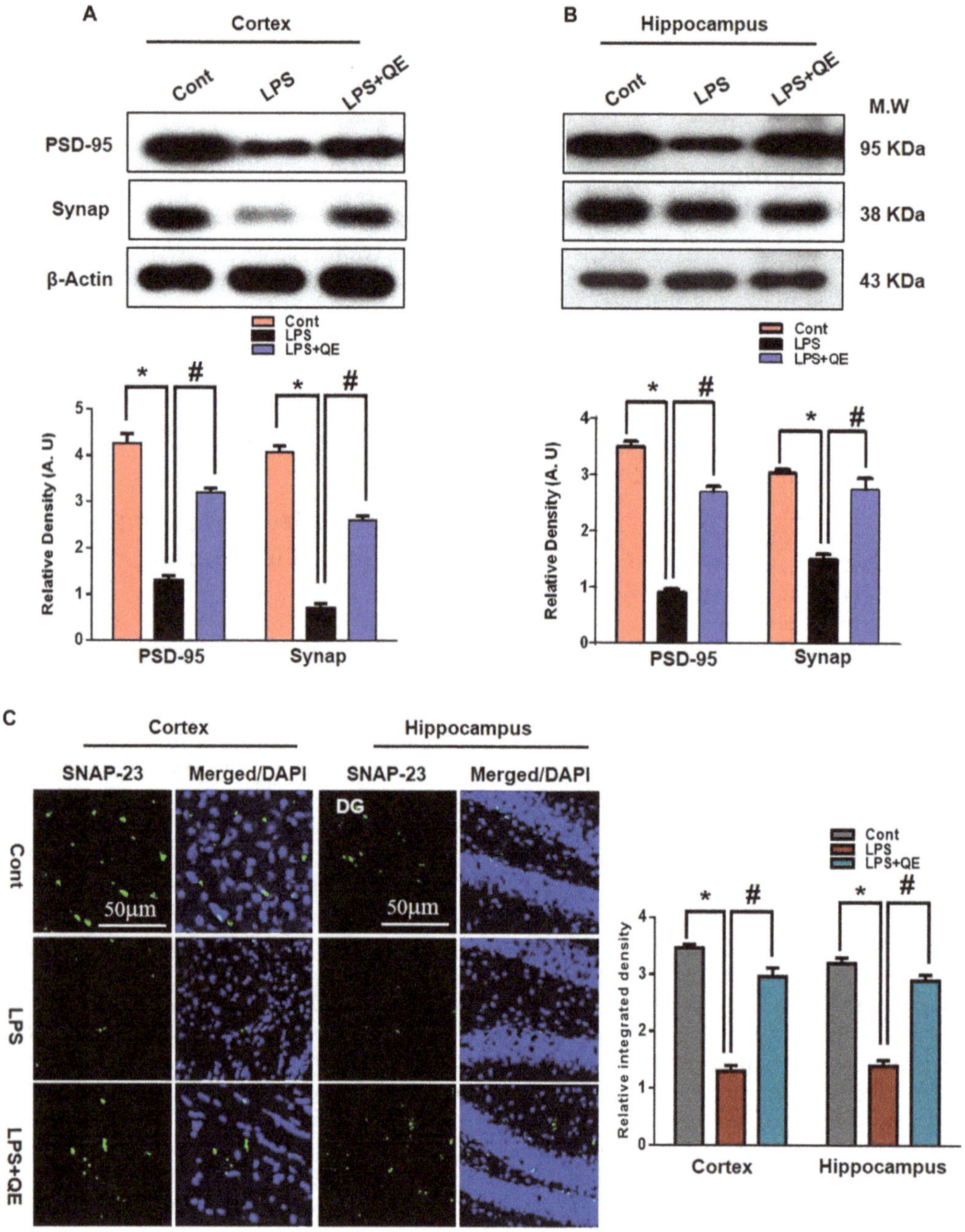

FIGURE 3 | Quercetin improved the pre- and postsynaptic markers in the LPS-treated mice. **(A,B)** Western blotting of the proteins Synap and PSD95; their differences in the cortex and hippocampus of mouse brains are represented by a histogram. β-Actin was used as a loading control. The quantified density values are shown in arbitrary units (A.U.) as the means ± SEM for the respective shown protein (8 mice/group). **(C)** Representative immunofluorescence images and the quantified histogram of SNAP-23 in the cortex and hippocampus of adult mice (5 mice/group). Magnified 10×. Scale bar = 50 μm. The expressed data are relative to the control. * Significantly different from the control; # significantly different from LPS-treated group. Significance: $P < 0.05$.

to neuroinflammation and neurodegeneration (Johansson et al., 2005; Badshah et al., 2016; Carvalho et al., 2017; Khan et al., 2017; Jung et al., 2017). TLR-4 is a primary receptor for LPS-activated microglia (Qin et al., 2006; Badshah et al., 2016; Rehman et al., 2018). Here, we also found through western blotting that systemic administration of LPS activated TLR-4 in the adult mouse cortex and hippocampus compared to the control group of mice. Quercetin treatment along with LPS significantly decreased the expression of TLR-4 in the mouse cortex and hippocampus compared to LPS-treated mice (**Figures 5A,B**). Activated TLR-4 is responsible for inflammatory signaling in the MyD88-dependent pathway, which is responsible for the up-regulation of p-NF-κB and ultimately leads to neuroinflammation

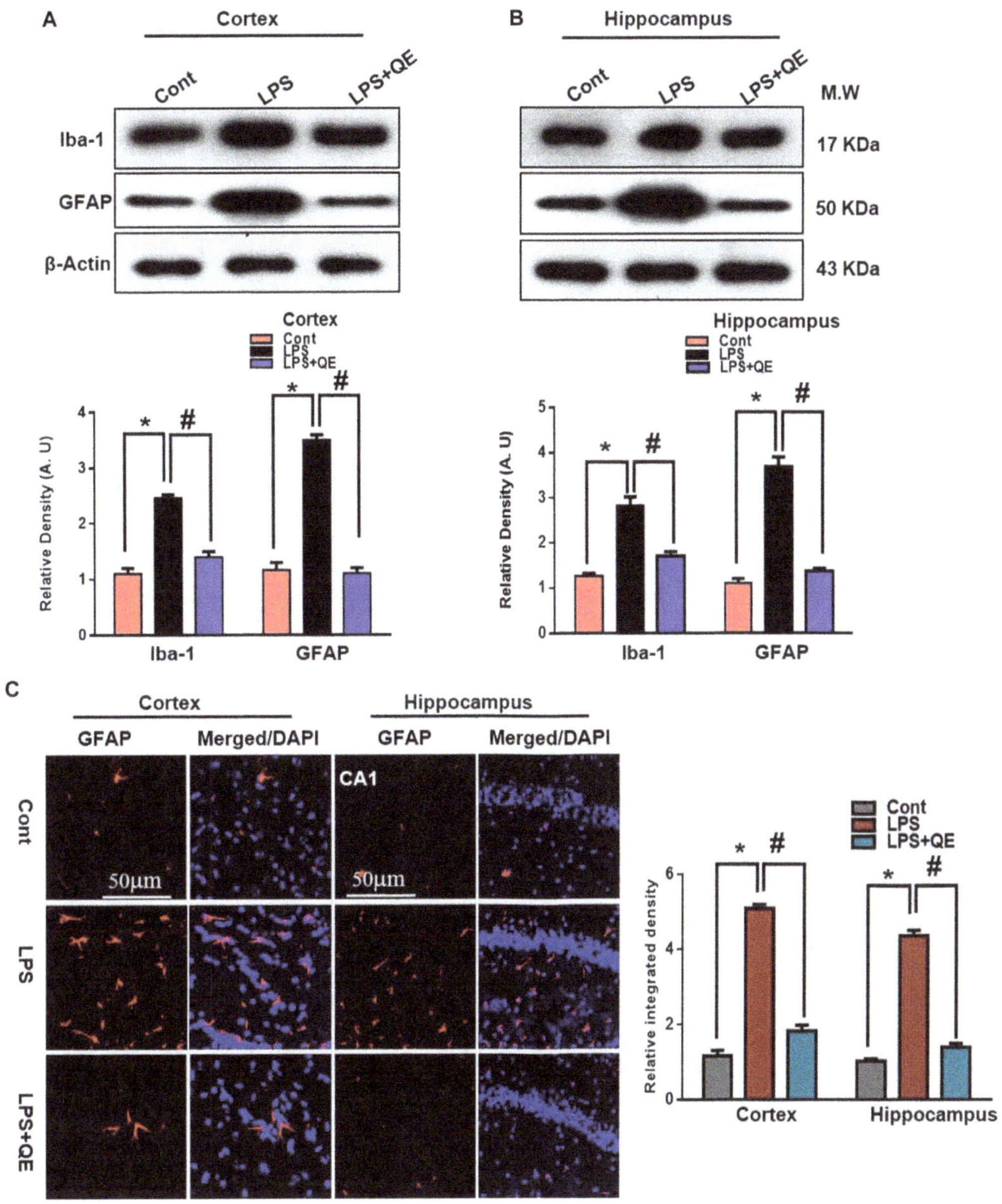

FIGURE 4 | Quercetin ameliorated LPS-induced activated gliosis in the cortex and hippocampus of adult mice. **(A,B)** Western blotting of the proteins GFAP and Iba-1; their differences in the cortex and hippocampus of mouse brains are represented by a histogram. β-Actin was used as a loading control. The quantified density values are shown in arbitrary units (A.U.) as the means ± SEM for the respective shown protein (8 mice/group). **(C)** Representative immunofluorescence images and the quantified histogram of activated GFAP in the cortex and hippocampus of adult mice (5 mice/group). Magnified 10×. Scale bar = 50 μm. The expressed data are relative to the control. * Significantly different from the control; # significantly different from LPS-treated group. Significance: $P < 0.05$.

and neurodegeneration (Yao et al., 2017). We also found through western blotting that LPS administration activated p-NF-κB expression in the cortex and hippocampus of adult mice compared to the control group of mice. Treatment with quercetin significantly reduced the expression of p-NF-κB in the cortex and hippocampus of adult mice (**Figures 5A,B**).

Furthermore, the immunofluorescence results of p-NF-κB showed immunofluorescence reactivity in the LPS-treated group compared to the control groups. Quercetin treatment along with LPS significantly reduced the immunofluorescence reactivity compared to LPS-treated mice (**Figure 5C**).

Quercetin Attenuated LPS-Induced Neuroinflammation-Associated Markers

Quercetin is a natural flavonoid found in many vegetables and fruits and possesses potential biological and health beneficial effects that have the ability to inhibit inflammatory mediators (Lesjak et al., 2018). It has been reported that LPS

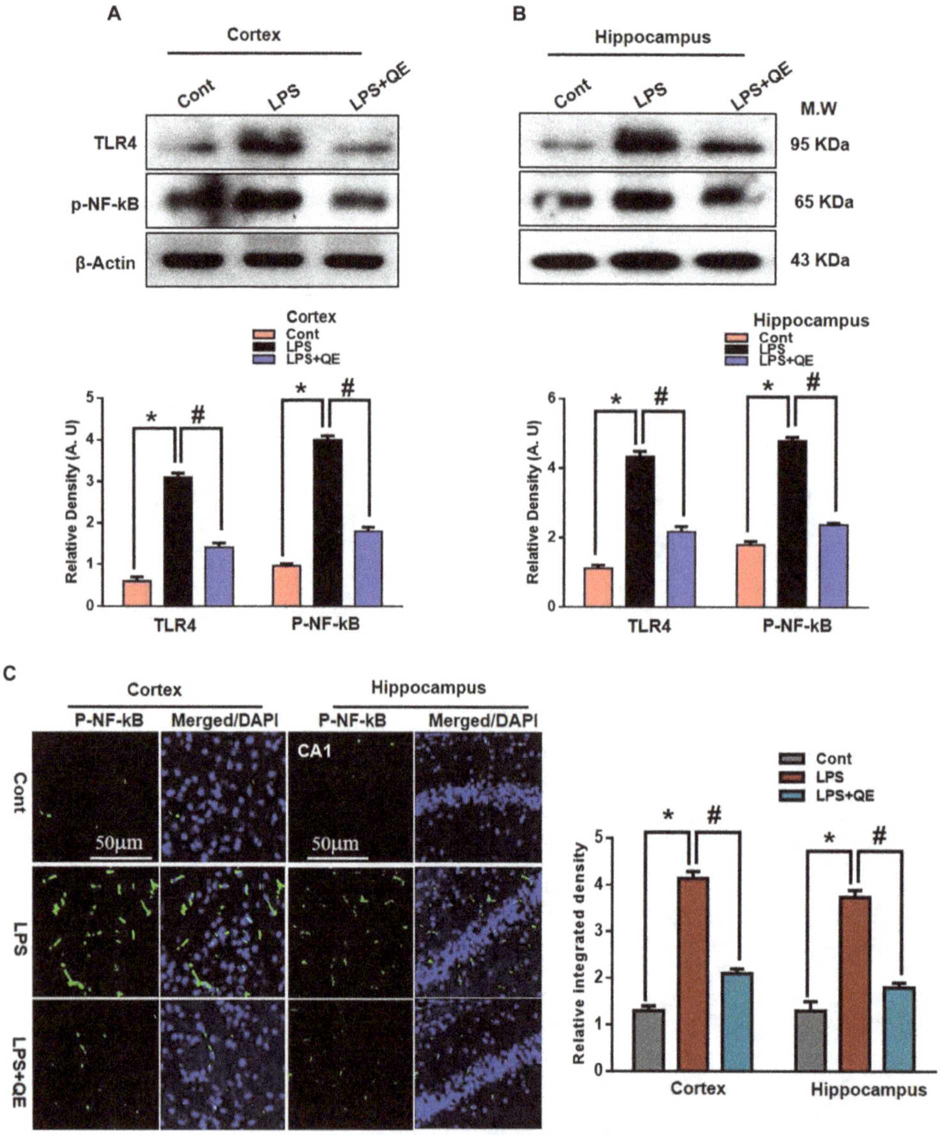

FIGURE 5 | Quercetin halts the LPS-induced activated TLR4/NFKB pathway. **(A,B)** Western blotting of TLR4 and p-NFKB proteins; their differences in the cortex and hippocampus of mouse brains are represented by a histogram. β-Actin was used as a loading control. The quantified density values are shown in arbitrary units (A.U.) as the means ± SEM for the respective shown protein (8 mice/group). **(C)** Representative immunofluorescence images and the quantified histogram of p-NFKB in the cortex and hippocampus of adult mice (5 mice/group). Magnified 10×. Scale bar = 50 μm. The expressed data are relative to the control. * Significantly different from the control; # significantly different from LPS-treated group. Significance: $P < 0.05$.

administration has the potential to increase the production of several inflammatory mediators, such as TNF-α, COX-2, NOS-2, and IL-1β (Badshah et al., 2015b, 2016; Khan et al., 2016, 2017). Here, we also ascertained through western blotting that LPS administration increased the expression of TNF-α, COX-2, and NOS-2 in the cortex and hippocampus of adult mice compared to the control group of mice. Quercetin treatment along with LPS significantly tempered and reduced the expression of these inflammatory proteins (**Figures 6A,B**). Similarly, the immunofluorescence results of IL-1β showed that LPS administration increased the number of IL-1β-positive cells compared to control mice in the cortex and DG region, but the group of mice that received quercetin along with LPS significantly downregulated the IL-1β-positive cells and fluorescence immunoreactivity in the cortex and DG region (**Figure 6C**).

Quercetin Prevented LPS-Induced Neuronal Degeneration

The mitochondrial apoptotic pathway plays a key role in neuronal degeneration. In the mitochondrial apoptotic pathway, the antiapoptotic Bcl-2 and proapoptotic Bax markers have a primary role in the apoptotic pathway. The Bax/Bcl-2 ratio is an important

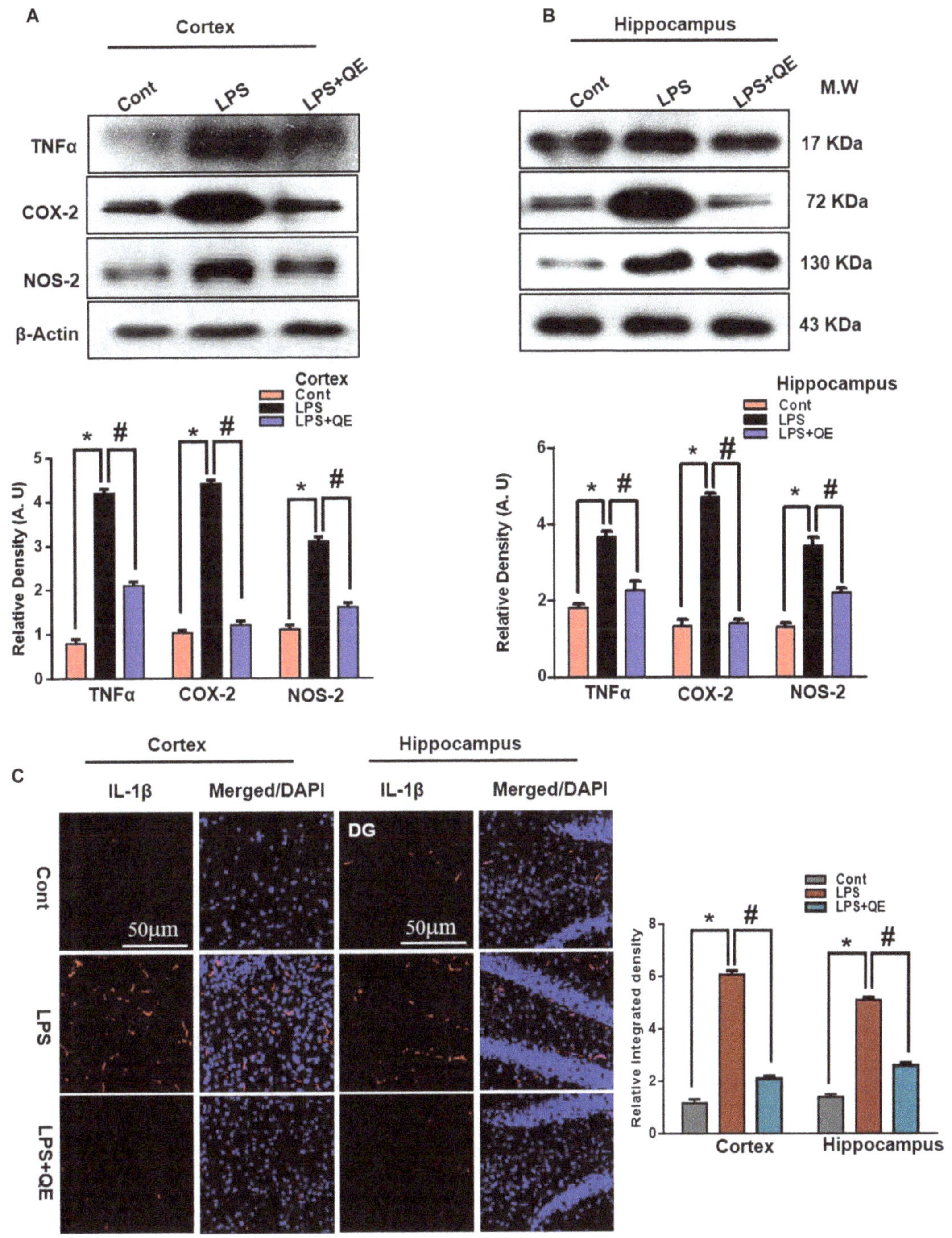

FIGURE 6 | Quercetin attenuated LPS-induced neuroinflammation-associated markers. **(A,B)** Western blotting of TNF-α, COX-2 and NOS2 proteins; their differences in the cortex and hippocampus of mouse brains are represented by a histogram. β-Actin was used as a loading control. The quantified density values are shown in arbitrary units (A.U.) as the means ± SEM for the respective shown protein (8 mice/group). **(C)** Representative immunofluorescence images and the quantified histogram of IL-1β in the cortex and hippocampus of adult mice (5 mice/group). Magnified 10×. Scale bar = 50 μm. The expressed data are relative to the control. * Significantly different from the control; # significantly different from LPS-treated group. Significance: $P < 0.05$.

indicator of the apoptotic pathway. Furthermore, increased Bax/Bcl-2 ratio induced overactivation of Cyto. c, an important mediator in the mitochondrial associated pathway, which leads to activation of caspases (Li et al., 1997; Chao and Korsmeye, 1998; Debatin et al., 2002; Badshah et al., 2015a). Previous studies (Badshah et al., 2015a; Khan et al., 2016) have indicated that flavonoids play a key role in regulating the mitochondrial apoptotic pathway; therefore, we also investigated the effect of

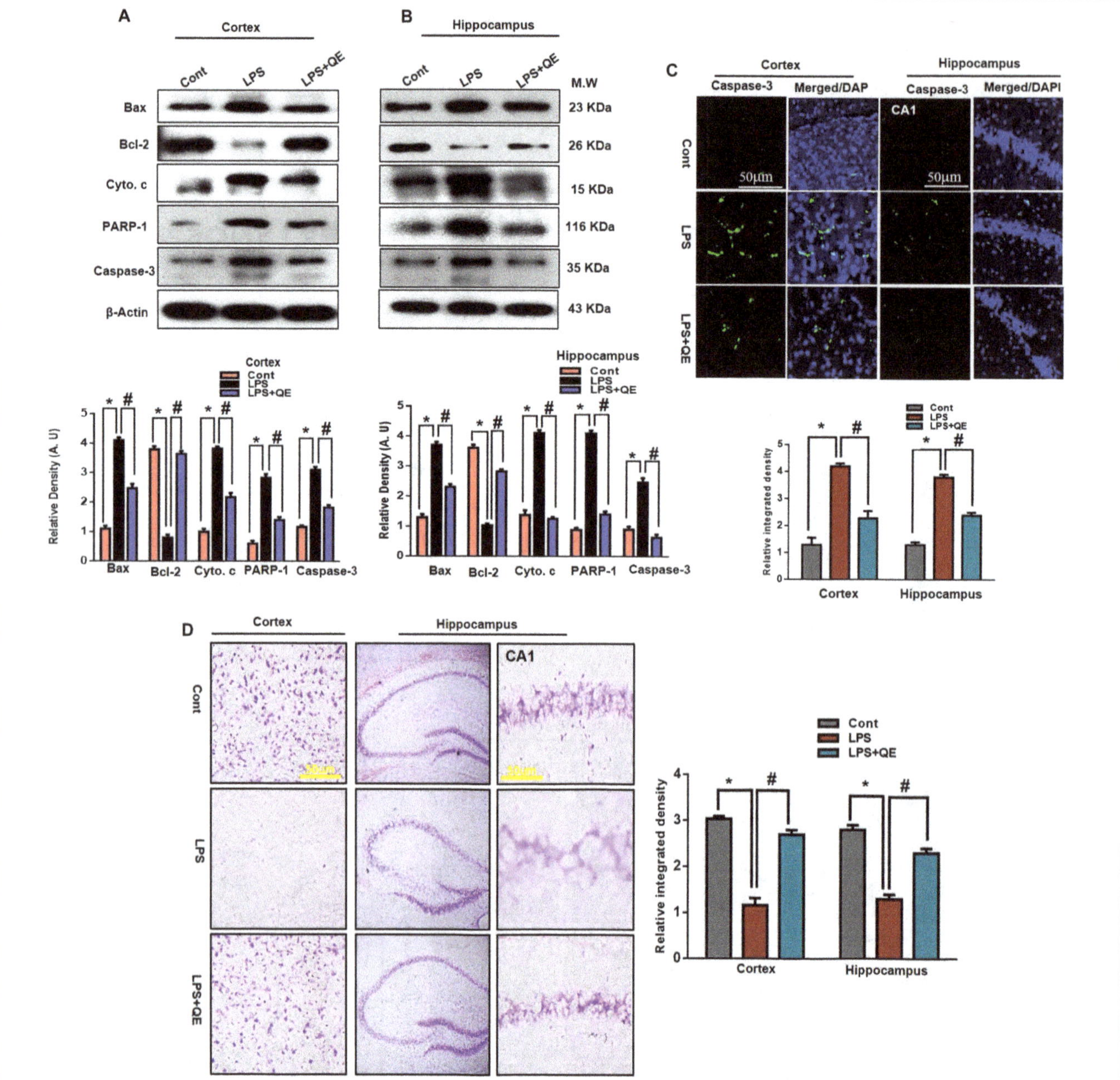

FIGURE 7 | LPS-induced neuronal apoptotic pathway prevented by quercetin in the cortex and hippocampus. **(A,B)** Western blotting of Bcl-2, Bax, Cyto. c, Caspase-3 and PARP-1 proteins; their differences in the cortex and hippocampus of mouse brains are represented by a histogram. β-Actin was used as a loading control. The quantified density values are shown in arbitrary units (A.U.) as the means ± SEM for the respective shown protein (8 mice/group). **(C)** Representative immunofluorescence images and the quantified histogram of Caspase-3 in the cortex and hippocampus of adult mice (5 mice/group). Magnified 10×. Scale bar = 50 µm. **(D)** Representative immunohistochemical images (Nissl staining) and the quantified histogram of the survival neuron reactivity and integrated density in the cortex and hippocampus region of adult mice. The expressed data are relative to the control. * Significantly different from the control; # significantly different from LPS-treated group. Significance: $P < 0.05$.

quercetin on the mitochondrial pathway. We ascertained through western blots that LPS triggers the Bax/Bcl-2 ratio and release of Cyto. c compared to the control group. Quercetin significantly reduced the Bax/Bl2 ratio and Cyto. c expression level compared to the LPS-treated group alone.

In apoptotic neurodegeneration, the caspase family plays an important role. Among caspase cascades, caspase-3 is the major player in apoptosis and plays a key role in apoptosis (Le et al., 2002; Carloni et al., 2004; Ali et al., 2015a; Badshah et al., 2015a, 2016). Therefore, we also evaluated caspase-3 activity by western blotting and confocal microscopy. Our western blot results show that LPS activated caspase-3 activity in the cortex and hippocampus of adult mice compared to the control group of mice. Treatment with quercetin along with LPS significantly reduced the activated caspase-3 activity compared to LPS-treated mice (**Figures 7A,B**). Similarly, the confocal microscopy results showed that there are more caspase-3-positive cells and fluorescence reactivity of caspase-3 in the cortex and CA-1 region of the LPS-received mice compared to the control group of mice. However, treatment with quercetin significantly reduced caspase-3-positive cells and fluorescence immunoreactivity in the cortex and CA-1 region of the brain (**Figure 7C**).

PARP-1is a nuclear enzyme with a wide range of physiological and pathological functions. In physiological function, it is involved in DNA repair and genomic stability. In pathological conditions, the over activation of PARP-1 leads to neuronal cell death (Berger, 1985; Chaitanya et al., 2010). It has been reported that activated caspase-3 increased the over activation of PARP-1 (Williams et al., 2008; Badshah et al., 2015a). Therefore, in this context, we also evaluated the expression of PARP-1 through western blotting in both the cortex and hippocampus of adult mice. Our western blotting results revealed that systemic LPS administration results in the overexpression of PARP-1 in the cortex and hippocampus of adult mice compared to the control group of mice. Treatment with quercetin along with LPS reduced the expression of PARP-1 in the adult mouse cortex and hippocampus (**Figures 7A,B**). Furthermore, the immunohistochemical Nissl staining results showed that LPS injection decreased the neuronal survival reactivity in the cortex and hippocampus of adult mouse brains compared to the control group of mice. Importantly, quercetin administration to LPS-injected mice enhanced the survival of neuronal cells in the cortex and hippocampus of adult mouse brains (**Figure 7D**).

DISCUSSION

The application and consumption of natural substances is a primary focus for the prevention of neurodegenerative diseases. Among natural substances, polyphenol-derived medicinal substances are important therapeutic agents for the slowing or prevention of neurological disorders (Dajas et al., 2003; Scapagnini et al., 2011; Prakash et al., 2013; Liu et al., 2014; Badshah et al., 2015a; Ahmad et al., 2016; Jung et al., 2017; Ali et al., 2018). Quercetin is a well-approved and recommended flavonoid that has medicinal properties and protective roles in different paradigms of CNS insult-induced detrimental effects (Lei et al., 2015; Chen S. et al., 2016; Kanter et al., 2016). In this study, we also investigated the neuroprotective effect of quercetin against LPS-induced detrimental effects such as neuroinflammation-mediated neurodegeneration and synaptic/memory deficits in the cortical and hippocampal regions of the adult mouse brain.

Chronic neuroinflammation is a pathological cascade that occurs during the progression of several neurological disorders, such as AD, PD, FTD, and amyotrophic lateral sclerosis (ALS) (Glass et al., 2010; Von Bernhardi et al., 2010; Chen W.W. et al., 2016; Hong, 2017). In chronic neuroinflammation, activated microglia and astrocytes disturb homeostasis and are implicated in all degenerative conditions of the CNS (Netea et al., 2003; Perry et al., 2003; Hoogland et al., 2015; Jung et al., 2017). Previous studies have shown that systemic administration of LPS activates microglia and astrocytes (Qin et al., 2007; Badshah et al., 2016). The TLR family has a promising and key role in the immune response. This family comprises 13 members in rodents and 11 members in humans. Furthermore, several studies have confirmed that TLR-4 is a primary target and receptor in glial cells (Shimazu et al., 1999; Aravalli et al., 2007; Block et al., 2007; Glass et al., 2010; Rehman et al., 2018). In both *in vivo* and *in vitro* evidence confirmed that LPS binds to TLR-4, inducing activated gliosis, which consequently mediates NF-kB cascade activation, which plays a serious role in the activation of inflammation and neurodegeneration processes (Chen et al., 2012; Catorce and Gevorkian, 2016). NF-kB has been considered a mediator between neuroinflammation and neurodegeneration. Several studies reported that natural flavonoids prevented activated gliosis by inhibiting completely or partially by inhibiting the TLR4 and NF-kB cascades (Lee et al., 2012; Badshah et al., 2016; Khan et al., 2016; Rehman et al., 2018). The inhibition of the TLR4 and NF-kB cascades confers desirable effects in any pathogenic and neurotoxic condition. Bureau et al., 2008, reported that quercetin inhibited LPS-induced activated glial cells. Likewise, we have found that quercetin administration prevents LPS-induced activated gliosis by reducing the expression of TLR4 and NF-kB cascades.

Activated microglia and astrocytes are responsible for the release of inflammatory molecules such as TNF-α, IL-1β, COX-2, and NOS2, which are responsible for neuroinflammation. Studies have reported that activated nuclear translocation of the NF-kB cascades pathway is implicated in the over production and release of the above proinflammatory mediators (Li and Verma, 2002; Lee et al., 2012; Song et al., 2014; Gu et al., 2015; Hong, 2017). In a literature review reported that transgenic rodents that overexpressed TNF-α exhibited inflammation and neurodegeneration, which lead to memory impairment. Over activation of TNF-α has been reported to induce neurotoxicity in human cortical neurons. Similarly, mounting studies have reported overexpressed immunoreactive IL-1β cells in pathogenic conditions, brain injuries and degeneration. Overexpressed IL-1β affects both neuronal and non-neuronal cells in the CNS Wyss-Coray and Rogers (2012). In addition, when murine BV2 microglial cells are exposed to LPS- and IFN-γ-induced NO production and iNOS gene expression, neuroinflammation-mediated neurodegeneration is triggered (Chen et al., 2005; Song et al., 2014). Interestingly, quercetin acts as an antioxidant and anti-inflammatory agent to inhibit NO and iNOS expression by regulating the NF-kB/HO pathway in LPS-exposed BV2 cells (Chen et al., 2005; Kao et al., 2010). TNF-α, IL-1β and reactive species such NO and iNOS induced the overexpression of COX2, which has a key role in the intensification of neuroinflammation-mediated neurodegeneration (Feng et al., 1995; Yamamoto et al., 1995; O'Banion et al., 1996; Salvemini, 1997). Recent attention has been given to natural compounds such as flavonoids that possess multiple neuroprotective activities, such as suppressing neuroinflammation and neuronal apoptosis, and promoting neuronal survival and memory enhancing effect (Lee et al., 2012; Dey et al., 2017; Shal et al., 2018). Flavonoids have been suggested as promising therapeutic agents for the reduction of neuroinflammation (Magalingam et al., 2015; Chen S. et al., 2016). Quercetin is found abundantly in onions and various berries. Studies have reported that quercetin shows strong activity against neuroinflammation (Spencer, 2008; Kanter et al., 2016; Matias et al., 2016; Duet al., 2016). In the present study, our results supported the previous findings and elucidated that quercetin suppressed the proinflammatory mediators as described above and consequently attenuated LPS-induced neuroinflammation in the adult mouse cortex and hippocampus.

Chronic neuroinflammation mediates the neuronal degeneration process in various diseases, such as AD, PD, and ALS. In both *in vivo* and *in vitro* studies, LPS-induced activated cytokines and chemokines as well as activated redox and nitrogen species, which further trigger apoptotic neurodegeneration (Li and Verma, 2002; Chen et al., 2005; Chen W.W. et al., 2016; Kao et al., 2010; Lee et al., 2012; Song et al., 2014; Gu et al., 2015; Kempuraj et al., 2016, 2017; Hong, 2017). Studies have reported that LPS induces the mitochondrial apoptotic pathway by interfering with Bax/Bcl-2 signaling (Badshah et al., 2015b, 2016; Khan et al., 2016, 2017). Activated Bax/Bcl-2 triggers the activation of Cyto. c, which further triggers the activation of caspase cascades. Caspase cascades, e.g., caspase-3, play a major role in apoptotic neuronal degeneration. The activation of caspase-3 induced neuronal cell death and has been considered a main feature of neurodegenerative diseases. Activated caspase-3 cleaves PARP-1, which leads to neuronal DNA damage (Le et al., 2002; Carloni et al., 2004; Ali et al., 2015a; Badshah et al., 2015a, 2016). The natural dietary flavonoid shows a protective role against CNS-insult-induced neurodegeneration. Quercetin is a natural flavonoid that inhibits neuronal apoptotic cell death (Bureau et al., 2008; Yang et al., 2014; Lei et al., 2015; Kanter et al., 2016; Shveta et al., 2016). Interestingly, quercetin also regulated the mitochondrial apoptotic pathway and prevented the activation of Cyto. c, activated caspase 3 and cleaved PARP-1 expression and subsequently prevents neuronal degeneration, demonstrating that neuroinflammation-mediated neurodegeneration is rescued by quercetin.

It has been studied that systemic administration of LPS triggers neuroinflammation-mediated neurodegeneration, which is responsible for synaptic and memory dysfunction (Qin et al., 2007; Lee et al., 2012; Badshah et al., 2016). Flavonoids have been investigated well for improving learning and memory functions in aberrant and detrimental conditions (Scapagnini et al., 2011; Prakash et al., 2013; Liu et al., 2014; Ahmad et al., 2016; Ali et al., 2018). Studies show that LPS administration is responsible for decreasing the level of presynaptic and postsynaptic proteins (Badshah et al., 2016; Khan et al., 2018; Rehman et al., 2018). Our results also claimed that the systemic administration of LPS decreased the level of presynaptic proteins synaptophysin and postsynaptic protein PSD-95 in the mouse cortex and hippocampus. Our results show that quercetin treatment alleviates the LPS-induced impairment of synaptic functions in the mouse cortex and hippocampus. Similarly, we also observed that systemic LPS administration induced memory dysfunction. This memory dysfunction in the LPS-treated mice was reversed by quercetin, indicating that quercetin would be beneficial to improve the memory functions associated with synaptic functions in CNS-insult-induced detrimental effects.

In conclusion, our results demonstrated that quercetin prevented LPS-induced detrimental effects, such as neuroinflammation-mediated neurodegeneration and synaptic/memory impairment, in adult mice. These results suggest that drugs of natural origin with significant potential biological activity would be beneficial against pathogenic and neuronal insults in neurological disorders.

AUTHOR CONTRIBUTIONS

AK designed and managed the experimental work, and wrote the manuscript. TA contributed in the manuscript writing. AK, HB, SR, SA, KS, MI, TM, and MSK performed the western blot and morphological experiments. MOK was the corresponding author, having reviewed and approved the manuscript, and holds all the responsibilities related to this manuscript. All authors reviewed the manuscript.

FUNDING

This research was supported by the Brain Research Program through the National Research Foundation of Korea (NRF) funded by the Ministry of Science, ICT & Future Planning (2016M3C7A1904391).

REFERENCES

Ahmad, A., Ali, T., Park, H. Y., Badshah, H., Rehman, S. U., and Kim, M. O. (2016). Neuroprotective effect of fisetin against amyloid beta-induced cognitive/synaptic dysfunction, neuroinflammation and neurodegeneration in adult mice. *Mol. Neurobiol.* 54, 2269–2285. doi: 10.1007/s12035-016-9795-4

Ali, T., Badshah, H., Kim, T. H., and Kim, M. O. (2015a). Melatonin attenuates D-galactose-induced memory impairment, neuroinflammation and neurodegeneration via RAGE/NF-K B/JNK signaling pathway in aging mouse model. *J. Pineal Res.* 58, 71–85. doi: 10.1111/jpi.12194

Ali, T., Yoon, G. H., Shah, S. A., Lee, H. Y., and Kim, M. O. (2015b). Osmotin attenuates amyloid beta-induced memory impairment, tau phosphorylation and neurodegeneration in the mouse hippocampus. *Sci. Rep.* 5:11708. doi: 10.1038/srep11708

Ali, T., Kim, T., Rehman, S. U., Khan, F. U., Khan M., Ikram M., et al. (2018). Natural dietary supplementaion of anthocyanins via PI3K/Akt/Nrf2/HO-1 pathways mitigates oxidative stress, neurodegeneration, and memory impairment in a mouse model of Alzheimer's disease. *Mol. Neurobiol.* 55, 6076–6093. doi: 10.1007/s12035-017-0798-6

Aravalli, R. N., Peterson, P. K., and Lokensgard, J. R. (2007). Toll-like receptors in defense and damage of the central nervous system. *J. NeuroImmune Pharmacol.* 2, 297–312. doi: 10.1007/s11481-007-9071-5

Ashrafpour, M., Parsaei, S., and Sepehri, H. (2015). Quercetin improved spatial memory dysfunctions in rat model of intracerebroventricular streptozotocin-induced Alzheimer's disease. *Nat. J. Phys. Phar.* 5, 411–415. doi: 10.5455/njppp.2015.5.2308201563

Badshah, H., Ali, T., Ahmad, A., Kim, M. J., Abid, N. B., Shah, S. A., et al. (2015a). Co-treatment with anthocyanins and vitamin C ameliorates ethanol-induced neurodegeneration via modulation of GABAB receptor signaling in the adult rat brain. *CNS Neurol. Disord. Drug Targets* 14, 791–803. doi: 10.2174/1871527314666150225142919

Badshah, H., Ali, T., Rehman, S. U., Amin, F. U., Ullah, F., Kim, T. H., et al. (2015b). Protective effect of lupeol against lipopolysaccharide-induced neuroinflammation via the p38/c-Jun N-terminal kinase pathway in the adult mouse brain. *J. Neuroimm. Pharmacol.* 11, 48–60. doi: 10.1007/s11481-015-9623-z

Badshah, H., Ali, T., and Kim, M. O. (2016). Osmotin attenuates LPS-induced neuroinflammation and memory impairments via the TLR4/NFK signalling pathway. *Sci. Rep.* 6:24493. doi: 10.1038/srep24493

Bahar, E., Kim, J. Y., and Yoon, H. (2017). Quercetin attenuates manganese-induced neuroinflammation by alleviating oxidative stress through regulation of apoptosis, iNOS/ NF-kB and HO/Nrf2 pathways. *Int. J. Mol. Sci.* 18:E1989. doi: 10.3390/ijms18091989

Berger, N. A. (1985). Poly(ADP-ribose) in the cellular response to DNA damage. *Radiat. Res.* 101, 4–15. doi: 10.2307/3576299

Biesmans, S., Meert, T. F., Bouwknecht, J. A., Acton, P. D., Davoodi, N., De Haes, P., et al. (2013). Systemic immune activation leads to neuroinflammation and sickness behavior in mice. *J. Mediat. Inflamm.* 2013:271359. doi: 10.1155/2013/271359

Block, M. L., Zecca, L., and Hong, J. S. (2007). Microglia-mediated neurotoxicity: uncovering the molecular mechanisms. *Nat. Rev. Neurosci.* 8, 57–69. doi: 10.1038/nrn2038

Bureau, G., Longpre, F., and Martinoli, M. G. (2008). Resveratrol and quercetin, two natural polyphenols, reduce apoptotic neuronal cell death induced by neuroinflammation. *J. Neurosci. Res.* 86, 403–410. doi: 10.1002/jnr.21503

Carloni, S., Mazzoni, E., and Balduini, W. (2004). Caspase-3 and calpain activities after acute and repeated ethanol administration during the rat brain growth spurt. *J. Neurochem.* 2004, 197–203. doi: 10.1111/j.1471-4159.2004.02341.x

Carvalho, F. B., Gutierres, J. M., Bueno, A., Agostinho, P., Zago, A. M., Vieira, J., et al. (2017). Anthocyanins control neuroinflammation and consequent memory dysfunction in mice exposed to lipopolysaccharide. *Mol. Neurobiol.* 54, 3350–3367. doi: 10.1007/s12035-016-9900-8

Catorce, M. N., and Gevorkian, G. (2016). LPS-induced murine neuroinflammation model: main features and suitability for pre-clinical assessment of nutraceuticals. *J. Curr. Neuropharmacol.* 14, 155–164. doi: 10.2174/1570159X14666151204122017

Chaitanya, G. V., Steven, A. J., and Babu, P. P. (2010). PARP-1 cleavage fragments: signatures of cell-death proteases in neurodegeneration. *J. Cell Commun. Signal.* 8:31. doi: 10.1186/1478-811X-8-31.

Chao, D. T., and Korsmeye, S. J. (1998). Bcl-2 family: regulators of cell death. *Annu. Rev. Immunol.* 1998, 395–419. doi: 10.1146/annurev.immunol.16.1.395

Chen, S., Jiang, H., Wu, X., and Fang, J. (2016). Therapeutic effects of quercetin on inflammation, obesity, and Type 2 diabetes. *J. Mediat. Inflamm.* 2016:9340637. doi: 10.1155/2016/9340637

Chen, W. W., Zhang, X., and Huang, W. J. (2016). Role of neuroinflammation in neurodegenerative diseases. *Mol. Med. Rep.* 13, 3391–3396. doi: 10.3892/mmr.2016.4948

Chen, Z., Jalabi, W., Shpargel, K. B., Farabaugh, K. T., Dutta, R., Yin, X., et al. (2012). Lipopolysaccharide-induced microglial activation and neuroprotection against experimental brain injury is independent of hematogenous TLR4. *J. Neurosci.* 32, 11706–11715. doi: 10.1523/JNEUROSCI.0730-12.2012

Chen J. C., Ho F. M., Pei-Dawn Lee, Chao., Chen, C. P., Jeng, K. C., Hsu, H. B., et al. (2005). Inhibition of iNOS gene expression by quercetin is mediated by the inhibition of IkappaB kinase, nuclear factor-kappa B and STAT1, and depends on heme oxygenase-1 induction in mouse BV-2 microglia. *Eur. J. Pharmacol.* 521, 9–20. doi: 10.1016/j.ejphar.2005.08.005

Costa, L. G., Garrick, J. M., Roque, P. J., and Pellacani, C. (2016). Mechanisms of neuroprotection by quercetin counteracting oxidative stress and more. *J. Oxid. Med. Cell Longev.* 2016:2986796. doi: 10.1155/2016/2986796

Dajas, F., Rivera-Megret, F., Blasina, F., Arredond, F., Abin-Carriquiry, J. A., Costa, G., et al. (2003). Neuroprotection by flavonoids. *Braz. J. Med. Biol. Res.* 36, 1613–1620. doi: 10.1590/S0100-879X2003001200002

Debatin, K. M., Poncet, D., and Kroemer, G. (2002). Chemotherapy: targeting the mitochondrial cell death pathway. *Oncogene* 21, 8786–8803. doi: 10.1038/sj.onc.1206039

Dey, A., Bhattacharya, R., Mukherjee, A., and Pandey, D. K. (2017). Natural products against Alzheimer's disease: pharmaco-therapeutics and biotechnological interventions. *Biotechnol. Adv.* 35, 178–216. doi: 10.1016/j.biotechadv.2016.12.005

Di Filipopo, M., Chiasserini, D., Tozzi, A., and Picconi, B., and Calabresi, P. (2010). Mitochondria and the link between neuroinflammation and neurodegeneration. *J. Alzheimer's Dis.* 20(Suppl. 2), S369–379. doi: 10.3233/JAD-2010-100543

Di Filippo, M., Sarchielli, P., Picconi, B., and Calabresi, P. (2008). Neuroinflammation and synaptic plasticity: theoretical basis for a novel, immune-centred, therapeutic approach to neurological disorders. *J. Trends Pharmacol. Sci.* 29, 402–412. doi: 10.1016/j.tips.2008.06.005

Feng, L., Xia, Y., Garcia, G. E., Hwang, D., and Wilson, C. B. (1995). Involvement of reactive oxygen intermediates in cyclooxygenase-2 expression induced by IL-1, TNF-alpha, and lipopolysaccharide. *J. Clin. Invest.* 95, 1669–1675. doi: 10.1172/JCI117842

Glass, C. K., Saijo, K., Winner, B., Marchetto, M. C., and Gage, F. H. (2010). Mechanisms underlying inflammation in neurodegeneration. *Cell* 140, 918–934. doi: 10.1016/j.cell.2010.02.016

Gopinath, K., Prakash, D., and Sudhandiran, G. (2011). Neuroprotective effect of naringin, a dietary flavonoid against 3-nitropropionic acid-induced neuronal apoptosis. *Neurochem. Int.* 59, 1066–1073. doi: 10.1016/j.neuint.2011.08.022

Gu, S. M., Park, M. H., Hwang, C. J., Song, H. S., Lee, U. S., Han, S. B., et al. (2015). Bee venom ameliorates lipopolysaccharide-induced memory loss by preventing NF-kappaB pathway. *J. Neuroinflamm.* 12:124. doi: 10.1186/s12974-015-0344-2

Haleagrahara, N., Radhakrishnan, A., Lee, N., and Kumar, P. (2009). Flavonoid quercetin protects swimming stress-induced changes in oxidative stress biomarkers in the hypothalamus of rats. *Eur. J. Pharmacol.* 621, 46–52. doi: 10.1016/j.ejphar.2009.08.030

Hong, J. T. (2017). NFKB as a mediator of brain inflammation inflammation in AD. *CNS Neurol. Disord. Drug Targets* doi: 10.2174/1871527316666170807130011 [Epub ahead of print].

Hoogland, I. C. M., Houbolt, C., van Westerloo, D. J., van Gool, W. A., and van de Beek, D. (2015). Systemic inflammation and microglial activation: systematic review of animal experiments. *J. Neuroinflamm.* 12:114. doi: 10.1186/s12974-015-0332-6

Hooper, L., Kroon, P. A., Rimm, E. B., Cohn, J. S., Harvey, I., Le Cornu, K. A., et al. (2008). Flavonoids, flavonoid-rich foods, and cardiovascular risk: a meta-analysis of randomized controlled trials. *J. Am. J. Clin. Nutr.* 88, 38–50. doi: 10.1093/ajcn/88.1.38

Hwang, S. L., Shih, P. H., and Yen, G. C. (2012). Neuroprotective effects of citrus flavonoids. *J. Agric. Food Chem.* 60, 877–885. doi: 10.1021/jf204452y

Johansson, S., Bohman, S., Radesäter, A. C., Oberg, C., and Luthman, J. (2005). *Salmonella* lipopolysaccharide (LPS) mediated neurodegeneration in hippocampal slice cultures. *J. Neurotox Res.* 8, 207–220. doi: 10.1007/BF03033974

Jung, J. S., Choi, M. J., Lee, Y. Y., Moon, B. I., Park, J. S., and Kim, H. S. (2017). Suppression of lipopolysacharide-induced neuroinflammation by morin via MAPK, PI3K/Akt, and PKA/HO-1 signaling pathway modulation. *J. Agric. Food Chem.* 65, 373–382. doi: 10.1021/acs.jafc.6b05147

Kanter, M., Unsal, C., Aktas, C., and Erboga, M. (2016). Neuroprotective effect of quercetin against oxidative damage and neuronal apoptosis caused by cadmium in hippocampus. *Toxicol. Ind. Health* 32, 541–550. doi: 10.1177/0748233713504810

Kao. T. K., Ou, Y. C., Raung, S. L., Lai, C. Y., Liao, S. L., and Chen, C. J. (2010). Inhibition of nitric oxide production by quercetin in endotoxin/cytokine-stimulated microglia. *Life Sci.* 86, 315–321. doi: 10.1016/j.lfs.2009.12.014

Kempuraj, D., Thangave, R., Selvakumar, G. P., Zaheer, S., Ahmed, M. E., Raikwar, S. P., et al. (2017). Brain and peripheral atypical inflammatory mediators potentiate neuroinflammation and neurodegeneration. *Front. Cell. Neurosci.* 11:216. doi: 10.3389/fncel.2017.00216

Kempuraj, D., Thangavel, R., Natteru, P. A., Selvakumar, G. P., Saeed, D., Zahoor, H., et al. (2016). Neuroinflammation induces neurodegeneration. *J. Neurol. Neurosurg. Spine* 1:1003.

Khan, M. S., Ali, T., Abid, M. N., Jo, M. H., Khan, A., Kim, M. W., et al. (2017). Lithium ameliorates lipopolysaccharide-induced neurotoxicity in the cortex and hippocampus of the adult rat brain. *J. Neurochem. Int.* 108, 343–354. doi: 10.1016/j.neuint.2017.05.008

Khan, M. S., Ali, T., Kim, M. W., Jo, M. H., Jo, M. G., Badshah, H., et al. (2016). Anthocyanins protect against LPS-induced oxidative stress-mediated neuroinflammation and neurodegeneration in the adult mouse cortex. *Neurochem. Int.* 100, 1–10. doi: 10.1016/j.neuint.2016.08.005

Khan, M. S., Ali, T., Kim, M. W., Jo, M. H, Chung, J. I., and Kim, M. O. (2018). Anthocyanins improve hippocampus-dependent memory function and prevent neurodegeneration via JNK/Akt/GSK3β signaling in LPS-treated adult mice. *Mol. Neurobiol.* doi: 10.1007/s12035-018-1101-1 [Epub ahead of print].

Le, D. A., Wu, Y., Huang, Z., Matsushita, K., Plesnila, N., Augustinack, J. C., et al. (2002). Caspase activation and neuroprotection in caspase-3 deficient mice after in vivo cerebral ischemia and in vitro oxygen glucose deprivation. *Proc. Natl. Acad. Sci. U.S.A.* 99, 15188–15193. doi: 10.1073/pnas.232473399

Lee, Y. J., Choi, D. Y., Choi, I. S., Kim, K. H., Kim, Y. H., Kim, H. M., et al. (2012). Inhibitory effect of 4-O-methylhonokiol on lipopolysaccharide-induced neuroinflammation, amyloidogenesis and memory impairment via inhibition of nuclear factor-kappaB in vitro and in vivo models. *J. Neuroinflamm.* 9:35. doi: 10.1186/1742-2094-9-35

Lei, X., Chao, H., Zhang, Z., Lv, J., Lis, S., Wei, H., et al. (2015). Neuroprotective effects of quercetin in a mouse model of brain ischemic/reperfusion injury via anti-apoptotic mechanisms based on the Akt pathway. *J. Mol. Med. Rep.* 12, 3688–3696. doi: 10.3892/mmr.2015.3857

Lesjak, M., Beara, I., Simin, N., Pintac, D., Majkic, T., Bekvalac, K., et al. (2018). Antioxidant and anti-inflammatory activities of quercetin and its derivatives. *J. Funct. Foods* 40, 68–75. doi: 10.1016/j.jff.2017.10.047

Li, P., Nijhawan, D., Budihardjo, I., Srinivasula, S. M., Ahmad, M., Alnemri, E. S., et al. (1997). Cytochrome c and dATPdependent formation of Apaf-1/caspase-9 complex initiates an apoptotic protease cascade. *Cell* 91, 479–489. doi: 10.1016/S0092-8674(00)80434-1

Li, Q., and Verma, I. M. (2002). NFKB regulation in the immune system. *Nat. Rev. Immunol.* 2:725. doi: 10.1038/nri910

Liao, Y. R., and Lin, J. Y. (2015). Quercetin intraperitoneal administration ameliorates lipopolysaccharide-induced systemic inflammation in mice. *Life Sci.* 137, 89–97. doi: 10.1016/j.lfs.2015.07.015

Liu, M., Chen, F., Sha, L., Wang, S., Tao, L., Yao, L., et al. (2014). (-)-Epigallocatechin-3-gallate ameliorates learning and memory deficits by adjusting the balance of TrkA/p75NTR signaling in APP/PS1 transgenic mice. *Mol. Neurobiol.* 49, 1350–1363. doi: 10.1007/s12035-013-8608-2

Magalingam, K. B., Radhakrishnan, A. K., and Haleagrahara, N. (2015). Protective mechanisms of flavonoids in Parkinson's disease. *J. Oxid. Med. Cell Longev.* 2015:14560. doi: 10.1155/2015/314560

Matias, I., Buosi, A. S., and Gomes, F. C. (2016). Functions of flavonoids in the central nervous system: astrocytes as targets for natural compounds. *Neurochem. Int.* 95, 85–91. doi: 10.1016/j.neuint.2016.01.009

Matias, I., Diniz, L. P., Buosi, A., Neves, G., Stipursky, J., and Gomes, F. C. A. (2017). Flavonoid hesperidin induces synapse formation and improves memory performance through the astrocytic TGF-β1. *Front. Aging Neurosci.* 9:184. doi: 10.3389/fnagi.2017.00184

Mennen, L. I., Sapinho, D., de Bree, A., Arnault, N., Bertrais, S., Galan, P., et al. (2004). Consumption of foods rich in flavonoids is related to a decreased cardiovascular risk in apparently healthy french women. *J. Nutr.* 134, 923–926. doi: 10.1093/jn/134.4.923

Netea, M. G., van der Meer, J. W., van Deuren, M., and Kullberg, B. J. (2003). Proinflammatory cytokines and sepsis syndrome: not enough, or too much of a good thing? *Trends Immunol.* 24, 254–258. doi: 10.1016/S1471-4906(03)00079-6

O'Banion, M. K., Miller, J. C., Chang, J. W., Kaplan, M. D., and Coleman, P. D. (1996). IL-1 beta induces prostaglandin G/H synthase-2 (cyclooxygenase2) in primary murine astrocyte cultures. *J. Neurochem.* 66, 2532–2540. doi: 10.1046/j.1471-4159.1996.66062532.x

Park, D. J., Shah, F. A., and Koh, P. O. (2018). Quercetin attenuates neuronal cells damage in a middle cerebral artery occlusion animal model. *J. Vet. Med. Sci.* 80, 676–683. doi: 10.1292/jvms.17-0693

Perry, V. H., Newman, T. A., and Cunningham, C. (2003). The impact of systemic infection on the progress of neurodegenerative disease. *Nat. Rev. Neurosci.* 4, 103–112. doi: 10.1038/nrn1032

Pogacnik, L., Pirc, K., Palmela, I., Skrt, M., Kim, K. S., Brites, D., et al. (2016). Potential for brain accessibility and analysis of stability of selected flavonoids in relation to neuroprotection in vitro. *J. Brain Res.* 1651, 17–26. doi: 10.1016/j.brainres.2016.09.020

Prakash, D., Gopinath, K., and Sudhandiran, G. (2013). Fisetin enhances behavioral performances and attenuates reactive gliosis and inflammation during aluminum chloride-induced neurotoxicity. *Neuromol. Med.* 15, 192–208. doi: 10.1007/s12017-8210-1

Prakash, D., and Sudhandiran, G. (2015). Dietary flavonoid fisetin regulates aluminium chloride induced neuronal apoptosis in cortex and hippocampus of mice brain. *J. Nutr. Biochem.* 26, 1527–1539. doi: 10.1016/j.jnutbio.2015.07.017

Qin, L., Wu, X., Block, M. L., Liu, Y., Breese, G. R., Hong, J. S., et al. (2007). Systemic LPS causes chronic neuroinflammation and progressive neurodegeneration. *Glia* 55, 453–462. doi: 10.1002/glia.20467

Rao, Y. K., Fang, S. H., and Tzeng, Y. M. (2005). Inhibitory effects of the flavonoids isolated from *Waltheria indica* on the production of NO, TNF-alpha and IL-12 in activated macrophages. *Biol. Pharm. Bull.* 28, 912–915. doi: 10.1248/bpb.28.912

Rehman, S. U., Ali, T., Ibrar, S. A., and Kim, M. O. (2018). Ferulic acid rescued LPS-induced neurotoxicity via modulation of the TLR4 receptor in the mouse hippocampus. *Mol. Neurobiol.* doi: 10.1007/s12035-018-1280-9 [Epub ahead of print].

Rinwa, P., and Kumar, A. (2013). Quercetin suppress microglial neuroinflammatory response and induce antidepressent-like effect in olfactory bulbectomized rats. *J. Neurosci.* 255, 86–98. doi: 10.1016/j.neuroscience.2013.09.044

Salvemini, D. (1997). Regulation of cyclooxygenase enzymes by nitric oxide. *Cell Mol. Life Sci.* 53, 576–582. doi: 10.1007/s000180050074

Scapagnini, G., Vasto, S., Abraham, N. G., Caruso, C., Zella, D., and Fabio, G. (2011). Modulation of Nrf2/ARE pathway by food polyphenols: a nutritional neuroprotective strategy for cognitive and neurodegenerative disorders. *Mol. Neurobiol.* 44, 192–201. doi: 10.1007/s12035-011-8181-5

Shal, B., Ding, W., Ali, H., Kim, Y. S., and Khan, S. (2018). Anti-neuroinflammatory potential of natural products in attenuation of Alzheimer's disease. *Front. Pharmacol.* 9:548. doi: 10.3389/fphar.2018.00548

Sheng, J. G., Bora, S. H., Xu, G., Borchelt, D. R., Price, D. L., Koliatsos, et al. (2003). Lipopolysaccharide-induced-neuroinflammation increases intracellular accumulation of amyloid precursor protein and amyloid beta peptide in APPswe transgenic mice. *J. Neurobiol. Dis.* 14, 133–145. doi: 10.1016/S0969-9961(03)00069-X

Shimazu, R., Akashi, S., Ogata, H., Nagai, Y., Fukudome, K., Miyake, K., et al. (1999). MD-2, a molecule that confers lipopolysaccharide responsiveness on toll-like receptor 4. *J. Exp. Med.* 189, 1777–1782. doi: 10.1084/jem.189.11.1777

Shveta, N., Rozy, K., and Devinder, K D. (2016). Neuroprotective role of quercetin against arsenic induced oxidative stress in rat brain. *J. Environ. Anal. Toxicol.* 6:359. doi: 10.4172/2161-0525.1000359

Song, S. Y., Jung, Y. Y., Hwang, C. J., Lee, H. P., Sok C. H., Kim, J. H., et al. (2014). Inhibitory effect of ent-Sauchinone on amyloidogenesis via inhibition of STAT3-mediated NF-κB activation in cultured astrocytes and microglial BV-2 cells. *J. Neuroinflamm.* 11:118. doi: 10.1186/1742-2094-11-118

Spencer, J. P. (2008). Flavonoids modulation of brain function? *Br. J. Nutr.* 99(E Suppl 1), ES60–ES77. doi: 10.1017/S0007114508965776

Sriraksa, N., Wattanathorn, J., Muchimapura, S., Tiamkao, S., Brown, K., Chaiswamongkol, K. (2012). Cognitive-enhancing effect of quercetin in a rat model of Parkinson's disease induced by 6-hyrodoxydopamine. *J. Evid. Based Complement. Alternat. Med.* 2012:823206. doi: 10.1155/2012/823206

Tajuddin, N., Moon, K. H., Marshall, S. A., Nixon, K., Naefsey, E. J., Kim, H. Y., et al. (2014). Neuroinflammation and neurodegeneration in adult rat brain from binge ethanol exposure: abrogation by docosahexaenoic acid. *PLoS One* 9:e101223. doi: 10.1371/journal.pone.0101223

Tichauer, J. E., and Eugenín, J. (2010). Aging-dependent changes of microglial cells and the irrelevance for neurodegenerative disorders. *J. Neurochem.* 112, 1099–1114. doi: 10.1111/j.1471-4159.2009.06537.x

Williams, B. L., Hornig, M., Yaddanapudi, K., and Lipkin, W. I. (2008). Hippocampal poly(ADPRibose) polymerase 1 and caspase 3 activationin neonatal bornavirus infection. *J. Virol.* 82, 1748–1758. doi: 10.1128/JVI.020 14-07

Witte, M. E., Geurts, J. J., de Vries, H. E., van der Valk, P., and van Horssen, J. (2010). Mitochondrial dysfunction A potential link between neuroinflammation and neurodegeneration? *Mitochondrion* 10, 411–418. doi: 10.1016/j.mito.2010.05.014

Wyss-Coray, T. and Rogers, J. (2012). Inflammation in Alzheimer disease- a brief review of the basic science and clinical literature. *Cold Spring Harb Perspect Med.* 2:a006346. doi: 10.110/cshperspect

Yamamoto, K., Arakawa, T., Ueda, N., and Yamamoto, S. (1995). Transcriptional roles of nuclear factor kappa B and nuclear factor- IL-6 in the TNF alpha-dependent induction of cyclooxygenase-2 in MC3T3-E1 cells. *J. Biol. Chem.* 270, 31315–31312. doi: 10.1074/jbc.270.52.31315

Yang, T., Kong, B., Gu, J. W., Kuang, Y. Q., Cheng, L., Yang, W. T., et al. (2014). Anti-apoptotic and oxidative roles of quercetin after traumatic brain injury. *Cell Mol. Neurobiol.* 34, 797–804. doi: 10.1007/s10571-014-0070-9

Yang, Y., Liu, X., Wu, T., Zhang, W., Shu, J., He, Y., et al. (2018). Quercetin attenuates AZT-induced neuroinflammation in the CNS. *Sci. Rep.* 8:6194. doi: 10.1038/s41598-018-24618-2

Yao, L. H., Jiang, Y. M., Shi, J., Tomas-Barberan, F. A., Datt, N., Singanusong, R., et al. (2004). Flavonoids in food and their health benefits. *Plant Foods Hum. Nutr.* 59, 113–122. doi: 10.1007/s11130-004-0 049-7

Yao, X., Liu, S., Ding, W., Yue, P., Jiang, Q., Zhao, M., et al. (2017). TLR4 signal ablation attenuated neurological deficits by regulating microglial M1/M2 phenotype after traumatic brain injury in mice. *J. Neuroimmunol.* 310, 38–45. doi: 10.1016/j.jneuroim.2017.06.006

Zhang, Z. J., Cheang, L. C., Wang, M. W., and Lee, S. M. (2011). Quercetin exerts a neuroprotective effect through inhibition of the iNOS/NO system and pro-inflammation gene expression in PC12 cells and in zebrafish. *J. Int. J Mol. Med.* 27, 195–203. doi: 10.3892/ijmm.2010

17

Moringa oleifera Seed Extract Alleviates Scopolamine-Induced Learning and Memory Impairment in Mice

Juan Zhou[1†], Wu-shuang Yang[2†], Da-qin Suo[3†], Ying Li[4], Lu Peng[3], Lan-xi Xu[3], Kai-yue Zeng[3], Tong Ren[3], Ying Wang[4], Yu Zhou[3], Yun Zhao[3], Li-chao Yang[1,3] and Xin Jin[3]**

[1] Department of Obstetrics and Gynecology, The First Affiliated Hospital of Xiamen University, Xiamen University, Xiamen, China, [2] Department of Neurosurgery, Xiamen Hospital of Traditional Chinese Medicine, Xiamen, China, [3] Xiamen Key Laboratory of Chiral Drugs, Medical College, Xiamen University, Xiamen, China, [4] Department of Pharmacy, Xiamen Medical College, Xiamen, China

***Correspondence:**
Li-chao Yang
yanglc116@xmu.edu.cn
Xin Jin
xinjin@xmu.edu.cn

† These authors have contributed equally to this work.

The extract of *Moringa oleifera* seeds has been shown to possess various pharmacological properties. In the present study, we assessed the neuropharmacological effects of 70% ethanolic *M. oleifera* seed extract (MSE) on cognitive impairment caused by scopolamine injection in mice using the passive avoidance and Morris water maze (MWM) tests. MSE (250 or 500 mg/kg) was administered to mice by oral gavage for 7 or 14 days, and cognitive impairment was induced by intraperitoneal injection of scopolamine (4 mg/kg) for 1 or 6 days. Mice that received scopolamine alone showed impaired learning and memory retention and considerably decreased cholinergic system reactivity and neurogenesis in the hippocampus. MSE pretreatment significantly ameliorated scopolamine-induced cognitive impairment and enhanced cholinergic system reactivity and neurogenesis in the hippocampus. Additionally, the protein expressions of phosphorylated Akt, ERK1/2, and CREB in the hippocampus were significantly decreased by scopolamine, but these decreases were reversed by MSE treatment. These results suggest that MSE-induced ameliorative cognitive effects are mediated by enhancement of the cholinergic neurotransmission system and neurogenesis via activation of the Akt, ERK1/2, and CREB signaling pathways. These findings suggest that MSE could be a potent neuropharmacological drug against amnesia, and its mechanism might be modulation of cholinergic activity via the Akt, ERK1/2, and CREB signaling pathways.

Keywords: ***Moringa oleifera*, Alzheimer's disease, scopolamine, acetylcholine, neurogenesis**

INTRODUCTION

Alzheimer's disease (AD) is a neurodegenerative disease characterized by deterioration of cognitive and behavior function due to cholinergic nervous system dysfunction (Scarpini et al., 2003). As primarily observed in patients with AD, decreased cholinergic function in the brain can lead to a decline in memory and cognitive function (Hasselmo, 2006). In clinical studies, a number of cholinergic drugs have been approved to treat or ameliorate AD, and they exert therapeutic effects by preventing acetylcholine (ACh) insufficiency and consequently increasing ACh levels in the brain (Drever et al., 2007). In fact, acetylcholinesterase (AChE) inhibitors are the most common class drugs for AD, such as galantamine, rivastigmine, and donepezil, which temporarily enhance the availability of ACh at cholinergic synapses (Lanctot et al., 2009). However, the number of drugs approved for the treatment of AD patients with cognitive impairment is limited due to their side effects, which include pain, nausea and hepatotoxicity (Lahiri et al., 2003). Therefore, an alternative treatment strategy for AD patients is required.

Scopolamine is a tropane alkaloid drug that produces competitive antagonism at muscarinic acetylcholine receptors (mAChRs) by interfering with cholinergic transmission, leading to impairing learning and short-term memory in rodents and humans (Iversen, 1997). Therefore, scopolamine administration is used in animals as an experimental model of the memory deficits and cognitive impairment observed in AD. This dementia model has been used to screen for drugs that have potential therapeutic value in AD-type dementia patients (Bartus et al., 1982). Scopolamine administration not only induces dysregulation of the cholinergic system and memory circuits in the brain but also decreases the expression of cAMP-response element binding protein (CREB) and brain-derived neurotrophic factor (BDNF) in the central nervous system (CNS). BDNF is responsible for synaptic plasticity and memory performance and is coupled to CREB activation. CREB is closely related to hippocampal learning and memory (Tyler et al., 2002). Moreover, hippocampal BDNF and CREB play vital roles in pathological conditions and neurodegenerative diseases such as AD. Therefore, the BDNF/CREB pathway may act as a novel therapeutic target to treat cognitive deficits.

Moringa oleifera (*M. oleifera*) is one of the Moringaceae (Abdull Razis et al., 2014). *M. oleifera*, by virtue of its high nutritional as well as ethno-medical values, has gained profound interest both in nutrition and medicinal research (Al-Malki and El Rabey, 2015). The leaves, roots, seeds, bark, fruits, flowers, and stem of *M. oleifera* have been shown to exert various pharmacological effects. Additionally, aqueous and ethanolic *M. oleifera* seed extract (MSE) has been shown to possess various pharmacological and commercial utility, such as metal antidote, anti-oxidant, anti-asthmatic, anti-arthritic, anti-bacterial, anti-tumor, and hepatoprotective effects (Abdull Razis et al., 2014). However, few reports have addressed the benefits of ethanolic MSE in diseases involving brain dysfunction. To elucidate the potential effects of MSE on cognitive function and the cholinergic system, we assessed learning and memory retention using the passive avoidance and Morris water maze (MWM) tests and evaluated cholinergic markers (ACh, AChE, and ChAT) in mice exposed to scopolamine.

MATERIALS AND METHODS

Animals

Male ICR mice (6 weeks old, 25–30 g) were purchased from Beijing Vita River Experimental Animal Co. (Beijing, China) and housed under a 12/12 h dark/light cycle and specific pathogen-free (SPF) conditions. The experimental protocols were approved by the Animal Care and Use Committee of the Medical College of Xiamen University in compliance with the NIH Guide for the Care and Use of Laboratory Animals (NIH Publications No. 80-23).

Drug Preparation

Dry *M. oleifera* seeds were purchased from LuYan Pharma Co. (Fujian Province, China). Fifty grams of dried *M. oleifera* seed were extracted with 0.5 L of 70% ethanol at 85°C for 2 h, and the suspension was filtered using 300-mesh 50-mm filter paper (Advantec, Toyo Roshi Kaisha, Tokyo, Japan). Filtrate was concentrated in a rotary evaporator and lyophilized. The final yield of the extract was stored at −80°C.

Drug Administration

Animals were randomly assigned to the following groups of 12 mice each: control (saline), scopolamine (4 mg/kg) plus saline (scopolamine-treated control), scopolamine plus MSE (250 mg/kg), and scopolamine plus MSE (500 mg/kg). MSE and scopolamine were dissolved in sterile saline containing 10% Tween-80. MSE was administered by oral gavage (*p.o.*) once a day for 7 or 14 consecutive days, according to the different treatment conditions listed in **Supplementary Figure S1**, and the mice in the control and scopolamine-treated (*i.p.*) groups were treated with the same volume of vehicle for the same duration. Behavioral tasks were performed 24 h after MSE administration daily for 7 days.

Step-Down Test

The bottom of the apparatus consisted of a cupreous grid, and a platform made of rubber was placed in the center of the apparatus. The mouse was placed on the apparatus without electric shock for 3 min to adapt to the environment before the trial. The mouse was subsequently placed on the platform, and the cupreous bottom received an intermittent electric shock. The mouse was shocked if it stepped down from the platform to the cupreous bottom; it would then step on the platform again. The number of errors (i.e., number of times the mouse stepped onto the platform and received an electric shock) and latency (i.e., time until the mouse first stepped down onto the cupreous bottom with four paws) was recorded in the training phase. Twenty-four hours after training, the retention task was administered to the mouse: it was placed on the platform, and the latency and the number of errors within 300 s were recorded as measures of learning.

Step-Through Test

The passive avoidance step-through task was also used to measure associative memory performance. The equipment for this test comprised 2 equal compartments (20 cm × 20 cm × 20 cm) separated by a grid door (5 cm × 5 cm). For the acquisition trial, mice were initially placed in the illuminated compartment, and the door between the two compartments was opened 20 s later. The time taken for a mouse to enter the dark compartment (step-through latency) was recorded. Upon entering the dark compartment, the door was closed, and an electrical foot shock (0.5 mA for 5 s) was delivered through the stainless-steel rods. On the second day, the same procedure was followed. The mice were again placed in the illuminated compartment to test retention. The step-through latency was measured as a measure of retention (Worms et al., 1989). If the mouse did not enter the dark compartment within 300 s, it was assumed that the mouse had remembered the single acquisition trial experience.

Morris Water Maze Test

The MWM was used to test spatial learning and memory (Morris et al., 1982) and was begun from day 8 to day 14 after MSE treatment. For acquisition trial, every mouse was trained four trials per day from days 9 to 13 after MSE administration. Mice were slightly placed into the water from the wall of the pool. The escape latency of finding the hidden platform was recorded during each acquisition trial. The whole time was 90 s. On the last day (day 14), all mice were subjected to probe test without platform, and were recorded for 90 s. The time spent in the target quadrant and the number crossed the platform position was measured for spatial memory.

ACh and AChE Estimation by Assay Kits

Mice were anesthetized with chloral hydrate (0.4 ml/kg), and their brains were removed. The hippocampus was taken out and was divided into two pieces. One piece was rapidly frozen in liquid nitrogen and stored at −80°C for subsequent Western blot analysis; the second piece was used to assess ACh and AChE using an assay quantification kit (Nanjing Jiancheng Biological Instrument Company, China). Half of the hippocampus was homogenized with assay buffer (0.1 g/0.9 ml) and centrifuged at 3200 r/min for 10 min; the supernatant was then removed. The supernatant was used for estimating ACh and AChE content according to the instructions for the acetylcholine assay kit.

Immunohistochemistry and Cell Counting

Mice were anesthetized with chloral hydrate and perfused transcardially with ice-cold saline followed by perfusion with 4% paraformaldehyde 24 h after reperfusion. The brains were removed and post-fixed overnight for 24 h in paraformaldehyde; they were then coronally sectioned (30 μm) using a vibrating microtome (Leica, Wetzlar, Germany). The sections were incubated in PBS containing 0.5% Triton X-100 and 10% normal goat serum for 1 h at room temperature, following by incubation with rat monoclonal anti-BrdU (1:400; Abcam, Cambridge, United Kingdom) at 4°C overnight. After several PBS rinses, sections were incubated with Alexa Fluor 594 donkey anti-rat IgG (1:200; Invitrogen, Carlsbad, CA, United States).

An experimenter (L-cY) coded all slides from the experiments before quantitative analysis. All BrdU-labeled cells in the DG of injured hemisphere were counted in each section by another experimenter (D-qS) blinded to the study coding. The total number of BrdU-labeled cells per section was determined and multiplied by 10 to obtain the total number of cells per DG using fluorescence confocal microscopy (EX61; Olympus, Tokyo, Japan).

Western Blot Analysis

Brain samples were obtained from the hippocampal tissue of mice 24 h after the MWM test. Hippocampal tissue was homogenized with lysis buffer (50 nM/L NaCl, 1 mM/L EDTA, 1% Triton X-100, 0.5% SDS, 0.5% sodium deoxycholate, and 20 mM/L Tris HCl; pH 7.5) and centrifuged at 15,000 × *g* for 20 min. Protein samples (50 μg) per lane were run on polyacrylamide gel, transferred to a PVDF membrane (Millipore, Billerica), and blocked with 5% milk solution (non-fat dry milk in PBST) for 2 h. The membrane was incubated at 4°C overnight with the following specific antibodies: rabbit polyclonal anti-ChAT (1:1000; Cell Signaling Technology, Boston, MA, United States), phospho-Akt (1:1000; Cell Signaling Technology), Akt (1:1000; Cell Signaling Technology), phospho-CREB (1:1000; Cell Signaling Technology), CREB (1:1000; Cell Signaling Technology), ERK1/2 (1:1000, Cell Signaling Technology), phospho-ERK1/2 (Thr202/Thr204) (1:1000, Cell Signaling Technology), BDNF (1:1000, Cell Signaling Technology), NR1 (1:1000, Cell Signaling Technology), NR2B (1:1000, Cell Signaling Technology), GAP-43 (1:1000, Cell Signaling Technology), and mouse monoclonal anti-β-actin (1:10000; Sigma). After washing with TBST five times, the membranes were then incubated with the corresponding conjugated anti-rabbit IgG (1:10000; Cell Signaling Technology) at room temperature for 1 h. Immunoreactive proteins were quantified using an enhanced chemiluminescence (ECL) kit (Millipore, Billerica), and the relative density of the protein bands was scanned using an LAS 4000 Fujifilm imaging system (Fujifilm, Tokyo, Japan) and analyzed by densitometric evaluation using Quantity-One software (Bio-Rad Hercules, CA, United States).

Statistical Analysis

All data are expressed as the mean ± SEM. We performed the statistical assay using two-way analysis of variance (ANOVA) and one-way ANOVA. The differences between the groups were analyzed by Bonferroni's *post hoc* test (Prism 5 for Windows, GraphPad Software, Inc., United States). $P < 0.05$ was considered statistically significant.

RESULTS

Effects of MSE on Scopolamine-Induced Memory Impairment in the Step-Down Avoidance Test

We assessed the effects of MSE on scopolamine-induced cognitive dysfunction using the step-through passive avoidance task. Compared with control mice, mice treated with scopolamine exhibited reduced escape latencies (**Figure 1A**) and increased errors (**Figure 1B**). In contrast, escape latencies of animals pretreated with 500 mg/kg of MSE for 7 days were significantly longer than those of scopolamine-treated animals

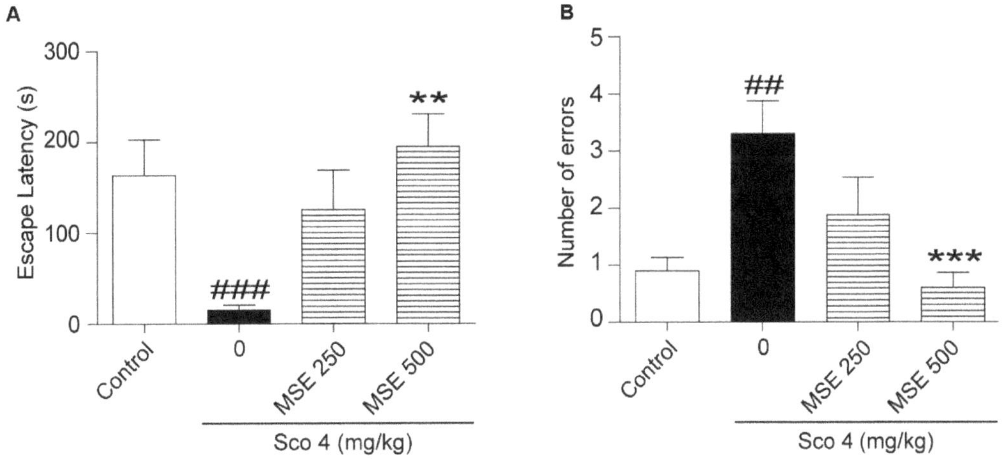

FIGURE 1 | Effects of *Moringa oleifera* seed extract (MSE) on scopolamine-induced memory impairments on the step-down test. MSE (250, or 500 mg/kg, *p.o.*) or the same volume of vehicle (10% Tween 80 solution) was administered to mice by oral gavage for 7 days before the acquisition trial. Memory impairment was induced by scopolamine (4 mg/kg, *i.p.*) 30 min before the acquisition trial. Twenty-four hours after the acquisition trial, a retention trial was conducted for 300 s. Escape latency **(A)** and number of errors **(B)** of mice were detected after training. Data are expressed as the means ± SEM. $N = 12$ for each group. $^{\#\#}P < 0.01$, $^{\#\#\#}P < 0.001$ vs. control group, $^{**}P < 0.01$, $^{***}P < 0.001$ vs. scopolamine+vehicle group.

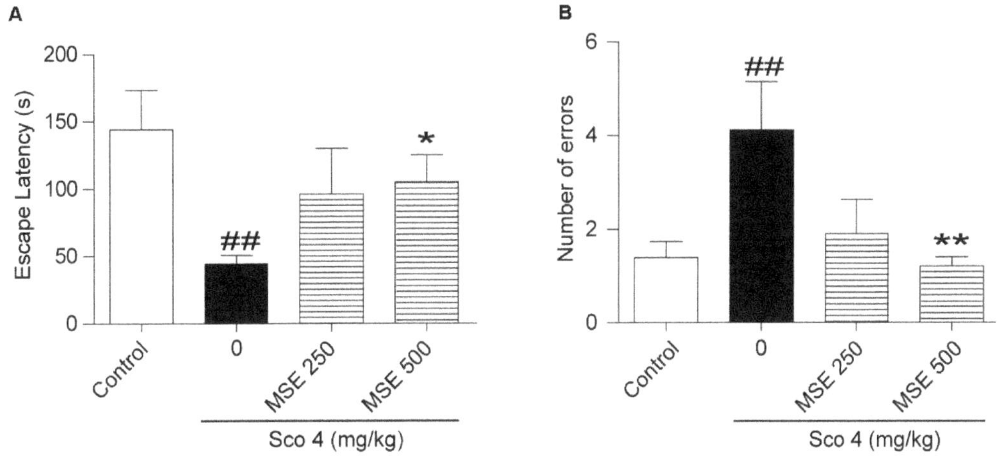

FIGURE 2 | Effects of MSE on scopolamine-induced memory impairments on the step-through test. MSE (250, or 500 mg/kg, *p.o.*), or the same volume of vehicle (10% Tween 80 solution) was administered to mice by oral gavage for 7 days before the acquisition trial. Memory impairment was induced by scopolamine (4 mg/kg, *i.p.*) 30 min before the acquisition trial. Twenty-four hours after the acquisition trial, a retention trial was conducted for 300 s. Escape latency **(A)** and number of errors **(B)** of mice were detected after training. Data are expressed as the means ± SEM. $N = 12$ for each group. $^{\#\#}P < 0.01$ vs. control group, $^{*}P < 0.05$, $^{**}P < 0.001$ vs. scopolamine+vehicle group.

(**Figure 1A**), but there was no significant difference between the 250 mg/kg MSE and scopolamine groups (**Figure 1A**). Meanwhile, the number of errors in the 500 mg/kg MSE group was lower than that in the scopolamine group (**Figure 1B**).

Effects of MSE on Scopolamine-Induced Memory Impairment in the Step-Through Avoidance Test

After the step-down test, we detected the effects of MSE on scopolamine-induced cognitive impairment by the step-through test. As shown in **Figure 2**, escape latencies of animals treated with scopolamine were decreased, and error frequency was increased in comparison with the control group (**Figures 2A,B**). In contrast, the effect of scopolamine on escape latencies and error frequency was reversed by 500 mg/kg of MSE (**Figures 2A,B**; $P < 0.05$, $P < 0.01$, respectively). However, 250 mg/kg of MSE had no effect on scopolamine-induced memory impairment (**Figures 2A,B**).

Effects of MSE on Scopolamine-Induced Memory Impairment in the Morris Water Maze Test

To further detect the influence of MSE on scopolamine-induced cognitive impairment, we exposed animals to the water maze task after 14 days of MSE treatment. Spatial learning was evaluated by the time required to find the hidden platform (escape latency). **Figure 3A** illustrates swim paths of animals on the sixth day of the water maze test. Scopolamine-treated mice spent nearly the same amount of time in the different quadrants of the pool, and swimming traces were uniformly distributed among the four zones. However, the swimming traces of the control group and scopolamine-treated mice that also received 500 mg/kg MSE were concentrated in the target zone, where the platform had been set. On day 13, group comparisons revealed that mice in the scopolamine-induced group displayed a longer latency in finding the platform than did animals in the control group (**Figure 3B**). These results indicated that scopolamine resulted in a significant impairment of cognitive acquisition and confirmed the usefulness of this model in detecting MSE effects on memory ability. After treatment with 500 mg/kg MSE, escape latency was markedly reduced on day 5 (**Figure 3B**). These data showed that pretreatment with 500 mg/kg MSE effectively ameliorated spatial learning across the 5-day training period. There were no significant differences between the 250 mg/kg MSE-treated and scopolamine-impaired mice in escape latency (**Figure 3B**). The platform was removed in the spatial probe trial, and scopolamine-impaired mice crossed the platform position less frequently and spent less time searching in the target quadrant than did control mice (**Figures 3C,D**). Compared with the scopolamine-impaired group, the 500 mg/kg MSE group exhibited obviously increased time in the target quadrant and more frequent crossing of the platform position (**Figures 3C,D**). Therefore, MSE treatment ameliorates scopolamine-induced spatial memory impairments. We additionally measured the swimming speed of all mice and found no differences, suggesting that these animals have normal motor function (data not shown).

Effects of MSE on ACh and AChE Levels and ChAT Protein Expression in the Hippocampi of Scopolamine-Impaired Mice

The central cholinergic system is well known to play a major role in cognitive function, which is strongly modulated by the neurotransmitter ACh. Therefore, samples of hippocampus taken from mice were used for evaluation of cholinergic system reactivity after MWM test. Scopolamine produced a significant decrease of ACh content in the hippocampus (**Figure 4A**). Moreover, pretreatment with 500 mg/kg MSE significantly reversed the decrease in ACh levels induced by scopolamine (**Figure 4A**). Compared with the control group, the scopolamine-treated group showed significant enhancement of AChE activity in hippocampal tissue (**Figure 4B**), while pretreatment with 500 mg/kg MSE completely inhibited the hyperactivation of AChE induced by scopolamine (**Figure 4B**). ChAT, a key enzyme modulating ACh content in brain, is considered the definitive

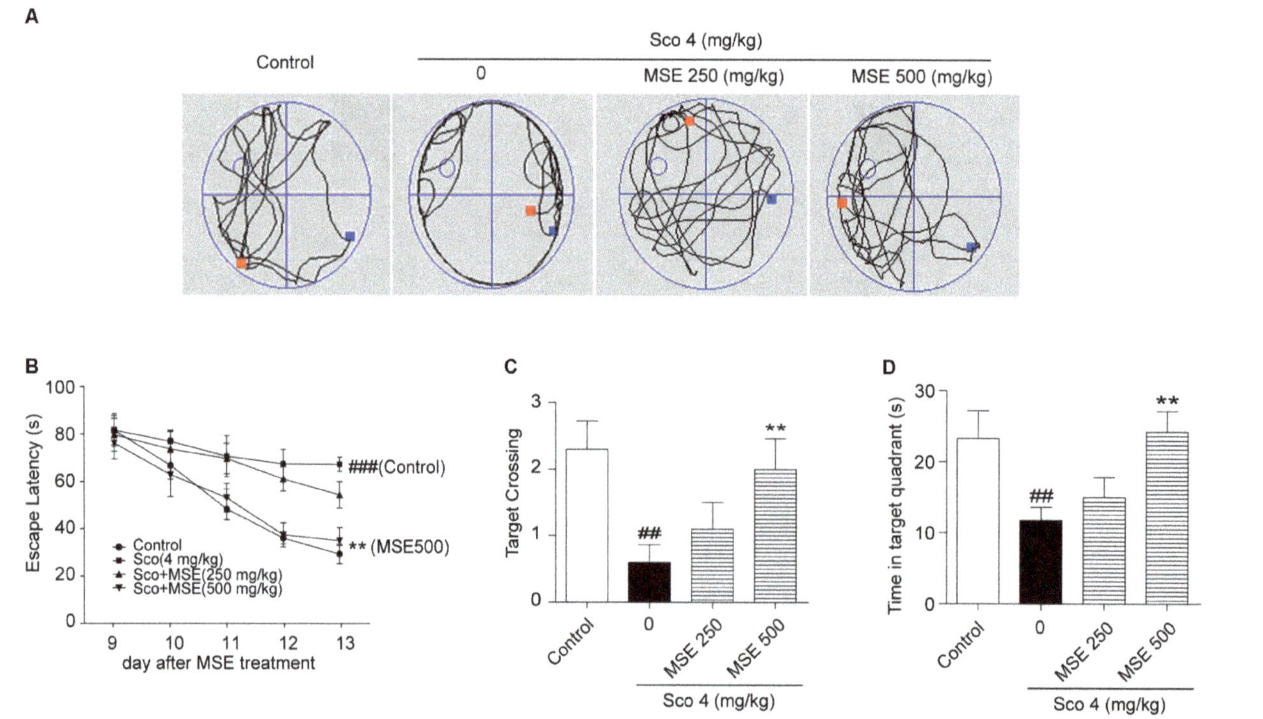

FIGURE 3 | *Moringa oleifera* seed extract ameliorated scopolamine-induced spatial cognitive deficits on the Morris water maze (MWM) test. MSE (250 or 500 mg/kg) was administered to mice by oral gavage for 14 days, and memory impairment was induced by intraperitoneal injection of scopolamine (4 mg/kg) for 6 days. **(A)** Representative swimming traces on the spatial probe trial for each group. **(B)** Escape latency in the hidden platform trials. **(C,D)** The number of target platform crossings and time spent in the target quadrant during spatial probe trials. Data are expressed as the means ± SEM. $N = 12$ for each group. $^{\#\#}P < 0.01$, $^{\#\#\#}P < 0.001$ vs. control group, $^{**}P < 0.01$ vs. scopolamine+vehicle group.

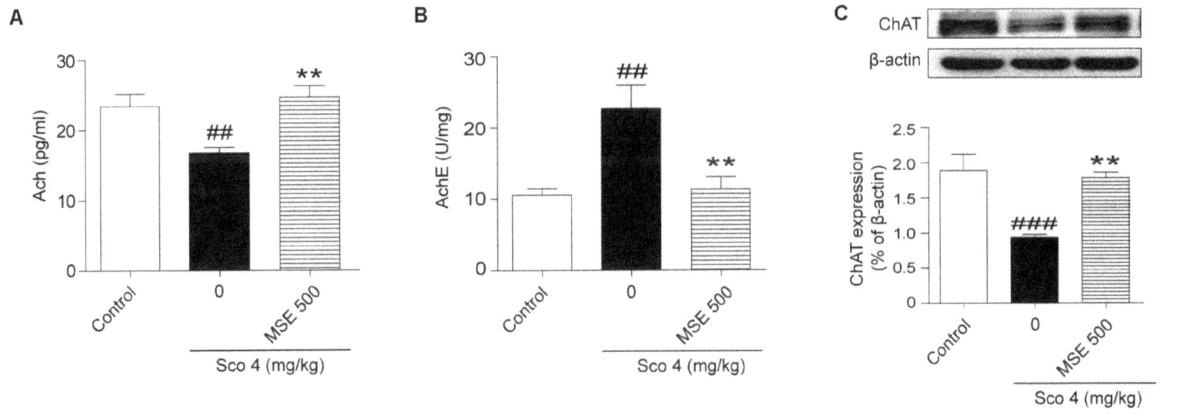

FIGURE 4 | Effects of MSE (500 mg/kg) on acetylcholine (ACh) levels, acetylcholinesterase (AChE) activity and ChAT expression in the hippocampi of scopolamine-impaired mice. Mice were decapitated immediately after the MWM test, and the hippocampi were removed to determine ACh level, AChE activity, and ChAT expression. **(A,B)** Densitometry analysis of ACh and ChAT protein levels and **(C)** representative western blot gel in the hippocampus. Quantified results were normalized to β-actin expression. Data are presented as the means ± SEM (n = 12). $^{\#\#}P < 0.01$, $^{\#\#\#}P < 0.001$ vs. control group, $^{**}P < 0.01$ vs. scopolamine +vehicle group.

marker of central cholinergic function. The scopolamine-treated group showed significantly less ChAT level in the hippocampus than did the control group (**Figure 4C**). However, pretreatment with 500 mg/kg MSE significantly increased ChAT expression (**Figure 4C**).

Effects of MSE on Neurogenesis and Synaptic Plasticity in the Hippocampus

Scopolamine injection significantly suppressed the birth of new neural precursor cells in the hippocampal DG region, particularly in the SGZ, as evidenced by reduced BrdU staining (**Figure 5A-a**). These effects in the 500 mg/kg MSE pretreatment group were significantly reversed compared with those in the scopolamine-impaired group (**Figure 5A-b**). In the hippocampus, NR1, NR2B, and GAP-43 levels in scopolamine-treated mice were significantly lower than in the control group (**Figures 5B-a–c**). In contrast, the 500 mg/kg MSE group had significantly higher NR1, NR2B and GAP-43 protein levels in the hippocampus than did the scopolamine group (**Figures 5B-a–c**).

Effects of MSE on Akt, ERK1/2, and CREB Signaling Pathways in Scopolamine-Impaired Mice

Compared with the control group, the scopolamine-treated group exhibited significant down-regulation of the phosphorylation levels of Akt at Ser473 and ERK1/2 at Thr202/Thr204 (**Figures 6A-a,B-a**). Compared with the scopolamine-treated group, 500 mg/kg MSE treatment significantly ameliorated these effects (**Figures 6A-a,B-a**). We did not observe a significant difference in total Akt or ERK1/2 levels among the groups (**Figures 6A-b,B-b**). Compared with control treatment, scopolamine treatment produced a robust decrease in the phosphorylation level of CREB (Ser133) and expression of BDNF in the hippocampus (**Figures 6C-a,C-c**). In contrast, compared with scopolamine treatment, pretreatment with 500 mg/kg MSE markedly increased phosphor-CREB (Ser133) and BDNF level (**Figures 6C-a,C-c**). Total CREB level did not differ between the groups (**Figure 6C-b**).

DISCUSSION

In the present study, we used scopolamine to investigate the effects of MSE on cognitive impairment. Our results demonstrated that MSE is able to protect mice from scopolamine-induced learning and memory dysfunction as assessed by the passive avoidance and MWM tests. MSE pretreatment significantly enhanced cholinergic system reactivity and neurogenesis in the hippocampus. Additionally, the levels of phosphorylated Akt, ERK1/2, and CREB in the hippocampus were significantly decreased by scopolamine, and these decreases were prevented by MSE treatment.

The effect of MSE on cognitive function in animal models of scopolamine-induced impairment was detected using the passive avoidance and MWM tests. These two behavioral tests are both hippocampus-dependent tasks. The passive avoidance task is a fear-motivated test to assess hippocampus-dependent associative memory function in rodents (Izquierdo et al., 2006). The MWM test is commonly used to assess hippocampus-dependent spatial memory (Vorhees and Williams, 2006). Therefore, the effects of MSE on associative and spatial learning and memory functions were evaluated following scopolamine-induced impairment. We performed a pilot dose-response experiment with MSE (250 or 500 mg/kg) and found that 500 mg/kg was effective in improving scopolamine-induced amnesic effects, including memory deficits on the passive avoidance and MWM tests. These data suggest that MSE ameliorates scopolamine-induced impairments on different types of memory tests. Therefore, the present results support the utility of MSE in models of memory impairment, such as the associative and spatial learning and memory deficits.

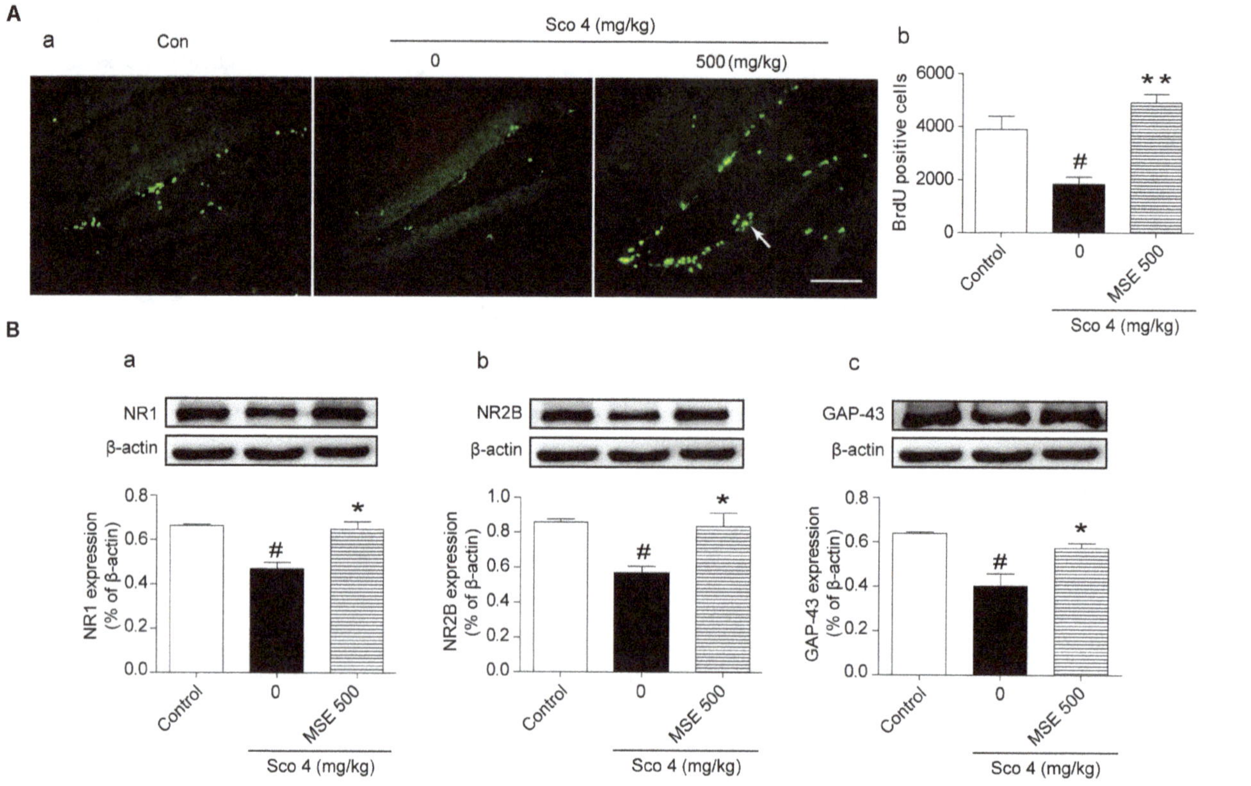

FIGURE 5 | *Moringa oleifera* seed extract (500 mg/kg) promoted proliferation of neural precursor cells in the DG of the hippocampus. Mice were decapitated immediately after the MWM test, and hippocampal BrdU immunoreactive cells were examined using immunofluorescence. **(A-a)** Representative fluorescence images of BrdU immunoreactive cells (white arrow) on day 14 after MSE pretreatment. **(A-b)** Quantitative analysis of BrdU positive cells on day 14 after MSE pretreatment. **(B)** Western blots of NR1 **(B-a)**, NR2B **(B-b)**, GAP-43 **(B-c)** in the hippocampus on day 14 after MSE pretreatment. Quantified results were normalized to β-actin expression. The values are represented as the means ± SEM. $N = 12$ mice were used for immunohistochemistry, and $n = 5$ were used for western blot per group. $^{\#}P < 0.05$ vs. control group, $^{*}P < 0.05$, $^{**}P < 0.01$ vs. scopolamine+vehicle group. Bar = 50 μm.

The cholinergic system plays a vital role in learning and memory. Inhibition of cholinergic transmission may be responsible, at least in part, for cognitive impairments in models of scopolamine-induced amnesia (Hirokawa et al., 1996). In the present study, we used scopolamine to detect the effects of MSE in the cholinergic system. ACh is an essential neurotransmitter related to learning and memory processes, and strategies to enhance ACh level can improve cognitive function (Pepeu and Giovannini, 2004). ACh is unique among the classical neurotransmitters because its synaptic action is terminated by ACh hydrolysis by AChE (Ballard et al., 2005). However, excessive AChE activity results in constant ACh deficiency and cognitive deficits (Deak et al., 2016). Therefore, inhibition of AChE activity serves as a therapeutic target for the treatment of senile dementia, AD and Parkinson's disease. ChAT is responsible for ACh biosynthesis and is essential for cholinergic neurotransmission in the CNS (Giacobini, 2002). The expression and activation of AChE and ChAT regulate the dynamic level of ACh in cholinergic synapses in the AD brain (Giacobini, 2002). We found that repeated scopolamine administration caused a reduction in ACh levels and ChAT expression as well as an increase in AChE activity in the hippocampus. However, MSE pretreatment significantly elevated ACh levels and ChAT expression and inhibit AChE activity in hippocampal tissues of the scopolamine-treated mice. These findings indicate that the anti-amnesic effects of MSE may be due to improvement of cholinergic neurotransmission system.

Adult hippocampal neurogenesis plays a vital role in hippocampal cognitive function (Vivar, 2015). BrdU is an analog of thymidine and can be incorporated into the DNA of cells during the S phase. Thus, it has been used to check cell proliferation (Doeppner et al., 2009). In the present study, we found that MSE treatment for 2 weeks by oral administration clearly increased the quantity of BrdU^{+} cells in the DG of the hippocampus, suggesting that MSE promoted basal neurogenesis in scopolamine-impaired mice. Learning and memory are not only closely related to cholinergic neurotransmission but also related to glutamatergic neurotransmission, which involves the *N*-methyl-D-aspartate (NMDA) receptor in the CNS (Whitlock et al., 2006). The effect of NMDA receptor signaling on learning and memory in the CNS is well established (Rao and Finkbeiner, 2007). Enhanced activation of NMDA receptor signaling results in facilitation of learning and memory in various behavioral tests (Shimizu et al., 2000). To investigate whether NMDA receptor signaling is involved in the effects of MSE on cognitive function, we evaluated the expression of

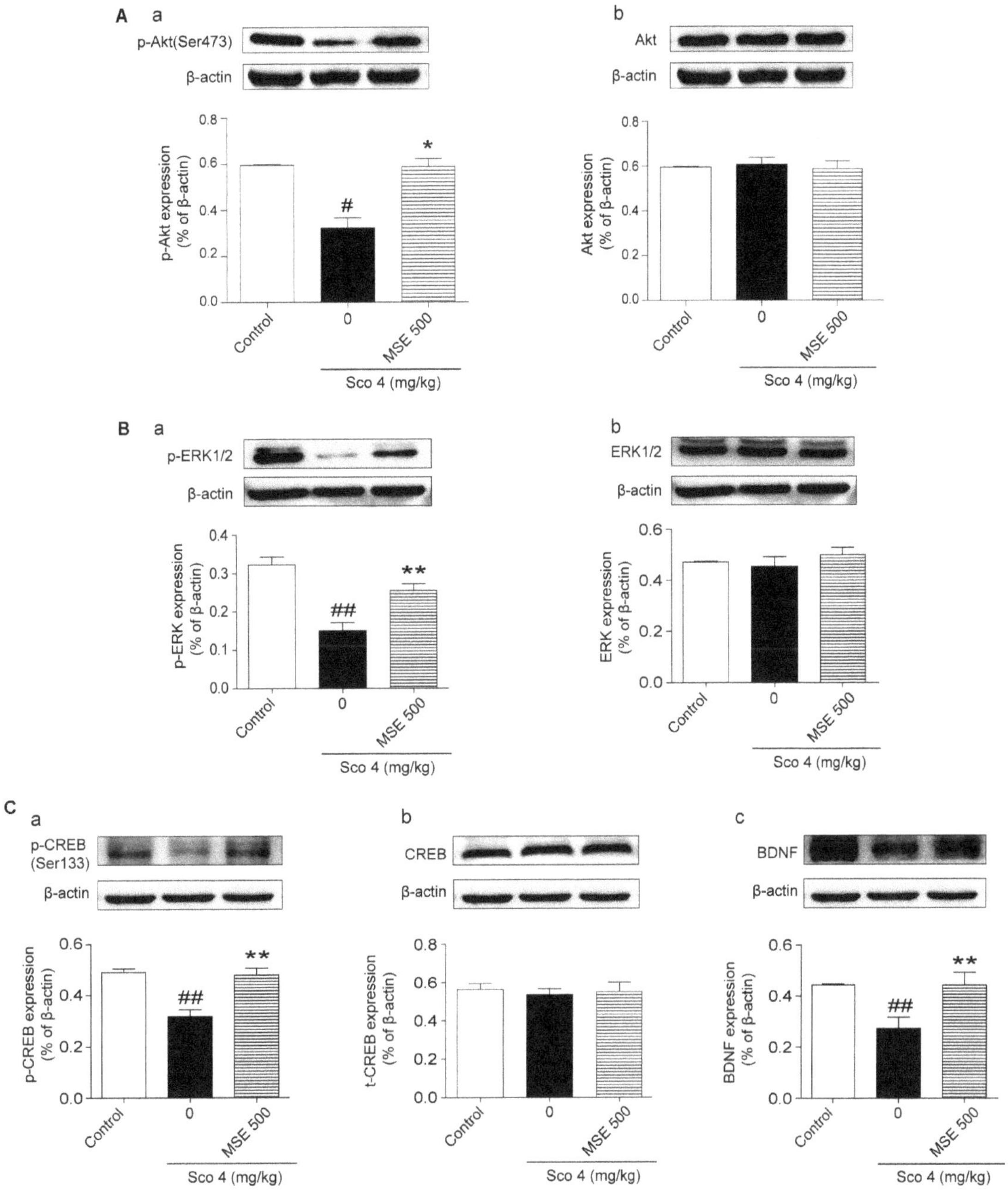

FIGURE 6 | *Moringa oleifera* seed extract (500 mg/kg) treatment increased the Akt, ERK1/2 and CREB signaling pathways. Western blots of phosphor-Akt **(A-a)**, total Akt **(A-b)**, phosphor-ERK1/2 **(B-a)** and total ERK1/2 **(B-b)**, phosphor-CREB **(C-a)**, total CREB **(C-b)**, and BDNF **(C-c)** in the hippocampus 14 days after MSE pretreatment. Quantified results were normalized to β-actin expression. The values are represented as the means ± SEM. $N = 5$ for each group. $^{\#}P < 0.05$, $^{\#\#}P < 0.01$ vs. control group, $^{*}P < 0.05$, $^{**}P < 0.01$ vs. scopolamine+vehicle group.

NR1 and NR2B using Western blots. Our results showed that MSE treatment significantly increased the expression of both NR1 and NR2B, suggesting that NMDA receptor signaling may be implicated in the beneficial effects of MSE on cognitive dysfunction. In particular, the NMDA receptor plays a vital role in synaptic plasticity, which has been implicated in learning and memory (Nakanishi, 1992). To better understand the effects of MSE on cognitive deficits in scopolamine-treated mice, we assessed the effects of MSE pretreatment on synaptic plasticity. GAP-43 is an intracellular growth protein that plays a vital role in the regulation of growth cone guidance, synaptic plasticity and neurite outgrowth (Aigner et al., 1995). Our results demonstrate a significant decrease in GAP-43 levels in hippocampal tissue after scopolamine treatment. However, MSE pretreatment significantly increased expression of GAP-43. Thus, the effect of MSE on cognitive functional recovery may be

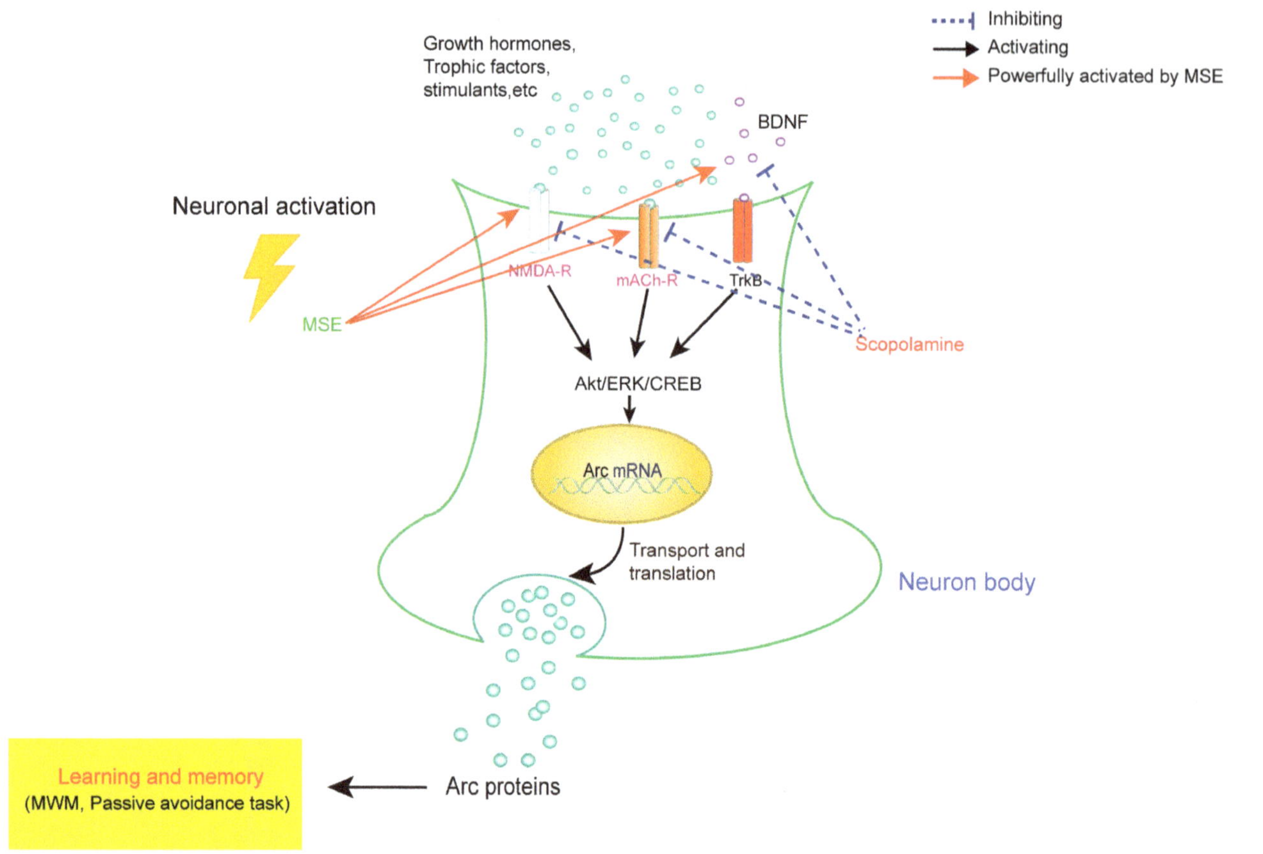

FIGURE 7 | Model for correlating the modulation of learning and memory with MSE-mediated changes in the scopolamine-induced amnesic mouse brain. In amnesic mice, MSE may promote cholinergic system reactivity through activation of the Akt, ERK1/2, and CREB signaling pathways.

attributable to MSE-induced neurogenesis and synaptic plasticity in the hippocampus.

The activation of mAChRs by ACh is known to induce the elevation of intracellular calcium levels, phosphoinositol turnover and activation of several kinases such as protein kinase A (PKA), protein kinase B (Akt), and ERK1/2(Bonner et al., 1987; Felder, 1995; Rosenblum et al., 2000). Akt activation leads to expression of learning-related proteins. Akt has been reported to play a vital role in synaptic plasticity. Inhibition of Akt activation causes impairments in fear-related learning, passive avoidance learning and spatial learning (Barros et al., 2001). ERK1/2, another signaling pathway, is involved in learning and memory (Giovannini, 2006). Because Akt and ERK1/2 are related to learning and memory processes, agents that affect activation of Akt and ERK1/2 may have potential benefits for the treatment of AD. To evaluate molecular mechanisms of MSE on improving cognitive functions, we measured phosphorylation levels of Akt and ERK1/2 in the hippocampus after MSE pretreatment. Our data showed that MSE pretreatment reversed the inhibition of Akt and ERK1/2 activation induced by scopolamine injection, suggesting that the cognitive improvements of MSE may be related to mitigation of scopolamine-induced Akt and ERK1/2 inactivation. CREB is a downstream nuclear factor of PKA and is essential for synaptic plasticity and memory in the CNS. Previous studies have shown that activation of CREB ameliorates cognitive impairment via the cholinergic system (Kotani et al., 2006). BDNF is known to improve learning function and neurogenesis via activation of CREB signaling (Bimonte-Nelson et al., 2008). To further evaluate the molecular mechanisms of MSE on learning and memory function, the effects of MSE on CREB activation and BDNF expression in the hippocampus were assessed. In accordance with previous studies (Kotani et al., 2008; Joh et al., 2012; Kim et al., 2013), our results showed that the phosphorylation level of CREB and the expression of BDNF in the hippocampus were inhibited by treatment with scopolamine. However, these changes were reversed by MSE pretreatment. Taken together, our results suggest that the beneficial cognitive effects of MSE may be related to activation of the Akt, ERK1/2, and CREB signaling pathways.

A previous report indicated that MSE extract primarily comprises either hydrocarbons or long chain polyunsaturated fatty acids and their derivatives, including polyunsaturated fatty acids (PUFAs) (Al-Asmari et al., 2015). Supplementation of PUFAs increases synaptic plasticity in the hippocampus and improves cognitive function (Das, 2008; Bazinet and Laye, 2014). The ability of MSE to improve learning and memory may be associated with PUFAs. However, determining which ingredients in MSE promote learning and memory function requires further experimentation.

CONCLUSION

As summarized in **Figure 7**, our data demonstrate that MSE has an anti-amnesic effect, which could be mediated by cholinergic activity, hippocampal neurogenesis and the Akt/ERK1/2/CREB signaling pathways. These findings suggest that the *M. oleifera* seed may be a promising treatment for patients with neurodegenerative disorders. Further studies should aim to confirm these neuroprotective effects and their corresponding mechanisms using active compounds of *M. oleifera* seed.

AUTHOR CONTRIBUTIONS

L-cY and XJ conceived and designed the experiments. JZ, W-sY, YL, LP, K-yZ, YW, and TR performed the experiments. YuZ and YunZ analyzed the data. JZ, W-sY, and D-qS wrote the paper. All authors reviewed and gave final approval.

FUNDING

We thank the Xiamen City Joint Research Project of Major Disease (3502Z20159018) for financially supporting this work.

SUPPLEMENTARY MATERIAL

FIGURE S1 | Experimental design and schedule. In experiment 1, mice were orally pretreated with *Moringa oleifera* seed extract (MSE) (250 or 500 mg/kg) for 7 days, and scopolamine (4 mg/kg) was injected intraperitoneally 30 min before the step-down test on day 8. Twenty-four hours after the acquisition trial, a retention trial was conducted for 300 s. In experiment 2, mice were orally pretreated with MSE (250 or 500 mg/kg) for 7 days, and scopolamine (4 mg/kg) was injected intraperitoneally 30 min before the step-through test on day 8. Twenty-four hours after the acquisition trial, a retention trial was conducted for 300 s. In experiment 3, MSE (250 or 500 mg/kg) was administered to mice by oral gavage for 14 days (days 1–14), and memory impairment was induced by intraperitoneal injection of scopolamine (4 mg/kg) for 6 days (days 9–14). BrdU (50 mg/kg, *i.p.*) was given twice daily during days 1–7. BrdU immunohistochemistry was performed on day 14 after MSE pretreatment.

REFERENCES

Abdull Razis, A. F., Ibrahim, M. D., and Kntayya, S. B. (2014). Health benefits of *Moringa oleifera*. *Asian Pac. J. Cancer Prev.* 15, 8571–8576. doi: 10.7314/APJCP.2014.15.20.8571

Aigner, L., Arber, S., Kapfhammer, J. P., Laux, T., Schneider, C., Botteri, F., et al. (1995). Overexpression of the neural growth-associated protein GAP-43 induces nerve sprouting in the adult nervous system of transgenic mice. *Cell* 83, 269–278. doi: 10.1016/0092-8674(95)90168-X

Al-Asmari, A. K., Albalawi, S. M., Athar, M. T., Khan, A. Q., Al-Shahrani, H., and Islam, M. (2015). *Moringa oleifera* as an anti-cancer agent against breast and colorectal cancer cell lines. *PLoS One* 10:e0135814. doi: 10.1371/journal.pone.0135814

Al-Malki, A. L., and El Rabey, H. A. (2015). The antidiabetic effect of low doses of *Moringa oleifera* Lam. seeds on streptozotocin induced diabetes and diabetic nephropathy in male rats. *Biomed Res. Int.* 2015:381040. doi: 10.1155/2015/381040

Ballard, C. G., Greig, N. H., Guillozet-Bongaarts, A. L., Enz, A., and Darvesh, S. (2005). Cholinesterases: roles in the brain during health and disease. *Curr. Alzheimer Res.* 2, 307–318. doi: 10.2174/1567205054367838

Barros, D. M., Mello e Souza, T., de Souza, M. M., Choi, H., DeDavid e Silva, T., Lenz, G., et al. (2001). LY294002, an inhibitor of phosphoinositide 3-kinase given into rat hippocampus impairs acquisition, consolidation and retrieval of memory for one-trial step-down inhibitory avoidance. *Behav. Pharmacol.* 12, 629–634. doi: 10.1097/00008877-200112000-00007

Bartus, R. T., Dean, R. L. III., Beer, B., and Lippa, A. S. (1982). The cholinergic hypothesis of geriatric memory dysfunction. *Science* 217, 408–414. doi: 10.1126/science.7046051

Bazinet, R. P., and Laye, S. (2014). Polyunsaturated fatty acids and their metabolites in brain function and disease. *Nat. Rev. Neurosci.* 15, 771–785. doi: 10.1038/nrn3820

Bimonte-Nelson, H. A., Granholm, A. C., Nelson, M. E., and Moore, A. B. (2008). Patterns of neurotrophin protein levels in male and female Fischer 344 rats from adulthood to senescence: how young is "young" and how old is "old"? *Exp. Aging Res.* 34, 13–26. doi: 10.1080/03610730701761908

Bonner, T. I., Buckley, N. J., Young, A. C., and Brann, M. R. (1987). Identification of a family of muscarinic acetylcholine receptor genes. *Science* 237, 527–532. doi: 10.1126/science.3037705

Das, U. N. (2008). Folic acid and polyunsaturated fatty acids improve cognitive function and prevent depression, dementia, and Alzheimer's disease–but how and why? *Prostaglandins Leukot. Essent. Fatty Acids* 78, 11–19. doi: 10.1016/j.plefa.2007.10.006

Deak, F., Kapoor, N., Prodan, C., and Hershey, L. A. (2016). Memory loss: five new things. *Neurol. Clin. Pract.* 6, 523–529. doi: 10.1212/CPJ.0000000000000314

Doeppner, T. R., Nagel, F., Dietz, G. P., Weise, J., Tonges, L., Schwarting, S., et al. (2009). TAT-Hsp70-mediated neuroprotection and increased survival of neuronal precursor cells after focal cerebral ischemia in mice. *J. Cereb. Blood Flow Metab.* 29, 1187–1196. doi: 10.1038/jcbfm.2009.44

Drever, B. D., Anderson, W. G., Johnson, H., O'Callaghan, M., Seo, S., Choi, D. Y., et al. (2007). Memantine acts as a cholinergic stimulant in the mouse hippocampus. *J. Alzheimers Dis.* 12, 319–333. doi: 10.3233/JAD-2007-12405

Felder, C. C. (1995). Muscarinic acetylcholine receptors: signal transduction through multiple effectors. *FASEB J.* 9, 619–625. doi: 10.1096/fasebj.9.8.7768353

Giacobini, E. (2002). Long-term stabilizing effect of cholinesterase inhibitors in the therapy of Alzheimer' disease. *J. Neural Transm. Suppl.* 62, 181–187. doi: 10.1007/978-3-7091-6139-5_17

Giovannini, M. G. (2006). The role of the extracellular signal-regulated kinase pathway in memory encoding. *Rev. Neurosci.* 17, 619–634. doi: 10.1515/REVNEURO.2006.17.6.619

Hasselmo, M. E. (2006). The role of acetylcholine in learning and memory. *Curr. Opin. Neurobiol.* 16, 710–715. doi: 10.1016/j.conb.2006.09.002

Hirokawa, S., Nose, M., Ishige, A., Amagaya, S., Oyama, T., and Ogihara, Y. (1996). Effect of Hachimi-jio-gan on scopolamine-induced memory impairment and on acetylcholine content in rat brain. *J. Ethnopharmacol.* 50, 77–84. doi: 10.1016/0378-8741(95)01332-6

Iversen, S. D. (1997). Behavioural evaluation of cholinergic drugs. *Life Sci.* 60, 1145–1152. doi: 10.1016/S0024-3205(97)00059-3

Izquierdo, I., Bevilaqua, L. R., Rossato, J. I., Bonini, J. S., Medina, J. H., and Cammarota, M. (2006). Different molecular cascades in different sites of the brain control memory consolidation. *Trends Neurosci.* 29, 496–505. doi: 10.1016/j.tins.2006.07.005

Joh, E. H., Lee, I. A., and Kim, D. H. (2012). Kalopanaxsaponins A and B isolated from *Kalopanax pictus* ameliorate memory deficits in mice. *Phytother. Res.* 26, 546–551. doi: 10.1002/ptr.3596

Kim, E. J., Jung, I. H., Van Le, T. K., Jeong, J. J., Kim, N. J., and Kim, D. H. (2013). Ginsenosides Rg5 and Rh3 protect scopolamine-induced memory deficits in mice. *J. Ethnopharmacol.* 146, 294–299. doi: 10.1016/j.jep.2012.12.047

Kotani, S., Yamauchi, T., Teramoto, T., and Ogura, H. (2006). Pharmacological evidence of cholinergic involvement in adult hippocampal neurogenesis in rats. *Neuroscience* 142, 505–514. doi: 10.1016/j.neuroscience.2006.06.035

Kotani, S., Yamauchi, T., Teramoto, T., and Ogura, H. (2008). Donepezil, an acetylcholinesterase inhibitor, enhances adult hippocampal neurogenesis. *Chem. Biol. Interact.* 175, 227–230. doi: 10.1016/j.cbi.2008.04.004

Lahiri, D. K., Farlow, M. R., Sambamurti, K., Greig, N. H., Giacobini, E., and Schneider, L. S. (2003). A critical analysis of new molecular targets and strategies for drug developments in Alzheimer's disease. *Curr. Drug Targets* 4, 97–112. doi: 10.2174/1389450033346957

Lanctot, K. L., Rajaram, R. D., and Herrmann, N. (2009). Therapy for Alzheimer's Disease: how effective are current treatments? *Ther. Adv. Neurol. Disord.* 2, 163–180. doi: 10.1177/1756285609102724

Morris, R. G., Garrud, P., Rawlins, J. N., and O'Keefe, J. (1982). Place navigation impaired in rats with hippocampal lesions. *Nature* 297, 681–683. doi: 10.1038/297681a0

Nakanishi, S. (1992). Molecular diversity of glutamate receptors and implications for brain function. *Science* 258, 597–603. doi: 10.1126/science.1329206

Pepeu, G., and Giovannini, M. G. (2004). Changes in acetylcholine extracellular levels during cognitive processes. *Learn. Mem.* 11, 21–27. doi: 10.1101/lm.68104

Rao, V. R., and Finkbeiner, S. (2007). NMDA and AMPA receptors: old channels, new tricks. *Trends Neurosci.* 30, 284–291. doi: 10.1016/j.tins.2007.03.012

Rosenblum, K., Futter, M., Jones, M., Hulme, E. C., and Bliss, T. V. (2000). ERKI/II regulation by the muscarinic acetylcholine receptors in neurons. *J. Neurosci.* 20, 977–985.

Scarpini, E., Scheltens, P., and Feldman, H. (2003). Treatment of Alzheimer's disease: current status and new perspectives. *Lancet Neurol.* 2, 539–547. doi: 10.1016/S1474-4422(03)00502-7

Shimizu, E., Tang, Y. P., Rampon, C., and Tsien, J. Z. (2000). NMDA receptor-dependent synaptic reinforcement as a crucial process for memory consolidation. *Science* 290, 1170–1174. doi: 10.1126/science.290.5494.1170

Tyler, W. J., Alonso, M., Bramham, C. R., and Pozzo-Miller, L. D. (2002). From acquisition to consolidation: on the role of brain-derived neurotrophic factor signaling in hippocampal-dependent learning. *Learn. Mem.* 9, 224–237. doi: 10.1101/lm.51202

Vivar, C. (2015). Adult hippocampal neurogenesis, aging and neurodegenerative diseases: possible strategies to prevent cognitive impairment. *Curr. Top. Med. Chem.* 15, 2175–2192. doi: 10.2174/1568026615666150610141524

Vorhees, C. V., and Williams, M. T. (2006). Morris water maze: procedures for assessing spatial and related forms of learning and memory. *Nat. Protoc.* 1, 848–858. doi: 10.1038/nprot.2006.116

Whitlock, J. R., Heynen, A. J., Shuler, M. G., and Bear, M. F. (2006). Learning induces long-term potentiation in the hippocampus. *Science* 313, 1093–1097. doi: 10.1126/science.1128134

Worms, P., Gueudet, C., Perio, A., and Soubrie, P. (1989). Systemic injection of pirenzepine induces a deficit in passive avoidance learning in rats. *Psychopharmacology* 98, 286–288. doi: 10.1007/BF00444707

Permissions

All chapters in this book were first published by Frontiers; hereby published with permission under the Creative Commons Attribution License or equivalent. Every chapter published in this book has been scrutinized by our experts. Their significance has been extensively debated. The topics covered herein carry significant findings which will fuel the growth of the discipline. They may even be implemented as practical applications or may be referred to as a beginning point for another development.

The contributors of this book come from diverse backgrounds, making this book a truly international effort. This book will bring forth new frontiers with its revolutionizing research information and detailed analysis of the nascent developments around the world.

We would like to thank all the contributing authors for lending their expertise to make the book truly unique. They have played a crucial role in the development of this book. Without their invaluable contributions this book wouldn't have been possible. They have made vital efforts to compile up to date information on the varied aspects of this subject to make this book a valuable addition to the collection of many professionals and students.

This book was conceptualized with the vision of imparting up-to-date information and advanced data in this field. To ensure the same, a matchless editorial board was set up. Every individual on the board went through rigorous rounds of assessment to prove their worth. After which they invested a large part of their time researching and compiling the most relevant data for our readers.

The editorial board has been involved in producing this book since its inception. They have spent rigorous hours researching and exploring the diverse topics which have resulted in the successful publishing of this book. They have passed on their knowledge of decades through this book. To expedite this challenging task, the publisher supported the team at every step. A small team of assistant editors was also appointed to further simplify the editing procedure and attain best results for the readers.

Apart from the editorial board, the designing team has also invested a significant amount of their time in understanding the subject and creating the most relevant covers. They scrutinized every image to scout for the most suitable representation of the subject and create an appropriate cover for the book.

The publishing team has been an ardent support to the editorial, designing and production team. Their endless efforts to recruit the best for this project, has resulted in the accomplishment of this book. They are a veteran in the field of academics and their pool of knowledge is as vast as their experience in printing. Their expertise and guidance has proved useful at every step. Their uncompromising quality standards have made this book an exceptional effort. Their encouragement from time to time has been an inspiration for everyone.

The publisher and the editorial board hope that this book will prove to be a valuable piece of knowledge for researchers, students, practitioners and scholars across the globe.

List of Contributors

Benjamin M. Bader, Konstantin Jügelt, Luise Schultz and Olaf H.-U. Schroeder
NeuroProof GmbH, Rostock, Germany

Ochuko L. Erukainure and Gloria N. Elemo
Nutrition and Toxicology Division, Federal Institute of Industrial Research Oshodi, Lagos, Nigeria

Nadia Ashraf
Faculty of Pharmacy, Barrett Hodgson University, Karachi, Pakistan

Asma S. Naqvi
Dr. Panjwani Center for Molecular Medicine and Drug Research, International Center for Chemical and Biological Sciences, University of Karachi, Karachi, Pakistan

Moses Z. Zaruwa
Department of Biochemistry, Adamawa State University, Mubi, Nigeria

Aliyu Muhammad
Dr. Panjwani Center for Molecular Medicine and Drug Research, International Center for Chemical and Biological Sciences, University of Karachi, Karachi, Pakistan
Department of Biochemistry, Ahmadu Bello University, Zaria, Nigeria

Adenike D. Odusote
Analytical Division, Federal Institute of Industrial Research Oshodi, Lagos, Nigeria

Mahmood Rasool, Kalamegam Gauthaman, Muhammad I. Naseer, Mohammed H. Al-Qahtani and Peter N. Pushparaj
Center of Excellence in Genomic Medicine Research, Faculty of Applied Medical Sciences, King Abdulaziz University, Jeddah, Saudi Arabia

Arif Malik, Sulayman Waquar, Qura Tul-Ain, Tassadaq H. Jafar, Rabia Rasool, Aasia Kalsoom and Muhammad A. Ghafoor
Institute of Molecular Biology and Biotechnology, The University of Lahore, Lahore, Pakistan

Sheikh A. Sehgal
Institute of Zoology, Chinese Academy of Sciences, Beijing, China

Gou-ping Ma
Tongde Hospital of Zhejiang province, Hangzhou, China

Qun Zheng, Meng-bei Xu, Xiao-li Zhou and Guo-Qing Zheng
Department of Neurology, The Second Affiliated Hospital and Yuying Children's Hospital of Wenzhou Medical University, Wenzhou, China

Lin Lu
School of Chinese Medicine, Hong Kong Baptist University, Hong Kong, China

Zuo-xiao Li
Department of Neurology, Affiliated Hospital of Southwest Medical University, Luzhou, China

Yi Zhang, Yuan-Yuan Wang, Wan-Di Feng, Hong-Mei Sun and Zhen-Yu Guo
Department of Anatomy, School of Traditional Chinese Medicine, Beijing University of Chinese Medicine, Beijing, China

Xiao-Gang Gong
Department of Anatomy, School of Traditional Chinese Medicine, Beijing University of Chinese Medicine, Beijing, China
College of Special Education, Beijing Union University, Beijing, China

Jing-Hong Hu
Center for Scientific Research, School of Traditional Chinese Medicine, Beijing University of Chinese Medicine, Beijing, China

Lin Li
Key Laboratory for Neurodegenerative Diseases of Ministry of Education, Capital Medical University, Beijing, China

Ping Li
Beijing Key Lab for Immune-Mediated Inflammatory Diseases, Institute of Clinical Medical Science, China-Japan Friendship Hospital, Beijing, China

Zhen-Zhen Wang
State Key Laboratory of Bioactive Substances and Functions of Natural Medicines, Neuroscience Center, Institute of Materia Medica, Chinese Academy of Medical Sciences, Peking Union Medical College, Beijing, China

Nai-Hong Chen
College of Pharmacy, Hunan University of Chinese Medicine, Changsha, China

Hammad Ullah and Haroon Khan
Department of Pharmacy, Abdul Wali Khan University Mardan, Mardan, Pakistan

Jong Hee Choi
Department of Science in Korean Medicine and Brain Korea 21 Plus Program, Graduate School, Kyung Hee University, Seoul, South Korea
Department of Convergence Medical Science, College of Korean Medicine, Kyung Hee University, Seoul, South Korea

Minhee Jang
Department of Convergence Medical Science, College of Korean Medicine, Kyung Hee University, Seoul, South Korea

Seikwan Oh
Department of Neuroscience and Tissue Injury Defense Research Center, School of Medicine, Ewha Womans University, Seoul, South Korea

Seung-Yeol Nah
Ginsentology Research Laboratory and Department of Physiology, College of Veterinary Medicine and Bio/ Molecular Informatics Center, Konkuk University, Seoul, South Korea

Ik-Hyun Cho
Department of Science in Korean Medicine and Brain Korea 21 Plus Program, Graduate School, Kyung Hee University, Seoul, South Korea
Department of Convergence Medical Science, College of Korean Medicine, Kyung Hee University, Seoul, South Korea
Institute of Korean Medicine, College of Korean Medicine, Kyung Hee University, Seoul, South Korea

Aamir Mushtaq and Mobasher Ahmad
Department of Pharmacology, Punjab University College of Pharmacy, University of the Punjab, Lahore, Pakistan
Gulab Devi Institute of Pharmacy, Gulab Devi Educational Complex, Lahore, Pakistan

Rukhsana Anwar
Department of Pharmacology, Punjab University College of Pharmacy, University of the Punjab, Lahore, Pakistan

Renan Barretta Gaiardo and Suzete Maria Cerutti
Departamento de Ciências Biológicas, Laboratório de Farmacologia Celular e Comportamental, Universidade Federal de São Paulo, Diadema, Brazil

Thiago Ferreira Abreu and Alexandre Keiji Tashima
Departamento de Bioquímica, Escola Paulista de Medicina, Universidade Federal de São Paulo, São Paulo, Brazil

Monica Marques Telles
Departamento de Ciências Biológicas, Laboratório de Fisiologia Metabólica, Universidade Federal de São Paulo, Diadema, Brazil

Bushra Shal, Hussain Ali and Salman Khan
Department of Pharmacy, Faculty of Biological Sciences, Quaid-i-Azam University, Islamabad, Pakistan

Wei Ding
Department of Neurosurgery, Rizhao Hospital of Traditional Chinese Medicine, Rizhao, China

Yeong S. Kim
College of Pharmacy, Seoul National University, Seoul, South Korea

Bin Liu
Cardiovascular Disease Center, First Hospital of Jilin University, Changchun, China

Zhaoqi He, Jingjing Wang and Jiaxin Wang
Department of Clinical Veterinary Medicine, College of Veterinary Medicine, Jilin University, Changchun, China

Zhuoyuan Xin and Fan Li
Department of Pathogenobiology, The Key Laboratory of Zoonosis, Chinese Ministry of Education, College of Basic Medicine, Jilin University, Changchun, China

Yunhe Fu
Department of Clinical Veterinary Medicine, College of Veterinary Medicine, Jilin University, Changchun, China
Department of Pathogenobiology, The Key Laboratory of Zoonosis, Chinese Ministry of Education, College of Basic Medicine, Jilin University, Changchun, China

Saatheeyavaane Bhuvanendran, Yatinesh Kumari, Iekhsan Othman and Mohd Farooq Shaikh
Neuropharmacology Research Laboratory, Jeffrey Cheah School of Medicine and Health Sciences, Monash University Malaysia, Bandar Sunway, Malaysia

Rizwana Sarwar, Umar Farooq, Sadia Naz and Syed M. Bukhari
Department of Chemistry, COMSATS Institute of Information Technology Abbottabad, Abbottabad, Pakistan

Ajmal Khan
Department of Chemistry, COMSATS Institute of Information Technology Abbottabad, Abbottabad, Pakistan
UoN Chair of Oman's Medicinal Plants and Marine Natural Products, University of Nizwa, Nizwa, Oman

Nasiara Karim
Department of Pharmacy, University of Malakand, Chakdara, Pakistan

Imran Khan
Department of Pharmacy, University of Swabi, Swabi, Pakistan

Wu-shuang Yang
Department of Neurosurgery, Xiamen Hospital of Traditional Chinese Medicine, Xiamen, China

Ahmed Al-Harrasi
UoN Chair of Oman's Medicinal Plants and Marine Natural Products, University of Nizwa, Nizwa, Oman

Hayate Javed
Department of Anatomy, College of Medicine and Health Sciences, United Arab Emirates University, Al Ain, United Arab Emirates

Mohamed Fizur Nagoor Meeran, Sheikh Azimullah, Abdu Adem, Bassem Sadek and Shreesh Kumar Ojha
Department of Pharmacology and Therapeutics, College of Medicine and Health Sciences, United Arab Emirates University, Al Ain, United Arab Emirates

Thaiane Coelho dos Santos, Bruno Araújo Serra Pinto and Antonio Marcus de Andrade Paes
Laboratory of Experimental Physiology, Department of Physiological Sciences, Biological and Health Sciences Centre, Federal University of Maranhão, São Luís, Brazil

Thaís Mota Gomes and Adriana Leandro Camara
Laboratory of Experimental Physiology, Department of Physiological Sciences, Biological and Health Sciences Centre, Federal University of Maranhão, São Luís, Brazil

Ying Li and Ying Wang
Department of Pharmacy, Xiamen Medical College, Xiamen, China

Amjad Khan, Tahir Ali, Shafiq Ur Rehman, Muhammad Sohail Khan, Sayed Ibrar Alam, Muhammad Ikram, Tahir Muhammad, Kamran Saeed, Haroon Badshah and Myeong Ok Kim
Division of Applied Life Science (BK 21), College of Natural Science, Gyeongsang National University, Jinju, South Korea

Juan Zhou
Department of Obstetrics and Gynecology, The First Affiliated Hospital of Xiamen University, Xiamen University, Xiamen, China

Ayaz Ahmed
Dr. Panjwani Center for Molecular Medicine and Drug Research, International Center for Chemical and Biological Sciences, University of Karachi, Karachi, Pakistan

Da-qin Suo, Lu Peng, Lan-xi Xu, Kai-yue Zeng, Tong Ren, Yu Zhou, Yun Zhao and Xin Jin
Xiamen Key Laboratory of Chiral Drugs, Medical College, Xiamen University, Xiamen, China

Li-chao Yang
Department of Obstetrics and Gynecology, The First Affiliated Hospital of Xiamen University, Xiamen University, Xiamen, China
Xiamen Key Laboratory of Chiral Drugs, Medical College, Xiamen University, Xiamen, China

Index

www.ingramcontent.com/pod-product-compliance
Lightning Source LLC
LaVergne TN
LVHW082210200926
848484LV00008B/2238

9798887402741